D0077197

How to access the supplemental web study guide

We are pleased to provide access to a web study guide that supplements your textbook, *Fitness and Wellness: A Way of Life.* This resource provides lab activities, 48 video clips, and practical learning exercises to provide real-life context to the material.

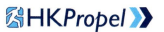 **HKPropel** »

IMPORTANT UPDATE REGARDING YOUR FREE DIGITAL PRODUCT

The digital content that is included free with this print copy of *Fitness and Wellness* has been migrated to HK's new learning platform, HK*Propel*.

Please disregard references inside the print book to www.HumanKinetics.com/FitnessAndWellness and INSTEAD use the instructions on this sheet to seamlessly access the learning content in HK*Propel*.

If it's your first time using HK*Propel*:

1. Visit HKPropel.HumanKinetics.com.
2. Click the "New user? Register here" link on the opening screen to register for an account and redeem your one-time-use access code.
3. Follow the onscreen prompts to create your HK*Propel* account. Use a **valid email address** as your username to ensure you receive important system updates and to help us find your account if you ever need assistance.
4. Enter the access code exactly as shown below, including hyphens. You will not need to re-enter this access code on subsequent visits, and this access code cannot be redeemed by any other user.
5. After your first visit, simply log in to HKPropel.HumanKinetics.com to access your digital product.

If you already have an HK*Propel* account:

1. Visit HKPropel.HumanKinetics.com and log in with your username (email address) and password.
2. Once you are logged in, click the arrow next to your name in the top right corner and then click **My Account**.
3. Under the "Add Access Code" heading, enter the access code exactly as shown below, including hyphens, and click the **Add** button.
4. Once your code is redeemed, navigate to your Library on the Dashboard to access your digital content.

> **Product:** Fitness and Wellness HKPropel Access
>
> **Access code:** LK2U-IMFI-YZOC-LCLD

NOTE TO STUDENTS: If your instructor uses HK*Propel* to assign work to your class, you will need to enter a class enrollment token in HK*Propel* on the **My Account** page. This token will be provided **by your instructor at no cost to you**, but it is required **in addition** to the unique access code that is printed above.

Helpful tips:
You may reset your password from the log in screen at any time if you forget it.

Your license to this digital product will expire **1 year** after the date you redeem the access code. You can check the expiration dates of all your HK*Propel* products at any time in **My Account**.

For assistance, contact us via email at HKPropelCustSer@hkusa.com.   06-2021

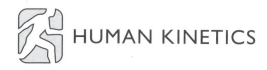 HUMAN KINETICS

Way of Life

guide

Key code: ARMBRUSTER-GXNRC3-OSG

This unique to the web study guide.

Access is provided if you have purchased a new book. Once submitted, the code may not be entered for any other user.

08-2018

Fitness and Wellness

A Way of Life

Carol K. Armbruster, PhD
Indiana University Bloomington

Ellen M. Evans, PhD
University of Georgia, Athens

Catherine M. Laughlin, HSD, MPH
Indiana University Bloomington

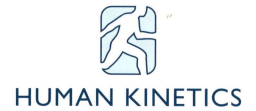

HUMAN KINETICS

Library of Congress Cataloging-in-Publication Data

Names: Kennedy, Carol A., 1958- author. | Evans, Ellen M., 1965- author. |
  Laughlin, Catherine M. 1965- author.
Title: Fitness and wellness : a way of life / Carol Kennedy-Armbruster, PhD,
  Indiana University, Bloomington, Ellen M. Evans, PhD, University of
  Georgia, Athens, Catherine M. Laughlin, HSD, MPH, Indiana University,
  Bloomington.
Description: Champaign, IL : Human Kinetics, [2019] | Includes
  bibliographical references and index.
Identifiers: LCCN 2018001419| ISBN 9781492552666 (print) | ISBN 9781492552673
  (e-book)
Subjects: LCSH: Physical fitness--Study and teaching (Higher) |
  Exercise--Study and teaching (Higher) | Health--Study and teaching (Higher)
Classification: LCC RA781 .K446 2019 | DDC 613.7076--dc23
LC record available at https://lccn.loc.gov/2018001419

ISBN: 978-1-4925-5266-6 (paperback)
ISBN: 978-1-4925-5645-9 (loose-leaf)

The web addresses cited in this text were current as of May 2018, unless otherwise noted.

Senior Acquisitions Editor: Amy N. Tocco
Senior Developmental Editor: Christine M. Drews
Managing Editor: Anna Lan Seaman
Copyeditor: Joy Hoppenot
Indexer: May Hasso
Permissions Manager: Dalene Reeder
Senior Graphic Designer: Nancy Rasmus
Cover Designer: Keri Evans
Cover Design Associate: Susan Rothermel Allen
Photograph (cover): andrest/Getty Images
Photographs (interior): © Human Kinetics, unless otherwise noted on the Photo Credits pages
Photo Asset Manager: Laura Fitch
Photo Production Coordinator: Amy M. Rose
Photo Production Manager: Jason Allen
Senior Art Manager: Kelly Hendren
Illustrations: © Human Kinetics, unless otherwise noted
Printer: Walsworth

Printed in the United States of America   10 9 8 7 6 5 4 3 2 1

The paper in this book was manufactured using responsible forestry methods.

Human Kinetics
P.O. Box 5076
Champaign, IL 61825-5076
Website: www.HumanKinetics.com

In the United States, email info@hkusa.com or call 800-747-4457.
In Canada, email info@hkcanada.com.
In the United Kingdom/Europe, email hk@hkeurope.com.

For information about Human Kinetics' coverage in other areas of the world, please visit our website:
www.HumanKinetics.com

E7089 (paperback) / E7102 (loose-leaf)

CONTENTS

Preface vii • Features of the Web Study Guide xi • Photo Credits xiii

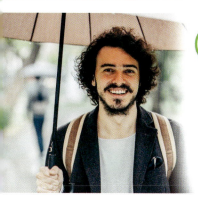

① Staying Healthy and Well Throughout Life 1

Staying Healthy Through the Life Span 2 • New Perspectives on Wellness 8 • Components of Wellness 11 • What Are Functional Movement and Wellness? 16 • Summary 24

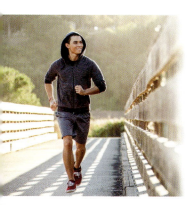

② Functional Fitness and Movement Choices 25

Understanding Physical Activity Recommendations 27 • Integrating Sedentarism, Physical Activity, and Exercise 31 • Fitting Movement Into Everyday Life 34 • Summary 37

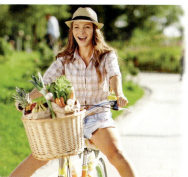

③ Successfully Managing Healthy Behavior Change 39

Are You Ready to Change? 41 • Personalizing the Behavior Change Process 53 • Goal Setting Revisited 54 • Safety First: Getting Started With a Personal Movement Program 55 • Summary 58

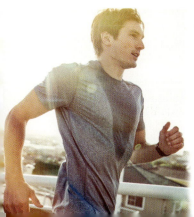

④ Cardiorespiratory Fitness 59

Your Energy Needs: Supply and Demand 60 • Evaluating Your Cardiorespiratory Function 71 • Cardiorespiratory Fitness Benefits You 73 • Your Plan to Improve Cardiorespiratory Fitness 75 • Safety First: Getting Started With Cardiorespiratory Fitness 83 • Summary 84

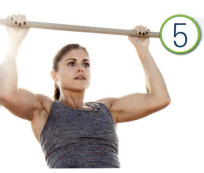

5 Muscular Fitness   85

Your Body Was Designed to Move 87 • Key Definitions 89 • Assessing Muscle Capacity 92 • Muscular Fitness Benefits Your Daily Life 95 • Designing Your Program for Muscular Fitness 95 • Analyzing Your Fitness Choices 101 • Safety Issues 102 • Summary 104

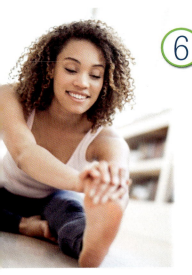

6 Flexibility, Neuromotor Fitness, and Posture   105

All About Flexibility 106 • Mind the Stretch Reflex! 112 • Neuromotor Exercise and Functional Fitness 113 • Physiological Teamwork for Flexibility and Neuromotor Fitness 114 • Preventing Low Back Pain 116 • Summary 119

SPECIAL INSERT

Functional Movement Training   120

Discover the purpose for strengthening specific muscles and how you might accomplish this both inside and outside a fitness facility. You'll learn how to train each muscle group using body weight, variable resistance machines, free weights, and stretching. Ideas for neuromotor training are also included.

Calves 122 • Quads 124 • Hams and Glutes 126 • Abdominals 128 • Lower Back 130 • Hip Abductors 132 • Hip Adductors 134 • Chest and Front of Shoulder 136 • Upper Back and Shoulders 138 • Lats and Middle Back 140 • Front of Upper Arm 142 • Back of Upper Arm 144

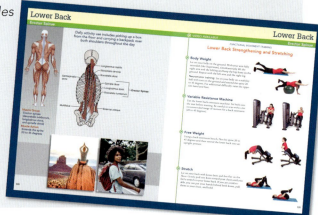

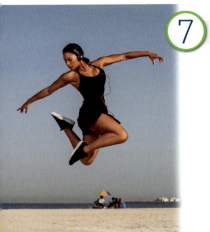

7 Body Composition   147

Body Composition Basics 148 • Assessing Body Composition 151 • Weight Status, Body Composition, and Your Risk of Chronic Disease 157 • A Healthy Body Composition Benefits You—Today and in the Future! 163 • Your Program for Managing Body Composition 164 • Summary 167

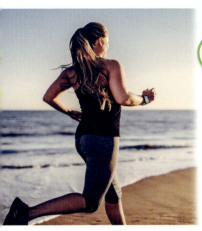

8 Fundamentals of Healthy Eating   **169**

Eating Well: Balanced and Clean 170 • The Many Benefits of a Healthy Diet 184 • Nutrition Recommendations and Resources 185 • Summary 196

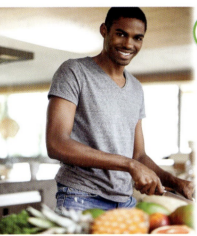

9 Weight Management   **197**

Weight Management: Our Greatest Modern Health Challenge 198 • Energy Balance Math 203 • Weight Management Strategies 207 • Daily Movement Is Essential for Weight Management 212 • Psychological Concerns Regarding Weight Management 213 • When Professional Help Is Needed 215 • Summary 216

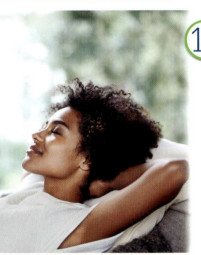

10 Stress Management   **217**

The Contemporary Stress Experience 218 • Common Stressors and Hassles of College Life 225 • Key Stress-Management Strategies 230 • Social, Stressed, and Sleepless 235 • Summary 238

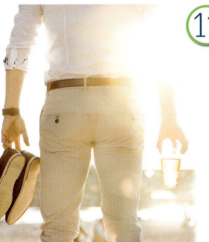

11 Remaining Free From Addiction   **239**

Types of Addictions 240 • What Is Substance Abuse Addiction? 244 • Psychoactive Drugs 249 • Alcohol 257 • Tobacco 264 • Summary 269

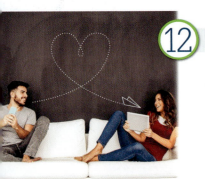

(12) **Sexuality and Health**   271

Sexuality as a Dimension of Health 272 • Reproductive System 273 •
Contraception and Birth Control Methods 279 • Sexually Transmitted
Infections 290 • Reducing the Risks 299 • Sexual Assault 302 •
Summary 305

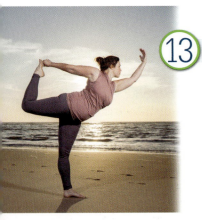

(13) **Reducing the Risks for Metabolic Syndrome**   307

Are You at Risk for Metabolic Syndrome? 308 • Evaluating Your Risk
for Diabetes Mellitus 310 • Cardiovascular Disease: Our Number One
Killer 315 • Prevention of CVD Starts Early in Life 326 • Summary 327

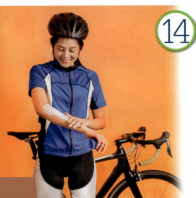

(14) **Reducing the Risks for Cancer**   329

The Nature of Cancer 331 • Who Gets Cancer? 333 • Detection,
Staging, and Treatment of Cancer 338 • Causes of Cancer 343 •
Most Commonly Diagnosed Cancers 349 • Summary 352

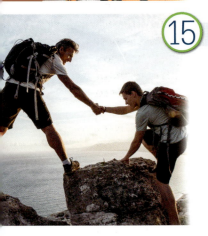

(15) **Fitness and Wellness: Today and Beyond**   355

Living Well Over the Life Span 356 • Differences Between Physiological
and Chronological Age 359 • Approaches to Medicine 361 • Finding
Resources to Enhance Your Fitness and Wellness 363 • Specific Wellness
Concepts and SMART Goals Revisited 367 • Healthy People 2030 and
Beyond 368 • Fitness and Wellness: A Way of Life 369

Glossary 371 • References 379 • Index 391 • About the Authors 400

PREFACE

Welcome to *Fitness and Wellness: A Way of Life*! We are glad you are joining us for this exciting journey of developing a lifetime of healthy living. Choices over time become habits that ultimately become your lifestyle. The steps you take now often determine what your lifestyle will be like after college. This book suggests healthy choices and patterns that you can use for the rest of your life. Our intent is to help you change your quality of life by intentionally applying evidence-based concepts of physical and mental health to your daily living practices. Our overall philosophy is that a healthy body is the key to a healthy mind and a life well lived.

This book is a labor of love between three professionals, academics, and mothers who have over 80 years of combined experience in health and wellness professional. We watched our children grow up in the internet age and saw outdoor play be replaced by organized activities and screen time. We also experienced personal conversations being replaced by email, text messages, tweets, and more. Therefore, we developed this book with you and our children in mind. We want to give you the tools you need to successfully manage healthy behaviors so you can live your life to the fullest.

Concepts in this book involve the following:

- Focusing on your personal behavior choices rather than following a prescription (We realize that everyone is unique and needs to develop his or her own plan.)
- Applying evidence-based research on physical activity, exercise, and sedentary living to functional movement outcomes through goal setting and behavior change concepts
- Understanding the complexity of healthy behavior change in terms of physical, mental, and emotional health
- Dealing with sensitive health issues related to sexuality, depression, anxiety, and stress that may influence your lives and those of the people you love

Fitness and Health Integrated

One of the major themes of this book is reducing stress by making choices that fit easily into your daily living activities. Instead of paying for a fitness facility membership and making time for an organized workout, you can focus on moving more throughout the day. Try taking the stairs instead of the escalator or going on a hike with your friends instead of going out to lunch. We call this functional training. Our Functional Movement Training section after chapter 6 is unique in that it shows you the purpose for strengthening specific muscles as well as how you might accomplish this, both inside and outside of a fitness facility. We hear regularly that students do not have enough time to take care of themselves. We hope that this book will help you change your thoughts about what it means to take care of yourself so that you can do so more simply.

How This Book Is Organized

Fitness and Wellness: A Way of Life has 15 chapters. Chapters 1 to 6 focus on the guidelines for exercise, physical activity, and sedentary living. We realize that many people begin their journey toward healthy practices with physical movement. Habitual movement can help us feel better, work better, and sleep better so that we can be the best version of ourselves. The beginning of the book helps you evaluate your physical health in terms of the human movement paradigm that is unique to this book. This paradigm stresses the importance of exercise, physical activity, and less sedentary living. Thinking about being more physically active can motivate you to incorporate movement into your day. Being aware of the consequences of sitting too much gets you focused on getting up frequently throughout the day. We also discuss what neuromotor exercise training is and how to incorporate it into your daily life.

Chapters 8 and 9 tackle healthy eating practices and weight management, which are often difficult to achieve with the college lifestyle. We provide you with the tools you need to be successful in your current environment. The later chapters help you round out your awareness and practice of wellness with information on stress, sleep, addictions, healthy sexuality, and reducing risks for metabolic syndrome and cancer.

Special Features of This Book

The book will help you reach your goals. Each chapter has key terms to help you focus your study

efforts and behavior check sidebars with specific ideas for integrating health concepts into your daily practices. These sidebars encourage small steps, which are helpful for removing barriers to change. Also included in each chapter are Now and Later sidebars, which help you realize that the positive choices you make today will lead to a healthier tomorrow.

Throughout the book, you will find infographics, figures, and evidence-based tables to reinforce the information you are learning in an easy-to-understand way. We make an extensive effort to connect research to practice and emphasize that making a healthier option the easy choice is often about simple daily decisions that make a huge difference in your health, today and in the future.

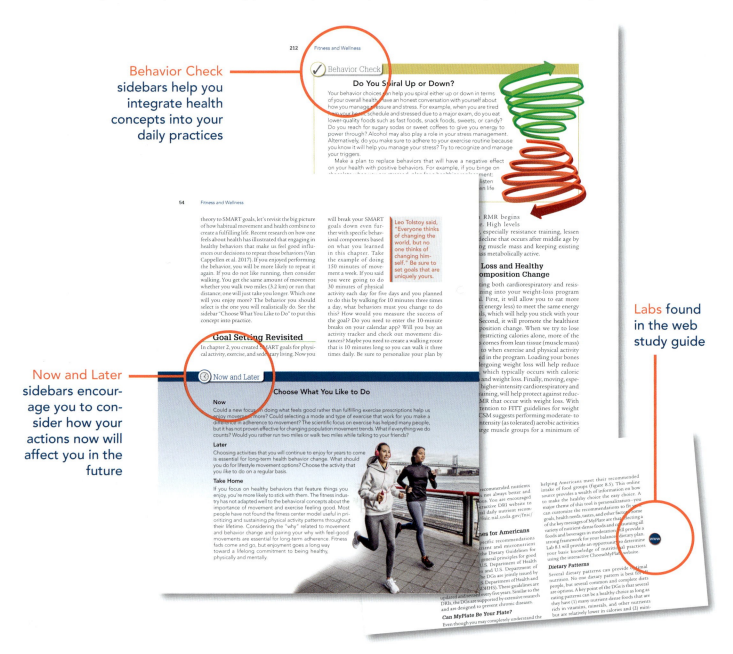

Behavior Check sidebars help you integrate health concepts into your daily practices

Now and Later sidebars encourage you to consider how your actions now will affect you in the future

Labs found in the web study guide

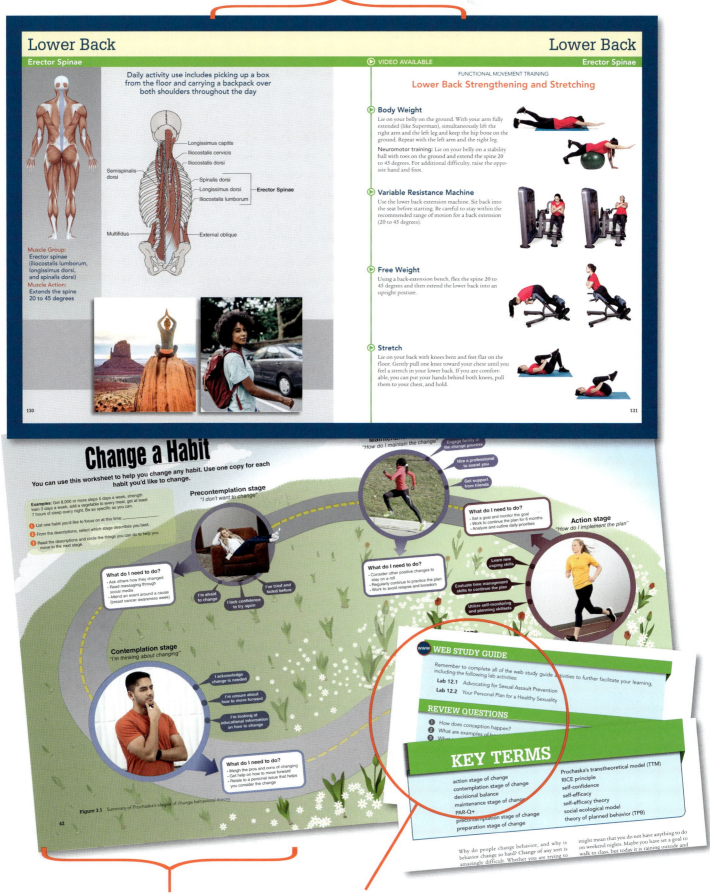

Infographics, evidence-based tables, and figures

Key terms and Review questions

Instructor Resources

Fitness and Wellness: A Way of Life is supported by a complete set of ancillaries: presentation package, image bank, instructor guide, test package, and chapter quizzes.

- The instructor guide contains semester- and quarter-based syllabi, chapter overviews, key concepts, chapter outlines, class activities to engage discussion and promote self-reflection among students, and answers to the in-text chapter review questions.

- The presentation package provides more than 700 PowerPoint slides with selected illustrations and tables from the text.

- The image bank contains most of the figures, tables, and content photos. You can use these images to supplement lecture slides, create handouts, or develop your own presentations and teaching materials.

- The test package contains more than 350 questions in a mix of true-or-false, multiple-choice, fill-in-the-blank, and essay formats.

- The ready-made chapter quizzes allow you to check students' understanding of the most important chapter concepts. Both the test package and chapter quizzes are available in a variety of formats and can be imported into most learning management systems.

All of these instructor ancillaries can be accessed at **www.HumanKinetics.com/FitnessAndWellness**.

Student Resources

Another powerful resource is the web study guide for students. The web study guide provides interactive study activities designed to help you strengthen your understanding of key chapter concepts. It also includes lab activities for every chapter, with video instructions and demonstrations for the labs that involve assessment of fitness components. These assessments focus on your individual scores and the goals you would like to set for yourself, rather than comparing to others' scores. The labs provide an opportunity for goal-setting over the course of a quarter, semester, or an entire year, even after you have finished the course. These labs can be downloaded, completed, and then submitted to your instructor through a learning management system. Finally, the web study guide contains a functional movement training section, which provides instructions, photos, and videos demonstrating exercise techniques for all major muscle groups.

Not only will this guide help you develop a full understanding of course content but also it will help you evaluate your own fitness and wellness behaviors. Through the activities in the web study guide, you will establish goals in the areas of physical activity, exercise, minimizing sedentarism, and health, and you will be encouraged to make plans that will keep you healthy and well for life!

See "Features of the Web Study Guide" on the next page for more information. The web study guide is available at **www.HumanKinetics.com/FitnessAndWellness**.

Final Thoughts

The primary goal of this book is to provide a personal, evidence-based interactive tool to help you lead and sustain a healthier, happier, and more productive life. Learning how to take care of yourself so you can take care of others is the first step in making a difference in the world. Our physicians have medical records that chart our path for preventing illness. We need to take responsibility for charting our own wellness paths. We are rarely encouraged to practice prevention early in our lifetime. Taking charge of your health, rather than expecting medicine to cure you after you've gotten sick, is an enlightening concept and one that we hope energizes you.

Living well is important to college students regardless of your major. Taking care of yourself will help you have the energy you need to be successful in college and beyond. People who love life and have a positive attitude are often those who are the healthiest and happiest, physically, mentally, and emotionally. We are excited to give you the tools you need to embrace healthy behavior changes in your life. Kudos to you for taking this class and being open to the possibilities of what healthy living can do for you, now and in your future. Let's do this!

FEATURES OF THE WEB STUDY GUIDE

The web study guide features a variety of engaging study activities designed to help you deepen your understanding of key chapter concepts by interacting with the content in unique ways. Activities include analyzing the goals, making decisions, and selecting exercises for virtual characters in preparation for setting your own goals, considering how to change a behavior, and designing your own movement plan. The web study guide is available at www.HumanKinetics.com/FitnessAndWellness.

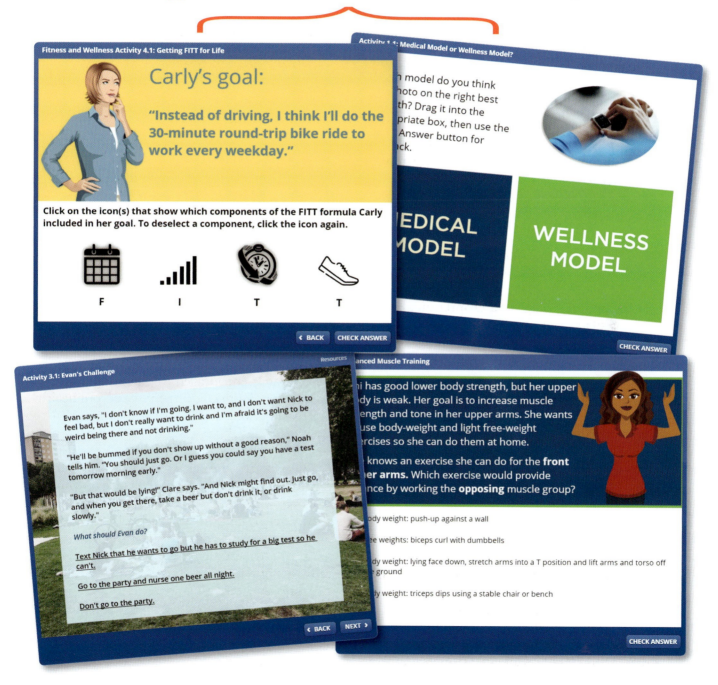

The functional movement training section, a resource filled with instructions, photos, and videos, can become your personal guide to selecting movement activities that work with your lifestyle and preferences. For every muscle group, we have included several videos demonstrating exercise technique. You can access video of 48 exercises in the web study guide!

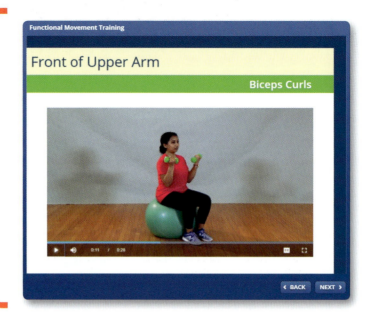

You'll also find 31 labs in the web study guide, which will help you personalize the content as you do such activities as create a family wellness history, consider pros and cons of changing habits, assess your fitness components and set individualized goals, consider aspects related to nutrition, and tackle tough subjects such as body image, addiction, sexual assault, and cancer.

Most self-assessment labs are accompanied by videos showing you how to perform tests to assess your strength, endurance, flexibility, and neuromotor capacity.

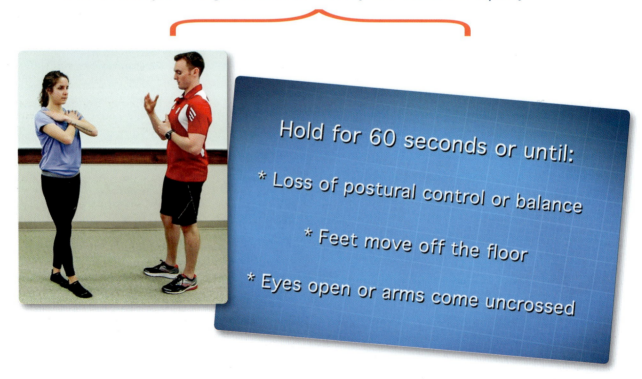

PHOTO CREDITS

Table of content photos in chronological order: Adam Hester/Blend Images/Getty Images; Azarubaika/E+/Getty Images; filadendron/E+/Getty Images; Hoxton/Ryan Lees/Getty Images; Kolostock/Blend Images/Getty Images; Kolostock/Blend Images/Getty Images; andresr/E+/Getty Images; Paul Aiken/EyeEm/Getty Images; Guido Mieth/Taxi/Getty Images; Klaus Vedfelt/DigitalVision/Getty Images; PeopleImages/DigitalVision/Getty Images; Todor Tsvetkov/E+/Getty Images Westend61/Getty Images; Mischa Keijser/Cultura/Getty Images; torwai/iStock/Getty Images Plus; Ascent Xmedia/Photographer's Choice/Getty Images

Page 1: Adam Hester/Blend Images/Getty Images

Page 2: Biggunsband/iStock/Getty Images

Page 6: PeopleImages/DigitalVision/Getty Images

Page 9: Andy Astfalck/Moment/Getty Images

Page 11 (from top to bottom): Ariel Skelley/DigitalVision/Getty Images; Caiaimage/Sam Edwards/OJO+/Getty Images

Page 12 (from left to right): Bettina Mare Images/Cultura/Getty Images; Kevin Kozicki/Image Source/Getty Images

Page 13: uschools/iStock/Getty Images

Page 14 (from left to right): Tom Merton/Caiaimage/Getty Images; Tom Merton/Caiaimage/Getty Images

Page 15: Hero Images/Getty Images

Page 16: JGI/Tom Grill/Blend Images/Getty Images

Page 17: Jordan Siemens/DigitalVision/Getty Images

Page 19: Westend61/Getty Images

Page 20: Petar Chernaev/E+/Getty Images

Page 21: Tetra Images/Getty Images

Page 22 (clockwise from top): skynesher/E+/Getty Images; Michael DeYoung/Blend Images/Getty Images; BryanRupp/iStock/Getty Images; oneinchpunch/iStock/Getty Images; Inti St Clair/Blend Images/Getty Images

Page 23: SolStock/iStock/Getty Images

Page 25: Azarubaika/E+/Getty Images

Page 26: Hero Images/Getty Images

Page 28: Artur Debat/Moment/Getty Images

Page 29: Sadeugra/iStock/ Getty Images

Page 31 (from left to right): Martin Novak/Moment/Getty Images; Wavebreakmedia/iStock /Getty Images Plus

Page 33: Blend Images - Peathegee Inc/Brand X Pictures/Getty Images

Page 39: filadendron/E+/Getty Images

Page 40: Hero Images/Getty Images

Page 45: olaser/E+/Getty Images

Page 46: Plume Creative/DigitalVision/Getty Images

Page 50: SKA/Cultura/Getty Images

Page 54: Xavier Arnau/E+/Getty Images

Page 55: IAN HOOTON/Science Photo Library/Getty Images

Page 56: Juanmonino/E+/Getty Images

Page 59: Hoxton/Ryan Lees/Getty Images

Page 60: Martin Novak/Moment/Getty Images

Page 63: Innocenti/Cultura/Getty Images

Page 64: PeopleImages/iStock/Getty Images Plus

Page 67 (clockwise from top): Mike Kemp/Blend Images/Getty Images; Wavebreakmedia/iStock/Getty Images Plus; Peathegee Inc/Blend Images/Getty Images; Guido Mieth/DigitalVision/Getty Images

Page 69: Hero Images/Getty Images

Page 70 (from left to right): Westend61/Getty Images; Image Source/DigitalVision/Getty Images; Jordan Siemens/Getty Images

Page 72: technotr/E+/Getty Images

Page 75: Hero Images/Getty Images

Page 76: Stanislaw Pytel/DigitalVision/Getty Images

Page 78: FS Productions/Blend Images/Getty Images

Page 79: Dirima/iStock /Getty Images Plus

Page 81: Idea Images/DigitalVision/Getty Images

Page 82: Westend61/Getty Images

Page 83: Tom Werner/DigitalVision/Getty Images

Page 85: Kolostock/Blend Images/Getty Images

Page 88: David Larson/iStock/Getty Images Plus

Page 89: Laurence Mouton/PhotoAlto Agency RF Collections/Getty Images

Page 90 (clockwise from top): gpointstudio/iStock/Getty Images Plus; diego_cervo/iStock/Getty Images Plus; Antonio_Diaz/iStock/ Getty Images Plus; Tom Merton/Caiaimage/Getty Images; patrickheagney/iStock/Getty Images Plus; skynesher/E+/Getty Images

Page 92: Image Source/Getty Images

Page 93 (from top to bottom): SolStock/E+/Getty Images; Hero Images/Getty Images; Peter Muller/Cultura/Getty Images; Hill Street Studios/Blend Images/Getty Images

Page 94 (clockwise from top): PeopleImages/DigitalVision/Getty Images; Dimitri Otis/DigitalVision/Getty Images; Copyright Christopher Peddecord 2009/Moment/Getty Images; MRBIG_PHOTOGRAPHY/E+/Getty Images

Page 95: JLPH/Image Source/Getty Images

Page 98: Marc Dufresne/E+/Getty Images

Page 101: Westend61/Getty Images

Page 103: Denkou Images/Cultura/Getty Images

Page 105: andresr/E+/Getty Images

Page 108 (clockwise from top): PeopleImages/DigitalVision/Getty Images; Endopack/iStock/Getty Images; Paul Bradbury/Caiaimage/Getty Images; Sam-Stock/iStock/Getty Images; Santa1604/iStock/Getty Images Plus

Page 110 (from left to right): Laurence Mouton/PhotoAlto Agency RF Collections/Getty Images; Wavebreakmedia/iStock/Getty Images Plus; kokouu/E+/Getty Images

Page 111: ZenShui/Frederic Cirou/PhotoAlto Agency RF Collections/Getty Images

Page 112: PeopleImages/DigitalVision/Getty Images

Page 114: Ryan McVay/DigitalVision/Getty Images

Page 115 (from left to right): Sam Edwards/OJO Images/Getty Images; Joos Mind/DigitalVision/Getty Images

Page 116: PeopleImages/E+/Getty Images

Page 121: Jupiterimages/Goodshoot/Getty Images Plus

Page 122 (from left to right): DaveLongMedia/E+/Getty Images; Philipp Nemenz/Cultura/Getty Images

Page 124 (from left to right): Trinette Reed/Blend Images/Getty Images; Peathegee Inc/Blend Images/Getty Images

Page 126 (from left to right): Klaus Vedfelt/DigitalVision/Getty Images; Slater King/Dorling Kindersley/Getty Images

Page 128 (from left to right): GROGL/iStock/Getty Images; Maskot/Getty Images

Page 130 (from left to right): Dave and Les Jacobs/Blend Images/Getty Images; Westend61/Getty Images

Page 132 (from left to right): stevecoleimages/E+/Getty Images; BERKO85/iStock/Getty Images

Page 134 (from left to right): laindiapiaroa/Blend Images/Getty Images; Sam Edwards/Caiaimage/Getty Images

Page 136 (from left to right): BJI/Blue Jean Images/Getty Images

Page 138 (from left to right): Bambu Productions/DigitalVision/Getty

Images; Westend61/Brand X Pictures/Getty Images

Page 140 (from left to right): Peathegee Inc/Blend Images/Getty Images; technotr/Vetta/Getty Images

Page 142 (from left to right): Tanya Constantine/Blend Images/Getty Images; Malorny/Moment/Getty Images

Page 144 (from left to right): iprogressman/iStock/Getty Images Plus; Sam Edwards/Caiaimage/Getty Images

Page 147: Paul Aiken/EyeEm/Getty Images

Page 150: Ming H2 Wu/Blend Images/Getty Images

Page 153 (from top to bottom): ©Ellen Evans; BSIP/Universal Images Group/Getty; ©Ellen Evans; ©Ellen Evans

Page 154 (top): CHRISTOPHE VANDER EECKEN/REPORTERSf/SCIENCE Source

Page 156: laflor/E+/Getty Images

Page 158: Mikolette/E+/Getty Images

Page 160: iancartwright/RooM/Getty Images

Page 161 (from left to right): ©Ellen Evans; ©Ellen Evans

Page 162 (clockwise from top): ©Ellen Evans; ©Ellen Evans; Westend61/Getty Images

Page 165: Meg Haywood-Sullivan/Getty Images

Page 166: nycshooter/iStock/Getty Images Plus

Page 169: Guido Mieth/Taxi/Getty Images

Page 171 (from left to right): Malcolm Hope/Icon Sportswire/Getty Images; roshinio/E+/Getty Images

Page 175: margouillatphotos/iStock/Getty Images Plus

Page 176: AshaSathees Photography/Moment/Getty Images

Page 177: Maskot/Getty Images

Page 178: Anthony Lee/Caiaimage/Getty Images

Page 180: Tyler Edwards/DigitalVision/Getty Images

Page 183: AJ_Watt/E+/Getty Images

Page 185: PeopleImages/DigitalVision/Getty Images

Page 186: Anthony Lee/Caiaimage/Getty Images

Page 187: Hero Images/Getty Images

Page 188: Bjorn Holland/Image Source/Getty Images

Page 191: Alain Schroeder/ONOKY/Getty Images

Page 192: Steve Debenport/E+/Getty Images

Page 193: Jay_Zynism/iStock/Getty Images Plus

Page 197: PeopleImages/Digital Vision/Getty Images

Page 200: Klaus Vedfelt/DigitalVision/Getty Images

Page 202: David Lees/ DigitalVision/Getty Images

Page 208: Tsvi Braverman / EyeEm/Getty Images

Page 210: Minette Hand/EyeEm/Getty Images

Page 213: Donald Iain Smith/Blend Images/Getty Images

Page 215: monkeybusinessimages/iStock/Getty Images

Page 217: PeopleImages/DigitalVision/Getty Images

Page 218: Hero Images/Getty Images

Page 219: Jacob Ammentorp Lund/iStock/Getty Images

Page 223: Jacob Ammentorp Lund/iStock/Getty Images

Page 226 (clockwise from top): National Archives; National Archives; National Archives; Pete Souza/National Archives; Ken Cedeno-Pool/Getty Images; Ken Cedeno-Pool/Getty Images

Page 227: Trokantor/E+/Getty Images

Page 228: PeopleImages/E+/Getty IMages

Page 229: AntonioGuillem/iStock/Getty Images

Page 231: Ginew/IStock/Getty Images

Page 232: Squaredpixels/E+/Getty Images

Page 234: caracterdesign/Vetta/Getty Images

Page 236: martin-dm/E+/Getty Images

Page 237: jacoblund/iStock/Getty Images

Page 239: Westend61/Getty Images

Page 240: zodebala/Vetta/Getty Images

Page 241: Monkeybusinessimages/iSTock/Getty Images

Page 243: Frankreporter/iStock/Getty Images

Page 246: sturti/E+/Getty Images

Page 248: ermingut/E+/Getty Images

Page 250: rstpierr/iStock/Getty Images

Page 251 (from top to bottom): Heath Korvola/DigitalVision/Getty Images; FotoMaximum/iStock/Getty Images

Page 252 (from top to bottom): Artem_Furman/iStock/Getty Images; Steve Bartholomew/Dorling Kindersley/Getty Images

Page 254: Andrew Burton/Getty Images

Page 256: Cogent-Marketing/iStock/Getty Images

Page 258: PeopleImages/E+/Getty Images

Page 263: Joe Raedle/Getty Images

Page 265 (from top to bottom): InkkStudios/iStock/Getty Images; ljubaphoto/iStock/Getty Images

Page 271: Todor Tsvetkov/E+/Getty Images

Page 273: jacoblund/iStock/Getty Images Plus

Page 281: jenjen42/E+/Getty Images

Page 286 (from top to bottom): BSIP/UIG Via Getty Images; Getty Images; BSIP/UIG Via Getty Images

Page 288: Blair_witch/iStock/Getty Images

Page 293 (from top to bottom): CDC/SCIENCE Source; lolostock/iStock/Getty Images

Page 297: Media for Medical/UIG via Getty Images

Page 298: BSIP/UIG Via Getty Images

Page 300: Portra/DigitalVision/Getty Images

Page 301: www.davingphotography.com/Moment/Getty Images

Page 303: JackF/iStock/Getty Images

Page 305: vm/E+/Getty Images

Page 307: Mischa Keijser/Cultura/Getty Images

Page 309: Peathegee Inc/Blend Images/Getty Images

Page 312: Paul Bradbury/Caiaimage/Getty Images

Pages 314-315: PeopleImages/E+/Getty Images

Page 320: Xsandra/E+/Getty Images

Page 322: Steve Debenport/E+/Getty Images

Page 323: Nina Stubicar/EyeEm/Getty Images

Page 325: macarosha/iStock/Getty Images

Page 329: torwai/iStock/Getty Images Plus

Page 330: Eugenio Marongiu/Cultura/Getty Images

Page 335: ferrantraite/E+/Getty Images

Page 339: monkeybusinessimages/iStock/Getty Images

Page 343: Caiaimage/Sam Edwards/OJO+/Getty Images

Page 344: Monkeybusinessimages/iStock/Getty Images

Page 345: serdjophoto/iStock/Getty Images

Page 347: Tom Merton/OJO Images/Getty Images

Page 348: Reprinted from National Cancer Institute (1990).

Page 349: Chatuporn Sornlampoo/EyeEm/Getty Images

Page 355: Ascent Xmedia/Photographer's Choice/Getty Images

Page 356: Blend Images - Dave and Les Jacobs/Brand X Pictures/Getty Images

Page 357 (from left to right): diego_cervo/iStock/Getty Images; B2M Productions/DigitalVision/Getty Images

Page 359: Blend Images - KidStock/Brand X Pictures/Getty Images

Page 361: PeopleImages/E+/Getty Images

Page 362: Ascent/PKS Media Inc./DigitalVision/Getty Images

Page 363: Phil Boorman/Cultura/Getty Images

Page 365: Mark Webster/Cultura/Getty Images

Page 366: Bojan89/iStock/Getty Images

Page 367: Westend61/Getty Images

Page 368: Caiaimage/Paul Bradbury/Getty Images

Staying Healthy and Well Throughout Life

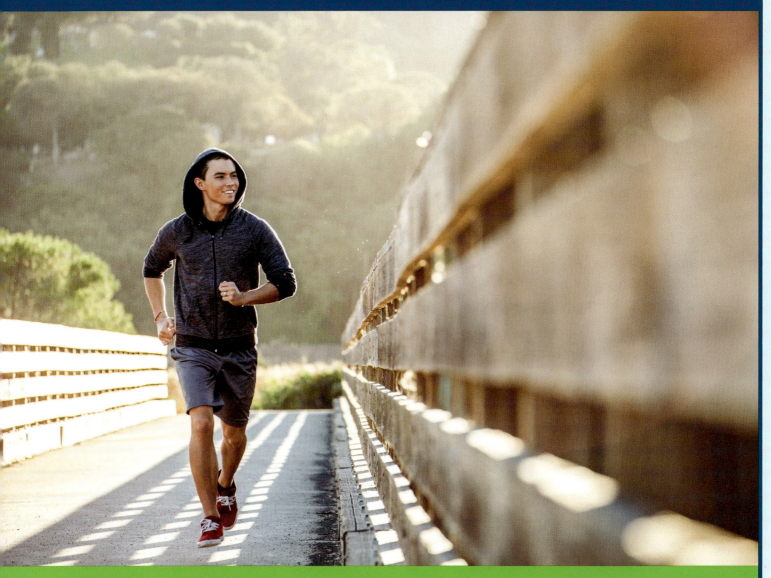

OBJECTIVES

❭ Explain the relationship between life expectancy and wellness practices.

❭ Describe the components of wellness and their interrelatedness.

❭ Differentiate between *functional movement* and *functional fitness training* in relation to healthy living.

❭ Create a personal wellness profile.

KEY TERMS

functional movement   life expectancy

functional fitness training   medical model

health span   wellness model

Wellness, well-being, health, and *fitness* are generally interchangeable terms that can be defined differently depending on your life circumstances. This book will help you to keep a positive outlook on what it means to be well. It will not offer prescriptions or scare you about what will happen if you don't practice healthy behaviors. Instead, this book emphasizes your personal lifestyle choices. After all, a lifestyle is a long-term process for which there are no quick fixes. The **medical model**, used by trained medical experts, focuses on prescribing drugs and procedures when illness is the cause of a lifestyle change. The **wellness model** empowers personal lifestyle choice and utilizes self-management skills for preventing disease through focusing on living well. Our overall vision for *Fitness and Wellness: A Way of Life* is to empower, educate, and encourage readers to practice productive and healthy lifestyle choices.

When you think of people who are healthy and well, what comes to mind? Getting eight hours of sleep? Not smoking? Eating broccoli and kale? You may picture hiking with friends. Do you think of people accomplishing incredible physical feats or just being generally active most of the time? Or maybe you're visualizing someone coming out of a yoga class with a deep sense of peace. Do the people you've thought of smile more or seem more positive to you than other people? Or is there something even deeper that marks the person as healthy and well?

Staying Healthy Through the Life Span

A life well lived starts with an understanding of productive health and wellness practices. This includes feeling good enough about your body to live well—to eat well, move more, and attend to all aspects of life (emotions, spirituality) that make you healthy. Recent books and articles report a new focus on wellness practices. People are more

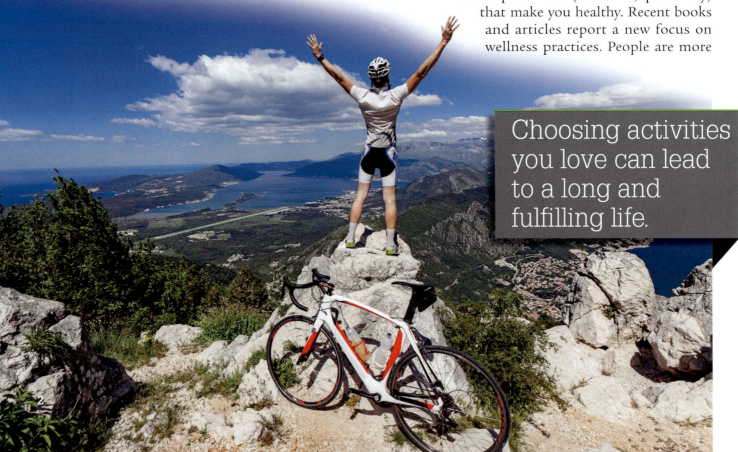

Choosing activities you love can lead to a long and fulfilling life.

> Be your best you! You are limited less by chance and nature than by your vision of yourself.

aware than ever that health can come in many sizes and so are losing interest in diet fads or extreme exercise programs. When people love their bodies, regardless of their size, they are prone to care for their bodies and eat healthy foods instead of buying diet foods (Schlossberg 2016). Michelle Segar (2015) believes that human decision making, motivation, and a behavior focus are the keys to healthy daily movement practices. She notes that prescribing a behavior (for example, a change in diet or exercise) comes out of a medical framework. The activity tracker craze is an example of this new focus on behavior. People are learning that moving more throughout the day can be as beneficial to health as going to a fitness facility for a workout. Seligman (2011), like Segar (2015), also focuses more on behavioral choices. He believes there are five keys to flourishing, which are positive emotions, engagement, relationships, meaning, and accomplishment.

In essence, staying healthy through the life span requires a focus on healthy habits, motivation, and behavioral choices. All these will help you fend off early preventable diseases and live your best life.

Life Expectancy and Wellness

For the first time since 1993, **life expectancy** (how long you live) in the United States has declined, from 78.9 years to 78.8 years (Xu et al. 2016), while global life expectancy has risen. People born in the United States in 2015 can expect to live an average of 71.4 years (73.8 years for women, 69.1 years for men; women still live, on average, longer than men). The longest life span is currently in Japan at almost 84 years. The shortest life expectancies are in Africa. However, in general, the U.S. population is seeing a turn toward overall longevity stabilizing.

The top 10 list of leading causes of death in the United States has not changed since 2014, and 7 of the causes are chronic diseases. The top two (heart disease and cancer) account for over 60 percent of deaths from those causes in the United States (figure 1.1).

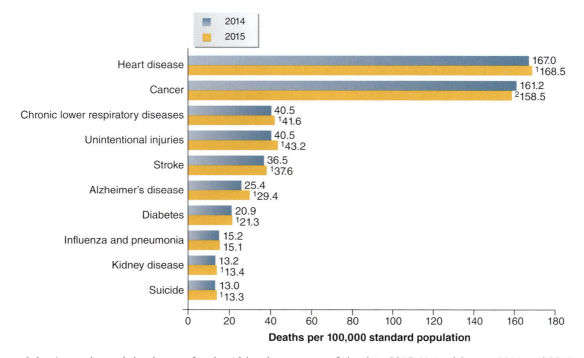

Figure 1.1 Age-adjusted death rates for the 10 leading causes of death in 2015: United States, 2014 and 2015.

[1]Statistically significant increase in age-adjusted death rate from 2014 to 2015 (p < .05).

[2]Statistically significant decrease in age-adjusted death rate from 2014 to 2015 (p < .05).

Notes: A total of 2,712,630 resident deaths were registered in the United States in 2015. The 10 leading causes accounted for 74.2 percent of all deaths in the United States in 2015. Causes of death are ranked according to number of deaths. Access data table for figure 1.1 at www.cdc.gov/nchs/data/databriefs/db267_table.pdf#3. SOURCE: NCHS, National Vital Statistics System, Mortality.

Reprinted from NCHS Data Brief N. 267, December 2016.

Contrast the decrease in U.S. life expectancy, despite the United States spending billions of dollars on health care, with the increase in world life expectancy (Boseley 2016). The U.S. government is not doing much to fund wellness, but U.S. companies are starting to help their employees be well because it is good for business. According to Springbuk (2017), almost one-third of worksites increased their overall benefits offerings in 2016, and health benefits (22 percent) and wellness benefits (24 percent) were the most likely to experience growth. Remember to ask about health and wellness benefits when you interview for a job.

Many factors affect longevity. Best-selling author Dan Buettner (2015) takes a unique approach to understanding how to increase the life span. He studied places in the world that had the longest life expectancy (he called them *blue zones*) and discovered that within these areas, people generally had healthy diets and moved more (figure 1.2). Therefore, where you live can affect your life span. Income also plays a part. Chetty and colleagues (2016) found that in the United States, the richest men live 15 years longer than the poorest men, and the richest women live 10 years longer than the poorest women.

Why are Americans not living as long as people from other countries around the world? Could this recent decrease in longevity (Xu et al. 2016) be due to technology and automation influencing sedentary lifestyles in our work and play? Is it because we sit too much, eat too much, or do most daily tasks (i.e., turn on the dishwasher) with a press of a button? Maybe these choices are made for us by the environment we choose to live in. Modern medicine has enhanced overall longevity, yet could technology and sedentary living be balancing out the influence of modern medicine in terms of overall life expectancy? Maybe the true meaning of being well has more to do with how we live our lives and where we choose to live and less to do with medical interventions. Maybe the key to living well is actually the life choices we make on a daily basis.

This book focuses on the wellness factors that influence longevity. Although the United States spends billions of dollars on health care (Boseley 2016), it is up to you to take care of yourself so you can prevent illness and be well. Good for you for reading this book! It will help you learn how to make decisions for yourself that will empower a wellness way of thinking and living.

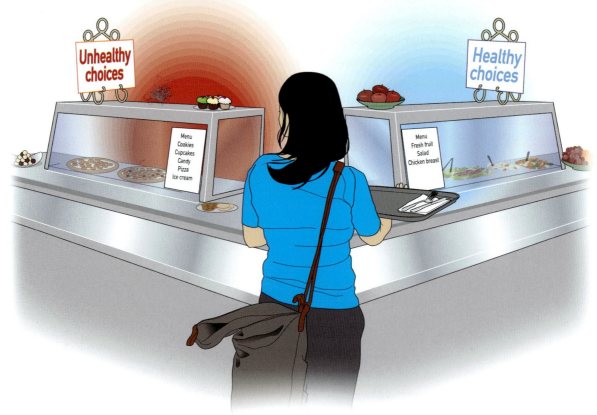

Figure 1.2   Life expectancy is influenced by many wellness factors, including making healthy choices.

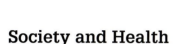

What's the Difference Between Life Span and Health Span?

Life span: The number of years we live from birth to death.

Health span: The number of functional and disease-free years we live from birth to death (period of life that does not include unhealthy years).

Society and Health

According to the U.S. National Prevention Health Promotion and Public Health Council (2016), Americans reaching the age of 65 today can expect, on average, to live an additional 19 years. One of the main focuses of this book is living well throughout the life span. Take a look at your older relatives and friends. Are they leading functionally successful lives as they age?

Is a longer life a better life? The term **health span** is a new one that describes how *well* those later years of life are. Life expectancy can be divided into healthy years and unhealthy years. Of course, you want to live more healthy years than unhealthy ones. Taking care of your body, mind, and soul is critical for adding more years to your health span. What you put into your body and how you take care of it now will increase the

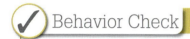

What's Your Family Health Span?

Now that you understand the difference between life span and health span, think about your grandparents and parents. Would you say they are living well as older adults? If yes, why do you think this? If no, why not? What habits do you possess that they too have? How do you envision your health span unfolding throughout your life span after watching your own relatives move through theirs?

Figure 1.3 shows life span extension from 60-year-olds through 90-year-olds. Note that living with disease from 60 to 90 years old is not a quality health span. In contrast, a morbidity period that is compressed to a few years in your 80s *does* indicate a high-quality health span. Your health and habits today dictate which of these paths you will go down later in life.

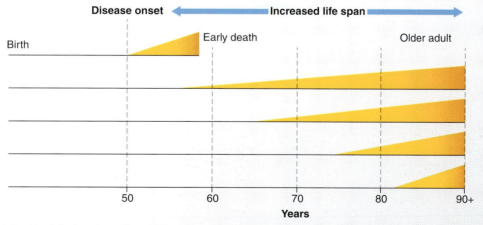

Figure 1.3 By delaying the onset of disease, you can delay death, increasing your life span and the quality of life in later years.

number of healthy years and reduce the number of unhealthy years. Wouldn't it be nice to quietly fall asleep at the end of life knowing that you gave it your best shot?

Most medical research is targeted at a disease in isolation, and yet evidence is mounting that physiological changes due to aging incorporate a large majority of chronic disease states, many of which could be prevented by making healthy lifestyle choices. We take great care investing in our 401(k) so we will be financially secure in our older years, investing in well-being is a sort of 401(k) for life. If you don't have your health, it will be difficult to enjoy your later years, even if you have a lot of money.

National Wellness Goals

Healthy People 2020 (HP 2020) and soon to be released Healthy People 2030 (HP 2030), government initiatives, set goals for improving the health and wellness in the United States. Their main goal is to provide data-driven decisions on improving quality of life and reducing preventable diseases and premature death. The reports provide science-based objectives for improving health and wellness on a global and individual basis. The major goals of HP 2020 and HP 2030 are to empower people to make informed health decisions and to measure the effect of prevention activities, with the support of government and community resources.

✓ Behavior Check

How Does Your Location Rank?

Think about where you live. When you compare it to figure 1.4, where does it rank in terms of happiness?

Now think about where you might like to live. Would this place help you move more, sit less, and live well? Does it have good walkability? Take the walkability test (www.walkscore.com) to see how walkable your current living area is. Compare it to where you grew up and where you might like to live. If the URL does not work for you, ask yourself these questions about the area in which you live:

- Can you walk to get to restaurants and grocery stores or do you need a car?
- How many parks are nearby?
- Can you get to places by bus, bike, or foot?
- What is the crime level? Is it safe to walk at all hours of the day or night?

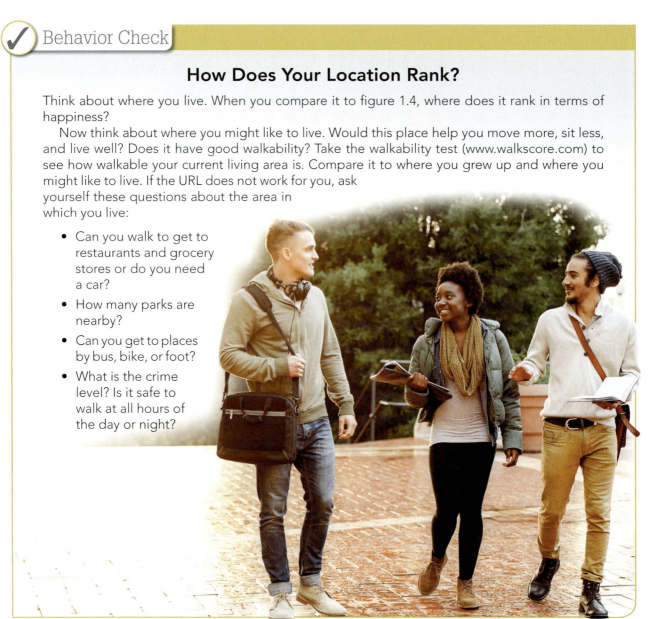

A private company called Healthways also sets well-being goals for companies and states in the United States. Understanding worksite wellness practices is important when picking a place to work. Gallup-Healthways has a well-being index that includes not only the major components of wellness but also social, community, physical, and financial aspects of life. Each year Gallup-Healthways surveys over 100,000 people by phone in all 50 states and in Washington, D.C.. Their 2016 survey revealed that 55.4 percent of Americans were thriving and that smoking rates had continued to decline. However, chronic diseases such as diabetes, obesity, and depression were at their highest points since 2008 (Gallup-Healthways 2017).

Choosing where to live is another important part of wellness. Companies have used the Healthways survey information, along with other factors such as crime, commute time, unemployment, and cost of living, to determine the happiest and saddest states. According to Hauser (2016), Hawaii was where the happiest people lived and West Virginia was where the saddest people lived. Khalid (2016) agreed that West Virginia was the saddest state and found Utah to be the happiest state. Figure 1.4 outlines the top 10 happiest states in the United States.

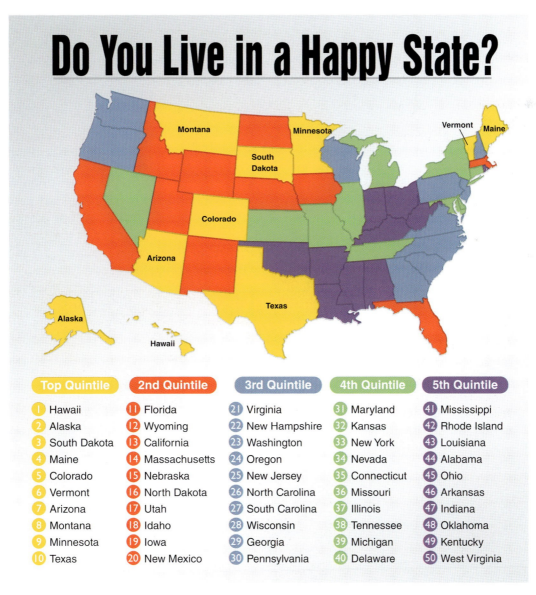

Figure 1.4   Top ten happiest states to live in, 2016.

Data from Gallup-Healthways (2017).

New Perspectives on Wellness

Past generations often defined the state of health as the absence of disease. But it's so much more than that. Arloski (2014) depicts wellness as a process of making choices for a more successful existence. His seven steps for lasting wellness are as follows:

1. Assessment
2. Foundational work on self
3. Setting the focus
4. Identifying habits developed in response to your environment
5. Initial behavior change
6. Deeper work on self
7. Lasting behavior or lifestyle change

You will see many of these steps in this book as we guide you through your own movement and wellness journey.

Dr. Jack Travis, an MD who created one of the first wellness inventory surveys in the mid-1970s, had a mission to shift the focus of the medical culture from authoritarianism and domination to partnership and cooperation. His vision was ahead of its time and also in line with being healthy throughout the health span. Travis's illness–wellness model (Well People 2011; see figure 1.5) depicts a paradigm where the neutral point is neither illness nor wellness. We move either right or left on this wellness continuum based on personal choices. To the right are high-level wellness and enhanced health and well-being. To the left are symptoms of disease and even disability, which

can cause premature death even before they take action on our physical or mental health. Dr. Travis is a pioneer in the creation of shifting our mindset beyond traditional medical and wellness practices.

Dr. Travis also believes that the current state of health is only the tip of the iceberg (Well People 2011). His vision of wellness is in line with contemporary research on aging, which tells us we have not studied wellness for as long as we have studied disease and pathology. Consider the iceberg model. The first level of the iceberg is the lifestyle or behavioral level. It includes what to eat, how to move, letting go of stress, and preventing accidents. If you chip away at the first level and start working on improving behavioral aspects of health, and then deepen further to the psychological or motivational level, you may improve your longevity. For true well-being, it is important to delve deeper into the connections between all the dimensions of wellness discussed in this book. Travis recommends diving below the surface to discover connections between eating well and moving, as well as socializing and enjoying a vacation. All of these options make up your health and wellness over the life span. To maintain a lifestyle change, we must understand why we are making the change. This requires research into the cultural, psychological, motivational, and even spiritual levels of well-being. Overall, changing wellness behaviors is complex. You will need concerted effort, focus, and balance to chip away at the iceberg and thus create a lasting healthy lifestyle focused on living long and living well.

A contemporary wellness focus encourages taking charge of one's health and wellness in order to enhance life expectancy. In addition to

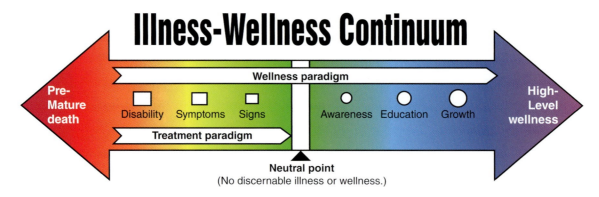

Figure 1.5   The illness–wellness continuum.
© 1972. 1988, 2004. John W. Travis, MD.

Dr. Travis's iceberg model, there are many other ways to break down wellness into workable pieces. See figure 1.6 for a progression of wellness models. The wellness pie and puzzle are commonly used to describe how wellness all comes together. These models are limiting because the pieces fit perfectly together and do not overlap or intermix. The reality of life is not this perfect. Habits from one piece roll over into the other pieces. Also, at any given time, we may be working more on one piece of wellness than another. For example, a college student's wellness focus would be more on the intellectual and social pieces of the pie, while the occupational and environmental pieces may take a backseat until graduation. In our 30s or 40s, our focus is on emotional and occupational wellness (marriage, kids, and work). In our 50s and 60s, when our kids leave home, there is more time for environmental discovery (e.g., cruises and hikes). Finally, in our 70s and 80s, the social and intellectual become more important to preserve toward the end of life. Throughout all of life, the physical, spiritual, and financial pieces are staples. Without these three pieces, it would be difficult to move through life and be happy, stable, and well. On another note, we all have our wellness model preferences—the components of wellness that are important to us at each particular stage in life.

Lifestyle change occurs during the transition of working on one or more wellness areas. The newest wellness model, with its focus on the ebb and flow of wellness components throughout the life span, depicts wellness not as a pie or puzzle piece but rather as what you value and want to bring with you throughout your life. Your own wellness model is closely aligned with your reality, where the significance of different areas ebbs and flows throughout life based on what you value and the life choices you make. Wellness is actually how you juggle all these life choices in order to live a fulfilling life and prevent early-onset lifestyle diseases. The decade of our 20s is where we make many life choices that affect our adult lives. Our personal assets from life include who we marry, our career choices, and what college we attend. Meg Jay, a psychologist who wrote a book on the 20s, calls this collection of our personal assets "identity capital" (2012).

Now and Later

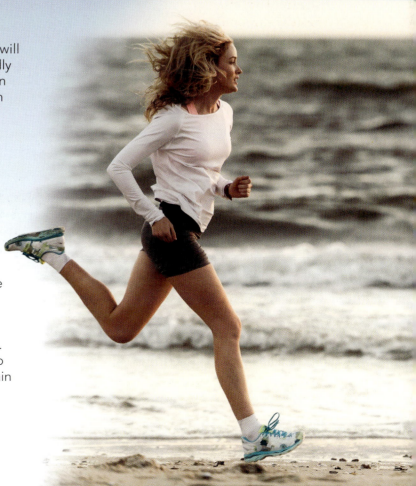

Wellness Preferences

You will see throughout this book that we will present Now and Later boxes that will continually remind you of the big picture of *why* a focus on your health in your earlier years will pay off in your later years.

Now

What are the main wellness pieces you are working on now?

Later

Think about your family, including your parents, grandparents, siblings, aunts, and uncles. Using their example as a guide, guess what your wellness focus will be as you age. Draw your wellness pieces throughout your life span as figure 1.6 depicts near the bottom.

Take Home

Wellness pieces and life values go hand in hand. List the main wellness pieces that you want to focus on throughout your life span and explain why these are important to you.

Progression of Wellness Models

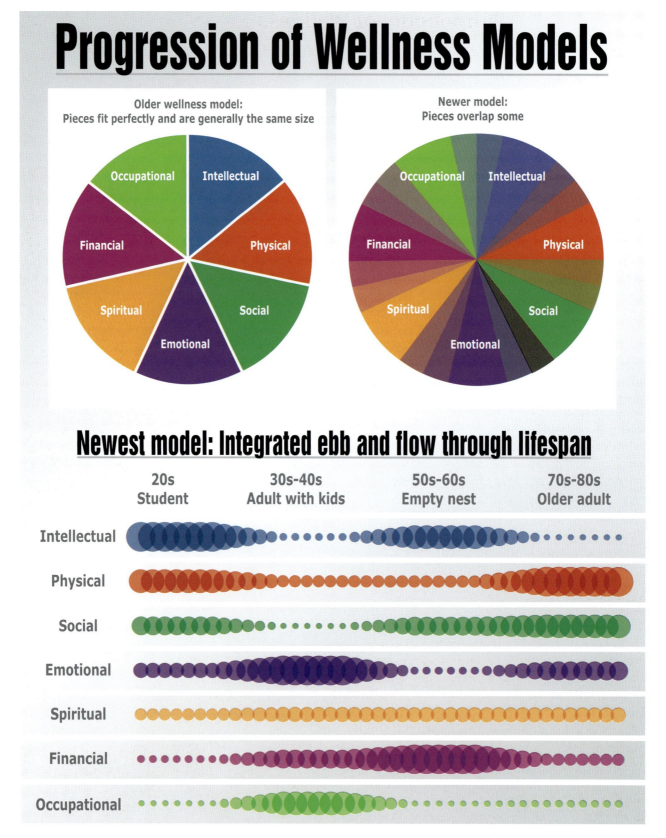

Figure 1.6 Our understanding of wellness has changed over time.

10

Components of Wellness

Wellness can be classified into eight major areas: physical, emotional, intellectual, social, environmental, occupational, financial, and spiritual. As you read about the eight major areas of wellness below, consider your own strengths and weaknesses. Then, write down a few ideas of wellness components you might want to focus on related to changing habits and lifestyle. Lab 1.1 in the web study guide will utilize knowledge of the wellness components and ask you to pick a few areas you want to work on.

Physical Wellness

Physical wellness is not only being active and fit but also being able to move and function effectively. It is carrying out daily tasks with vigor and energy or enjoying leisure-time pursuits without getting tired or sore. For example, someone who is physically well can go on a one- to two-mile (1.6 to 3.2 km) run and not feel sore the next day. It includes having enough physical health to perform adequate functional daily living activities because you are eating well and moving enough throughout the day. Physical wellness also involves making informed health decisions for your safety. It includes getting enough sleep, using alcohol and drugs responsibly, not texting while driving, and using sunscreen. Finally, it can also include intentional and responsible sexual choices and managing injuries and illnesses effectively by practicing good self-care. A large portion of this book is dedicated to the physical aspect of wellness. Often, having adequate physical wellness opens up the door to working on other aspects of wellness with energy and enthusiasm.

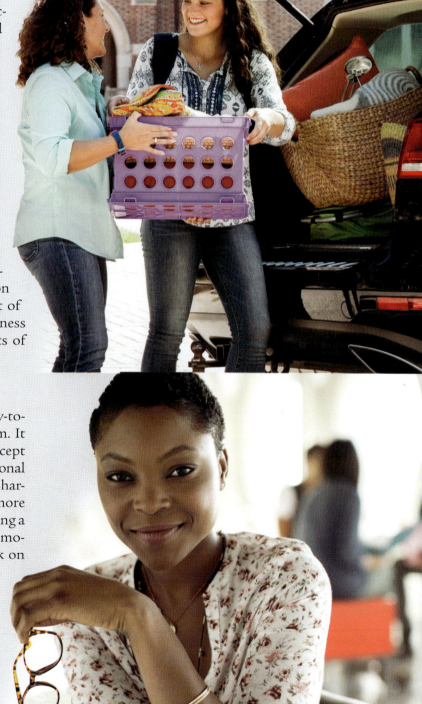

Emotional Wellness

Emotional wellness is your ability to carry on day-to-day activities with self-confidence and optimism. It means having the ability to understand and accept your feelings. It is also about being free from emotional and mental illnesses such as clinical depression. Sharing feelings with others and going through life more often happy than depressed are important to having a fulfilling life. People who possess a high level of emotional wellness generally have a positive outlook on life and are easily content. They are stable, dependable, positive, and persistent. They also can live and work independently while reaching out to others when in need. Achieving this type of wellness also involves finding professional help when needed.

Intellectual Wellness

People who possess good intellectual wellness are lifelong learners who focus on growing throughout the life span. Enjoying intellectual wellness involves constantly being challenged mentally. Instead of choosing a television show for background noise, sort through the offerings to find an educational program that is also entertaining. Intellectual wellness involves thinking logically and solving problems in order to meet life's challenges with creative ideas. It is reading books for pleasure and enjoyment and being open to learning new ways of thinking and working. If you are curious and motivated to master new skills or learn new things, you have high intellectual wellness. Finally, critical thinking and the courage to question the status quo are also aspects of high intellectual wellness.

> U.S. adults who have masters, doctoral, or professional degrees have been shown to exhibit even lower mortality rates than those who have bachelors degrees (Rogers et al. 2010).

Social Wellness

Do you know the difference between illness and wellness? Illness begins with "I" and wellness begins with "we."

Human beings are generally social. We strive to maintain positive and satisfying interpersonal relationships, which requires effective communication skills. Social wellness involves the ability to interact with others in meaningful ways that help establish long-term relationships. A person with a strong level of social wellness is generally characterized as being engaged in life rather than lonely. The ability to communicate effectively and develop a capacity for intimacy are also important elements of social wellness. The most critical skills for social wellness are finding social relationships, giving support, being assertive, practicing self-disclosure and emotional expression, and managing conflict. Finally, engaging in community activities, helping others, and listening are important in building positive social wellness. If you sense the need to improve your social wellness, consider seeking out clubs and groups that share your same interests!

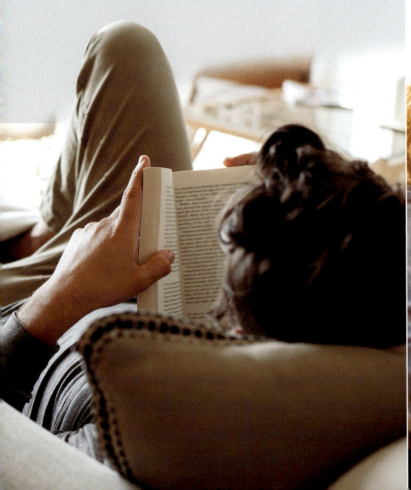

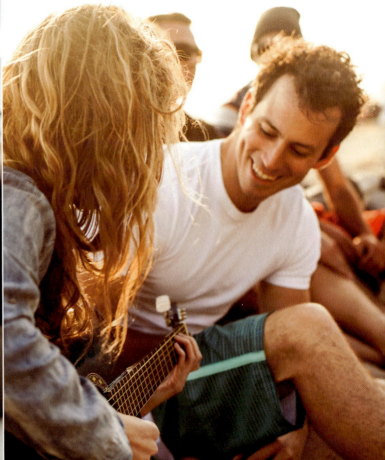

Environmental Wellness

Your sense of place in your surroundings includes your comfort within the environment where you live. For example, when you moved into your college space, did you bring some items that made you feel more at home? If you did, you were creating your own sense of place so you could feel comfortable in a new environment. This work of settling in is important no matter where you live or work. This concept has a lot to do with your environmental wellness on a day-to-day basis.

Sociologists and urban planners study why certain *places* hold special meaning to people. They call this process *place mapping*. The term has been identified as a way to observe human behavior. Buettner's blue zones (2015) are an example of place mapping. Having a strong *sense of place* will help you carefully select the place you live, since it will influence your environmental wellness. Remember the states where people were the happiest? Sense of place also relates to deeply feeling an emotion or sense of identity when you go to a particular place.

Think about how it feels to go home from college to your familiar family home. All your things are in place where you put them, the family dog comes to greet you, and you feel comfortable, safe, and relaxed in this space. Now think about where you will live when you leave college. Is there a history of violence where you choose to live? Is your environment walkable? Can you take steps to make sure your lifestyle is respectful of the environment and helps create sustainable human and ecological communities? Are recycling and gardening space available? Essentially, what is the livability of your surroundings, and do they meet your expectations for a happy and healthy environment? If not, then how can you make sure you live in an environment that meets your expectations? What is your plan to make this happen?

Many college alumni revisit their alma maters. As they explore campus again, they relive both positive and negative experiences. Thus, they experience their own place-mapping process.

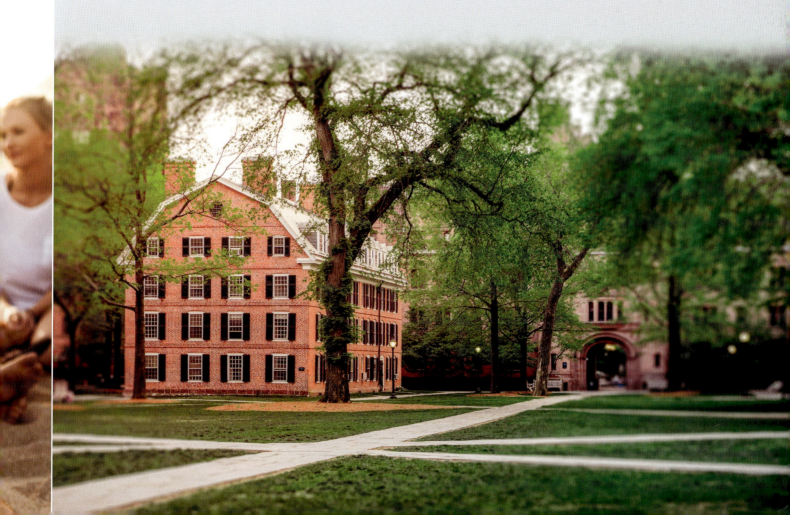

Occupational Wellness

Occupational wellness refers to the level of happiness and satisfaction you gain from the work you choose. Considering the many days you will spend at work, job choices are essential to health and wellness. Your well-being is connected to having a job that is meaningful and fulfilling, gives you personal satisfaction, and allows you to use your skills to contribute to your community. Having good occupational wellness is more than being paid well. If you don't value the work or gain personal satisfaction from it, it does not matter how well you are paid. In an ideal job, your supervisors recognize your work, you generally enjoy your coworkers, and the work is satisfying. Look for a job, but hunt for a career. Finding fulfilling work right out of college is often tough. However, if you are hunting for a fulfilling career rather than chasing money and prestige, you are heading in the right direction for an occupation you might enjoy for years to come.

> The only way to do great work is to love what you do. Hunt for a job; search for a career.

Financial Wellness

Managing finances is often a task that requires critical thinking, self-discipline, and financial planning. It involves living within your means, working to stay out of debt, and being realistic about spending habits. Keeping emotions in check related to your financial transactions is also important. Using several credit cards, letting friends make your decisions on finances for you, gambling, or having unrealistic expectations can cause emotional stress. Having a budget can help set realistic expectations and keep monetary spending under control. Just as tracking your movements can help you know how many steps you take in a day, so too will tracking your expenditures give you an idea of where your money goes. We often think that making more money will help us feel happier. However, research shows that once you make between $50,000 and $75,000, the correlation between income and well-being slopes off (Gilbert 2007). Check out the eight principles that bring you the most happiness for your money (Baer 2014):

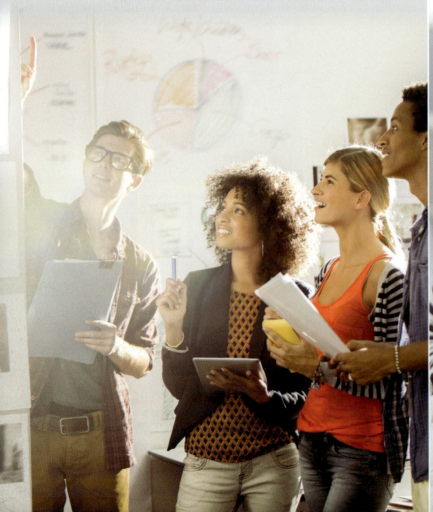

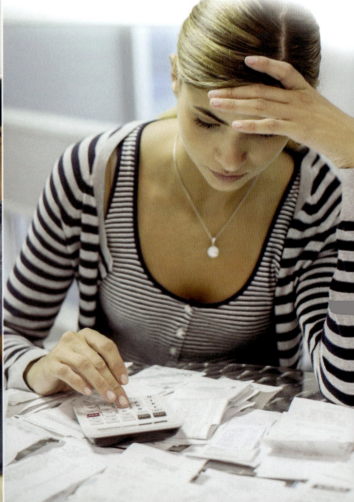

Principles That Bring You the Most Happiness for Your Money

1. Buy experiences instead of things.

2. Spend money to help others instead of yourself.

3. Buy many small pleasures instead of a few big ones.

4. Buy less insurance.

5. Pay now, consume later.

6. Think about what it's really like to own the thing you want to buy.

7. Stop the comparison shopping.

8. Ask your friends.

Spiritual Wellness

Wellness often focuses on the physical aspects of life, but a sense of purpose and a feeling of belonging can be just as important for overall well-being. A spiritually well person knows how to make the best of a bad situation and fend off naysayers by focusing on the positive. Spiritual wellness is also about possessing values, beliefs, and life principles to live by. It's the ability to recover from loss and forgive and forget with gratitude and gratefulness. Organized religion often helps with the development of spirituality, but it is not the only source of strength in times of need. Meditation, a walk in the forest with a friend, drawing, listening to music, and yoga can all help you gain spiritual wellness.

> You cannot teach people anything; you can only teach them to find it within themselves.

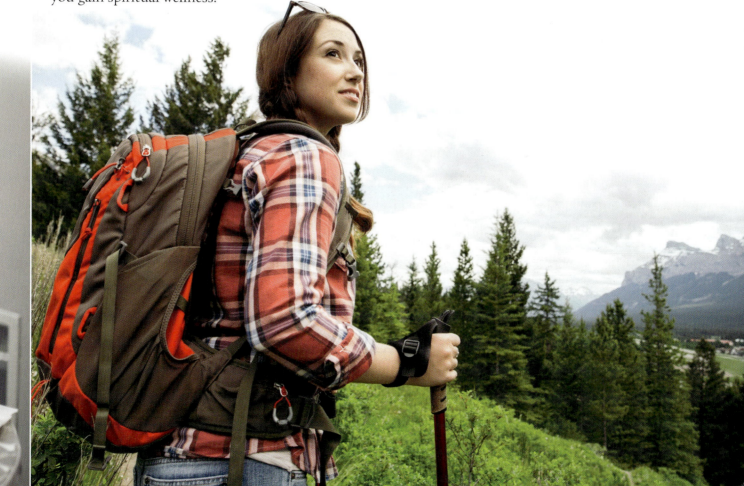

To Sum It Up

Making good wellness choices beginning in your 20s, some of which include the following:

- *Social wellness*. You might meet a significant other in a wellness setting (eating at a healthy restaurant or working out at the student recreation center).
- *Intellectual wellness*. Take a part-time job that helps you figure out what you want to do in life.
- *Spiritual wellness*. Find the job or leisure activities that you do well enough or long enough that they become who you are, not just what you do.
- *Physical wellness*. Making the healthy choice the easy choice in your 20s goes a long way toward creating regular healthy habits that ultimately become who you are.

What Are Functional Movement and Wellness?

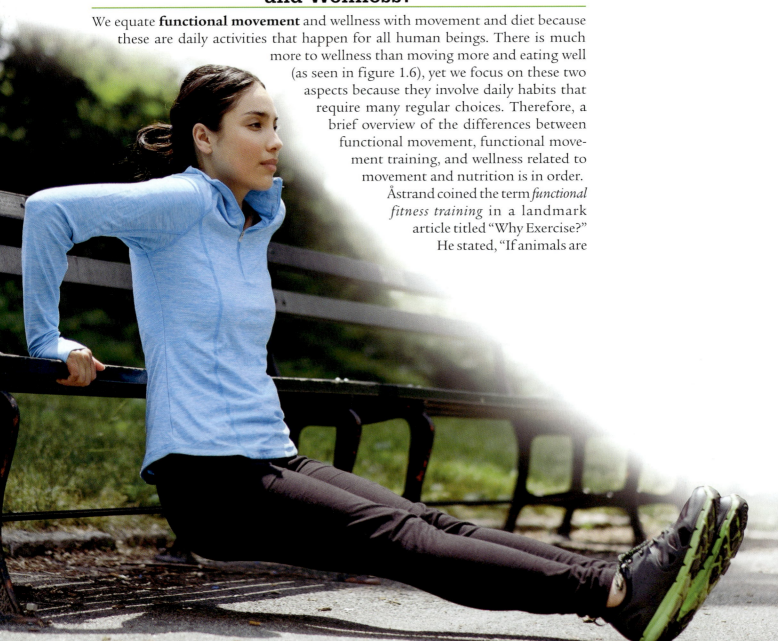

We equate **functional movement** and wellness with movement and diet because these are daily activities that happen for all human beings. There is much more to wellness than moving more and eating well (as seen in figure 1.6), yet we focus on these two aspects because they involve daily habits that require many regular choices. Therefore, a brief overview of the differences between functional movement, functional movement training, and wellness related to movement and nutrition is in order. Åstrand coined the term *functional fitness training* in a landmark article titled "Why Exercise?" He stated, "If animals are

⏱ Now and Later

Your Daily Choices Matter!

Now

In terms of staying healthy through the life span, the choices made in your 20s matter.

Later

Imagine this eulogy: "She passed away peacefully in her sleep after having walked her last one-mile route in the morning at 97 years old."

Take Home

Now that's a lifetime of living well! Living well requires behavior analysis, perseverance, and the joy of taking care of yourself throughout life so you can also take care of others. Going beyond physical aesthetics and empowering an internal well-being sense of place will make life tolerable and enjoyable on most days of the week.

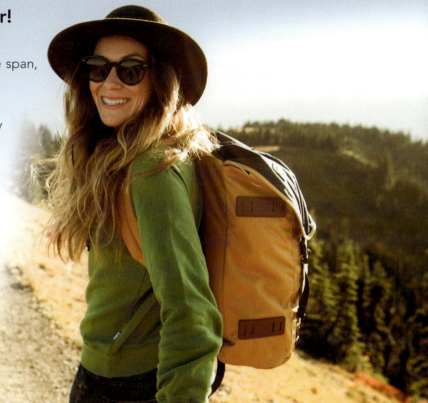

built reasonably, they should build and maintain just enough, but not more structure than they need to meet functional requirements" (1992, page 153). Dr. Åstrand was ahead of his time in predicting that people would soon be focusing more on why they should move than on how exercise changes their physique. Archer (2007) suggested that people need more of a sense of purpose for why they exercise and predicted that soon there will be a blending of fitness and wellness. Using data from a Harvard alumni study, Ming (1999) found that the demographic with the best chance of living the longest was those men who gained the most weight since college *and* expended 2,000 calories per week in physical activity. Men who gained at least 15 pounds (6.8 kg) since college but were very sedentary had mortality rates 53 to 96 percent higher than men who gained a similar amount of weight but were physically active. Rather than exercising to improve how we look, why not move to improve our lives? The term *functional movement* is often used to explain this change of focus from aesthetics to movement that matters for life's daily tasks.

For the purpose of this book, we will define **functional movement training** as what you do in an organized workout with the objective of improving your daily functional movement. This book includes a special functional movement training insert section after chapter 6 to help you better understand how to incorporate functional movement training in your workout schedule to improve your functional movement. In that special section, you'll find exercises that use body weight, resistance variable machines, free weights, and stretches. You can find videos demonstrating these exercises in the web study guide!

Functional movement is about the choices you make on a regular basis related to incorporating movement into daily living activities. It is choosing to walk to class rather than getting dropped off by a friend, taking the stairs instead of the elevator, or wearing your backpack over both shoulders to strengthen your core muscles as you walk to class. Neither functional movement training nor functional movement is better than the other; they are just different. A combination of the two is what makes for healthy physical activity for life.

Fitness Is More Than Going to a Fitness Facility

It makes sense to look at daily patterns of physical activity in order to better understand functional movement throughout the day. Let's look at movement intensity over time. Notice in figure 1.7 how Busy Bob (orange line), who sits at his desk all day and gets very little movement throughout his day, rarely rises above the low movement intensity. He even takes an afternoon nap because he is tired. Is that mental fatigue or physical fatigue? Could a short walk instead of a nap help him move more, sit less, and have more energy to do his work? On the other hand, Moving Mary (blue line) parks farther away from her building and walks in, takes the stairs while at work, walks to lunch and back, and takes frequent breaks throughout the day by walking to the printer or delivering messages in person. Finally, Moving Mary takes her dog on an after-dinner walk. Moving Mary expends much more energy in her daily activities than Busy Bob, but she does not have a planned movement experience. Then there is Running Roy (green line). His work is much like Busy Bob's, but he takes a break at lunch to work out. He drives to the local fitness facility and gets a good run in, then goes back to work and sits at his desk all day.

Ideally, a combination of Running Roy (functional fitness training) and Moving Mary (functional movement) is a way to envision healthy movement through the lifetime. If you cannot get to a fitness facility or you do not like to run, then be like Moving Mary. If you know you will sit at your desk all day, then Running Roy's day might work for you. The message here is that going to a fitness facility or running is not the only way to get movement into your day. You have many different ways to acquire daily movement, just as you can make many different choices about the doctor you see for your health needs or which foods you eat daily. All movement (whether in a fitness facility or throughout the day) is *good* movement and improves your health and well-being.

Sedentary living is another aspect of a healthy lifestyle to analyze when considering whether or not to go to the fitness facility today. A current topic within the physical domain of wellness is sedentarism, which is often termed "sitting time." The growing consensus among many public health experts is that sitting may be the new smoking (Levine 2014). Engaging in sedentary

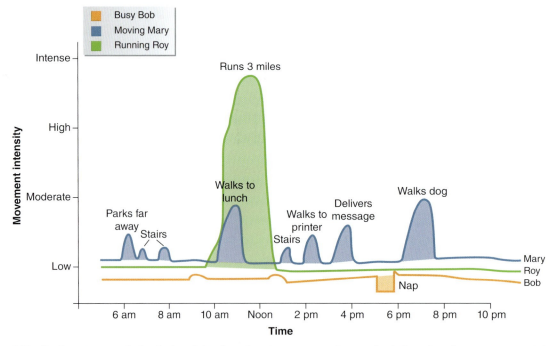

Figure 1.7   Basic patterns of physical activity: functional movement (green line), functional movement training (black line), and sedentary living (red line) (Blair, 1992).

Based on Blair, Kohl, III, and Gordon (1992).

behaviors was once thought of as the opposite of being physically active. However, emerging research suggests that people can visit fitness facilities and still engage in sedentary behaviors to the point of adversely affecting their health. A study on sedentary time and its association with risk for disease in adults concluded that prolonged sedentary time was associated with poor health outcomes regardless of physical activity levels (Biswas 2015). Daily movement has decreased because we sit while we work, while we commute to work, and when we get home. A single activity break each day is likely not enough movement to offset the harmful physiological and psychological effects of sitting so much. You can read more about this in chapter 2.

The increasing popularity of the standing desk is a social testimony that we are trying to maintain screen productivity but also get out of our chairs more. A study by Katzmarzyk (2014) indicated that standing may reduce mortality in those who are physically inactive, suggesting that it may be a health-

ier alternative to excessive periods of sitting. Interventions in the workplace to reduce sitting time are becoming the norm. In fact, a study by Healy (2016) discovered that intervening in employee sitting time can make a difference in their overall movement throughout the day when compared to controls. To keep up with the current literature on sitting time, check out the website www.JustStand.org, which contains evidence-based studies on sitting time that are updated regularly. Debate about this workplace sitting issue will continue, and we may see work spaces change dramatically in the future due to the health risk of being too sedentary for long periods of time.

We wonder why we are gaining weight when we go to a fitness facility and work out. We think it is because we have gained more muscle. A 60-minute workout in a fitness facility burns calories and can potentially improve heart health. After all, the heart is a muscle. However, what we are learning from the research on sedentary time is that working out is not the only solution. Paying attention to functional movement throughout the day is also essential. Therefore, the idea of working out to offset daily inactivity is no longer enough to maintain physical health. We need more functional movement in our days to be healthy physically.

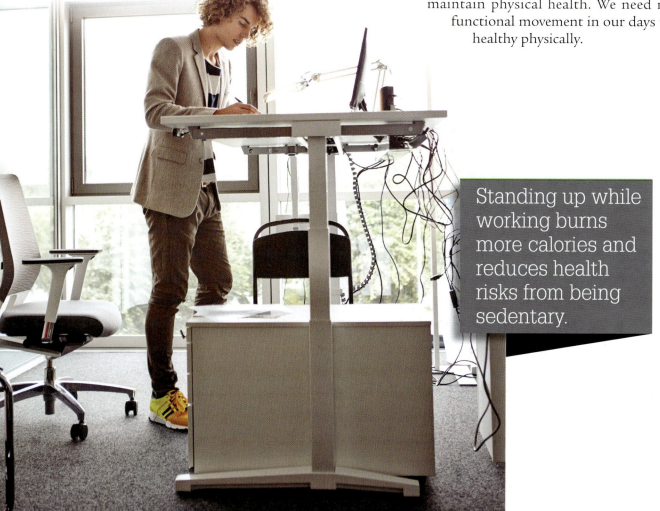

Standing up while working burns more calories and reduces health risks from being sedentary.

Wellness Is More Than Eating Healthy

Just as with movement and fitness, eating healthy is about making the healthy choice the easy choice. Nourishing the body is a very important part of wellness. What we eat, when we eat it, and who we are with make all the difference in terms of our daily nutritional choices. Consumer interest is growing in the health-enhancing role of specific foods that some experts call functional foods. Functional foods are simply foods that make you feel good. How do you feel physically after you eat a hamburger, French fries, and a milkshake? Most likely, you want to take a nap and allow your body to process a meal high in fat and calories. Equate this to sitting at a desk all day instead of getting up and moving around. The internet is abuzz with talk of functional foods. An article on Google food trends shows that people are now focusing not on eating less but on adding nutritionally sound foods to their daily diet (Pina 2016). Eating functional foods, like doing functional movement, is having a conscious awareness of what you are eating and how it makes your body feel and then choosing to eat well so you will feel well. There is more information on nutrition in later chapters to provide more specific nutritional recommendations.

Of course, occasionally we all celebrate and eat a bit more than we ought to or sit more than we would like to. Making good choices 80 percent of the time is a good goal for functional movement and nutrition. The intention of this book is not to make you feel guilty when you do not move or eat healthy food but rather to teach you how to treasure your body and be kind to it 80 percent of the time. This practice will help you live life with zest, joy, and a healthy attitude toward moving more and eating well.

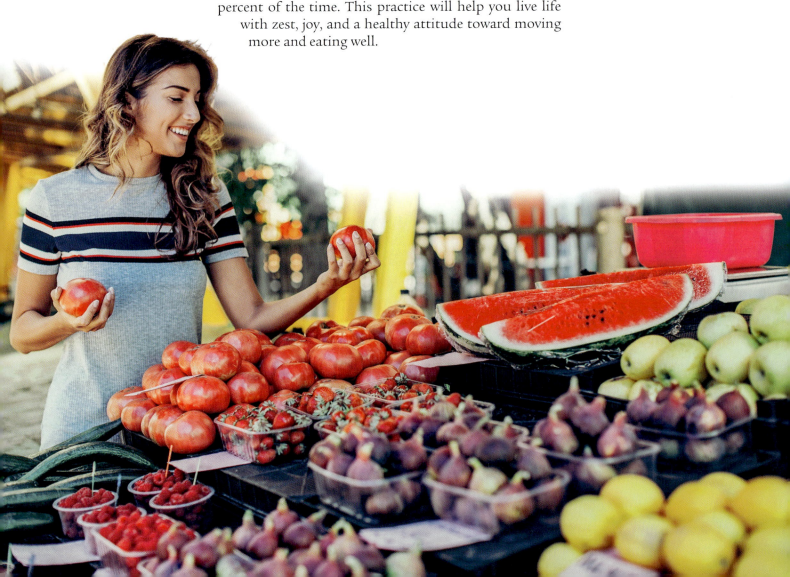

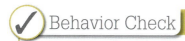

Daily Choices and the Calories You Burn

To help put this idea of movement and wellness into practical terms, let's think about the calories a 150-pound (68 kg) person will burn doing basic life tasks such as mopping the floor, grocery shopping, and vacuuming (table 1.1). You could hire most of these tasks out and then go to a fitness facility for a workout. From a wellness perspective, this might affect your financial wellness. It would also eliminate daily tasks that help you move more. Of course, the fitness facility membership might be your social outlet for wellness, so maybe that's okay. There's so much to consider when you make daily health and wellness choices.

Table 1.1 Calories Burned by a 150-Pound Person in Daily Activities

Activity	Calories
Raking leaves	147
Gardening or weeding	153
Moving (packing and unpacking)	191
Vacuuming	119
Cleaning the house	102
Playing with the kids (moderate activity level)	136
Mowing the lawn	205
Strolling	103
Sitting and watching TV	40
Biking to work (on a flat surface)	220

Based on McCoy (2009).

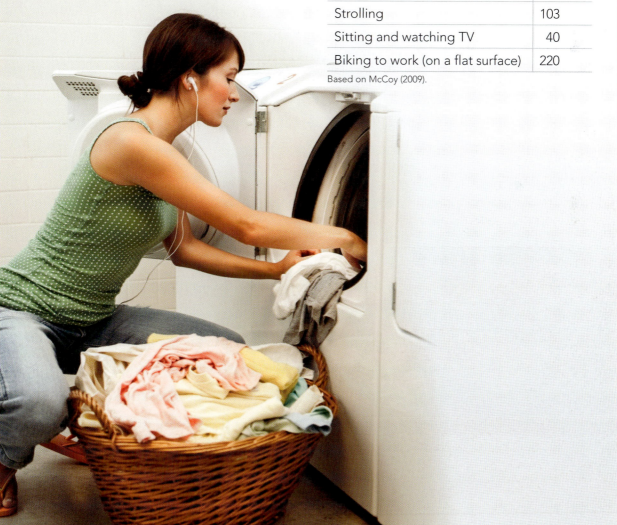

Lifestyle Choices of Real People

What gets in your way when it comes to being healthy and well?

Take a moment and make a list of habits versus healthy lifestyle choices. Begin to think about the real choices you make.

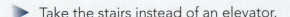

- ▶ Take the stairs instead of an elevator.
- ▶ Walk home instead of having a friend pick you up.
- ▶ Go to a local restaurant known for growing their own food instead of an all-you-can-eat local food chain for dinner.
- ▶ Park far away instead of finding the closest parking space when shopping.
- ▶ Shovel snow or rake leaves instead of using a blower to clean the yard.
- ▶ Instead of sitting to have coffee or tea with friends, walk and talk while enjoying your drinks.
- ▶ Go on a hike with friends instead of going out to dinner together.
- ▶ Walk your dog outside or go to a fitness facility instead of playing a video game.

These are just a few examples of typical functional movement choices we make on a daily basis that could be changed to enhance our health and wellness. We often schedule unhealthy moments in our lives because we feel we don't have enough time to take a walk, hike, or find a new healthy place to eat.

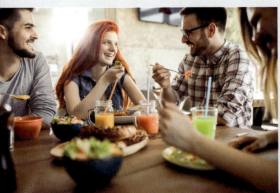
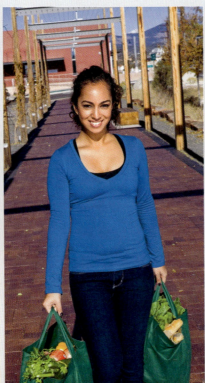
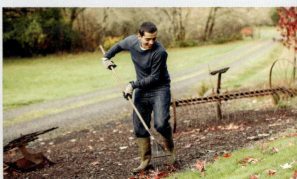
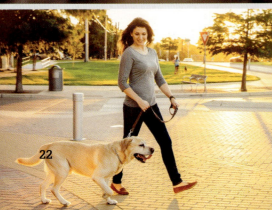
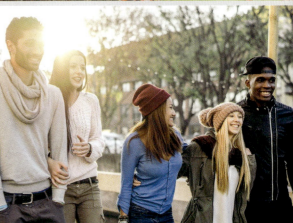

Life, Be in It!

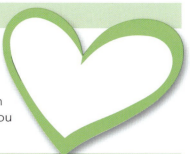

In 1975, the Australian government coined the slogan "Life. Be in it." The corresponding campaign featured cartoon characters moving, playing, eating well, and basically following good wellness practices. Australia did this in order to encourage its citizens to enjoy and embrace life rather than take it for granted. Do an internet search for "Life. Be in it" and see if you can find a character photo that portrays your lifestyle.

It is the little things that matter the most over time when it comes to evaluating a lifestyle. Think of life as a game and then ask yourself how you want to play it over the long term. A life well lived is one in which you come sliding into home plate at the end. It doesn't matter whether or not you are called "out." What you will remember is how you played the game.

In his 2009 book *Making Learning Whole: How Seven Principles of Teaching Can Transform Education*, David Perkins talks about how you take classes in college that build on one another to create a learning experience that will one day culminate into a career. You may wonder why taking chemistry will make you a better doctor or how a psychology class will make you a better accountant. The point is that you will one day put the cumulative effect of learning into a career and it will all make sense. The same is true with wellness. The little choices you make along the way compose your wellness life. It might seem like taking the stairs instead of the elevator each time you are greeted with this choice cannot mean much, but over a lifetime, it can make a huge difference for your health.

> A great life is not about great huge things—it's about small things that make a big difference.

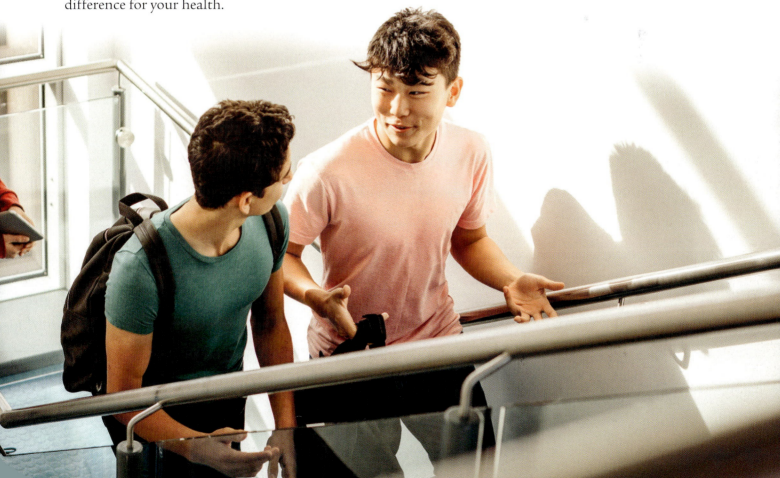

Summary

Stairs are becoming harder and harder to find because of the choices people regularly make. Will your children even know what stairs are, or will they grow up thinking elevators and escalators are how we get from one level to another? This book will help you think about the daily functional movement choices you make and how they will affect you for a lifetime. To continue with the baseball metaphor, aim to slide into home plate and be safe by a mile because you did all the right things while playing the game: You listened to the coach, worked hard to be a team player, and showed up with energy and enthusiasm to play the game.

To see how well you are playing the game of wellness, you will now fill out a wellness profile. This will help you inventory your wellness strengths and identify areas where you might focus your energy within. Complete lab 1.1 in the web study guide.

 WEB STUDY GUIDE

Remember to complete all of the web study guide activities to further facilitate your learning, including **Lab 1.1 Your Wellness Baseline**.

REVIEW QUESTIONS

1. What is the difference between life span and health span?

2. Name six of the eight components of wellness. Which three are you doing well? How do you know you are doing well in these areas? Make a list that shows your successes in these areas and a list to work on over time.

3. Describe the neutral point of the illness–wellness continuum created by Dr. Jack Travis.

4. Explain the difference between functional movement and functional fitness training.

5. List three ways to get functional movement in daily living.

6. Is there a difference in energy expenditure between working out in a fitness facility and taking a walk with a friend? Why or why not?

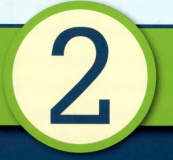

Functional Fitness and Movement Choices

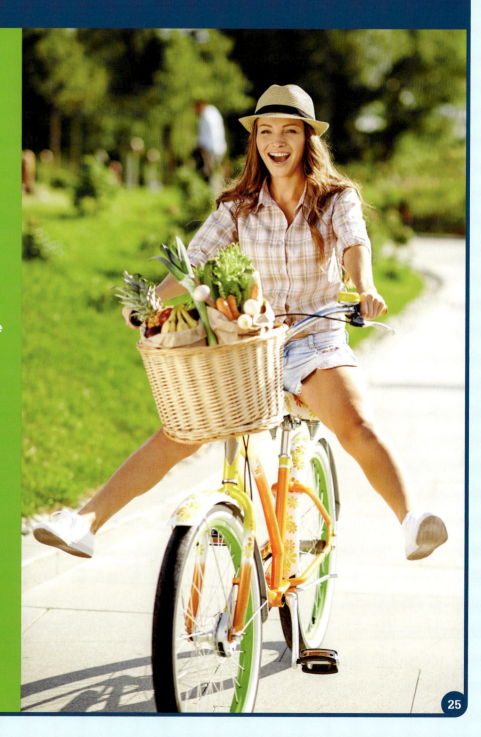

OBJECTIVES

》 Compare and contrast the U.S. Department of Health and Human Services (HHS) Physical Activity Guidelines (PAG) and the ACSM exercise guidelines.

》 Explain the emerging risk factor of sedentarism, or sedentary behavior.

》 Understand how the ACSM exercise guidelines and the HHS PAG complement one another.

》 Design a life-span functional fitness, movement, and health plan using the three-part human movement paradigm.

》 Analyze how environmental choices and daily movement opportunities affect your health investment for life.

》 Set SMART goals related to physical activity, exercise, and sedentary living.

KEY TERMS

ACSM exercise guidelines
HHS Physical Activity Guidelines
exercise
human movement paradigm

life span
physical activity
sedentarism
SMART Goals

The benefits of a physically active lifestyle are well established. Unfortunately, Americans have not kept pace with other nations in terms of advances in population health, instead focusing more resources on disease care than on chronic disease prevention and wellness (U.S. Burden of Disease Collaborators 2013). Chapter 1 discusses how life expectancy in the U.S. has recently decreased for the first time since 1993 (Xu et al. 2016). There are many reasons for this change; just like life, it is complex.

This chapter explores research on physical activity, exercise, and sedentarism and relates historical accounts of physical activity and exercise in order to understand how the intentional fitness movement began. It focuses on how daily movement and exercise choices can blend and contribute to healthy living. Your physical activity and functional movement training choices affect your quality and length of life as well as how you look and feel. Moving functionally trains the body, enhancing fitness, health, and well-being. Walking to class instead of taking the bus is an example of a functional movement choice. (See the sidebar What Is Functional Movement?)

What Is Functional Movement?

As stated in chapter 1, incorporating consistent functional movements into your day helps make daily movement easier and more enjoyable. Training the body using movements rather than individual muscle groups is the focus. Walking briskly to a ball game rather than taking the car is functional movement. We need more than a beautiful body to have a long, healthy life. What's going on inside your body matters just as much as what you look like on the outside. Results of daily functional movement could be the ability to get out of a chair quickly or go on a hike without feeling sore the next day.

Group hiking is one way to enjoy a functional movement experience.

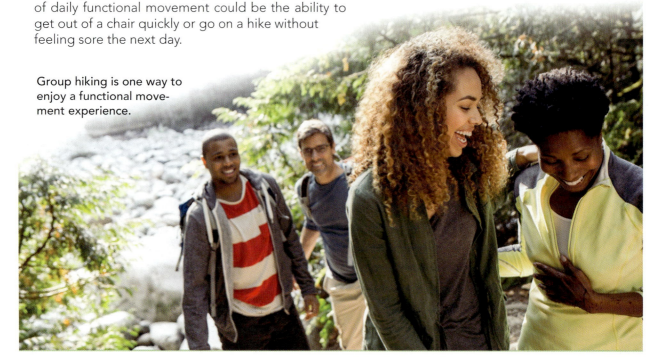

Exercise and **physical activity** combined matter over your lifetime. Our hope is that after reading this book, you will think twice before choosing a parking spot close to a building entrance because you know that choice does not enhance your health and well-being. This chapter also discusses traditional exercise in a fitness facility. At the end of this chapter, you will reflect on your current day-to-day movement choices and create a movement plan, considering your physical activity, exercise, and sedentary living habits, as well as your family history of disease and wellness.

Understanding Physical Activity Recommendations

This chapter also discusses the **HHS Physical Activity Guidelines**, the **ACSM exercise guidelines**, and the new emerging risk factor of **sedentarism**, or sedentary behavior (Matthews et al. 2015). This three-part **human movement paradigm** (figure 2.1) of physical activity, exercise, and sedentarism is directly linked to health and well-being. Kohl and colleagues (2012) reported that although evidence on the benefits of physical activity has been available since the 1950s, Americans have not kept up with movement guidelines. Experts suggest that a better way of solving the current physical inactivity crisis is to look beyond guidelines and recommendations and focus more on behavioral aspects of movement. Others in the physical activity field advocate changing the environment to help you make better daily choices, such as creating walking paths in place of bus routes (Trost et al. 2002). To integrate consistent movement into your daily movement choices, focus on your choices and behaviors as well as how you interact with the environment around you.

The notion of human movement has expanded beyond exercise to include distinct components

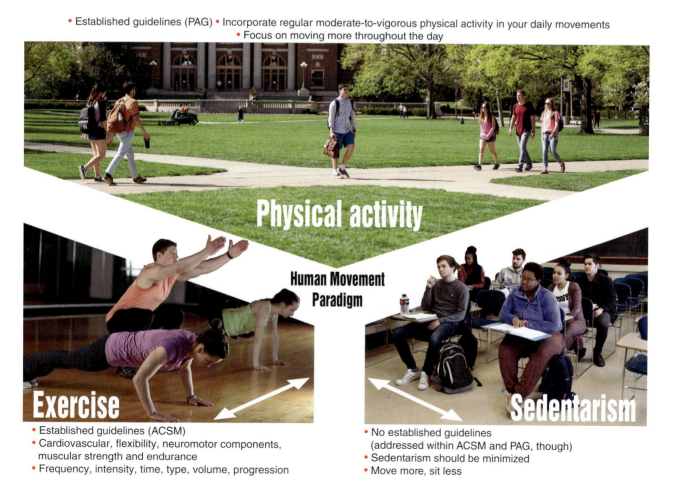

- Established guidelines (PAG) • Incorporate regular moderate-to-vigorous physical activity in your daily movements
- Focus on moving more throughout the day

Physical activity

Human Movement Paradigm

Exercise

- Established guidelines (ACSM)
- Cardiovascular, flexibility, neuromotor components, muscular strength and endurance
- Frequency, intensity, time, type, volume, progression

Sedentarism

- No established guidelines (addressed within ACSM and PAG, though)
- Sedentarism should be minimized
- Move more, sit less

Figure 2.1   The human movement paradigm, incorporating physical activity, exercise, and minimal sedentary living.

of physical activity and also sedentarism (also called sedentary behavior or sitting time). We have much work to do to change current physical activity adherence rates for adults. Only 20 percent of adults exercise regularly (Centers for Disease Control and Prevention 2016). Additionally, most adults in the United States spend approximately 55 percent of most days in a seated position (Matthews et al. 2008). This lifestyle was created over time, in part, by viewing exercise as a solution to the problem of sitting all day.

History of Intentional Exercise Practices

The term *prescription* is often defined as a written order by a physician or clinician for the administration of medicine. The definition of a prescription is simple. It is a piece of advice. The expression "exercise prescription" has been a staple of many fitness and medical professionals for decades. In more practical terms, the prescription might read more like, "Move more, sit less, and be well." Or as the Nike slogan states, "Just do it!"

This chapter focuses on the human movement paradigm, which is inclusive of all movement types (physical activity, exercise, and the minimization of time spent in sedentary behaviors). It provides a framework for movement prescription. Combining functional movement with functional movement training (exercise) and reducing sedentarism by sitting less are ideal for providing the energy needed to enhance your health and longevity for a lifetime.

We do not need to have a prescription to move. Moving is common sense because it makes us feel better. Our minds are broadening to include exercise habits beyond historical intentional movement practices. In the past, fitness prescriptions often left out the physical activity that we do just for the joy of moving. Why did we initially believe that going to a fitness facility and getting 60 minutes of daily movement was enough to compensate for a society dominated by sedentary living? Change is hard, especially in light of the health consequences that have arisen from the intentional fitness revolution.

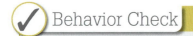 Behavior Check

Stairs Versus the Escalator

Think about the last time you were greeted with a scene like the one below. Would you choose those glorious stairs in the middle to charge up, or would you find your way to the escalator on the side of the stairs? Often we see crowds of people taking the escalator. Perhaps you can be the one who chooses the stairs next time. Remember, small decisions like choosing to take the stairs add up over time. Lots of small movement decisions throughout the day can equate to better overall health.

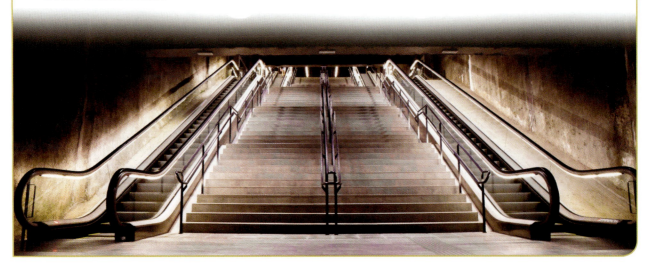

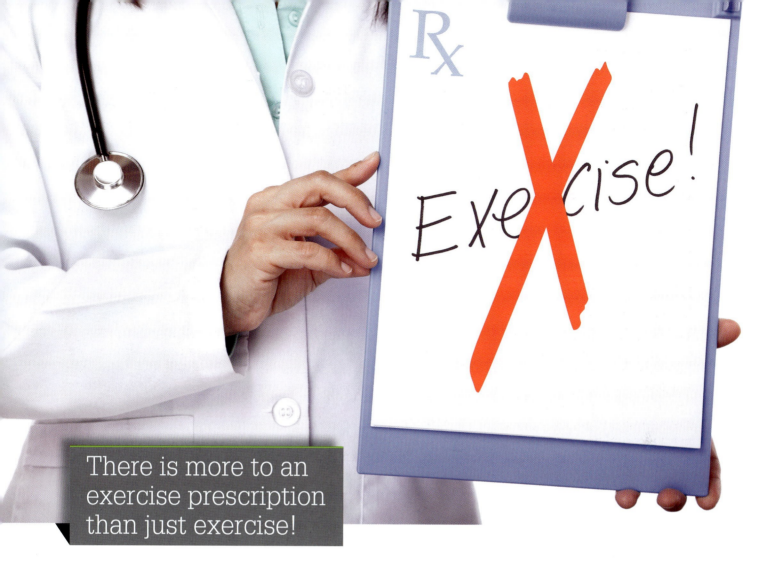

The Early Years

The history of the exercise prescription is best seen through updates from the American College of Sports Medicine (ACSM), specifically their *Guidelines for Exercise Testing and Prescription*. Often referred to as the best evidence-based source for exercise prescription, the various revisions of the ACSM position statement provide a chronological record and contextualization for the changes to the specifics of the exercise prescription. The acronym FITT (frequency, intensity, time, and type) initially proved useful for organizing an exercise prescription.

Although the details of the past position statements are not of primary interest, several changes in focus are important to note. The first ACSM position statement was published in 1978. Its primary focus was cardiorespiratory (aerobic) training due to the increase in the number of Americans diagnosed with heart disease in the 1970s and 1980s. This statement also advocated for performing movements that involved large muscle groups and doing sessions of moderate- to high-intensity activity for 15 to 60 continuous minutes three to five times per week (American College of Sports Medicine 1978).

1990s to present

In 1990, a major revision occurred to the ACSM position statement with the addition of muscular strength and endurance training (twice per week for all major muscle groups). Science continued to advance, and more substantial changes were recommended with the 1998 ACSM position stand (American College of Sports Medicine 1998). The time prescription for cardiorespiratory exercise sessions could be either 20 to 60 continuous minutes or more frequent 10-minute bouts that accumulated to make up 20 to 60 minutes. The muscular strength and endurance training prescription was altered to reflect different intensities for individuals younger or older than 50 years. Flexibility training was also added as a new mode of exercise. The 2006 ACSM position stand provided more detailed guidance with regard to intensity and duration for the primary modes of cardiorespiratory, resistance, and flexibility training (American College of Sports Medicine 2006). Notably, the initial FITT frame was preserved, with the addition of a musculoskeletal focus.

Figure 2.2 provides a visual summary of the 2018 ACSM guidelines for exercise. Less information from the scientific literature is related to flexibility and neuromotor practices because they are relatively new and have not been studied as much as the cardiorespiratory and muscular strength components of movement.

Future of Fitness for Real Life

The baby boomers, those born between 1946 and 1964, had the most influence on intentional fitness practices. They are still active participants in the fitness facility model because they invented it. This generation often used fitness facilities as a social outlet for getting out of the house and also for improving how they looked and felt. They were also the first generation to show us that we needed to modify our intentional movement choices as we age.

In the 1970s, the boomers were in their 20s. They participated in high-impact aerobics and ran 10K races in droves. In the 1980s and 1990s, boomers transitioned to low-impact aerobics, running 5Ks, step and slide classes, water exercise, indoor cycling, and yoga. The next two decades, when boomers were in their 50s and 60s, led to exercise with stability balls, balance devices, core strength, and TRX devices to improve neuromuscular and proprioceptive fitness. As boomers age into their 70s, look for them to be more involved in walking, corrective exercise, and pool water walking. Just as baby boomers changed their choices of fitness activities across their life span, so will your generation!

You may be a runner in your 20s, but you might need to move to gentler activities such as cycling or walking later in life. Your body is a treasure. It's the vehicle that drives your health and well-being throughout your **life span**. Listening to your

Becoming and Staying Fit

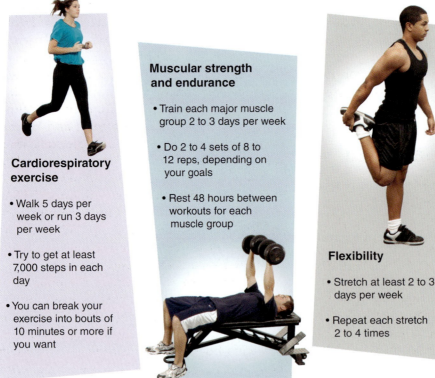

Cardiorespiratory exercise

- Walk 5 days per week or run 3 days per week
- Try to get at least 7,000 steps in each day
- You can break your exercise into bouts of 10 minutes or more if you want

Muscular strength and endurance

- Train each major muscle group 2 to 3 days per week
- Do 2 to 4 sets of 8 to 12 reps, depending on your goals
- Rest 48 hours between workouts for each muscle group

Flexibility

- Stretch at least 2 to 3 days per week
- Repeat each stretch 2 to 4 times

Neuromotor movement

- Do movements that focus on balance, agility, and coordination at least 2 to 3 days per week
- No known guidelines for volume and progression at this time

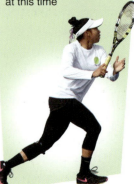

Figure 2.2   The best advice for improving your fitness, based on guidelines from the American College of Sports Medicine.

Data from *ACSM's Guidelines for Exercise Testing and Prescription* (2018).

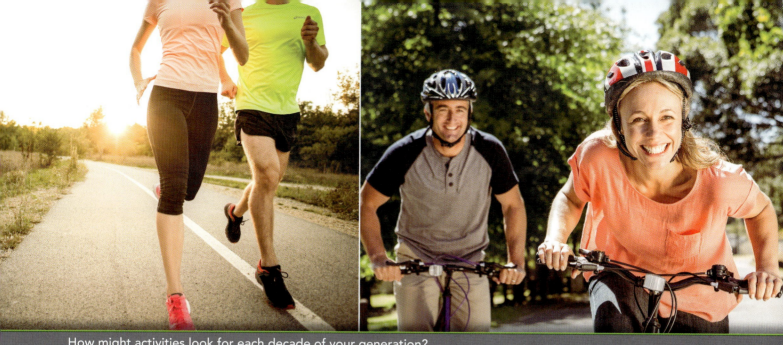

How might activities look for each decade of your generation?

body and changing your preference of movement options based on what it is telling you is the secret to a long, healthy life. If you are not moving, you may run into issues later in life. How many of your older relatives have had hip or knee replacements? If you take care of "your car," you can get many miles out of it without replacing parts.

To help you consider this topic, complete lab 2.1 in the web study guide. In this lab, you'll draw a timeline and record your movement history, along with that of your family and significant others. You'll also look to your future, projecting how your timeline might be different from or the same as those of the people who influenced you as you grew up.

Integrating Sedentarism, Physical Activity, and Exercise

Since 1978 the initial ACSM statement on how much exercise is enough, much more detailed research has been done. The exercise prescription is now so complex it can be overwhelming, even with our simplified version (see figure 2.2). Many exercisers have struggled to determine what to do, how intensely to do it, and how often to do it. Some started running and then learned walking was okay; some ran continuously for 30 minutes and learned that 10-minute increments were okay.

In 1995, Pate and colleagues published a landmark recommendation on behalf of both the HHS and ACSM advocating that every adult in the United States accumulate at least 30 minutes of moderate-intensity physical activity on most, preferably all, days of the week. No intensity, duration, or sets or reps were included in this public health statement. The message was intended to increase public awareness of the health-related benefits of moderate-intensity physical activity. The 1996 Surgeon General's report on physical activity and health (U.S. Department of Health and Human Services [HHS] 1996) aligned with the ACSM statement, emphasizing that health benefits occur at a moderate level of physical activity (moving approximately 150 minutes per week).

Hence, the first Physical Activity Guidelines (PAG, U.S. Department of Health and Human Services 2008) recommended a simple explanation stating that all movement counts no matter what intensity you choose. The 2018 Physical Activity Guidelines build upon the first edition of the PAG and form recommendations for federal physical activity and education programs. What's most important is that you move more and sit less daily.

The ACSM guidelines were focused on exercise, which only 20 to 25 percent of the population determined they could fit into their busy lifestyles. The HHS's 2008 PAG's emphasized 150 minutes of weekly movement and a lifestyle approach that highlights how leisure and recreational activity choices can be incorporated into a weekly physical activity plan. The 2018 Scientific Report, used to inform the most recent Physical Activity Guidelines demonstrates that, in addition to disease prevention benefits, regular physical activity provides a variety of benefits that help individuals sleep better, feel better, and perform daily tasks more easily (Office of Disease Prevention and Health Promotion 2018). The most recent Physical Activity Guidelines advise that you can achieve substantial health benefits simply by increasing your activity level and reducing your sedentary behavior. In short, do something and sit less!

We are getting back to finding joy in movement without a detailed prescription so that movement is more a part of life rather than "another thing we have to fit into an already busy schedule." Would you stick with an activity that is higher intensity, or is moving throughout the day over your life span a better option for your health? Think about it.

Physical Activity Guidelines and the National Physical Activity Plan

The ACSM exercise guidelines, written by scientists and intended for delivery by fitness professionals, are highly comprehensive and accurately detailed but can be hard to understand and translate to the general public. The HHS Physical Activity Guidelines (PAG) were developed by public health professionals and agencies who joined together to adopt physical activity as a force in preventing illness and enhancing quality of life. The HHS PAG may be more accessible to those working in the public health field, which prioritizes recommendations that are comprehensible for all members of society.

The current PAG align closely with the current ACSM guidelines with a noticeable lack of detail and complexity. One major goal of the PAG is to offer the general public an understandable method for implementing physical activity into daily practices with many options that may or may not include intentional structured exercise. Importantly, similar to the initial Surgeon General's report, the ACSM guidelines and the HHS PAG encourage reducing sedentary behaviors. The ACSM guidelines encourage people to take physical activity breaks throughout their day. The

> The National Physical Activity Plan (NPAP) is based on a vision that "one day, all Americans will be physically active, and they will live, work and play in environments that encourage and support regular physical activity" (NPAP n.d.).

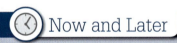

Now and Later

Everybody Walk

Now

Kaiser Permanente, in collaboration with many partners, created a 30-minute documentary called *The Walking Revolution*. It outlines the evidence-based practices of physical activity and why it is important to think about moving differently than we have in the past. Take half an hour and watch this important documentary: http://everybodywalk.org/documentary. Note that you can choose the short film version, which is only 8 minutes long. Approximately how many minutes do you walk per day?

Later

Now let's analyze how many minutes you think you will be walking per day when you are 50 to 60 years old. What are your parents or guardians currently doing for movement experiences? What about your grandparents? Will you be similar to your parents and grandparents or will you be more or less active?

Take Home

Now that you have watched the video and thought about your family movement history, what are your goals for walking and moving more throughout the day? How will you accomplish this goal? If you own technology that tracks your steps, such as an app on your phone or an activity tracker, what will your daily step goal be?

PAG provides ideas for how to incorporate physical activity more throughout the day, such as suggestions using a minimum of weight training equipment, using brisk walking to work the cardiorespiratory system, and incorporating body weight movements or work and leisure activities (e.g., garden or household chores) to provide muscular overload.

The National Physical Activity Plan (NPAP) was initiated by a group of health and wellness professions who sought to foster a culture that supports physically active lifestyles that enhance quality of life. This plan was developed by a coalition of national organizations that came together to form the NPAP Alliance. The Alliance is governed by a board of directors with representatives from each of the organizational partners. The NPAP was initiated in 2007. The first plan was released in 2010 and then updated in 2016. The plan includes policies, programs, and initiatives that increase physical activity in the U.S. population. Although the Alliance is based outside of the government, its overall plan has benefitted from a close partnership with HHS. Take a look at the NPAP plan specifics, and sign up for their free newsletter at www.physicalactivityplan .org.

With the guidance of the ACSM, the HHS Physical Activity Guidelines, and the NPAP, you can work to spread the goal of moving more and sitting less daily by starting to improve your own healthy habits and encouraging others to embrace a life of moving more and sitting less!

Health Effects of Too Much Sitting

Sedentarism (or sedentary behavior) is the last part of the human movement paradigm. The rise in importance of this part is linked to our culture's increasingly sedentary screen-based work and leisure. Although the 2018 ACSM exercise guidelines outline

You can reap significant health benefits from staying active throughout your day.

the components of the exercise prescription, the recommendations regarding sedentary behavior are less detailed due to a lack of comprehensive research. Even physically active adults can benefit from reducing the total time they engage in sedentary pursuits by interspersing frequent, short bouts of standing and physical activity between periods of sedentary activity. Physiological studies on being sedentary (Young et al. 2016) have taught us that inactivity is not the absence of physical activity (i.e., being physically inactive) or exercise.

Sedentary behavior recommendations are based on the following issues:

1. Spending significant time in sedentary behaviors increases disease risk; therefore, sedentary behavior is distinctly different from lack of physical activity and exercise.

2. Prolonged sitting can further increase disease risk in people who are already insufficiently physically active.

3. The molecular and physiological responses to too much sitting are not opposite, nor are they the same as responses that follow a bout of physical activity or exercise.

4. Physical activity and exercise cannot make up for the consequences of too much sitting. Physiologically, they are different and have unique health outcomes.

Hamilton and colleagues (2008) suggested that being sedentary has independent effects on key metabolic enzymes and risk for metabolic syndromes. Katzmarzyk and others (2009) concurred that extended sitting results in metabolic alterations that cannot be compensated for by an isolated exercise session. Similarly, Levine's (2014) work at Mayo Clinic determined that the negative effects of six hours of sedentary time were similar in magnitude to the benefit of one hour of exercise on fitness levels. There is more research coming out on sedentary behavior that will provide more guidance as to future recommendations.

The time spent engaged in sedentary behavior is the largest part of an average day for most of us. This new way of thinking about movement emphasizes the distinctions between not exercising, physical inactivity, and the health consequences of sedentary behavior (Young et al. 2016). Up until now, the expression "sedentary behavior" has misleadingly been used as a synonym for not exercising. But the two are not synonymous.

Sedentary behavior has serious consequences that are different than those from not exercising. Notably, in 2013, the American Medical Association (Brown 2013) adopted a policy recognizing the potential risks of prolonged sitting and suggested that employers make alternatives to sitting, such as standing desks, available to their employees. Standing (as opposed to exercise) interventions are currently being investigated. For example, Pronk (2012) determined that the "Take-a-Stand Project" reduced time spent sitting by 224 percent (66 minutes per day), lowered upper back and neck pain by 54 percent, and improved mood states. Notably, removal of the program largely negated all observed improvements within two weeks.

> Workers who use sit-to-stand desks are 78 percent more likely to report a pain-free day than those who do not have these desks (Ognibene et al. 2016).

Fitting Movement Into Everyday Life

Regular movement helps you stay healthy and maintain healthy physical function and independent living as you get older. A large literature base investigating physiological adaptations to exercise and physical activity training, including cardiorespiratory, resistance, flexibility, and neuromotor movement, documented that movement matters for independent living later in life (American College of Sports Medicine 2018). Chronic conditions are more likely to develop for middle-aged and older individuals who do not move daily and who sit a lot. Regular exercise and physical activity also play key roles in the management of most conditions, including anxiety and depression. Finally, the goal at the end of a long life is to preserve the capabil-

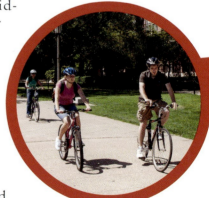

Let's roll!

Biking saves gas, reduces emissions, and keeps you moving!

ity for independent living and optimal social engagement. Regular physical movement is necessary, not only to look better, but also so you can enjoy leisure activities well into your 80s and even 90s. Some actually call exercise a miracle drug (Carroll 2016). Figure 2.3 presents ways you can fit purposeful movement into everyday life. In lab 2.1 in the web study guide, you will reflect on your personal fitness and movement history and get a better understanding of your movement history and preferences.

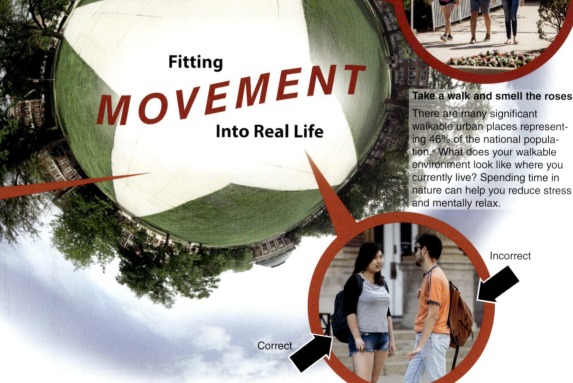

Stand or walk while you work

Sedentary time, or sitting, occupies more than half of adults' waking hours.[a] Use a standing desk, take your breaks on your feet, or use walking meetings. Steve Jobs of Apple favored walking meetings for creative thinking and movement.[b]

Take the stairs

Office workers constitute the largest single occupational sector in the U.S., and office work has been identified as a key setting in which to target reductions in prolonged sitting time.[c] Taking the stairs is actually faster than taking an elevator![d]

Fitting

MOVEMENT

Into Real Life

Take a walk and smell the roses

There are many significant walkable urban places representing 46% of the national population.[e] What does your walkable environment look like where you currently live? Spending time in nature can help you reduce stress and mentally relax.

Incorrect

Correct

Wear backpacks over both shoulders

Wearing a backpack correctly over both shoulders strengthens your postural muscles.

Figure 2.3 You can get creative with how to fit movement into your everyday life.

[a]Matthews 2008; [b]Isaacson 2011; [c]Healy 2012; [d]Shah et al. 2011; [e]Smart Growth America 2016

Setting SMART Goals for Fitness and Movement

Setting **SMART goals** (ones that are specific, measurable, attainable, relevant, and time bound) is an efficient way to begin any new behavior (see figure 2.4). Let's briefly review how to set a SMART goal so you can set physical activity goals based on where you are with your movement and where you want to be.

Following is an example of how one person set a SMART movement goal based on steps:

Specific. I would like to increase my steps per day so I get a weekly average of 10,000 steps a day during the last four weeks of the semester.

Measurable. I'll use my fitness tracker to calculate my steps per day and get a weekly average.

Attainable. Currently, I am getting 7,800 steps per day, so I believe that 10,000 steps per day is attainable as a goal.

Relevant. I get on the nearest bus to get to campus. I will walk to campus two times a week when I do not have early classes.

Time bound. I'm giving myself the entire semester to work up to my steps goal. By the last four weeks of the semester, I will get an average of 10,000 daily steps.

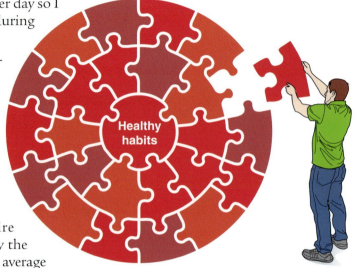

Figure 2.4 Building healthy habits through conscious goal setting one piece at a time.

 Now it's your turn. Use lab 2.2 in the web study guide to set SMART goals for physical activity, exercise, and sedentary living. Take the same

---

Now and Later

Movement: Your 401(k) of Life!

Now

In your 20s: Let's say you start to move more and sit less by walking to classes and getting some regular exercise in when you can. You are also aware of sitting too much of the time. You might even ask your professors for a break to stand and stretch in the middle of class!

Later

In midlife—your 30s to 50s—you can keep these habits going, maybe adding in some exercise bouts for insurance. When you reach your mid-50s, you will still be in good health!

In your 60s and beyond, you will have more time! In these years, you will be able to schedule your days around movement, enjoying others' company, and visiting family. You will have the energy to do this because of your lifelong investment in movement.

Take Home

Could movement be a miracle drug that helps you enjoy your later years, much like saving money for retirement does? How could you see the world if you were not physically able to travel? Think about plans to both save money and invest in your movement wellness—could they go hand in hand? Every time you get 7,000 steps a day, you might deposit $10 in your 401(k). That would add up to a nice retirement over your lifetime if you keep moving and saving at the same rate.

process mentioned in the previous example and make sure your goal meets the SMART criteria.

Summary

Although the evidence is clear that physical movement is essential to health, the benefits cannot be realized if you don't choose to move regularly. Both the ACSM and the HHS acknowledge that maintenance of movement behavior is challenging, since society has largely engineered movement out of our daily lives. Currently, only 20 to 25 percent of adults in the United States move 150 minutes a week (Centers for Disease Control and Prevention 2016). Even more interesting is that well over 90 percent of older adults lead a completely sedentary lifestyle (Matthews et al. 2008). In the past 50 years, we have gotten better at unlocking the behavioral keys to moving more and sitting less. Chapter 3 presents much more about behavioral concepts. To get regular physical activity, embrace the concept that healthy physical movement does not have to include intentional exercise in a fitness facility. Indeed, as the human movement paradigm in this chapter clearly shows, the opportunities and options for movement are numerous, enabling you to design a personal weekly movement plan based on your choices.

WEB STUDY GUIDE

Remember to complete all of the web study guide activities to further facilitate your learning, including the following lab activities:

Lab 2.1   Your Fitness and Movement History

Lab 2.2   SMART Goals for Physical Activity, Exercise, and Minimizing Sedentarism

REVIEW QUESTIONS

1. What is functional training? How is it different from intentional movement in a fitness facility setting?

2. What's the difference between the ACSM evidence-based guidelines for exercise and the HHS's Physical Activity Guidelines recommendations?

3. Intentional exercise practices (going to a fitness facility) were an early solution for getting more movement into one's day. Does exercise make up for sitting too much during the day? Why or why not?

4. What age group led the charge of the intentional movement focus? How have their exercise choices changed over their life span?

5. What are three ways you can incorporate intentional movement practices into your day?

6. What does the SMART acronym mean, and why do we use it to set goals?

Successfully Managing Healthy Behavior Change

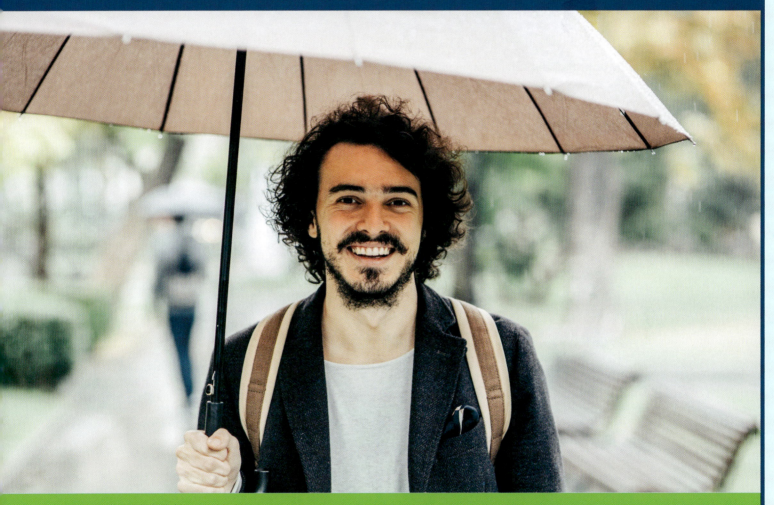

OBJECTIVES

❭ Identify how behavior influences health and well-being.

❭ Develop behavior change strategies.

❭ Analyze barriers and challenges to behavior change.

❭ Set up goals and strategies for integrating movement and health behavior change.

❭ Use movement goals from chapter 2 and behavioral theories from this chapter to choose and integrate a health-based behavior change.

❭ Combine SMART goals with behavior change strategies.

❭ Perform a personal screening and safety inventory prior to starting your program.

KEY TERMS

action stage of change

contemplation stage of change

decisional balance

maintenance stage of change

PAR-Q+

precontemplation stage of change

preparation stage of change

Prochaska's transtheoretical model (TTM)

RICE principle

self-confidence

self-efficacy

self-efficacy theory

social ecological model

theory of planned behavior (TPB)

Why do people change behavior, and why is behavior change so hard? Change of any sort is amazingly difficult. Whether you are trying to move more, change unhealthy eating practices, or create change in a relationship, it is quite natural to resist this change if you do not see an immediate reward or if you perceive the outcomes as negative. Leaving an unhealthy relationship might mean that you do not have anything to do on weekend nights. Maybe you have set a goal to walk to class, but today it is raining outside and you cannot locate your rain-proof gear. Do you get out your rubber boots, look for your umbrella or waterproof jacket, and walk to class, or do you find a ride because you do not have rubber boots, an umbrella, or a waterproof jacket?

Eating healthy takes preparation.

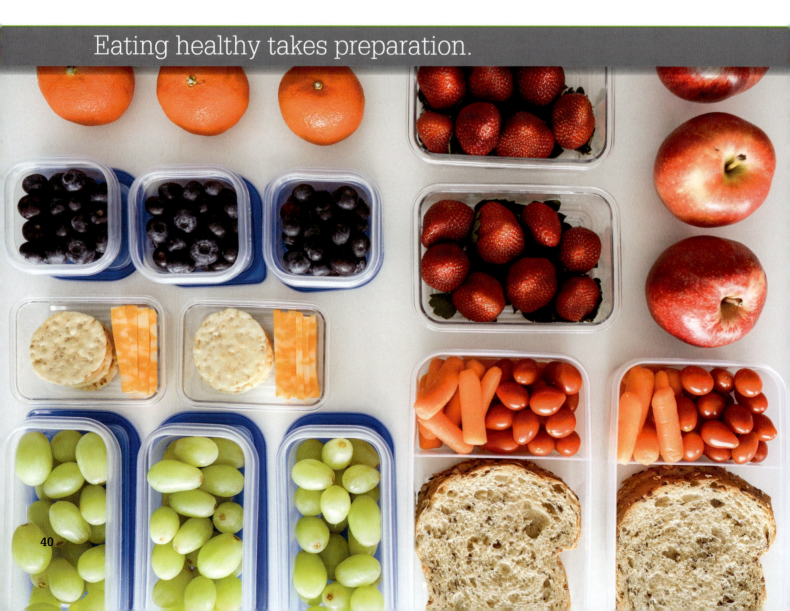

> The key to changing a behavior is understanding how habits work. If you want to sleep more but can't find the time, then focusing on where you use your time, rather than working on sleeping more, may be the start of changing that habit (Duhigg 2014).

Changing behavior often requires planning in order to be successful. The cumulative choices you make each minute, hour, or day have consequences for your overall health and well-being. Do you want or need to become more physically active, eat healthier, get more sleep, or change a bad habit? Health behavior is complicated and takes planning, thought, action, and reinforcement in order to create sustainable healthy lifetime practices. In simpler terms, it is difficult to change habits.

This chapter introduces a few theories of behavior change and provides practical examples of how to integrate these theories into practice to get you thinking about the process of behavior change. It quickly looks at personal screening prior to participation in physical activity or exercise to help you prevent injuries. The chapter also addresses how to treat injuries if they occur.

Having a lot of energy—physical, mental, social—is very important for success in college. Think about the things that zap your energy and bring you energy. Begin to focus on ways to enhance your energy level. What behaviors might you add or change to have more zest in your life?

At the end of the chapter, you will apply behavioral methods to your functional movement goals and create a health goal. Our hope is that the behavioral theory review will help you figure out if you are ready to tackle a specific change and decide where to begin habit modification in order to start on your movement and health goals.

Are You Ready to Change?

It addition to how complicated it can be to change, we should not underestimate the difficulty of *wanting* to change a behavior. Fortunately, health behaviorists have done research that can help guide the change process and show you how to begin. Prochaska's transtheoretical model, behavioral theories grounded in social psychology (the theory of planned behavior and self-efficacy theory), and the social ecological model are several theories discussed in this chapter that provide evidence-based insights and ideas on the behavior change process. As you learn about these theories, keep in mind that no one theory is perfect. You might benefit from combining multiple theories.

Before we dive into these theories, take a moment to reflect on a process for behavior change that has worked for you. Close your eyes and think of a behavior that you wanted to change in the past. Perhaps you wanted to make a habit of flossing your teeth or eating the recommended daily servings of vegetables. Whatever the change was, think for a moment: Why were you successful or not successful? What strategies helped facilitate the change process for you? What barriers made the change process difficult? Keep your previous experiences in mind as you review the theories that follow and start to formulate a plan to use the next time you are attempting to change a behavior.

Prochaska's Transtheoretical Model

Prochaska's transtheoretical model (TTM) of behavior change can help you conceptualize where you are in the change process (Prochaska and DiClemente 1984). This stages of change model initially came from research centered on smoking cessation, but it has been modified and applied to other behaviors. Because the main health behavior focus in this book is on physical activity, we use the TTM model as a way to outline beginning a physical activity or exercise plan.

Figure 3.1 summarizes the TTM. If you are not currently thinking about being physically active or exercising regularly, you are in the **precontemplation stage of change**, where moving more is not on your immediate radar. If you begin researching ways to move more, you are more likely in the contemplation stage because you are thinking about making a positive change. If you determine how you might create this change (for example, tomorrow I might go for a short walk), then you are in the **preparation stage**. If you start to walk three or four times per week for 30 minutes daily, you are in the **action stage of change**. If you continue to walk three of four times per week for 30 minutes a day for six months, you are in the **maintenance stage of change**.

Change a Habit

You can use this worksheet to help you change any habit. Use one copy for each habit you'd like to change.

Examples: Get 8,000 or more steps 5 days a week, strength train 3 days a week, add a vegetable to every meal, get at least 7 hours of sleep every night. Be as specific as you can.

1 List one habit you'd like to focus on at this time: _____ .

2 From the descriptions, select which stage describes you best.

3 Read the descriptions and circle the things you can do to help you move to the next stage.

Precontemplation stage
"I don't want to change"

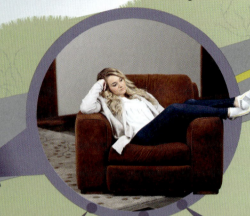

What do I need to do?
- Ask others how they changed
- Read messaging through social media
- Attend an event around a cause (breast cancer awareness week)

I'm afraid to change

I lack confidence to try again

I've tried and failed before

Contemplation stage
"I'm thinking about changing"

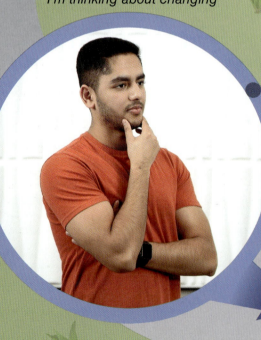

I acknowledge change is needed

I'm unsure about how to move forward

I'm looking at educational information on how to change

What do I need to do?
- Weigh the pros and cons of changing
- Get help on how to move forward
- Relate to a personal issue that helps you consider the change

Figure 3.1 Summary of Prochaska's stages of change behavioral theory.

Maintenance stage
"How do I maintain the change"

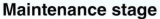

Engage family in the change process

Hire a professional to assist you

Get support from friends

What do I need to do?
- Set a goal and monitor the goal
- Work to continue the plan for 6 months
- Analyze and outline daily priorities

Action stage
"How do I implement the plan"

What do I need to do?
- Consider other positive changes to stay on a roll
- Regularly continue to practice the plan
- Work to avoid relapse and boredom

Learn new coping skills

Evaluate time management skills to continue the plan

Utilize self-monitoring and planning skillsets

Preparation stage
"How do I move from thinking to doing"

What do I need to do?
- Make a plan to reach your goals
- Evaluate where you are in relation to where you want to be
- Begin to move from thinking about the action to actually doing it

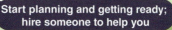

Start planning and getting ready; hire someone to help you

Make a plan and detail it out for a few months

Seek out information and get educated

43

Figure 3.1 provides a quick summary of the stages of change. Note that sometimes things happen that cause you to move from maintenance back to precontemplation. Maybe your running friend transfers to a different school, you can't afford a fitness facility, or you move and need time to learn about your new environment. After a life change, it is easy to move from maintenance all the way back down to precontemplation. After moving back to precontemplation, it is quite a process to get back to the maintenance stage of change. Change is never quick or permanent; it is usually a constant work in progress! You will most likely move back and forth through the stages of change before this behavior change becomes an accepted practice in your daily life.

Beginning a new behavior starts with increasing knowledge, caring about the effect of your health on yourself and others, and understanding the benefits gained. Once you begin to prepare for this change, looking for options, finding social support, and using reminders and rewards become important. The TTM guides the change process by helping you consider action items for various stages of change. Figure 3.2 contains a list of action items that may help with your change process, depending on your stage of change. For example, if you are not even thinking about becoming physically active, you are in the precontemplation stage of change, and you can help move your thinking along by increasing knowledge of physical activity, becoming aware of the risks of remaining inactive, and considering the consequences of your inactivity on others.

Developing Tools for Processes of Change Using the TTM

To help you get started on your own physical activity and health goals, let's integrate the TTM theory into practice. Bridging the gap between theory and practice is how you take research-based information and apply it to your own life. Let's use Prochaska's TTM theory to help you understand where you are in the behavior change process.

If you are not thinking about change, you are in the precontemplation stage of change. To encourage yourself to start to think about change, you might use these processes: Increase your knowledge (for example, learn more about eating healthier or doing more physical activity), think about what kind of role model you want to be to others, examine your attitudes and self-talk, or do some research about the benefits of this change.

To move to the **contemplation stage of change**, where you are thinking about changing but are not yet acting on it (see figure 3.3), weigh the pros and cons of this behavior change. You might also journal about your behavior, imagine the effects of this change on your life overall, and link the benefits of changing with what you want for yourself long term.

Once you are in the preparation stage of

> Robin Sharma said, "Change is hard at first, messy in the middle, and gorgeous at the end." In reality, change is never quick or permanent; it is usually a constant work in progress.

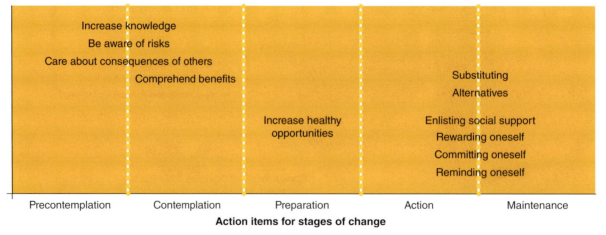

Precontemplation   Contemplation   Preparation   Action   Maintenance

Action items for stages of change

Figure 3.2 Action items for different stages of change. This figure outlines beneficial behaviors for each stage of change using the TTM.

✓ Behavior Check

Get Your Steps In!

Research suggests that 7,900 steps per day for men and 8,300 steps per day for women translate into approximately 30 minutes per day of moderate to vigorous physical activity and that 49,000 steps per week is around 150 minutes per week of moderate to vigorous physical activity (Tudor-Locke et al. 2011).

- How many steps do you take on most days?
- What is your goal for steps per day?

Whether you move more throughout the day for 30 minutes or exercise continuously for 30 minutes three or four times per week in an organized class or program, you will meet the weekly guidelines for physical activity.

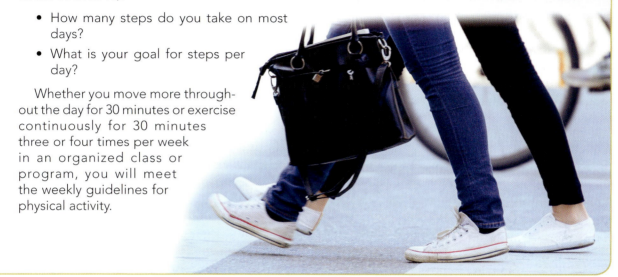

Thinking About Change

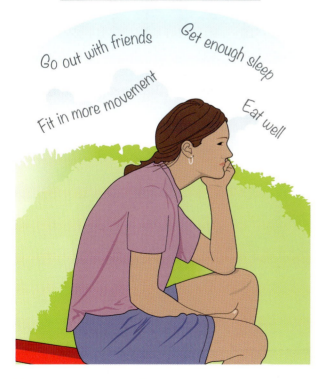

Figure 3.3   Thinking about change is a process.

change, sign a contract with yourself, your friends, and your family about your commitment to making a behavior change, and find tools and information that will help you change. For the action and maintenance stages of change, find a partner who will work with you, ask friends and family members to send you reminders or cues to work on your behavior change, and find a support group.

Another tool that you can use as you move through the stages of change is problem solving around or through barriers (figure 3.4). How will you stay active if the weather prevents you from exercising outdoors or if you can't afford a membership to a fitness center? What if your friends aren't supportive of the changes you want to make, or what if you can't seem to find time to exercise? Planning strategies in advance to overcome barriers is highly effective in making changes in your life.

Behavioral Theories Grounded in Social Psychology

Three behavioral theories grounded in social psychology, the self-efficacy theory (Bandura 1977;

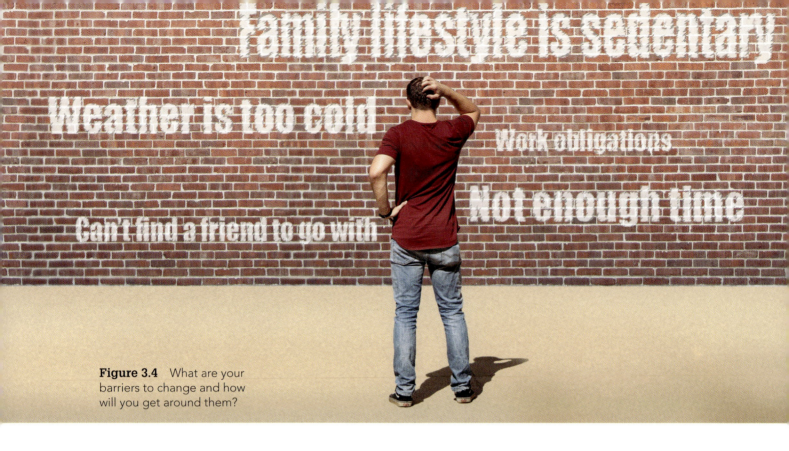

Family lifestyle is sedentary

Weather is too cold

Work obligations

Not enough time

Can't find a friend to go with

Figure 3.4 What are your barriers to change and how will you get around them?

McAuley 1994), the theory of planned behavior (Ajzen 1992), and the social ecological model (Sallis et al. 2012), are helpful for understanding and making behavior change. Let's take a minute and review each social psychology theory individually. We'll then note how several of these behavioral theories overlap.

Self-Efficacy Theory

Self-efficacy theory includes measures of what some would call confidence. What is **self-efficacy**? It is your belief in your ability to perform specific behaviors in order to produce the outcomes you desire. General self-efficacy is your confidence in your ability to control your motivation, behavior, and social environment. Self-efficacy theory suggests that the higher your self-efficacy (i.e., confidence), the more likely you are to be able to make a change in a habit or behavior (Nigg 2014). Specific self-efficacy is your belief in your ability to succeed at a designated task, such as walking three days per week to class instead of taking the bus.

Self-confidence is a more common term than self-efficacy. The two terms differ slightly in meaning. Self-confidence refers to your belief in your ability to succeed at what you put your mind to. It is a combination of self-esteem and general self-efficacy. For example, people with high self-confidence who decide they will not go out partying on a Saturday because they have an important exam on Monday will complete this task

46

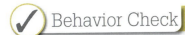
Behavior Check

Your Confidence in Meeting Your Goals

Stop for a minute and take a brief inventory of your confidence in the specific goals you set in chapter 2, lab 2.2.

1 Write down one of those goals here: _____

_____

2 How are you doing on this goal? This week, did you meet this goal? Why or why not? If you did not meet your goals, what happened? What were the barriers?

_____

_____

3 Now on a scale of 1 to 10, with 1 being not confident and 10 being very confident, how confident are you that you will succeed at meeting this goal by the end of the semester? Why do you think you will succeed or not succeed? Are your thoughts related to your self-efficacy, your self-confidence, or both? If you did not meet your goals last week, write down why in one sentence.

_____

_____

4 Finally, write down one thing you will do to increase your confidence in your ability to complete your goals by the end of the semester.

_____

_____

whether their friends pressure them to go or not. In contrast, people with low self-confidence may believe that their friends will stop liking them if they do not go out over the weekend. They would go out to make friends happy and risk not having enough time to study for the exam.

Theory of Planned Behavior (TPB)

The **theory of planned behavior (TPB)** links beliefs and behavior. This theory comes from the theory of reasoned action, which states that intention often predicts actual behavior outcomes. A meta-analysis applying these two theories to exercise (Downs and Hausenblas 2005) suggests that your intention is the strongest determinant of your behavior and your attitude strongly influences your intention. The knowledge that exercise does not have to be hard, continuous, or uncomfortable or happen in a facility in order to provide health benefits can change your attitude about movement. Let us take a positive intentions journey:

1. *Behavioral attitude.* I like to move; it makes me feel better.

2. *Subjective norm.* My friends like to move. I know a few people I can ask to go running or walking with me.

3. *Perceived behavioral control.* I can walk to class on my own, and it counts as exercise.

These three constructs help us predict our intentions and are similar to self-efficacy theory in that they require you to be confident in order to act on a behavior. The TPB can also apply to any other health practice you decide to focus on; for example, it's difficult in college to focus on healthy sleeping patterns. Let's work through an example using sleep as the health behavior you want to improve or change:

1. *Behavioral attitude.* I feel and think better when I get eight hours of sleep.

2. *Subjective norm.* I will let my roommates know sleep is important to me and ask

them to enter the room quietly if they see me sleeping.

3. *Perceived behavioral control.* I will wear earplugs to prevent my roommates from distracting or interrupting my sleep on the weekends.

Social Ecological Model

Another behavioral theory called the **social ecological model** reminds us that changes to physical activity and other health behaviors will require modifications to environments and policies (figure 3.5). Ecological models portray many levels of influence on behavior, from individual and social factors to institutional, community, built environment, and policy systems (Sallis, Owen, and Fisher 2015). A key principle of the social ecological model is that interventions are most effective when they change the person, the social environment, the physical (or built) environments, and policies.

Could our choices of the city we live in and our friends predispose us to health risks? This concept is one reason that the social ecological model was introduced as a behavioral theory. Figure 3.6 outlines the constructs of the social ecological model. The model begins with the individual but then ripples out into relationships, institutions and organizations, the community, and then even policies and systems. Who would have thought

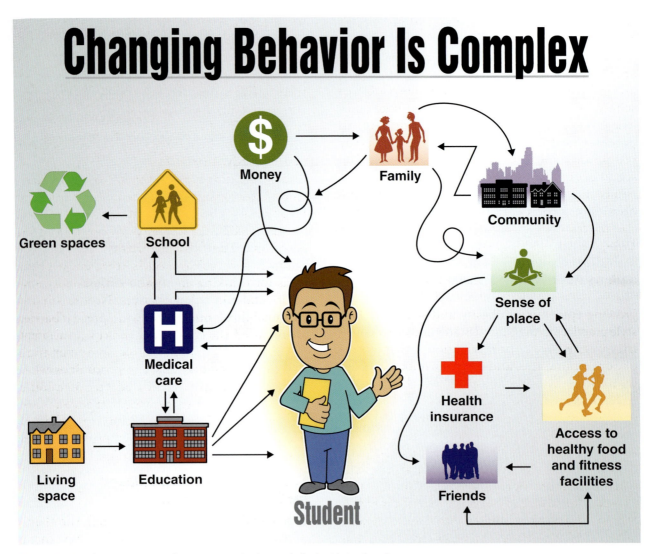

Changing Behavior Is Complex

Figure 3.5   There are many factors to consider and deal with in the change process.

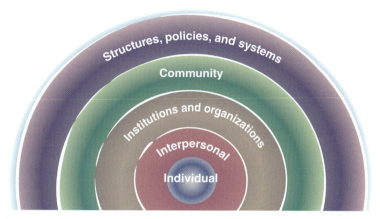

Figure 3.6   Example of the ripple effect of the social ecological model of behavior change (Sallis, Owen, and Fisher 2015).

the ripple effect outside our personal space might cause benefits and consequences to our health choices?

As you determine where you want to live, work, and play, carefully consider the environment around you. Do you avoid riding your bike to school or work because there are no bike lanes where you feel safe? Do you find it difficult to purchase healthy food because all of the nearby restaurants are fast food establishments? The social ecological model goes beyond personal choice to focus on the broader perspective of the physical environment, including where you live and the facilities available to you (Deci and Ryan 1985). This model suggests that urban planning, including transportation systems, parks, and walking trails, is a key contributor to increasing physical activity (Bauman et al. 2012). Given the growing epidemic of obesity and sedentary lifestyle practices in the United States and other countries, we need to pay more attention to the features of our communities and neighborhoods in order to make the healthy choice the easy choice.

Ecological models also consider the social environment when examining what determines behavior choice. Think about the company you keep, especially close friends and romantic partners. If your best friend leads a sedentary lifestyle, you may be more sedentary as well. Consider this 75-year Harvard study of adult development. It followed Harvard graduates with a mean income of $105,000 at age 50 and an inner-city cohort that had a mean income of $35,000 at age 50. It also followed a cohort of women. The study found that social well-being was more important than financial success. Specifically, good relationships, the quality (not quantity) of close relationships, and stable supportive marriages led to a happy life. (If you are interested in the details of the study, search for Robert Waldinger's TED talk, "What Makes a Good Life? Lessons From the Longest Study on Happiness." The study's initial author, George Valliant (2002), also wrote a book called *Aging Well* based on the study's outcomes.)

> When you like the activity you've chosen and you feel like you can do it well, you will be more likely to stick with it.

Finally, ecological models are the conceptual basis for thinking about and emphasizing environmental and policy changes. Health behavior sustainability is much more widespread if barriers are removed and convenient choices are available (Sallis et al. 2012). For example, some communities are starting bike share opportunities where you can use an app to rent a bike for 30 minutes for a set cost. You can leave the bike at your destination instead of having to return it to a bike rack. According to Fishman (2016), convenience is the major motivator for bike share use.

Summary of Theories Based on Social Psychology

Prochaska's transtheoretical model, the theory of planned behavior, and the self-efficacy theory are all individually based behavioral theories for making good life choices. The social ecological model has personal choices at its center but reminds us that there is much more to making good lifestyle choices than our own motivation. Where we choose to live, work, and play influence our happiness and contribute to healthy lifestyle practices.

Decisional Balance

This section discusses tools that can help us make good individual decisions. For example, advertising can strongly influence our choices. Berry and Howe (2004) looked at the effects of certain types of advertising on attitudes, social physique anxiety, and self-presentation. Health-based advertising had significant positive effects on social physique anxiety and self-presentation for exercisers, while appearance-based advertising had negative effects on nonexercisers' attitudes toward exercise. We look at things differently based on where we come from, what we know, and how we look at the world.

Decisional balance is a method of weighing the pros and cons of making an individual change to see if you are ready to invest the time and effort to do it. Once you have identified more advantages than disadvantages to making a change, you are more likely to be successful at making that change.

Complete the sidebar Using Decisional Balance to Help Set Goals to see how you are feeling about your fitness goals.

Let's use another set of constructs and see if you prefer another type of activity for understanding change. Reflect on the same goal you used with the decisional balance activity. Kilpatrick, Hebert, and Jacobsen (2002) came up with five guidelines and questions for you to consider regarding success with goal setting when focusing on a movement or exercise goal:

1. **Have choices of activities (autonomy).** What activities do you like and what would you realistically choose to do that would enhance your exercise or movement goal?

2. **What reasons did you select for choosing your activity?** What is your main purpose for choosing these activities? Look at your pros and cons from the decisional balance matrix.

3. **Who will provide you with positive feedback so you gain competence?** Can you inform close friends or family members about your goal so they can help hold you accountable?

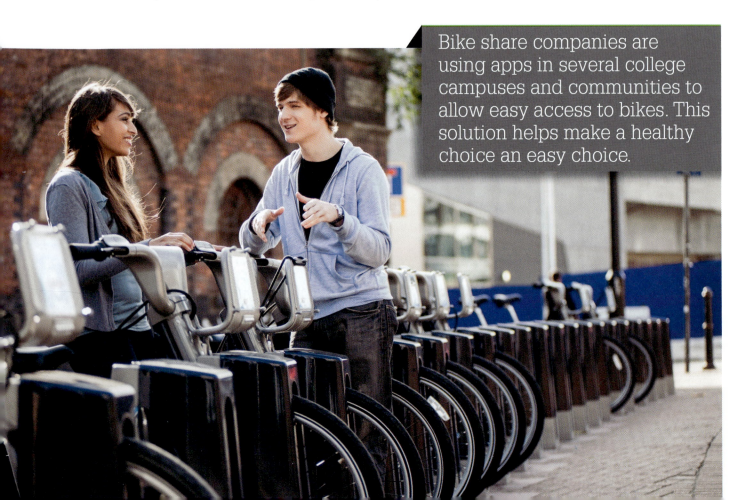

Bike share companies are using apps in several college campuses and communities to allow easy access to bikes. This solution helps make a healthy choice an easy choice.

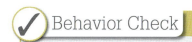

Using Decisional Balance to Help Set Goals

Answer the following questions to see how ready you are to meet the challenges of one of the SMART movement or exercise goals you set in chapter 2.

First, choose one of your movement or exercise SMART goals from lab 2.2:

_____

List your movement goal below and answer the questions in table 3.1. Examples are listed to give you an idea of where to begin.

Goal: _____

Example: Get 150 minutes of movement weekly and include this movement throughout the day in little blocks of time.

Table 3.1 Decisional Balance Matrix

	Not changing movement behavior	Changing movement behavior
Pros	What is something **good** that could come from *not* taking action to meet your goal? _____ _____ _____ Examples • No effort needed. • I'd rather watch my recorded shows in my spare time. • I need time for myself to relax and sleep. • I don't want to share my personal health struggles with others.	What is something **good** that could come from taking action to meet your goal? _____ _____ _____ Examples • I'd have more energy to do schoolwork. • I may lose a few pounds. • I'd feel better overall. • When I look better, I feel more confident. • I will get outside and move more, which improves my thinking.
Cons	What is something **bad** that could come from *not* taking this action? _____ _____ _____ Examples • I would not get healthier. • I might gain the "freshmen 15." • I won't be able to keep up with my roommates (they walk fast). • I might end up like my parents, with health conditions at an early age.	What is something **bad** that could come from taking this action? _____ _____ _____ Examples • I might get muscle aches and pains if I start too quickly. • I have to purchase some comfortable shoes that are also stylish. • I take more time to walk to classes, which might cut into my sleep time.

Did filling out this decisional balance matrix help you clarify whether you have selected the right goal? If you had a hard time filling this out, change your goal and try again. It is important to recognize (as depicted in the TTM of change) whether you are *ready* to make a change. Setting a goal is one aspect of the change process; analyzing that goal to be sure you are ready is the next phase in the behavior change process.

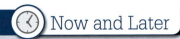

Now and Later

The National Physical Activity Plan

Now

The National Physical Activity Plan is based on a vision that one day all Americans will be physically active and will live, work, and play in environments that encourage and support regular physical activity. However, daily physical activity is on the decline. A 2016 report gave an overall activity rating of a D– to youth and young adults. Concern is growing about what the future will hold if we do not increase our movement and reduce sedentary time (National Physical Activity Plan n.d.; table 3.2).

Table 3.2   Summary of 2016 Report Card Indicators and Grades

Indicator	Definition	Data source*	Prevalence	Grade
Overall physical activity	The proportion of U.S. children and youth attaining 60 or more minutes of moderate to vigorous activity on at least 5 days per week.	2005-06 NHANES	6-11 yr: 43% 12-15 yr: 8% 16-19 yr: 5%	D–
Sedentary behaviors	The proportion of U.S. youth engaging in 2 hours or less of screen time per day.	2013-14 NHANES	6-11 yr: 47% 12-15 yr: 39% 16-19 yr: 31%	D–
Active transportation	The percentage of U.S. children and youth who usually walk or bike to school.	2009 NHTS	5-14 yr: 13%	F
Organized sport participation	The proportion of U.S. high school students participating on at least 1 school or community sports team.	2015 YRBSS	Boys: 62% Girls: 53%	C–

*Complete references available in the 2016 Long Form Report Card.
NHANES: National Health and Nutrition Examination Survey; NHTS: National Household Travel Survey; YRBSS: Youth Risk Behavior Surveillance System; NNYFS: NHANES National Youth Fitness Survey; NSCH: National Survey of Children's Health.

Reprinted from *National Physical Activity Plan* (2016, pg. 3).

4. **Set a goal that is moderately difficult so you challenge yourself.**

   Is your goal too easy? Challenge yourself enough that you will be able to spend three to six months working on the goal.

5. **Find a friend who might be able to work with you.**

   Can share your goals with someone who would be supportive and check in with you?

Reflect on these questions and statements to see if you are truly ready to begin to work on changing your habit in order to enhance your health and well-being. How did this survey compare to your decisional balance review? When you get an assignment for a class, you finish it because you are required to do so to get a good grade. Changing a behavior is a work in progress, so it's easier to let a behavior goal slip by the

Later

Before our society became glued to screens and chairs, natural movement happened throughout the day (figure 3.7), and there was no need to have physical activity ratings for youth and young adults. In addition to increased screen time, in some communities, playing outside is no longer safe.

Take Home

As you consider your physical activity or exercise goals, remember to include reducing sedentary time in your overall movement plan. As we have learned from the cumulative research on sitting time (Levine 2014), it is not enough to exercise; you also have to increase physical activity and decrease sedentary behaviors. Consider this as you work on your movement goals.

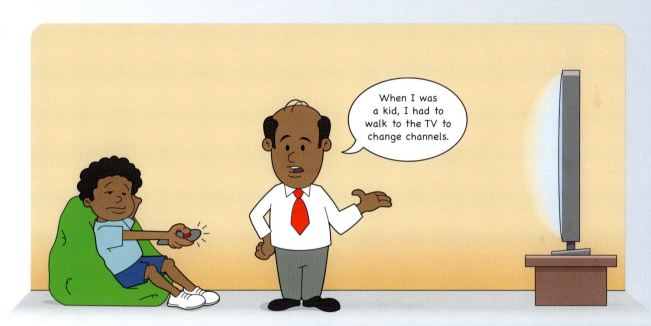

Figure 3.7   The progression toward sedentary living seems unstoppable.

wayside when you have time challenges. You may justify this by rationalizing that you will work on it later, but then later becomes next week, next week becomes next month, and before you know it, next month becomes never. Remember, *you* are important! Putting yourself first in the behavior change process is essential.

Personalizing the Behavior Change Process

In chapter 2, lab 2.2, you were asked to set SMART (specific, measurable, attainable, realistic, time-bound) goals for three specific behaviors you wanted to change. To best apply behavior change theory to SMART goals, let's revisit the big picture of how habitual movement and health combine to create a fulfilling life. Recent research on how one feels about health has illustrated that engaging in healthy behaviors that make us feel good influences our decisions to repeat those behaviors (Van Cappellen et al. 2017). If you enjoyed performing the behavior, you will be more likely to repeat it again. If you do not like running, then consider walking. You get the same amount of movement whether you walk two miles (3.2 km) or run that distance; one will just take you longer. Which one will you enjoy more? The behavior you should select is the one you will realistically do. See the sidebar "Choose What You Like to Do" to put this concept into practice.

Goal Setting Revisited

In chapter 2, you created SMART goals for physical activity, exercise, and sedentary living. Now you will break your SMART goals down even further with specific behavioral components based on what you learned in this chapter. Take the example of doing 150 minutes of movement a week. If you said you were going to do 30 minutes of physical activity each day for five days and you planned to do this by walking for 10 minutes three times a day, what behaviors must you change to do this? How would you measure the success of the goal? Do you need to enter the 10-minute breaks on your calendar app? Will you buy an activity tracker and check out movement distances? Maybe you need to create a walking route that is 10 minutes long so you can walk it three times daily. Be sure to personalize your plan by

> Leo Tolstoy said, "Everyone thinks of changing the world, but no one thinks of changing himself." Be sure to set goals that are uniquely yours.

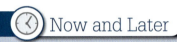

Now and Later

Choose What You Like to Do

Now

Could a new focus on doing what feels good rather than fulfilling exercise prescriptions help us enjoy movement more? Could selecting a mode and type of exercise that work for you make a difference in adherence to movement? The scientific focus on exercise has helped many people, but it has not proven effective for changing population movement trends. What if everything we do counts? Would you rather run two miles or walk two miles while talking to your friends?

Later

Choosing activities that you will continue to enjoy for years to come is essential for long-term health behavior change. What should you do for lifestyle movement options? Choose the activity that you *like* to do on a regular basis.

Take Home

If you focus on healthy behaviors that feature things you enjoy, you're more likely to stick with them. The fitness industry has not adapted well to the behavioral concepts about the importance of movement and exercise feeling good. Most people have not found the fitness center model useful in prioritizing and sustaining physical activity patterns throughout their lifetime. Considering the "why" related to movement and behavior change and pairing your why with feel-good movements are essential for long-term adherence. Fitness fads come and go, but enjoyment goes a long way toward a lifelong commitment to being healthy, physically and mentally.

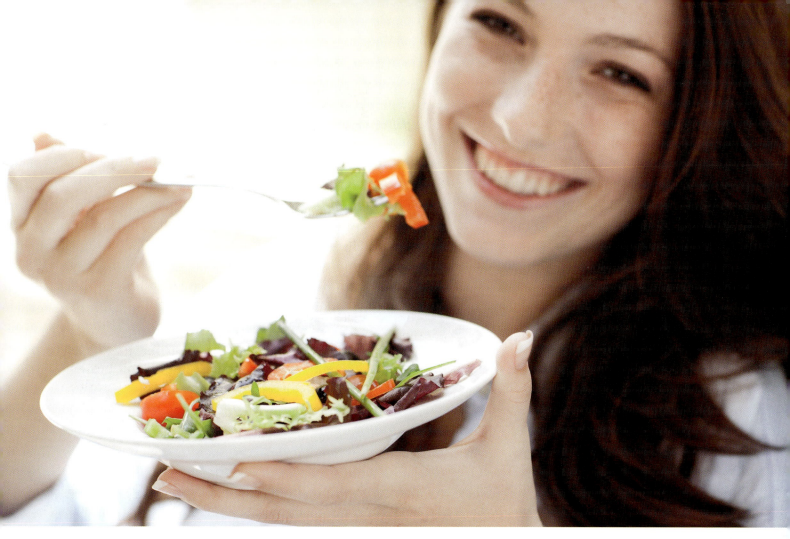

choosing options that are going to feel good for you.

Let's start with the movement goals you set in chapter 2. Using lab 3.1 in the web study guide, look over these goals again. As in the previous example, write in the main behavior you think you need to change to meet these movement goals.

Next, set a health goal that is not movement based. This could include more sleeping, changing your eating patterns, or doing inventory on your relationship with your significant other. Choose a goal that feels important to address now. If you want ideas on health goals outside of the physical activity realm, other chapters in this book discuss sexuality, chronic diseases, such as cancer and diabetes, stress, and addiction issues. Feel free to look ahead for inspiration.

Again, choose behaviors you'll need to change to meet the health goal. If your health goal is to eat more vegetables, what strategies will help you do that? Maybe you'll want to add vegetables you like to eat to your shopping list or change which aisles of the grocery store you choose to walk down.

In lab 3.2 in the web study guide, you'll work through a decisional balance process for each of your goals. You'll also prioritize your goals, choosing which ones to work on first.

Safety First: Getting Started With a Personal Movement Program

This chapter looks at how behavior change theories apply to any type of healthy change you would like to make. You can use them to become more physically active, eat healthier, make a habit of wearing your seatbelt, or get enough sleep. Before you design a personal movement or exercise program, make sure you can do it safely to prevent injury. Injuries, especially ones that become chronic, can hinder your ability to stick with your daily movement program. Prevent injuries in the short term to enable lifelong movement. Strategies for injury prevention start with screening, are enhanced by good planning and practices, and end with care strategies if you do suffer an acute or chronic injury.

Screening for Major Challenges to Moving Safely

The major challenge to moving safely is related to heart and lung function. Most young adults have healthy cardiorespiratory systems, but some people experience conditions such as a heart murmur or asthma that make it more challenging to move safely. Lab 3.3 in the web study guide includes a preparticipation screening questionnaire (Warburton et al. 2011) that will help you understand whether you need to consult your physician before initiating a movement or exercise program. As part of lab 3.3 in the web study guide, access http://eparmedx.com and work through the questions on the Physical Activity Readiness Questionnaire for Everyone (**PAR-Q**+) to see if you are healthy enough to begin a movement or exercise program without consulting a physician. If you have a chronic medical condition or must use certain medica-

tions on a regular basis, you should consult your personal physician to talk through the specific details.

You may have musculoskeletal limitations that are not covered as thoroughly in this screening process. If you have pain in your muscles or joints with movement, consult your physician to have a thorough evaluation before engaging in moderate- or vigorous-intensity movement or exercise. The "no pain, no gain" mentality simply does not work. If you experience pain, listen to these signals and seek professional medical assistance so you can continue to move throughout your lifetime injury free.

Injury-Prevention Strategies

How you plan and execute your movement plan can have a major effect on your risk for injuries. Of course, the type of activity you want to do will determine which strategies are most appropriate. An intense weightlifting session requires different strategies than an all-day hike. Figure 3.8 illustrates the keys to moving safely.

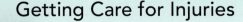

Getting Care for Injuries

If you need to manage a minor exercise injury to a soft tissue such as muscles or tendons, use the **RICE principle**: rest, ice, compression, and elevation:

Rest. Try to rest the injured body part. Stay off your feet if any part on your leg is injured.

Ice. In the first 24 hours after an injury, apply a cold compress for 20 to 30 minutes and remove it for 20 to 30 minutes. Repeat as needed. Do not apply heat.

Compression. Wrap a sprain or strain in a compression bandage for the first day or two after an injury. Make sure toes or fingers have some blood flow.

Elevation. If possible, try to keep the injured part above the heart.

Other important strategies include seeking professional help when needed (i.e., consult your personal physician or an athletic trainer or physical therapist) and using reputable resources for information such as WebMD (www.webmd.com) or the National Athletic Training Association (www.nata.org). Finally, do not ignore chronic nagging injuries, which often progress into serious situations that are more challenging to resolve.

Injury Prevention Strategies

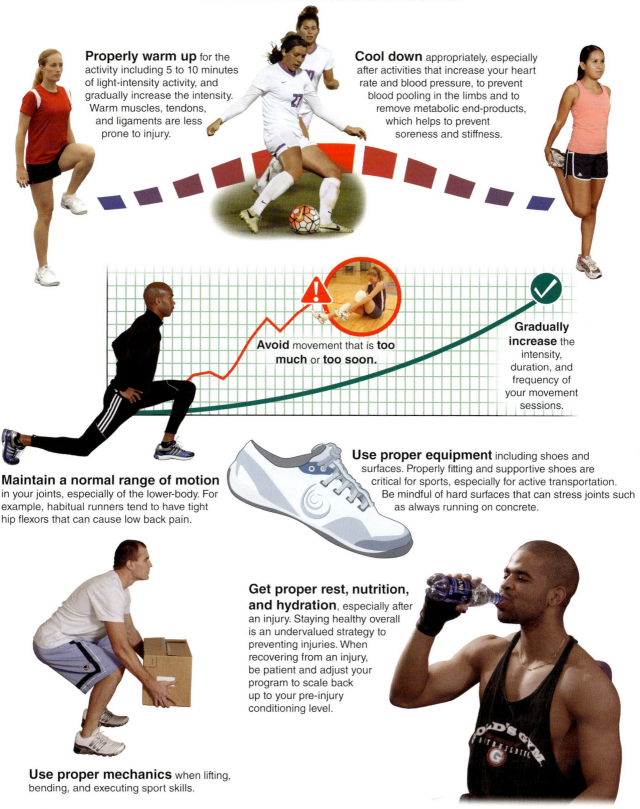

Properly warm up for the activity including 5 to 10 minutes of light-intensity activity, and gradually increase the intensity. Warm muscles, tendons, and ligaments are less prone to injury.

Cool down appropriately, especially after activities that increase your heart rate and blood pressure, to prevent blood pooling in the limbs and to remove metabolic end-products, which helps to prevent soreness and stiffness.

Avoid movement that is **too much** or **too soon.**

Gradually increase the intensity, duration, and frequency of your movement sessions.

Maintain a normal range of motion in your joints, especially of the lower-body. For example, habitual runners tend to have tight hip flexors that can cause low back pain.

Use proper equipment including shoes and surfaces. Properly fitting and supportive shoes are critical for sports, especially for active transportation. Be mindful of hard surfaces that can stress joints such as always running on concrete.

Get proper rest, nutrition, and hydration, especially after an injury. Staying healthy overall is an undervalued strategy to preventing injuries. When recovering from an injury, be patient and adjust your program to scale back up to your pre-injury conditioning level.

Use proper mechanics when lifting, bending, and executing sport skills.

Figure 3.8 Plan well to avoid injury as you become more active.

Summary

Chapters 1 and 2 discuss wellness and the importance of functional movement goals. Chapter 3 reminds us that incorporating behavior change aspects into our functional movement and wellness goals will require us to dig deeper into why we may have started and stopped exercise or other movement choices in the past. We may have a better chance at lasting success in our wellness goals if we also consider research-based implications for behavior as a piece of successful goal-setting practices. Using personal behavior change constructs such as self-efficacy, self-confidence, and awareness of where we are in the change process prior to beginning our journey will help overall success. Also, the TPB reminds us that our attitude, the support of friends and family, and our perceived control over the change are also essential.

Research shows the importance of a behavior change idea being *your* idea instead of one your friend had or one you decided to work on with a friend (Zenko, Ekkekakis, and Kavetsos 2016). A good personal trainer will coach you by asking what *you* want out of the program. Trainers who give you *their* workout are not doing their job of helping you enjoy the experience and continue it on your own. The medical profession has taught us to prescribe behavior, but the human aspect of decision making is critical for ongoing behavior change (Segar 2015). Therefore, if you want to move, make the decision to move, and choose a movement that you enjoy, you will have a much better chance of regular participation in exercise and you will experience outcomes that matter for a lifetime of healthy living.

WWW WEB STUDY GUIDE

Remember to complete all of the web study guide activities to further facilitate your learning, including the following lab activities:

Lab 3.1   Incorporating SMART Behavioral Goals Into Your Goals for Physical Activity, Exercise, Minimizing Sedentarism, and Health

Lab 3.2   Decisional Balance

Lab 3.3   Preparticipation Screening Questionnaire

REVIEW QUESTIONS

1   What are the five stages of change in Prochaska's transtheoretical model?

2   List one or two behavioral action items for each of the five stages of change in the Prochaska model.

3   Compare and contrast the self-efficacy theory and the theory of planned behavior.

4   Explain the social ecological model of behavior change and apply it to your personal goal setting for exercise or movement.

5   How might the decisional balance tool help the goal-setting process?

6   Why is it important to consider behavior goals when setting specific SMART goals for exercise or movement?

7   What are five injury prevention strategies that are important to use before beginning a healthy movement or exercise program?

8   When it comes to getting injured while moving or exercising, the acronym RICE is used for first aid. What does RICE stand for?

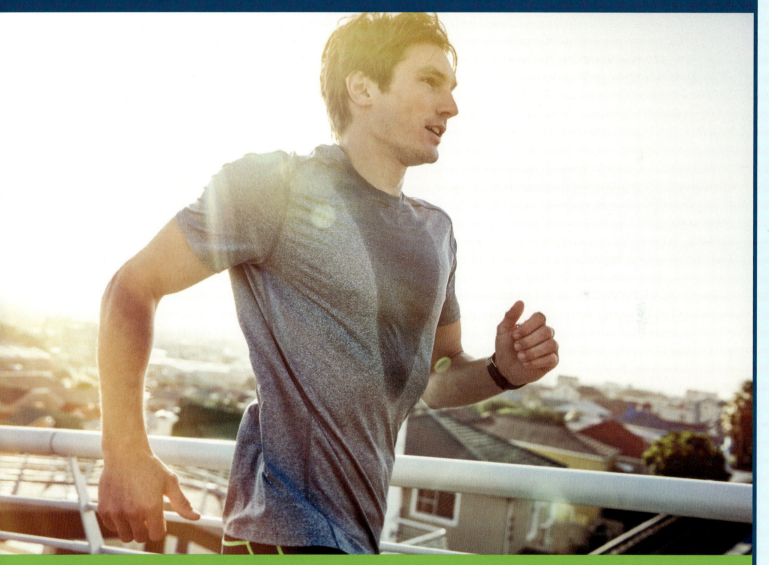

4

Cardiorespiratory Fitness

OBJECTIVES

❭ Understand how your body obtains and uses energy for physical movement.

❭ Describe methods for assessing your cardiorespiratory fitness.

❭ Appreciate ways in which cardiorespiratory fitness can enhance your health and make you feel better.

❭ Design a personalized plan to improve your cardiorespiratory fitness.

KEY TERMS

adenosine triphosphate (ATP)

adenosine triphosphate–phosphocreatine (ATP-PC) system

carbohydrates

cardiorespiratory endurance

cardiorespiratory fitness

diastole

dietary fats

dose–response association

glucose

glycogen

heart rate reserve (HRR) method

high-intensity interval training (HIIT)

maximal oxygen consumption ($\dot{V}O_2$max)

metabolic equivalents (METs)

metabolism

nonoxidative (anaerobic) energy system

oxidative (aerobic) system

protein

rating of perceived exertion (RPE)

specificity of training

systole

talk test

Cardiorespiratory endurance (also called cardiorespiratory fitness) is a key component of health-related fitness. To acquire cardiorespiratory fitness, you must challenge your cardiovascular and respiratory systems. A trained cardiorespiratory system helps you enjoy recreational pursuits and complete your daily activities with greater ease. After all, the heart is a muscle. The heart and lungs need to be challenged regularly in order to effectively deliver oxygen to the working muscles. Cardiorespiratory fitness plays an important role in the prevention of chronic diseases and helps you live a life filled with energy and zest.

Your Energy Needs: Supply and Demand

The human body's ability to adapt is amazing. Energy systems provide muscles with the fuel needed to contract and produce movement. The cardiorespiratory system produces the majority of energy for general day-to-day movement. This chapter will help you design a safe and effective program to enhance your cardiorespiratory fitness so you can go through life with a smile on your face and a bounce in your step.

Cardiorespiratory System

The cardiovascular and respiratory systems, commonly referred to together as the cardiorespiratory system, are responsible for many critical functions. These can be classified into the following primary categories:

1. *Delivery* of oxygen, nutrients, and hormones and other chemical messengers
2. *Removal* of carbon dioxide and waste products
3. *Maintenance* of body temperature and acid–base balance (pH)
4. *Prevention* of infection as assisted by the immune function

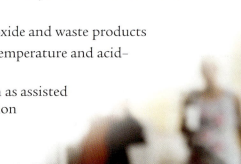

The cardiorespiratory system is made up of the heart, blood vessels, and lungs. Of course, the blood flowing through the cardiorespiratory system is also of primary importance. As covered in chapter 13, cardiovascular diseases are the number one cause of death in most countries in the world. A healthy cardiorespiratory system makes you feel good now and prevents an early death later.

The Heart as Your Pump

The heart is a large muscle located just behind and slightly to the left of your breastbone. It has four chambers and two circulatory systems that miraculously work in nearly perfect harmony. This system sends a volume of oxygen-poor blood to the lungs to be loaded with oxygen. It also sends a nearly identical volume of oxygenated blood to the body for use by various organs and tissues, including the muscles. The right side, or pulmonary circulation, accepts oxygen-poor blood returning from the body and then delivers it to the lungs for waste removal and reoxygenation. The left side, or systemic circulation, has a more strenuous job, relatively speaking. It distributes the oxygenated blood to the rest of the body (see figure 4.1).

The heart can be thought of as a powerful muscular pump. As such, with every beat of the heart, a healthy heart performs a perfectly choreographed dance. The cells within the heart muscle undergo electrical depolarization, which causes each cell of the heart muscle to contract. This perfectly synchronized depolarization–contraction sequence sends nearly equal volumes of blood to the lungs and the rest of the body. This contraction phase is termed **systole**. In the relaxation phase, or **diastole**, the chambers fill in preparation for the next heart cycle, or heartbeat. Therefore, although the left-pulmonary and right-systemic circulations are separate, they must work together for healthy

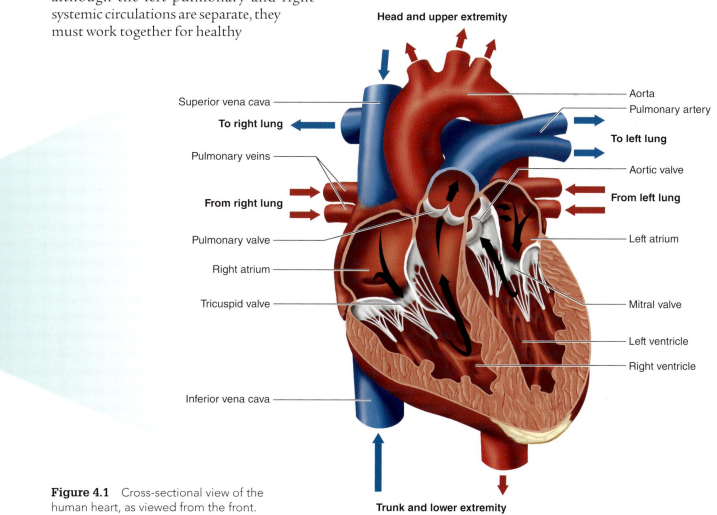

Figure 4.1   Cross-sectional view of the human heart, as viewed from the front.

heart function. Each of the heart chambers has valves that must function well, serving as doors through which the blood moves in and out. The heart muscle must also be strong. Each contraction has to generate enough pressure to move the blood volume from the left ventricle and deliver it to the rest of the body. Thus, a healthy left ventricle is especially important during exercise, when the muscles have a greater need for oxygenated blood.

Vessels Provide Blood Delivery

The blood vessel system within the body is an amazing arrangement of paths for blood delivery. Just as a city has a variety of roadways, such as large interstate highways, state routes, and one-way city streets, the human body has vessels that vary in function and size (figure 4.2). Arteries carry oxygenated blood away from the heart and deliver it to the body. The aorta leaving the heart just next to the left ventricle absorbs the highest pressure within the circulatory system.

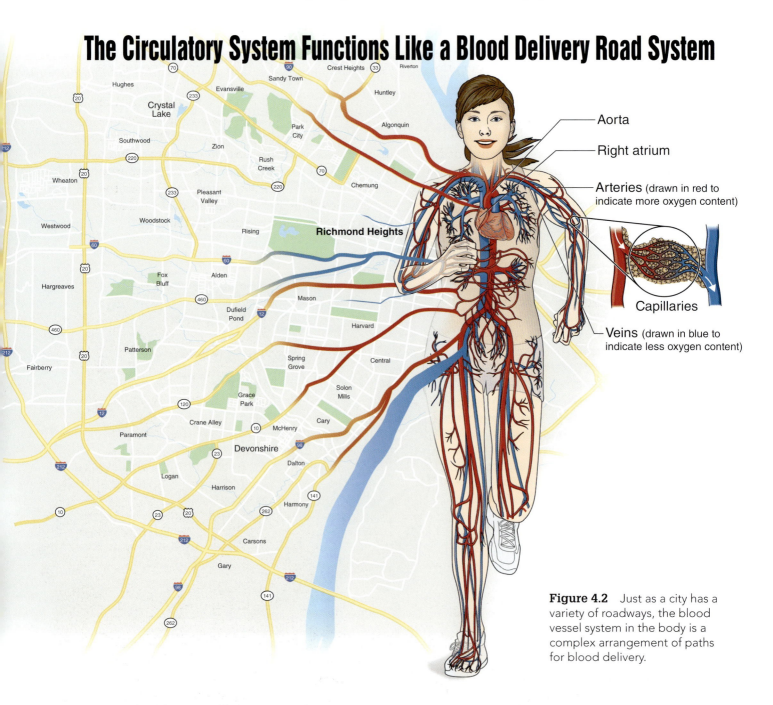

The Circulatory System Functions Like a Blood Delivery Road System

Figure 4.2 Just as a city has a variety of roadways, the blood vessel system in the body is a complex arrangement of paths for blood delivery.

The aorta branches into smaller and smaller vessels, ultimately ending at the capillaries that are located in all tissues of the body. The arterial system is characterized by thick elastic walls that can expand or contract to direct blood to tissues that need it. In this manner, the arterial system acts like a traffic director for blood delivery within the body. The capillaries are very tiny. They are the site of oxygen, nutrient, and carbon dioxide waste product exchange within the body.

After this exchange in the individual muscle cell (capillary level), blood travels to small veins called *venules* and then progresses through veins that increase in size until the blood reaches the heart, emptying into the right atrium. There, the cycle begins again. Veins have thin, stretchy walls that allow them to expand and hold larger volumes of blood. When we have blood drawn from our arms, the thin walls of the veins allow the needle to easily puncture them. Veins also have valves that help keep blood flowing in the right direction back to the heart with minimal pressure in the system. If you have ever stood in a warm environment for a long period of time, you might have noticed that the veins in your legs became larger and sometimes bumpy due to the valves.

Hence, the cardiovascular system, especially the veins, plays a critical role in thermoregulation of the body.

A well-designed and managed road system (i.e., the vascular system) is important, but if there is no transportation vehicle, delivery will not occur. Therefore, blood can be thought of as the cars and trucks of the vascular road. An average-sized person has approximately 5 liters of blood that circulate around the body once every minute during rest. Imagine the contents of two and a half 2-liter soda pop bottles circulating through your system every minute. During maximal strenuous exercise, the working muscles can require as much as 25 liters per minute (see figure 4.3)—that's 12-1/2 large pop bottles per minute!

Blood pressure is defined as the pressure exerted on the arteries. An average blood pressure is 120 over 80 measured in millimeters of mercury (mmHg). The systolic blood pressure (the first number; 120) occurs during the heart's contraction. Diastolic blood pressure (the second number; 80) occurs during its relaxation phase. Pressure is higher when the blood is ejected into the aorta (the main artery of the body) from the left ventricle. Pressure decreases as the blood travels throughout the circulatory system.

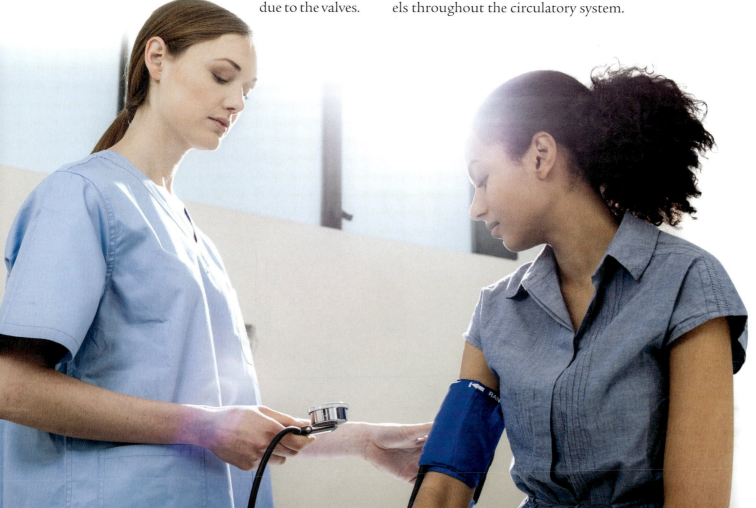

Amount of Blood Circulating Per Minute

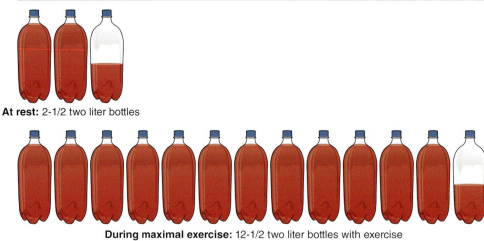

At rest: 2-1/2 two liter bottles

During maximal exercise: 12-1/2 two liter bottles with exercise

Figure 4.3 The amount of blood needed to circulate *per minute* at rest and during maximal exercise.

Blood pressure management is a common health topic due to the negative health consequences of hypertension, or high blood pressure, which are described in chapter 13. However, low blood pressure is also very serious. If blood pressure is too low, blood will not flow appropriately and in the correct direction. A major role of the muscular pumping heart is to generate enough pressure so that the pumped blood will flow through the arterial system. Signs of low blood pressure are fainting spells, especially when standing or working in hot environmental conditions, and feeling light-headed or seeing stars when quickly standing up. Typically, low blood pressure in young healthy individuals is due to dehydration, an issue described in chapter 8.

Respiratory System

The respiratory system, including all the passages from the nose and mouth to the lungs, is a critical partner to the heart for delivery and removal of oxygen and maintenance functions of the cardiorespiratory system (figure 4.4). The diaphragm and abdomen muscles (during more intense exercise only) contract and relax, changing pressure within the chest cavity. This pressure change allows air to flow in and out. As blood flows from the right ventricle to the capillaries in the lungs, carbon dioxide and oxygen are exchanged. Oxygen-rich blood returns to the heart to be pumped to the body. Carbon dioxide passes from the capillaries into the lungs and leaves the body through the nose and mouth during exhalation.

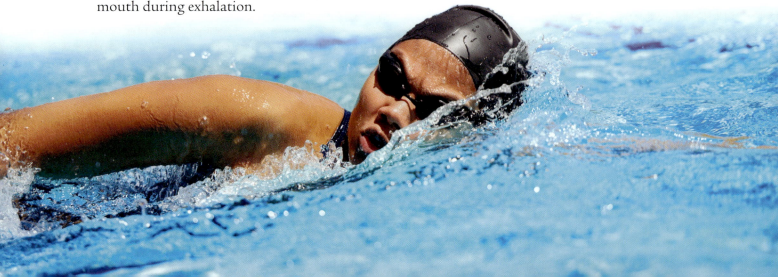

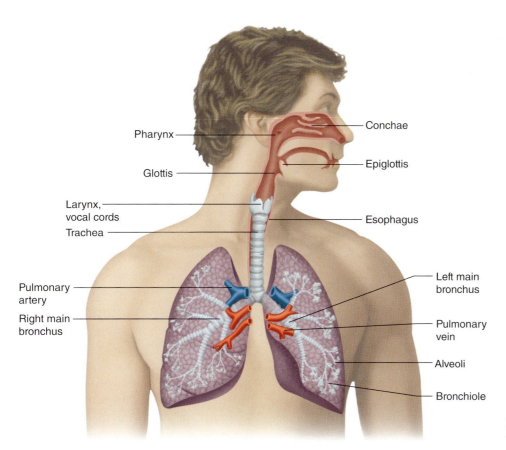

Pharynx

Glottis

Larynx,
vocal cords

Trachea

Pulmonary
artery

Right main
bronchus

Conchae

Epiglottis

Esophagus

Left main
bronchus

Pulmonary
vein

Alveoli

Bronchiole

Figure 4.4 Anatomy of the respiratory system.

Cardiorespiratory Systems Are Challenged by Exercise

When you are at rest or doing light activity, your cardiorespiratory system functions easily. A healthy person has a fairly steady resting heart rate of 60 to 100 beats per minute, breathing rate of 12 to 20 breaths per minute, and blood pressure at or near 120/80 mmHg (systolic/diastolic). However, when you are exercising or engaging in physical activity at a moderate or vigorous intensity, these systems must provide your working muscles with oxygen and fuel to perform the work. This requires a coordinated effort by the nervous and hormone systems, both of which are controlled by the brain, to increase breathing and heart rate. Blood supply is redistributed to the working muscles. Figure 4.5 summarizes the many changes that occur when the body goes from rest to maximal exercise.

Energy Production Systems

People often talk about metabolism in reference to weight management. For example, a person who can regularly take in excessive calories without any weight gain is said to have high metabolism. What exactly does this term mean? **Metabolism** refers to the breakdown of food and its transformation into energy through various chemical processes. This available energy fuels muscle contraction and moves the human body during physical activity.

The unit of energy used to describe the energy available in various foods or expended by the human body is the kilocalorie (kcal). The total energy need for the body is a person's metabolic rate and is expressed in kcal per day. As described in chapter 9, many factors influence your energy balance equation on both the food intake side and the energy expenditure side.

Food: The Energy for Life

The food and drink you consume is converted through complex biochemical processes into a substance the body can use to do biological work or store energy for later use. Energy transfer is never completely perfect: A lot of heat is lost during this conversion from chemical energy to

How the Cardiorespiratory System Responds to Exercise

Lungs
- Breathing depth increases and the rate of breathing typically increases up to 50 breaths per minute moving to 10 to 120 L/min.

Vascular system
- Systolic blood pressure increases from 120 to ~200 mmHg.
- Diastolic blood pressure remains steady or slightly decreases.

Leg muscles
- Blood flow increases from ~15%-20% to 85%-90% of the amount circulated on a per minute basis. More oxygen is taken up by the muscles and used to produce energy.

Heart
- Heart rate increases, on average, to ~200 beats per minute.
- More blood is ejected into the body per beat, increasing, on average, from 70 to 120 beats per minute.
- The total amount of blood pumped out and circulated to the body increases from 5 L/min at rest to ~25 L/min.

Gut
- Blood flow is reduced to the stomach, intestines, liver, and kidneys, reducing digestion and urine production.

Skin
- Increased blood flow to the skin and sweating assist with the maintenance of body temperature.

Figure 4.5 Responses of the cardiorespiratory systems to maximal exercise for a typical healthy college student.

biological energy. Also, there are times in the day when we are not eating. If some energy wasn't stored for future use, we would have to continuously eat to maintain life.

The three food components that provide energy for movement are carbohydrate, fat, and protein. They are burned as fuel in the metabolic furnace within the cells. These components, termed macronutrients, are described in chapter 8.

Think back over your day. What movement activities have you done? For example, you might have sat in your room or in class for a number of hours, slowly walked between classes or to lunch, and then walked briskly from building to building, ran to catch the bus, or played a sport. Each macronutrient and energy system contributed in specific ways to help you accomplish these tasks. Your body relied primarily on fat for energy when you slowly walked between classes but used carbohydrate when you ran to catch the bus.

Carbohydrates, either simple or complex, are a ready energy source. They are easily digested, especially simple sugars, and converted to glucose and released into the blood. Glucose can be stored in the form of glycogen within muscles and the liver and then made available later. If immediate needs are met and glycogen storage needs are at maximal capacity, the extra carbohydrate will be stored as body fat.

In today's world of struggles with weight management, **dietary fats** have a bad reputation, but they are a great energy source. Plus, fat provides nutrients

Although the term *calorie* often has a negative connotation, it is just a unit of energy that allows your body to move!

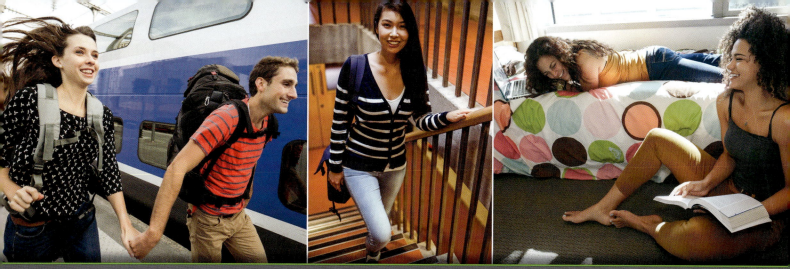

Carbohydrate, fat, and protein contribute in specific ways to help you accomplish a range of physical movement activities.

that make foods taste good. Dietary fats are a great choice when energy is needed for long-duration, lower-intensity movement. For example, trail mixes often contain nuts because they contain lots of energy (due to their fat content) and are easy to carry when hiking for hours. However, similar to carbohydrate, once immediate energy needs have been met, any extra dietary fat will be stored as body fat.

Protein provides amino acids, which are the building blocks of tissues for new growth and repair. It also can be used for energy production, although this is typically as a last resort when carbohydrate and fat are lacking. As with carbohydrate and fat, any excess protein consumed is stored as body fat.

If we think of body fat as stored energy, it can have a positive connotation. If we store too much energy, we gain weight.

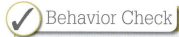 Behavior Check

Is Sweating Sexy?

In today's showered and groomed world, it is often not acceptable to be sweaty unless working out. Because humans are machines that are not very efficient, when we move, we give off heat. In fact, we have about a 22 percent efficiency, which is not very good compared to contemporary refrigerators or wood-burning stoves! This means that nearly three quarters of our energy is given off as heat.

Our bodies have adaptive ways to get rid of this extra heat through sweating. If you try to avoid sweating, you are missing out on chances for movement opportunities. Plan to sweat a little throughout the day. For example, in the morning, put a small toiletry kit and perhaps some extra undergarments into your backpack. Or stay cooler while walking across campus by going through air-conditioned buildings. Thinking strategically can give you lots of daily steps.

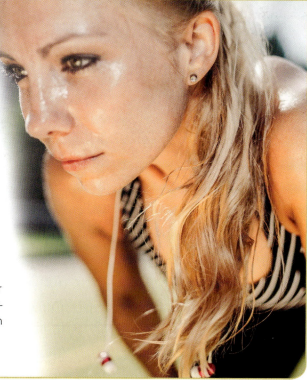

ATP: The Energy Bucks of the Human Body

All cells need energy for biological work. Muscle cells gain their energy for work through the bond breaking of **adenosine triphosphate** (**ATP**). Cells must use ATP directly to gain the energy they need. Thus, the body is constantly using ATP to get energy for biological functions like muscle contraction and gaining it back through the metabolism of food—carbohydrate, fat, and protein. Therefore, ATP can be thought of as the energy bucks of the human body, as illustrated in figure 4.6. Similar to your bank account, the ATP dollar is constantly being deposited (generated) in the cells and then withdrawn (used) for energy production. If we have too much saved energy, it becomes excess body weight or stored energy.

Three Energy Systems

Muscle cells within the body are fueled by three energy systems that cooperate to provide ATP. These three systems vary in their metabolic machinery, the fuel they use, and the types of physical activities that use them (based on time and intensity, as summarized in table 4.1). Flexibility in fuel source and the range of energy production options are critical to our daily function.

In our evolutionary past, a hunter–gatherer might have been walking with no particular destination when stumbling upon an animal intent on eating him or her. This would require the hunter–gatherer to either run quickly or turn and fight, both of which would

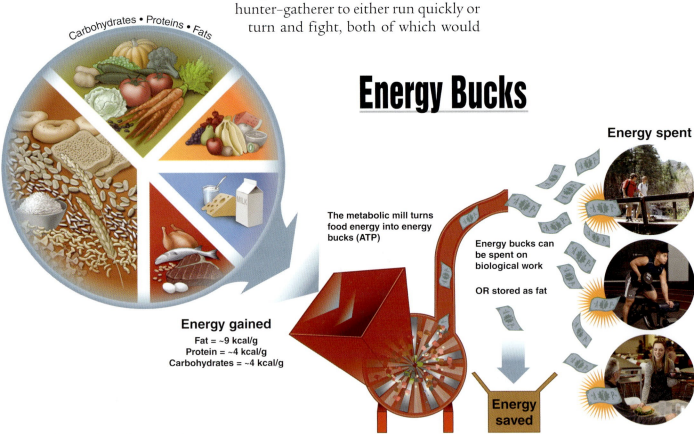

Carbohydrates • Proteins • Fats

Energy Bucks

Energy spent

The metabolic mill turns food energy into energy bucks (ATP)

Energy bucks can be spent on biological work

OR stored as fat

Energy gained

Fat = ~9 kcal/g
Protein = ~4 kcal/g
Carbohydrates = ~4 kcal/g

Energy saved

Figure 4.6   The human body creates and uses energy from ATP stored in cells, much like we earn and spend money from our bank accounts.

Table 4.1 Movement Energy Systems: Summary and Comparison

Characteristic	Immediate (ATP-PC)	Nonoxidative (anaerobic)	Oxidative (aerobic)
		ENERGY SYSTEMS	
Rate of ATP production	Immediate	Rapid	Slow
Duration of activities where system is most used*	≤10 seconds	10 seconds to 2 minutes	>2 minutes
Intensity of activities where system is most used*	High	High	Low to moderate
Fuel source	ATP and PC	Muscle glucose and glycogen	Liver stores of glycogen (glucose), fat, protein
Example sports	Golf swing Weightlifting	200-meter hurdles 50-meter swim	Running a marathon Distance cycle race
Example leisure activities	Playing catch with a football or baseball	Intense gardening and yard work	Hiking at moderate pace
Example daily-life activities	Carrying shopping bags	Running through the airport to catch a flight	Walking on campus

*All three energy systems contribute to almost all activities, but usually one or two systems are used the most.

require rapid access to a large supply of ATP for muscle contraction. In the present day, these collaborative energy systems allow our activities of daily living and provide fuel for many sports, especially those that require explosive movements interspersed with low-intensity activities (e.g., soccer, basketball).

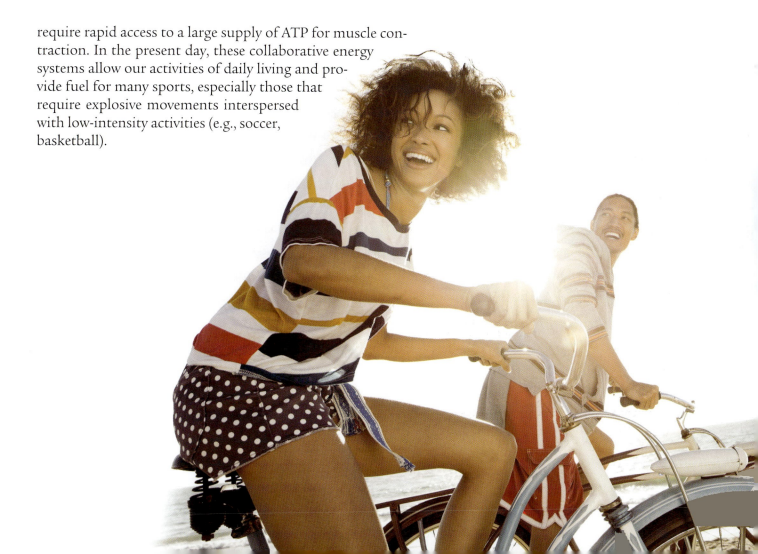

The immediate energy system, or the **adenosine triphosphate–phosphocreatine (ATP-PC) system** is fueled by a small amount of ATP stored in the cells. The benefit of this system is that it provides energy very quickly. The downside of this system is that it has a very short supply of ATP, so activities that are fueled by this system can last only a few seconds (about 10 seconds maximum). After that, unless other systems provide the energy, muscle fatigue and failure will occur and movement will stop.

The **nonoxidative (anaerobic) energy system** is critical at the beginning of activity and for higher-intensity movement lasting from ~10 seconds to ~2 minutes. The fuel source used for this system is sugar—**glucose** or **glycogen**. Because this system does not require oxygen, it is often termed *anaerobic*. (It is also sometimes called the glycolytic system because it uses glycogen.) The positive aspect of this system is that energy is readily available at a relatively high supply. The negatives for this system are that (1) the body does not store much glucose or glycogen, so fuel supply is limited, and (2) bioproducts of this pathway result in metabolic acids, such as lactic acid (lactate), that reduce your muscles' ability to contract and contribute to muscle fatigue and discomfort. A real-life example of this physiology in action is high-intensity interval training (HIIT). Although highly effective, HIIT activities are not always very comfortable because the byproduct of lactic acid causes discomfort during the exercise bout.

Finally, the system most often used is the **oxidative (aerobic) system**, termed so because it requires oxygen. This system is used during activities that last longer than two minutes and are of low to moderate intensity. This system has many advantages, including the use of numerous fuel sources (carbohydrate, fat, and protein) and the ability to supply a large amount of ATP. The only major downside to this energy system is that it cannot provide ATP very quickly. Therefore, this system powers most of our activities of daily living, including when muscles are used for posture during sitting and standing. Remember, this system is not used to fuel the first few minutes of movement or any activity of high intensity such as sprinting for the campus bus.

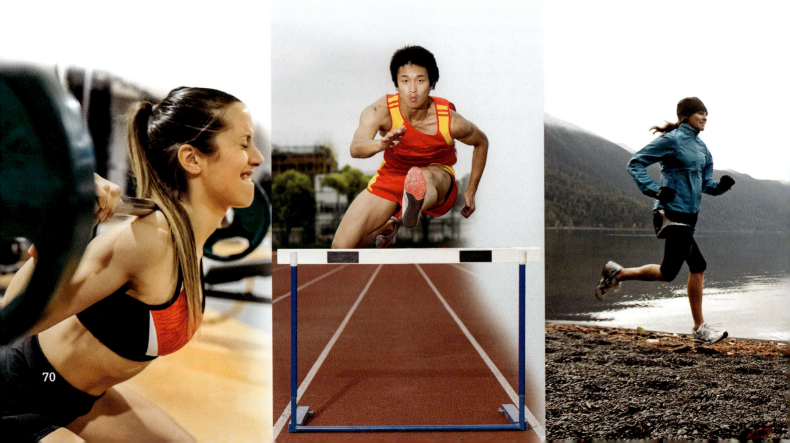

Energy Expenditure for Human Movement: The Continuum

Although the three energy systems appear to have distinct time frames when they contribute to energy production (i.e., less than 10 seconds, 10 seconds to 2 minutes, more than 2 minutes), they do not necessarily turn on and off with a timer. These energy systems have great teamwork to provide ATP. We use all three of the energy systems during daily movement and especially when we exercise. Therefore, in determining the energy system being used for a given activity or movement bout, it is useful to think of the *relative contribution of the system*. Very few activities actually obtain 100 percent of their ATP from a single energy system in order to generate movement. One example is a powerlifter during one specific lift. Another might be a 100-meter sprinter, but even then, the aerobic and anaerobic systems both contribute. When considering which energy system is predominately being used for an activity bout, think about both time and intensity.

If your energy systems are working well, you likely won't need to worry about them much. However, what if you want to train for a specific activity to improve your performance? A major concept in the field of exercise science is **specificity of training**. Specificity can apply to many aspects of conditioning and fitness, but it is particularly important for energy systems. If you want to enhance performance in a given activity, train the system that supports the energy production for that activity. Also, training one system can reduce the performance of another system. For example, sprinters in training who add distance running to their training program will experience reduced sprinting performance. The same is true for a distance runner who adds sprinting. A sprinter relies on well-conditioned anaerobic systems, whereas a distance runner uses a trained aerobic system. Training to enhance all of your energy systems is important for optimal health; however, it is most important to train the aerobic energy systems, since this enhances cardiorespiratory fitness and prevents chronic diseases.

> If you want to enhance performance in a given activity, train the muscles and the energy system that support that activity. For example, if you want to run better, run often!

Evaluating Your Cardiorespiratory Function

Regularly engaging in physical activities that stress the cardiorespiratory system is important. If you are sedentary, you will have low levels of cardiorespiratory fitness regardless of your age, even if you are otherwise healthy. Assessing your cardiorespiratory endurance will establish a baseline, motivate you to improve it, and help you track progress. Embarking on a program to improve your cardiorespiratory fitness brings you closer to a wellness lifestyle that can make you feel better and live longer. But first, what exactly are cardiorespiratory fitness and endurance?

Cardiorespiratory Fitness Defined

Cardiorespiratory fitness is the ability to perform large muscle movements for a prolonged period of time. This concept is also referred to as **cardiorespiratory endurance**. The greater your cardiorespiratory fitness, the longer you can perform an activity at a given intensity (American College of Sports Medicine 2018). Cardiorespiratory fitness is the ability to provide oxygen to the working muscles to supply the contracting muscles with ATP. In real-life terms, if you are winded after walking up a set of stairs, you need to train your cardiovascular system. Physical exertion takes a coordinated effort between the cardiovascular, respiratory, and muscular systems.

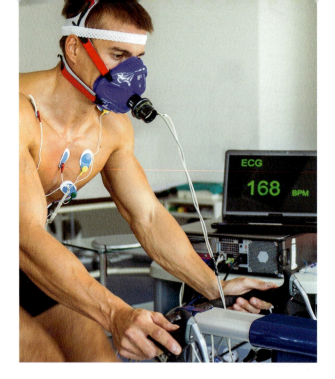

The higher the intensity of your exertion, the more oxygen you'll consume until you have to stop the activity. The point at which you have to stop activity is termed **maximal oxygen consumption ($\dot{V}O_2$max)**. This is the maximum amount of oxygen a person can take in and use to perform dynamic exercise with large muscle groups. Maximal oxygen consumption is considered an objective measure of cardiorespiratory fitness. The relationship between exercise intensity and heart rate is similar to the one between exercise intensity (or relative work capacity) and oxygen uptake. Both are linear (see figure 4.7). This helps us use field methods of cardiorespiratory fitness assessment—from measuring heart rate, we can make good estimates about a person's oxygen consumption and overall cardiorespiratory fitness (American College of Sports Medicine 2018).

Laboratory Methods of Assessment

Maximal oxygen uptake ($\dot{V}O_2$max) is well accepted in the exercise science field as the gold standard measure of cardiorespiratory fitness. The most common laboratory method uses a system, often generally called a metabolic cart, which measures

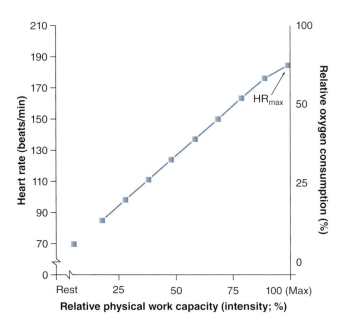

Figure 4.7   The relationship of physical work capacity or exercise intensity to oxygen consumption and heart rate.

Reprinted by permission from W.L. Kenney, J.H. Wilmore, and D.L. Costill, *Physiology of Sport and Exercise*, 6th ed. (Champaign, IL: Human Kinetics, 2015), 197.

the amount of air a person inhales, the oxygen that is used from that air, and how much carbon dioxide is then exhaled. Typically, a person runs or walks on a treadmill for 2-minute stages of increasing intensity for 8 to 12 minutes total. Although subjects inhale air from the room, they exhale into a mouthpiece system connected to the metabolic cart, which then analyzes the air. Metabolic carts are costly, and tests need to be conducted by professionals trained in exercise science, especially if the person being tested has chronic health conditions. Because of these challenges, numerous simpler assessment processes have been developed that rely on the relationship between oxygen consumption and heart rate, which is much easier to measure. These tests are considered field methods (American College of Sports Medicine 2018).

Field Methods of Assessment

Field methods do not require a laboratory and special equipment. They can be performed at home, in a fitness facility, or on an outdoor track. There are two main types of field methods for estimating cardiorespiratory fitness (American College of Sports Medicine 2018):

- *Run/walk tests*. You complete the greatest distance in the allotted time period (e.g., 12 minutes) or you complete a defined distance (e.g., 1.5 miles) in the shortest period of time. You then use an equation to estimate $\dot{V}O_2$max from either time or distance.

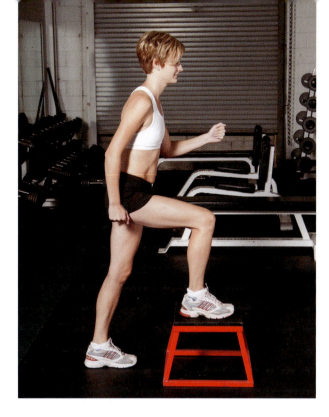

- **Step tests**. In these tests, you step at a fixed rate, at a fixed height, or both. The lower your HR response during or after exercise, the greater your cardiorespiratory fitness.

Lab 4.1 in the web study guide provides detailed directions on how to conduct these run/walk tests. You will have an opportunity to assess your own cardiorespiratory fitness.

Cardiorespiratory Fitness Benefits You

Maintaining your cardiorespiratory fitness will not only prevent chronic diseases later in life but also give you more energy for daily life tasks. A high level of aerobic fitness adds life to your years. The following sections summarize how optimal cardiorespiratory fitness can help you feel better in the short and long term.

Reduced Risk of the Big Metabolic Three

Three major diseases affect most people, either personally or through the caretaking of someone they love. These diseases are cardiovascular disease, type 2 diabetes, and cancer. Although genetics play a role, the common risk factor for all three diseases are lifestyle choices. The human body is designed to move. Nonmovement is not a normal state and results in unhealthy use of metabolic fuels. Although it may appear that mainly older people get these diseases, many of the disease processes for the *Big Metabolic Three* begin in young adulthood.

- **Cardiovascular diseases**. Being sedentary is a major risk factor for many cardiovascular diseases (CVDs), which are the number one cause of death. As described in chapter 13, habitual endurance activities, especially of moderate to vigorous intensity, can enhance the health of the cardiovascular system, positively affecting the heart itself, the blood vessels, and the quality of the blood in the circulatory system.

- **Type 2 diabetes**. Because CVD and type 2 diabetes have so many common risk factors, they are often thought of together as *cardiometabolic diseases*. Regular contraction causes muscles to move glucose from the blood into the cells more easily. Too much glucose in the blood is the definition of type 2 diabetes. Movement is a key treatment for both the prevention and management of this disease.

- **Cancer**. Although the literature is less clear regarding the benefits of physical activity for prevention of cancer compared to that of CVD and type 2 diabetes, movement is protective for some types of cancers, with a key role in preventing colon and breast cancers. Chapter 14 provides detailed information on how healthy lifestyle choices can help prevent cancer.

> The disease process for CVDs, type 2 diabetes, and cancer begins in young adulthood. Get moving, and take action now to prevent these diseases.

Weight Management

Do you equate exercise and physical activity with weight management? Many people do. In fact, a common goal for an exercise program is to become and stay lean. As explained in chapter 9, regular movement, especially moderate- to high-intensity exercise, is very important for managing body composition, which is the proportion of fat, muscle, and bone in your body. Energy expenditure through movement allows you to splurge on a few calories with your favorite foods and drinks and still remain in energy balance.

Daily Physical Tasks Get Easier

When you have a high level of cardiorespiratory fitness, the physical tasks you do each day, like walking and going up and down stairs, will be easier. With cardiorespiratory fitness, you will reap the following benefits:

- For any given physical challenge, your heart rate and breathing rate will be lower.
- Your muscles will produce less lactate and lactic acid, which means that physical challenges will feel easier and stress your body less.
- You will need less time to recover from physical tasks. For example, carrying a full backpack from point A to point B in a given period will not be as tiring.

Enhanced Work, Recreation, or Sport Performance

The better your cardiorespiratory fitness, the less stress your body will experience from physical work, recreation, and sports:

- If you have a service job that requires you to be on your feet for many hours doing light to moderate activity, you will experience less physical stress and fatigue by the end of your shift.
- You can enjoy the outdoors during hiking without undue fatigue or performance worry.
- You will enjoy recreational sport activities and group fitness classes more when you can keep up with the team or the class.

Better Immune Function

Regular exercise and physical activity usually have positive effects on the immune system. The exception to this rule is in conditions of overtraining or in response to an intense challenge such as a marathon. An enhanced immune function is important for both longer-term immune challenges such as cancer and short-term daily

challenges such as bacterial infections and cold and flu viruses. If you are physically fit, you get fewer colds and upper respiratory tract infections compared to people who are sedentary (Martin, Pence, and Woods 2009). On college campuses, upper respiratory illnesses are regular occurrences. One study found that 91 percent of students at a large Midwestern university experienced symptoms of an upper respiratory infection or flu in a given semester (Nichol, Heilly, and Ehlinger 2005). This study reminds us that other key behaviors to enhance immune function, such as healthy dietary choices, optimal sleep, stress management, and good hygiene practices like hand washing, are essential for better immune function.

Better Brain Function and Academic Achievement

Cardiorespiratory fitness is positively associated with cognition and enhanced brain structure and function, especially in children and adolescents (Donnelly et al. 2016). In other words, cardiorespiratory fitness helps your brain work better. It has been linked to better academic performance (Ratey 2008). The college years by definition are cognitively challenging—you have to think hard and study for long hours! For optimal personal performance, regular physical activity, especially at an intensity that improves cardiorespiratory fitness, can greatly enhance your academic life.

Feeling Better: Improved Sleep and Psychosocial Well-Being

The many benefits of regular cardiorespiratory exercise include stress management, better sleep, and prevention of depression, as described in chapter 10. Regular physical movement, especially training that results in improvements in cardiorespiratory fitness, can improve the following aspects of daily life.

- You will sleep better. Good restorative sleep is critical for many physiological and psychological processes that are important to daily life. Being tired is a primary complaint from students of all ages—better quality of sleep will help you feel better.
- You will be less affected by daily stressors and have less anxiety.

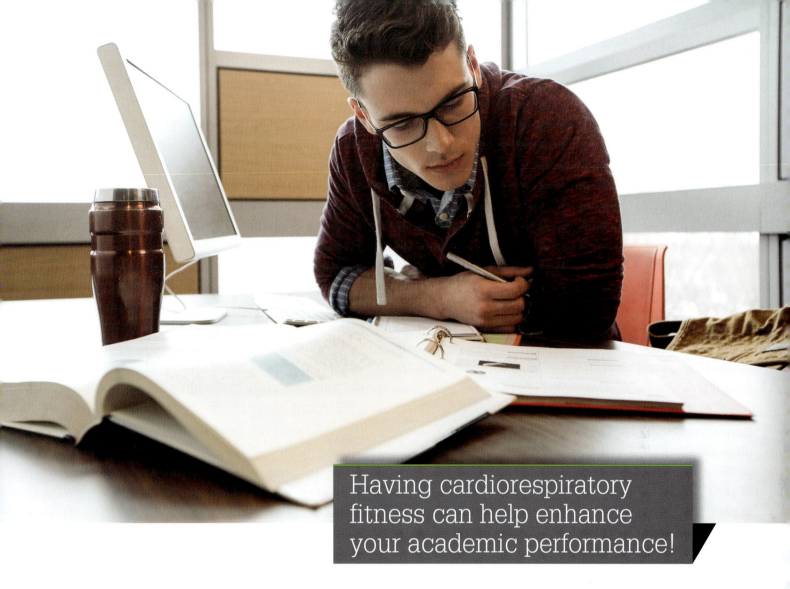

Having cardiorespiratory fitness can help enhance your academic performance!

- You can help prevent depression at a time when the prevalence of anxiety and depression, unfortunately, is increasing on college campuses.
- Good movement habits can provide vitality and energy to your day. Having enough energy to complete your daily tasks is critical to success as a student.

In summary, we admire people of all ages who have lots of energy and a high engagement in their lives. By investing in your health, you will have more energy to do the things you have to do, *plus* energy to do all the things you want to do. A healthy cardiorespiratory fitness ultimately helps you live your best life.

> **Having good cardiorespiratory fitness not only makes you healthier, it also helps you feel better!**

Your Plan to Improve Cardiorespiratory Fitness

Now that you know how your cardiorespiratory system and muscles collaborate and you understand the benefits of improving your cardiorespiratory fitness, the next step is to formulate a personal plan so that you can develop and maintain cardiorespiratory fitness throughout your life.

The Plan Depends on the Goal

Your plan to develop cardiorespiratory fitness is highly dependent on your goal. Your personal goals may be influenced by your recreational interests. For example, maybe you want a conditioning level that will allow you to enjoy rigorous hiking in nearby mountains. You might want to participate in a fun run with your friends or family. Or perhaps you play on a recreational basketball league and your performance would benefit from a good conditioning base. Alternatively, you may want to manage your weight and be lean so that you look good and feel good. Maybe you want your cardiorespiratory program to reduce your anxiety about your academic performance and help you sleep better. Your goals may cross several domains of sport performance, health, body image, and academic performance.

Regardless of your goals, at a minimum, strive to meet the guidelines put forth by various agencies such as the 2008 physical activity guidelines (U.S. Department of Health and Human Services 2008) and the American College of Sports Medicine (ACSM) position statement (Garber et al. 2011). These are summarized in figure 4.8. If you want to reach other goals, such as for sports performance or weight management, you will need to use slightly different strategies.

FITT: Frequency, Intensity, Time, and Type

The fundamental frame for your program will follow the acronym FITT, which is a way to organize your movement program to gain and maintain cardiorespiratory fitness. The FITT components interact with each other in terms of their benefits. Additionally, the best program for you depends on your goals and interests. Selecting activities you enjoy is very important, because if you don't stay with your program, you won't be able to both achieve and maintain your cardiorespiratory fitness.

Frequency

The U.S. Department of Health and Human Services (2008) and ACSM (Garber et al. 2011) agree that most people need to engage in moderate- to vigorous-intensity endurance activities three to

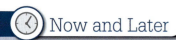 Now and Later

401(k) Versus 401(H)

Most college students want to study hard, earn a high GPA, and build their resumes so they can make a good living. However, on the way to financial success and security, you would be wise to think about your 401(H), where *H* stands for health. Often, people invest heavily in their financial success—their 401(k)—but not enough in their health. Financial health and physical and emotional health are often very intertwined.

Now

Adding movement into your daily life might look like this: Higher levels of fitness are related to better cognitive performance and better academic achievement. Lower levels of anxiety and depression and better sleep quality will help you concentrate.

Later

These same benefits will be present when you are a multitasking professional. Most college students do not have cardiovascular diseases, diabetes mellitus, or cancer caused by lifestyle choices. Indeed, these chronic conditions—the Big Metabolic Three—typically occur in middle age. However, the biological processes underlying these conditions typically start in young adulthood. For example, plaque buildup in the coronary arteries, which causes many heart attacks, begins in young adults.

Take Home

Engaging in moderate- and vigorous-intensity activities over your life span will make you feel better and perform better and will prevent many chronic diseases. Your fitness just might help you have a great 401(H) and 401(k)!

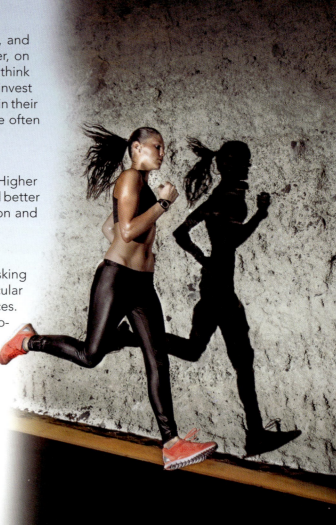

five days per week. Expert guidelines recognize that frequency is influenced by intensity level. For example, cardiorespiratory fitness benefits are similar for performing moderate-intensity activity five times per week and vigorous-intensity activity three times per week. More than five bouts of exercise per week may increase risk for musculoskeletal injury, especially if the activity stresses the same joints repeatedly. Cross-training, which involves using several different modes (e.g., three days of running and two days of cycling), may reduce risk of injury. Very deconditioned individuals may benefit from breaking a workout session into shorter bouts and repeating them throughout the day.

Intensity

Intensity is a major factor influencing cardiorespiratory fitness. The cardiorespiratory system and muscles adapt in response to a repeated stress. Thus, the greater the intensity of training, the greater the benefit. However, risk of injury also increases, especially in people with unhealthy cardiorespiratory or musculoskeletal systems. The actual intensity needed for improving cardiorespiratory fitness is influenced by age, health status, recreational activity, and other factors. Adjust intensity in response to environmental stress (e.g., hot and humid conditions) or when recovering from an illness or injury. You can use several methods of varying complexity to monitor endurance exercise intensity. You might want to consider mixing and matching them depending on your activity and how you feel.

One method for monitoring intensity is called the **heart rate reserve (HRR) method**, which is the difference between resting heart rate (RHR) and maximal heart rate (MHR). Heart rate (HR) can be used to estimate exercise intensity and is often prescribed using a target HR zone. According to the American College of Sports Medicine (2018), moderate-intensity exercise is 40 to 60 percent of HRR and vigorous exercise is 60 to 90 percent of HRR. Maximal heart rate is calculated by subtracting age from the number 220. For example, for a typical 20-year-old:

MHR = ~200 beats per minute (bpm), RHR = ~70 bpm, and HRR is 140 bpm.
A target HR zone for moderate-intensity endurance exercise (40 to 60 percent) would be estimated as follows:

(140 bpm × 40 percent) + 70 bpm = 126 bpm
(140 bpm × 60 percent) + 70 bpm = 154 bpm

Figure 4.8 Make a weekly to-do list that includes the FITT recommendation to enhance cardiorespiratory fitness.

To do this week

1. Take Muffy to the vet.
2. Get birthday present for Mom – new running shoes?
3. Return overdue library book!
4. Follow the FITT principles for cardiorespiratory fitness.
 ·**Frequency:** At least 5 days of moderate intensity or at least 3 days of vigorous intensity, or a combination.
 ·**Intensity:** Moderate or vigorous intensity based on heart rate or rating of perceived exertion.
 · **Time:** 30 to 60 minutes a day of moderate intensity or 20 to 60 minutes a day of vigorous intensity activities.
 ·**Type:** Large muscle group activities that are rhythmic and (somewhat) continuous.
5. Go to bed earlier than I did last week.

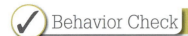

Behavior Check

Both Physical Activity and Exercise Matter: Just Move!

When was the last time you worked up a sweat? To be specific, when is the last time you broke a sweat from physical work that did not involve working out in a fitness facility or playing a sport? Our technologically based society has successfully engineered nearly all physical exertion out of our lives, so we must intentionally plan to exercise or move to gain health benefits (see the short video at www.designedtomove.org).

Many students cannot recall sweating from performing any manual labor except for moving in and out of college housing. The majority of people cannot offset their sedentary time (i.e., sitting time) by a small amount of exercise or physical activity. To remain physically and mentally healthy, we must commit to regular movement.

It is useful to think of physical activity in the four categories of occupational, domestic chores, transportation, and leisure. Challenge yourself to identify ways to increase your movement in these four categories by replacing a sedentary activity. As a professor, my homework might look like this:

- Replace my work chair with a standing desk
- Mow the yard with a push mower instead of a riding lawn mower
- Walk to a meeting across campus instead of driving (same time spent too!)
- Choose hiking instead of going to see a movie

Your turn! How can you increase movement in various areas of your life?

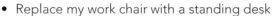

A second way to measure exercise intensity is through the use of **metabolic equivalents (METs)**. A MET can be used to express the rate of energy expenditure during an activity in comparison to the rate of energy expended at rest. Therefore, an activity that is 2 METs is twice the resting metabolic rate. In general, activities less than 3 METs are considered low intensity, in the range of 3 to 5 METs are moderate intensity, and 6 METs or greater are vigorous (American College of Sports Medicine 2018). For example, for most people, jogging or running is vigorous at 8 to 12 METs and hiking is moderate to vigorous at 3 to 7 METs.

A third way to monitor intensity is to use the **rating of perceived exertion (RPE)**, or your perception of your exertion level (American College of Sports Medicine 2018). When you become accustomed to exercising, especially habitually doing the same activity such as jogging or hiking, you will begin to feel how hard you are working subjectively. Additionally, it can be inconvenient to monitor HR, especially during some activities and without a wearable monitor. Table 4.2 depicts a common RPE scale ranging from 1 (near rest) to 10 (maximal effort). To learn this technique, start to associate an RPE rating with exercise in your target heart rate zone. Over time, this can be an easy way to monitor intensity.

Finally, the easiest method of all for estimating exercise intensity is called the **talk test**. Because higher levels of exertion require greater oxygen demand, respiration rate increases as intensity

An easy fitness test is to walk quickly up a hill on campus with a full backpack and see how out of breath you get!

increases. At higher intensities, your breathing rate becomes more labored. During moderate-intensity exertion, a person can typically talk; however, at vigorous intensities, most people can speak only in small phrases. Thus, the talk test can help you gauge your intensity and prevent yourself from overexertion.

Time

The recommended duration of the activity in a given bout is influenced by intensity. Physical activity guidelines indicate that a person should accumulate *at least* 150 minutes per week of moderate-intensity activity or 75 minutes of vigorous-intensity activity per week (U.S. Department of Health and Human Services 2008). Most adults should strive to get 30 to 60 minutes per day of moderate-intensity activity, 20 to 60 minutes per day of vigorous-intensity activity, or a combination of moderate and vigorous activities (American College of Sports Medicine 2018). However, if a person is deconditioned, moving for less than 10 minutes per day may be adequate to gain benefits and is a safe place to start. Pattern of time within the activity can also vary. For example, an exercise could be performed in a continuous session or in multiple sessions of 10 minutes or more to reach the desired duration or volume for a given day (American College of Sports Medicine 2018). As explained in chapter 9, longer durations of exercise (60 to 90 minutes per day) may be needed for weight management, especially if the rest of your day is spent sitting.

Type

You can use many modes of activities to enhance cardiorespiratory fitness. Rhythmic aerobic exercise that requires little skill and involves large muscle groups, especially the legs, is recommended for all adults for health. Sports that require a higher level of skill or fitness are options for people who have the training and conditioning

Table 4.2 Rating of Perceived Exertion (RPE) Scale

Rating	Description
1	Nothing at all (lying down)
2	Extremely little
3	Very easy
4	Easy (could do this all day)
5	Moderate
6	Somewhat hard (starting to feel it)
7	Hard
8	Very hard (making an effort to keep up)
9	Very, very hard
10	Maximum effort (can't go any further)

Reprinted by permission from NSCA, Aerobic Endurance Training Program Design, by P. Hagerman. In *NSCA's Essentials of Personal Training*, 2nd ed., edited by J.W. Coburn and M.H. Malek (Champaign, IL: Human Kinetics, 2012), 395.

You can estimate your exercise intensity by monitoring your heart rate.

> There are many ways to move to gain cardiorespiratory fitness—the key is to move at least at a moderate intensity on a nearly daily basis!

base to safely engage in these activities (American College of Sports Medicine 2018). The most popular activity is walking, since it is easily accessible to nearly everyone and requires only a good pair of shoes. Other common choices are running, cycling, swimming, and the use of exercise equipment. Doing cross-training and finding many ways to move will add variety and keep you interested and motivated. Figure 4.9 provides examples of common cardiorespiratory endurance activities that vary in skill and fitness requirements.

VP: Volume and Progression

The FITT framework provides a great approach to developing a cardiorespiratory fitness pro-

gram. Frequency, intensity, and time can interact when you organize your weekly movement plan and when combined with a variety of activities. No one person's program will be the same. After determining the program that is right for you and your interests, schedule constraints, and so on, your next step is to think about volume and progression. As mentioned previously, the pattern of how you exercise may also influence the other components.

Volume

Exercise volume is the product of frequency, intensity, and time. For example, if you exercise vigorously, you can move for less time and get health benefits similar to those of a longer program at moderate intensity. This concept is known as a **dose–response association**. The greater amounts of physical activity you do, the greater the health and fitness benefits you will obtain; however, it is less clear if there is a minimum or maximum amount. A total amount of energy expenditure of

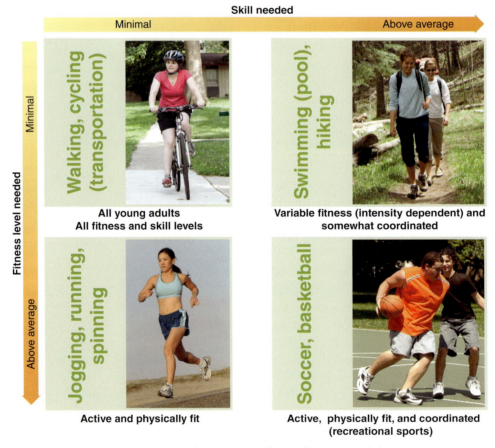

Figure 4.9   Common activities to promote cardiorespiratory fitness for young adults.

about 1,000 kcal per week is associated with the prevention of cardiovascular disease and thus is a reasonable target for most adults for heart health. This level of energy expenditure is approximately equal to 150 minutes per week of moderate-intensity activity (American College of Sports Medicine 2018).

Activity trackers and pedometers can be useful for estimating physical movement volume in steps per day. Although 10,000 steps per day is often cited as a health goal, if the steps are taken at a moderate intensity, approximately 5,400 to 7,900 steps per day can meet the recommended physical activity targets (Tudor-Locke et al. 2011). The math might look like this:

- Walking 100 steps per minute is generally a moderate-intensity activity.
- Walking one mile (1.6 km) is approximately 2,000 steps.
- Walking 30 minutes per day at a moderate intensity generates 3,000 to 4,000 steps per day.

It is best to use a combination of step counts and frequency, intensity, and time components when designing your exercise or physical activity program.

Progression

Progression of the cardiorespiratory endurance program is highly dependent on a person's health status, current fitness level, and exercise program goals. You can accomplish progression by advancing any of the FITT components. Generally, increasing time first is often the best option: Increases of 5 to 10 minutes per session every few weeks are recommended. You can then gradually advance other components over four to eight months (American College of Sports Medicine 2018). Most importantly, progression should be slow and planned to avoid muscular soreness, injury, and undue fatigue. The risk of going too hard, too fast, too long, and too soon is not just related to physiological outcomes. If you experience a lot of muscle soreness and fatigue, you will not feel motivated to stick to your fitness program. Therefore, progress slowly, listen to your body, and think of this adventure as something you will maintain your entire life with modifications as needed.

Pattern: Interval Training

Although it is not a formal component of the ACSM guidelines, pattern of movement can be altered by the week, day, or even the workout session. The daily accumulation of time spent in moderate-intensity activity aligns well with the typical day in the life of a college student, where class changes occur nearly every hour and the opportunity to move is built into the daily schedule. From a weekly perspective, since time and other demands of life often change day to day, you can plan your activity to fit within a week. For example, some days can have longer, more intense sessions and others will accommodate only intermittent bouts of moderate walking.

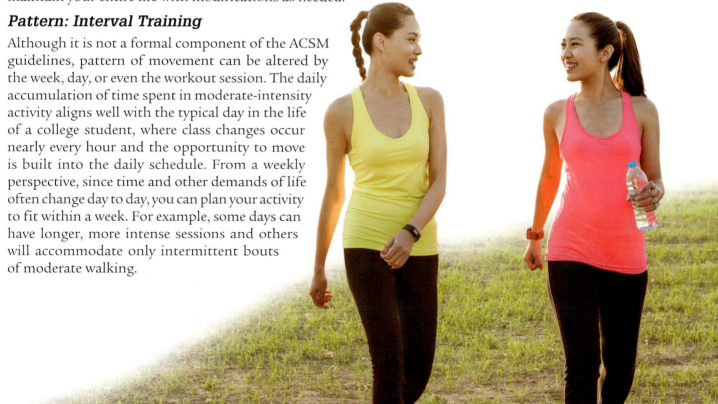

Applying interval training to a workout session brings us to the training technique called **high-intensity interval training** (**HIIT**), a hot topic in exercise research labs (Milanovic, Sporis, and Weston 2015). HIIT is one of the most effective methods for increasing cardiorespiratory fitness in a short period. Essentially, short, high-intensity bursts of activity are completed and then interspersed with longer low-intensity or rest periods. It does not matter what type of activity you use for this type of training, but the most common types are running, cycling, rowing, and swimming. Research studies document the effectiveness of HIIT used protocols of 30 seconds of near-maximal exercise followed by a rest period of three to five minutes of lower activity. For example, a runner might sprint very vigorously for 30 seconds, then jog or walk fast for four minutes to recover, and then repeat the cycle four to seven times in a given workout.

Research suggests that using a HIIT workout for longer than two weeks in healthy young adults can improve cardiorespiratory fitness better than a conventional endurance training protocol (Milanovic, Sporis, and Weston 2015). Thus, HIIT workouts are a very time-efficient way to enhance cardiorespiratory fitness. They can also be quite useful for adding variety to an exercise routine. The potential drawback of HIIT is the risk of injury. It is dangerous for people with health con-

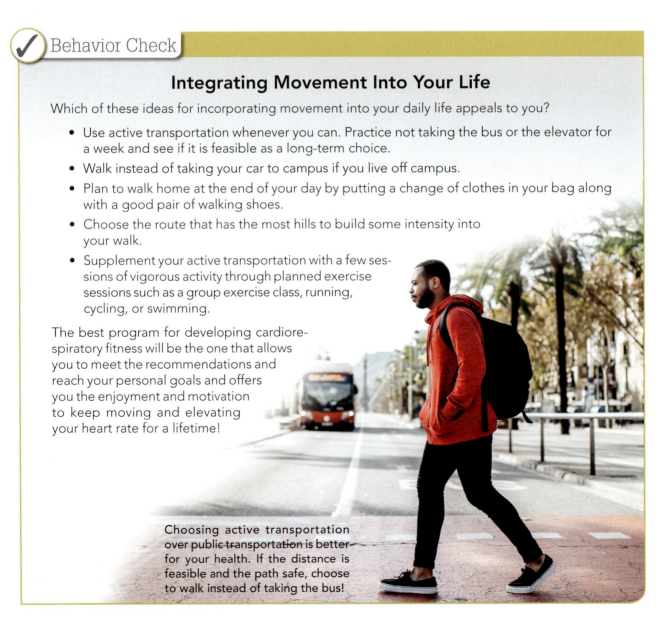

✓ Behavior Check

Integrating Movement Into Your Life

Which of these ideas for incorporating movement into your daily life appeals to you?

- Use active transportation whenever you can. Practice not taking the bus or the elevator for a week and see if it is feasible as a long-term choice.
- Walk instead of taking your car to campus if you live off campus.
- Plan to walk home at the end of your day by putting a change of clothes in your bag along with a good pair of walking shoes.
- Choose the route that has the most hills to build some intensity into your walk.
- Supplement your active transportation with a few sessions of vigorous activity through planned exercise sessions such as a group exercise class, running, cycling, or swimming.

The best program for developing cardiorespiratory fitness will be the one that allows you to meet the recommendations and reach your personal goals and offers you the enjoyment and motivation to keep moving and elevating your heart rate for a lifetime!

Choosing active transportation over public transportation is better for your health. If the distance is feasible and the path safe, choose to walk instead of taking the bus!

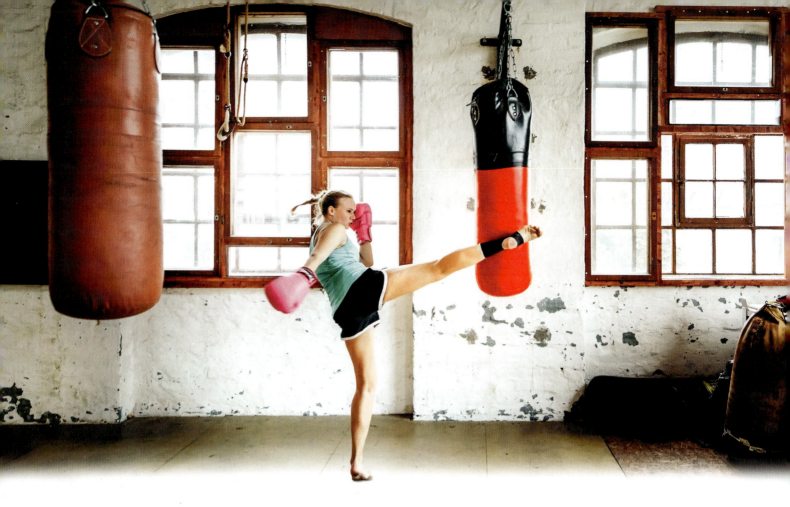

ditions involving the cardiorespiratory systems to train this intensely. Even healthy people might trigger abnormal heart rhythms with intense exercise of this nature. Intense exercise can also greatly strain the joints, tendons, and muscles and therefore poses a high risk for musculoskeletal injuries. Finally, HIIT can be extremely fatiguing. Therefore, this type of training is best for people who already have a very good conditioning base. If you do decide to try this type of training, start slowly, build slowly, and listen to your body and adjust accordingly.

Your Plan + Modern Life = Creativity Required

The FITT-VP principle of cardiorespiratory training outlined in this chapter provides a great framework for designing an individual program. The components of frequency, intensity, time, type, volume, and progression can be mixed and matched to produce a lifestyle movement program that is both effective and enjoyable. Find activities that keep you motivated to keep moving—elevating your heart rate—and working hard to obtain and maintain your fitness level. If you can figure out how to incorporate these behaviors into your days and weeks, you will experience the conditioning benefits. In today's highly sedentary world with long commutes and hours spent in front of a screen, you will need to be creative to obtain the volume of activity needed to improve cardiorespiratory fitness and positively influence your health. Use lab 4.2 in the web study guide to design your own program for developing cardiorespiratory fitness.

Safety First: Getting Started With Cardiorespiratory Fitness

Recall from chapter 3 the topics of safe movement and the importance of screening forms. In addition to doing an adequate prescreening with the PAR-Q, other primary keys for moving safely include a proper warm-up and cool-down. When heart rate, blood pressure, and breathing rate are elevated during moderate or vigorous activity, keep a few other considerations in mind.

- *Check your air quality*. Depending on where you live, watch your air quality. Poor-quality air can hinder your performance and enjoyment of aerobic-type activities. This is especially true if you have a chronic lung condition such as asthma. On poor air days, you may need to exercise indoors.

- *Hot weather*. Because the body is an inefficient machine, when you move, you give off heat. This causes your blood to move toward the surface of your body and also produces sweating. If you perform intense or longer-term exercise in the heat, you could be at risk of a hyperthermic event such as a heat cramps, exhaustion, or stroke. Proper hydration and clothing are keys to prevention.

- *Cold weather*. Hypothermia and frostbite are two common challenges when exercising outside in cold environments. Proper clothing is essential. This includes layering clothing that does not hold moisture. Also, avoid wearing wet clothing in the cold for long periods of time.

Summary

Cardiorespiratory endurance is a key component of health-related fitness. Your body's energy systems work with your cardiorespiratory system to supply energy for muscle contractions of all types. When you challenge these systems, they adapt, allowing you to meet physical challenges with less stress. Cardiorespiratory fitness is important not only for sport performance but also for activities of daily living. Cardiorespiratory fitness also plays a key role in the prevention of several important chronic diseases that typically arrive later in life. A regular movement program that you enjoy and are motivated to do on a weekly basis will help you feel great, perform your academic work better, and avoid illness now. It will also increase your chances for a long, healthy life.

WWW WEB STUDY GUIDE

Remember to complete all of the web study guide activities to further facilitate your learning, including the following lab activities:

Lab 4.1   Cardiorespiratory Fitness: The 1-Mile Walk Test or the 1.5-Mile Run Test

Lab 4.2   Daily Physical Activity: Using a Pedometer to Track Your Steps!

REVIEW QUESTIONS

1. List and describe the four critical functions that the cardiorespiratory systems perform in the human body.

2. Compare and contrast the three movement energy systems with regard to (a) rate of ATP production, (b) duration and intensity of activities where the system dominates, and (c) sample sport, leisure, and daily-living activities that primarily rely on the system.

3. Explain why heart rate can be used as a measure of cardiorespiratory fitness when measured in response to a step test.

4. Having a healthy cardiorespiratory fitness helps prevent the Big Metabolic Three. Name these three diseases and describe the primary way that fitness prevents them.

5. Name three key ways that cardiorespiratory fitness benefits the typical college student.

6. Describe how the physical activity guidelines and ACSM exercise recommendations are similar with regard to frequency, intensity, time, and type of physical movement to enhance cardiorespiratory fitness.

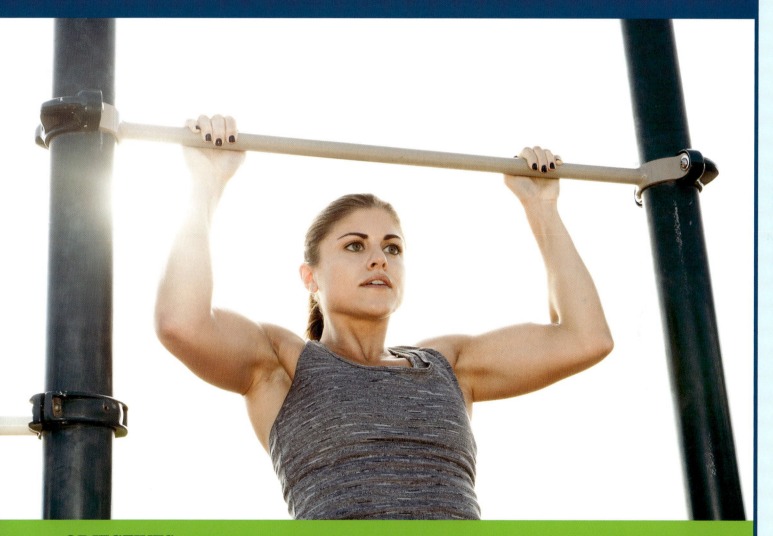

Muscular Fitness

OBJECTIVES

❯ Understand how muscles work.

❯ Know what the major muscle groups are.

❯ Design progressive workouts for muscular strength, endurance, neuromotor movement, and power.

❯ Recognize the importance of muscular fitness for looking good and aging well.

❯ Design a personalized plan to improve muscular fitness based on your health and fitness goals.

KEY TERMS

anabolic-androgenic steroids (AAS)

ergogenic

fast-twitch fiber

isometric

isotonic concentric

isotonic eccentric

muscle capacity

muscle fiber

muscular endurance

muscular power

muscular strength

slow-twitch fiber

Muscular strength and **muscular endurance** are two health-related components of physical fitness. You might also want to develop **muscular power**, which is the product of speed and strength. This chapter focuses on these three aspects of muscular fitness, which are important for sport performance, functional fitness (helping you with your daily activities), and living well for a lifetime. You need strong muscles to lift heavy furniture in your residence hall or apartment, muscles with endurance to walk long distances carrying a heavy load of books, and muscles with power to bicycle quickly up a hill. According to Aagaard and colleagues (2010), strength training increases muscle size and neuromotor function in elderly people, even after age 80. Muscles are simply waiting for us to understand their need to move more in order to stay fit over the life span.

In addition, flexibility, neuromotor fitness (which includes balance, agility, posture), and proprioceptive training are important for sport performance and daily activities. Both flexibility and neuromotor fitness are discussed in chapter 6.

All of these health-related components of fitness are particularly important for living injury free. You don't want to throw out your back moving furniture in your residence hall, causing you to hobble around campus! Joint pain may be the furthest thing from your mind right now; however, as people get older, joint replacements become common. If you are still skeptical, talk with your parents or grandparents to gain their perspective on how their joints are feeling these days. Remember, caring for your muscular structure now may help you prevent surgeries to replace your bones and joints later in life. Besides, having strong and long muscles can give your body tone, which is always a bonus (figure 5.1).

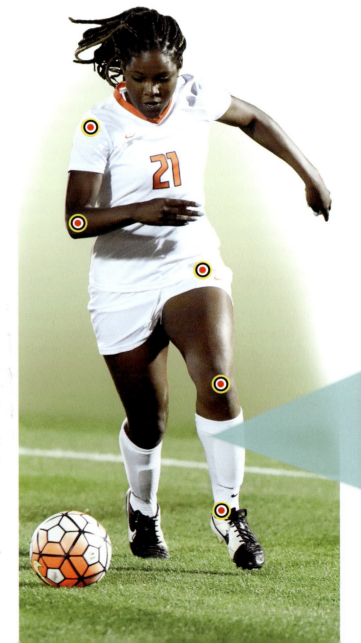

Figure 5.1 Keep your joints and muscles healthy through muscular strength, endurance, and flexibility training.

Your Body Was Designed to Move

We move less for survival than our ancestors did, but we still need to move for our health and quality of life. The muscles, bones, and joints in the human body provide us with an amazing ability to move in big and small ways and in various directions. Muscles in the body range from very large to very small. For example, walking is a large motor movement with little skill required and eye tracking requires small fine movements. The human body has many different bones, which muscles pull on when they contract. The purpose of this chapter is to help you understand basic muscle physiology so you can design an effective muscular fitness program for yourself.

Muscle Anatomy and Contraction Physiology

Although the body is complex, the fundamentals of movement are quite simple. Muscles are attached to bones by tendons. When they contract and produce force, the lever systems cause movement. Muscles generally pull on the tendons connected to bones; they cannot push. Thus, muscles are typically arranged in pairs to allow movements in both directions. Muscles differ in their force production abilities, which is the rate at which they can produce force and how long they can produce force based on their physiology.

Muscle Fibers

Individual muscle cells are the building blocks of all muscles. These cells are called **muscle fibers** and are clustered into bundles called fascicles (figure 5.2). A given muscle, no matter how small or large, is made up of many bundles of muscle fibers that are combined into a unit called a myofibril. Finally, myofibrils are arranged into sarcomeres. From a molecular perspective, sarcomeres are nearly entirely made up of actin

Between 2005 and 2030, the number of hip and knee revisions and replacements is projected to grow exponentially—137 percent for hips and 601 percent for knees (Kurtz et al. 2007). What will you do to help prevent this from happening to you? Answer: Work on your muscular strength, endurance, and flexibility!

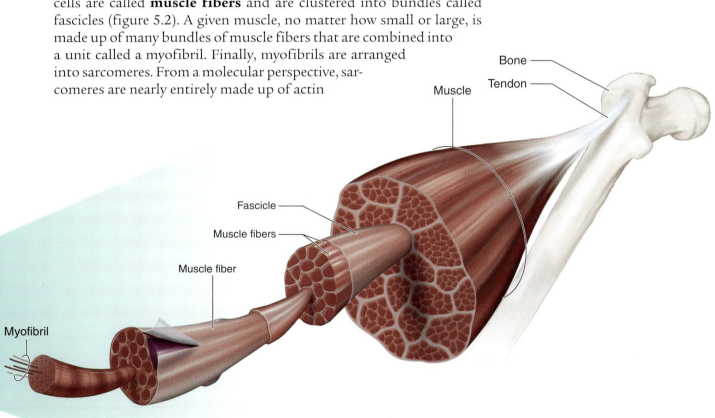

Bone

Tendon

Muscle

Fascicle

Muscle fibers

Muscle fiber

Myofibril

Figure 5.2   The basic structure of muscle.

and myosin. Muscle shortening occurs when muscle contracts and pulls on the tendons. During this process, actin attaches to the myosin molecules in a power stroke motion that is the fundamental basis of the sliding filament theory. Muscle shortening comes from a coordinated effort by many muscle cells arranged in work teams.

Not all muscle fibers are created equal. They are often broadly categorized as **slow-twitch** or **fast-twitch fibers** based on their speed of contraction, force output, and the primary energy source used to fuel the contraction. Slow-twitch fibers contract more slowly and resist fatigue better. They also primarily use the oxidative (aerobic) system to gain their ATP, or energy bucks. ATP (or energy bucks) provides a lot of energy at a slow rate. Slow-twitch fibers are often reddish (darker) in color due to the myoglobin stored in the muscles fibers that provide a quick source of oxygen. In contrast, fast-twitch fibers contract more forcefully and rapidly but fatigue more quickly than slow-twitch fibers. The primary fuel system for these fibers is the nonoxidative (anaerobic) energy system. Fast-twitch fibers are often whitish in color. Each fiber type has a preferred work output in terms of force production and rate of force production that is often matched to the job requirements.

The turkey and duck example is a relative comparison that is applicable to humans. Nearly all muscles contain a mixture of both slow-twitch and fast-twitch fibers, with the relative balance varying by the muscle and the individual as well as the person's needs and wants for daily movement. Fiber-type distribution is largely fixed at birth, but changes can occur with shifts in exercise or physical activity as well as through the aging process. Essentially, when given muscle fibers and their related energy system are overloaded, they will adapt to meet the demands placed on them. This is often referred to as the specificity of training principle.

Because our daily muscle demands are variable in terms of force production needs, this difference in jobs for each fiber type allows us greater flexibility to meet our movement demands. To use an analogy, think of the slow-twitch fibers as a car like a Hybrid Toyota Prius, which gets great gas mileage but does not accelerate very fast. In contrast, fast-twitch fibers could be represented by a Lamborghini, which accelerates very quickly but gets very poor gas mileage. Most cars blend these factors so that they get good gas mileage. However, if you need to accelerate rapidly (for example, when passing), you are able to do so safely. In a typical day on campus, you might need your slow-twitch fibers to walk across campus and maintain your sitting and standing postures. You might also need to grab your heavy backpack and dash to catch the campus bus; this primarily taxes your fast-twitch fibers.

Turkeys walk and do not fly much, heavily using slow-twitch fibers in their legs. For this reason, they have dark meat in their legs and white meat in their breasts. In contrast, ducks fly and do not walk much; therefore, they have dark meat in their breasts, which are affected by the repetitive nature of their flapping wings and white meat in their legs.

Motor Units

For a muscle to contract, it must be stimulated by the nervous system. This communication is accomplished by the motor unit, which is a nerve connected to a number of muscle fibers. Motor units can range from very small to very large with a ratio of one motor nerve to two muscle fibers or to several hundred fibers. Slow-twitch fibers are generally smaller motor units, whereas fast-twitch fibers are generally larger motor units. All motor units, regardless of size, abide by the all-or-none principle. This means that if they receive an adequate stimulus from the nervous system, all muscle fibers associated with that motor nerve and unit contract. In this way, the magnitude of force produced is determined by the number and type of motor units recruited. For example, you use smaller and fewer motor units when picking up a pencil compared to a large box of books. Keep in mind when we talk about neuromotor movement in subsequent chapters that the nervous system is number one when it comes to being in charge of how, when, and if we move.

Key Definitions

Designing an effective program for muscular fitness involves a thorough understanding of muscle terms. It's important to understand these terms and examples of the movements connected with them so you have the tools to build your own plan.

Muscle Contractions

The three main types of muscle contractions differ by length of the muscle and movement of the joint: **isometric**, **isotonic concentric**, and **isotonic eccentric**.

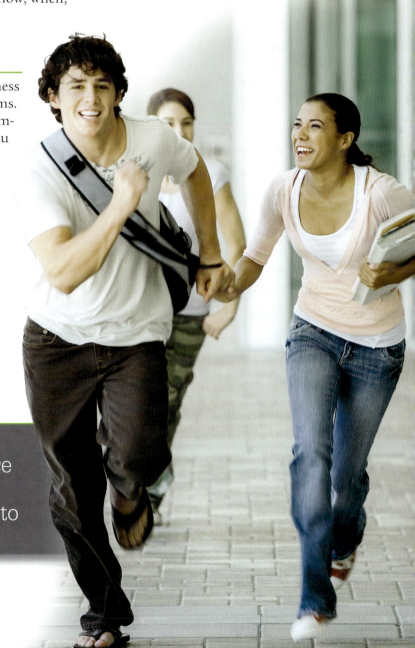

You use slow-twitch fibers when you are walking at a leisurely pace and fast-twitch fibers when you are running to catch a bus or get to class on time.

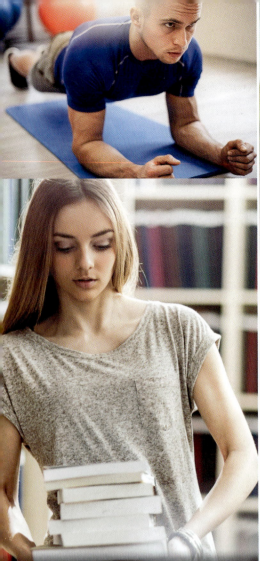

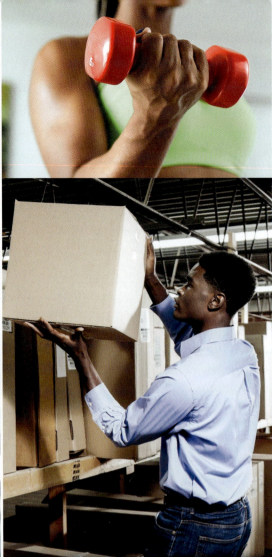

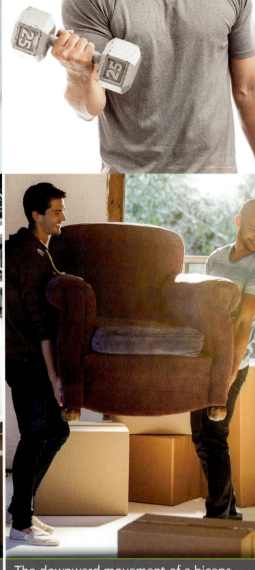

Holding a plank and carrying a pile of books in a fixed position are examples of isometric muscle contractions.

The up phase of a biceps curl and lifting a box to a shelf are examples of an isotonic concentric muscle action.

The downward movement of a biceps curl and moving furniture are examples of activities that use isotonic eccentric muscle action.

- *Isometric*. A static muscle contraction where the muscle length or the joint angle does not change. This type of contraction is important for core muscle development. The core muscles involve the torso and hip muscles, which provide important stabilization functions for daily movements.

- *Isotonic concentric*. This type of muscle contraction is used to build muscle capacity. The most common type of isotonic muscle action use is for nonpostural muscles. The up phase of a basic biceps curl using a dumbbell and the functional movement of putting a box on a shelf both use an isotonic concentric muscle action. In both of these examples, when the muscle contracts, it shortens and the joint angle decreases.

- *Isotonic eccentric*. This type of muscle contraction is the opposite action of an isotonic concentric contraction. As the muscle contracts, it lengthens and the joint angle increases. This type of contraction is often called a *negative* in the strength and conditioning room. Most resistance training programs that use free weights have an eccentric component when the weight is lowered to the ground against gravity in a controlled manner. Intense eccentric training can cause rapid strength gains but can also cause much muscle soreness if it is not done properly.

Muscle Capacity

Muscle capacity is the ability of your muscles to perform different types of movements at different speeds and levels of force. It is comprised of muscular strength, muscular endurance, muscular power, and flexibility. See the sidebar Definition of Muscle Capacity for definitions of each of those terms.

Which muscle capacity measure is the most important for your health and well-being? Think about what muscle actions you use daily. Sports such as wrestling need muscular strength, endurance, flexibility, and power to perform well during a competition. If you hike wearing a backpack for several hours, you tax all muscle capacities on various parts of the trail. Your postural muscles need endurance to sit and stand as you move through your days on campus. You might need muscular strength to lift boxes and furniture but muscular endurance to carry objects when moving in and out of your apartment. You may need flexibility to bend over and pick up something you dropped. Finally, you might need muscular power to jump out of the way of a cyclist coming quickly down the street.

Similar to cardiorespiratory fitness, the importance of your muscle capacity depends on your movement goals, which are influenced by how you live. For example, if you are a restaurant server and regularly carry large trays of food, you need good muscular strength and endurance in your arms and upper body. As you age, muscle capacity becomes increasingly important, especially as an older adult, because muscular fitness is essential for performing activities of daily living and living independently for as long as possible.

Adaptation to Muscular Overload

If you begin a muscle conditioning program, muscular strength, endurance, and power will all improve, with the greatest relative improvements dependent on how you overload your muscles. For example, if you mainly overload your muscles by lifting heavy weights very quickly, you will be training to enhance muscular power. Do you need muscular power for daily living? Muscular power can help you lift objects quickly. Is this essential to your life? Combining your needs with the muscle movement is important when building a program to enhance muscle capacity in general.

Muscle Learning

Muscle learning occurs in response to training, especially at the beginning of the training program. Resistance and flexibility training improve neural control even without changing muscle fiber size. Remember the first time you lifted a weight? You had to think about how to do it correctly. Once your muscle learned how to lift a weight or perform a specific stretch, it was much easier for you to perform the movement. As you age, the majority of muscle capacity increases in response to strength training are due to changes in neural control. Strength and flexibility training during your later years might not give you bigger muscles or increase your flexibility as an older adult, but it will certainly help you prevent falls.

Muscle Hypertrophy

Resistance training programs that provide overload with heavy weights and low repetitions increase the size and number of myofibrils, which results in larger muscles. When your muscles

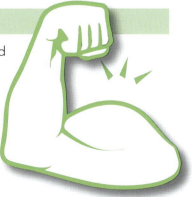

Definition of Muscle Capacity

Muscle capacity is categorized into the following health- and skill-related physical fitness components.

- **Muscular strength**—The amount of force that can be produced with a single maximum effort.
- **Muscular endurance**—The ability of the muscle to hold or repeat a contraction without fatigue.
- **Muscular power**—The rate at which muscle force can be executed; alternatively, muscle force production (strength) expressed relative to time.
- **Flexibility**—The range of movement in a joint or series of joints and length in muscles that cross the joints to induce a bending movement or motion.

get bigger, their increase in muscle fiber size is called hypertrophy. When you first start resistance training, you might not notice an increase in your muscle size, but over time, depending on how you train, your muscles may increase in size and strength.

All pumped up! Temporary hypertrophy, or the increase in muscle size during and immediately after an exercise bout, mainly results from fluid accumulation in the extracellular fluid spaces and between the muscle cells.

Assessing Muscle Capacity

Similar to assessing cardiorespiratory fitness, the various components of muscle capacity can be assessed using both laboratory equipment and less complicated field tests. However, instead of whole-body measures, assessments of muscle capacity are typically completed for one movement pattern (e.g., a squat) or joint action (e.g., knee extension), which may not be representative of the muscle capacity of other muscle groups. In a clinical setting, advanced dynamometers are used to assess all aspects of muscle capacity, especially muscular strength and endurance. This information informs training regimens and rehabilitation programs for people of all ages and fitness levels.

Hypertrophy is the increased size of a muscle, and it is often due to increases in muscle fiber size. Not all strength gains lead to hypertrophy.

Muscular Strength

Strength is assessed by measuring the maximal amount of weight a person can lift or move in a single effort, commonly called a one-repetition maximum (1RM). You could assess your 1RM for all of your muscle groups using free weights or machines. However, the 1RM can be intense for your muscles, tendons, and joints. You might risk getting injured. Thus, an alternative strength test is a submaximal effort using repetitions that can help predict your strength.

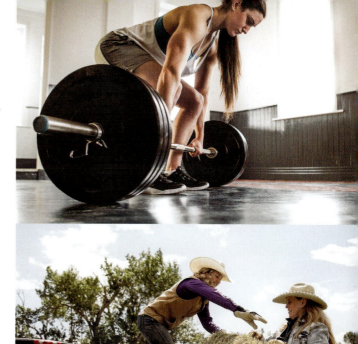

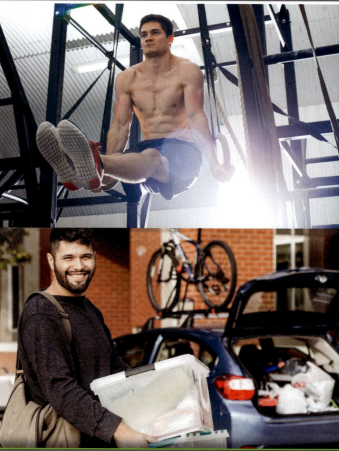

Both performing a deadlift in a strength and conditioning room and lifting a bale of hay require muscular strength.

Muscular Endurance

Muscle endurance is the ability to hold a muscle action or to repeat contractions that are not maximal. This component of muscle capacity is assessed by either the maximum number of repetitions that can be performed (e.g., push-ups) or the length of time a position can be held (e.g., planks). Similar to muscular strength, good muscular endurance is important for both sport performance and daily living. An example of this is carrying fewer items and making more trips because objects are heavy. Muscular endurance is key to having good posture. Labs 5.1 and 5.2 in the web study guide provide different assessment options you can use to assess your muscular endurance.

Both holding an iron cross position during gymnastics and carrying boxes while moving involve muscular endurance.

93

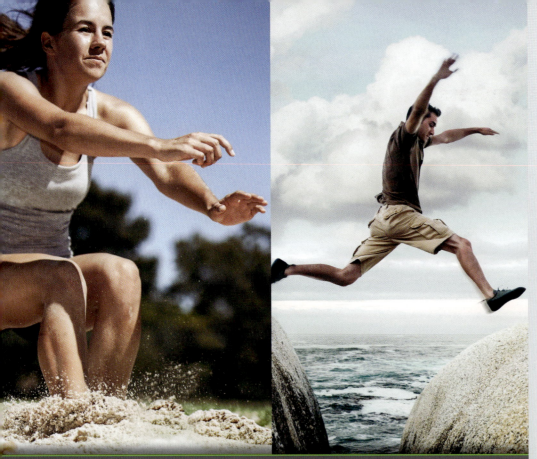

Muscular Power

Muscular power is not assessed as often as muscular strength and endurance are for health and fitness; however, it deserves mention for its role in daily functional movement. Muscular power is the ability of a muscle or muscle group to move a force quickly. The definition of muscular power is force multiplied by distance divided by time. Its contribution to optimal functional movement on a daily basis is less critical for young adults; however, the role muscular power plays in daily function for older adults is very important. Muscle power can be assessed by using a broad jump test for an athlete or measuring how quickly an older adult gets out of a chair.

Performing a broad jump and jumping from one rock to another are both examples of a muscular power movement.

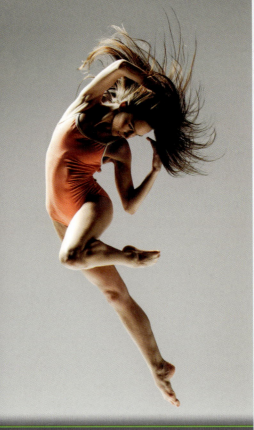

Muscle Size and Tone

Many people are interested in resistance training for aesthetic or physique reasons. Some people want to have large muscles, be lean, or tone their muscles. A regular program of strength and resistance training can enhance muscle size and definition and help you look and feel better. While having muscle tone and looking lean are qualitative assessments, muscle and fat mass can be quantitatively measured in the research laboratory or clinic.

Bodybuilders work on muscle size and tone through weight training, while dancers acquire muscle size and tone by lifting their body weight repeatedly through dance training.

Muscular Fitness Benefits Your Daily Life

Most of us are not competitive athletes and do not need to have high muscle capacity to make a living or function in our daily lives. Indeed, in our knowledge society, working on a keyboard in front of a screen does not require much muscle work except perhaps some muscular endurance for good sitting or standing posture. However, similar to cardiorespiratory fitness, good muscular fitness provides more benefits in your daily life than you may realize. In a study published out of John Hopkins University (Varma et al. 2017), researchers used activity trackers to measure daily activity at various life spans and found that the activity levels of 19-year-olds were comparable to those of 60-year-olds (i.e., very low). The authors concluded that physical activity levels during adolescence were lower than they expected. This study points out the need to pay attention to activity levels outside of a fitness setting, as discussed in earlier chapters related to the human movement paradigm. The same holds true for muscular fitness benefits. Just as the dancer gets muscular endurance from dancing and the hiker gets muscular power from jumping from rock to rock, you can integrate muscular training into your daily activities. Using a strength and conditioning room is one option, but if you don't have access to such a facility, you can find other ways to fit muscular conditioning into your daily life.

Designing Your Program for Muscular Fitness

Now that you know how muscles work and adapt to overload, you are ready to reflect on your own strength training program. Formulating a plan to

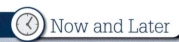

Now and Later

Benefits of Resistance Training

Now

In addition to the many benefits already described, a regular program of resistance training can help you lose inches off your body and greatly enhance your muscle tone. Combined with the benefits for posture and self-confidence, resistance training is a key to looking good and feeling good!

Later

Having muscular fitness is one of the primary keys to aging well, especially in your 70s and beyond. Starting a regular program for your muscular fitness early in life can enhance your bone health and physical functional capacity as you age. It is never too late to start a program and realize the benefits.

Take Home

Women and older adults are especially in need of maintaining a regular strength routine because they are more susceptible to osteoporosis and they live longer than men in general. There are more women in assisted care than men. Help the women in your life find the motivation to engage in strength training. Gone are the days of "Let me do that for you." Instead, say, "Grandma, you can lift that. I want you to be independent as long as you can. I know you love living in your own house, so think of it as a fitness center. What can you lift every day?"

help you realize the benefits of muscular fitness is next.

The Plan Depends on the Goal

Similar to cardiorespiratory fitness, your personal plan depends on your goal. For example, your muscular fitness might be primarily targeting aesthetic values—you want larger muscles or muscle tone in order to look good. Or perhaps you need a regular program to help your posture so you don't have back and neck pain from lots of computer screen time. Or maybe your intramural sport performance would benefit from a targeted program. You might want to be able to carry a large, heavy backpack while hiking on the weekends. To enhance your health and well-being over time, work on meeting the CDC and ACSM recommendations to make your daily life activities less stressful physiologically and prevent chronic diseases later in life. Content in this section is not targeted to strength training programs for the athlete, specific performance goals, or advanced strength training techniques such as periodization. If you are interested in moving beyond the general guidelines, we encourage you to consult a strength coach who has specific expertise for your sport or goal.

Overloading Options: Variable Resistance Machines, Free Weights, and Body Weight

Increasing muscular fitness requires you to overload the muscles in a consistent, progressive manner. Muscles respond to the overload, regardless of what is providing the stimulus. The most popular options are variable resistance machines, traditional free weights, and body weight. Table 5.1 lists the primary pros and cons for each of these choices. You can overload a muscle in many ways and can mix and match them to provide cre-

Table 5.1   Primary Overloading Options and Considerations

Overload option	Positives	Negatives	Considerations
Variable resistance machines	• Safe • Require no spotter • Easy to understand and use • Isolate muscle groups • Contain instructional placards on machines • Require little knowledge	• Expensive • Typically require membership at a fitness facility • Isolate muscle groups, which is not as applicable to real-life functional movement	• Train muscle groups and not movement • One machine typically works 1 or 2 muscle groups • Most movements performed in a seated position • Require maintenance
Free weights	• Movements are adaptable to real life • Various free weights can be used for many different exercises	• Potential for injury is greater • Relatively expensive to purchase equipment for a home • May require a spotter for some movements	• Easy to personalize a program • Home use is convenient but requires space
Body weight	• Inexpensive • Always available wherever you go; the equipment is portable	• Overload for strength may be limited depending on goals and baseline levels	• Resistance bands are inexpensive and travel well • Stability balls are inexpensive and work the core well

ative workouts. Note that you can work on your muscular fitness without ever going to a strength and conditioning facility.

FITT: Frequency, Intensity, Time, and Type

The fundamental frame for your muscular fitness program should follow the FITT acronym, which is an easy way to organize your overload to gain and keep muscular fitness. FITT stands for frequency, intensity, time, and type. Figure 5.3 shows how you can fit the guidelines of leading organizations, including those from the CDC and the ACSM, into your weekly schedule. The best program for you depends on your goals and interests. Select activities that you enjoy. The key is to find a method that works for you to both achieve and maintain muscular fitness. Unless you enjoy using a strength and conditioning room or attending a group exercise class, try not to become dependent on a facility. Relying on facility use for movement goals can hinder your adherence, particularly over your life span.

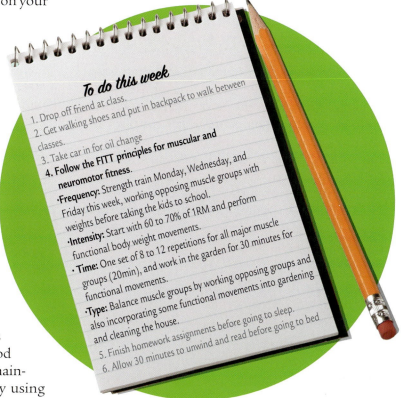

To do this week

1. Drop off friend at class.
2. Get walking shoes and put in backpack to walk between classes.
3. Take car in for oil change
4. Follow the FITT principles for muscular and neuromotor fitness.
   - **Frequency:** Strength train Monday, Wednesday, and Friday this week, working opposing muscle groups with weights before taking the kids to school.
   - **Intensity:** Start with 60 to 70% of 1RM and perform functional body weight movements.
   - **Time:** One set of 8 to 12 repetitions for all major muscle groups (20min), and work in the garden for 30 minutes for functional movements.
   - **Type:** Balance muscle groups by working opposing groups and also incorporating some functional movements into gardening and cleaning the house.
5. Finish homework assignments before going to sleep.
6. Allow 30 minutes to unwind and read before going to bed

Figure 5.3   Make a weekly to-do list that includes the recommended levels of muscular fitness training.

Frequency: How Many Days Do I Need to Strength Train?

Current recommendations are to strength train two or three days per week at moderate to high intensity with at least 48 hours between exercise training sessions for a given muscle group (American College of Sports Medicine 2018; Garber et al. 2011). If you train your quadriceps on Monday, you wouldn't do so again until at least Wednesday. Depending on your schedule and preference, you could train all the major muscle groups in a single session or separate them by splitting the body into regions and alternating your training. For example, many regular strength trainers alternate working the upper body and the lower body for a total of four days of training a week (e.g., lower body trained on Mondays and Thursdays, upper body trained on Tuesdays and Fridays). Whole-body or split-body routines are equally effective as long as each muscle group is trained two or three days per week. You can also choose more functional movements that require balance, stability, strength, and endurance. These types of workouts do not require splitting the body; rather, you would perform total-body functional movements that work several muscle groups simultaneously.

Intensity: How Hard Do I Work Out?

Your goal will influence the intensity of resistance training. Similar to other systems, the greater the intensity (i.e., overload) of training, the greater the benefit. However, a greater risk of injury also occurs, especially in people with aged or vulnerable musculoskeletal systems. The required intensity is also affected by age, health status, recreational activity, and baseline fitness. For beginners or intermediates, 60 to 70 percent 1RM is considered moderate to vigorous intensity (American College of Sports Medicine 2018). As you gain a conditioning base, you can increase up to 80 percent or more of 1RM to continue to improve strength. Deconditioned people might start at 40 to 50 percent 1RM. Increasing muscular endurance requires performing movements of lower intensities (such as less than 50 percent 1RM, which is considered light to moderate intensity) at a greater volume. Likewise, increasing power requires completing lower-intensity movements quickly.

Time: How Long Do I Spend on Strength and Endurance Training?

Your time depends on your goals in a strength and conditioning session. You can spend up to an hour or you can perform the minimum to keep you healthy, which is one set of 10 to 15 repetitions for all major muscle groups. Incorporating func-

tional movements that combine muscle groups will also save you time. According to the American Council on Exercise (2014), training volume is what is important. The cumulative work completed is referred to as training volume. Volume is equal to sets times repetitions. If you perform 10 repetitions of squats with two 25-pound (11 kg) dumbbells in your hands, your volume of work is lifting 250 pounds (113 kg). If you reduce the repetitions and increase the weights, you can do fewer repetitions, which will take you less time. Therefore, the time you spend in your session depends on how you perform your strength and conditioning routine and what your goals are.

Type: What Type of Movements Should I Choose?

Lots of options—many in your own home—can effectively provide an overload to your muscles. Cook (2010) recommends focusing more on daily functional movement than on exercises that work individual muscle groups. The American Council on Exercise (2014) also suggests that trainers make the client's movement efficiency and ability to

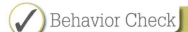

Behavior Check

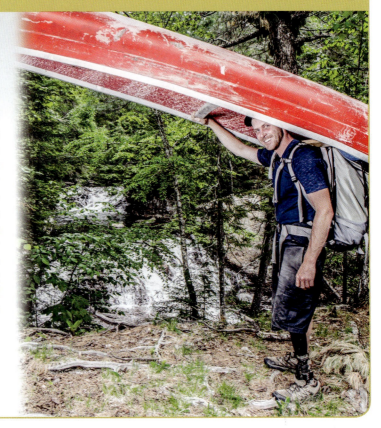

What is your why for strength training?

Which of your muscles do you think need to be strong and long? Why? Which of your muscles are already strong and flexible? Why is that? Think about the types of movements that you would like to do effectively. Would you like to be able to run two miles in under 18 minutes, enjoy a yoga class, eliminate back pain, or walk across campus without your shins hurting? Which muscles do you need to strengthen or lengthen to prevent pain and enhance quality of life? These are different questions than how much weight will you lift to get big arms or how do you get six-pack abs?

perform daily activities the staple of any workout routine. Recommendations for strength training include the following (American College of Sports Medicine 2018):

- Multijoint or compound exercises that affect more than one muscle group (e.g., squats, chest press)
- Single-joint exercises that target major muscle groups (e.g., leg curl, bicep curl)
- Core muscle training (e.g., planks and bridges) due to the key role these major muscles play in preventing low back pain
- Balancing opposing muscle groups (e.g., if you work the biceps, also work the triceps; see figure 5.4)

When incorporating a combination of exercises into your routine, be mindful of order of movement choice. In general, plan to perform exercises for large muscle groups or multijoint exercises before doing smaller-muscle or single-joint exercises. Fatiguing the small muscle groups first limits your ability to overload the larger muscle groups or complete compound exercises. Thus, you should first perform sets for squats, then leg extensions (compound versus single-joint exercise), followed by calf raises (larger versus smaller muscle groups).

How: Volume, Pattern, and Progression (VPP)

The FITT approach provides a framework for muscular fitness, but volume, pattern, and progression (VPP) inform your how and your why—how you will start and your motivation. Take a minute to think about what you want out of strength training by looking at some common muscle imbalances that occur due to daily living practices (see table 5.2).

Volume = Repetitions and Sets

Most muscular fitness programs are defined primarily by repetitions ("reps") and sets. The combination of them is the volume of your workout. According to Westcott (1996), two or three strength training sessions a week produce excellent results for most people. The ACSM recommends training two or three times per week with at least 48 hours separating the exercise training sessions

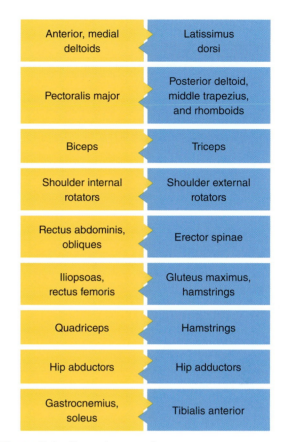

Figure 5.4 Opposing muscle groups.

Reprinted by permission from C. Kennedy-Armbruster and M.M. Yoke, *Methods of Group Exercise Instruction*, 3rd ed. (Champaign, IL: Human Kinetics, 2014), 44.

for the same muscle group (American College of Sports Medicine 2018; Garber et al. 2011). Each muscle group can be trained for a total of one to four sets. One or two sets will improve muscular endurance, and two to four sets are recommended for improving strength and power (American College of Sports Medicine 2018). You can do sets of the same exercise or of different exercises. For example, if you do two sets of leg squats and then two leg extensions on a machine on the same day, you will be giving your quadriceps muscles four sets of overload. Different exercises can provide variety in the overload and add motivation in terms of mental stimulation for those who get bored with routine.

In resistance training, intensity and reps are inversely related. They influence muscle capacity outcomes, specifically muscular strength and endurance. The greater the intensity (i.e., resistance), the fewer the number of reps you will need

Table 5.2 Common Muscle Imbalances

Muscle	Problem	Typical cause	Correction
Pectoralis major	Tight	Poor posture when sitting and standing	Stretch
Posterior deltoids, middle trapezius, rhomboids	Weak, over-stretched	Poor posture when sitting and standing	Strengthen
Shoulder internal rotators	Tight	Poor posture, carrying and holding objects close to body	Stretch
Shoulder external rotators	Weak	Poor posture	Strengthen
Abdominals	Weak	Poor posture, obesity	Strengthen
Erector spinae	Tight (and often weak)	Poor posture, obesity	Stretch (and strengthen)
Hip flexors	Tight	Poor posture, sedentary lifestyle	Stretch
Hamstrings	Tight	Sedentary lifestyle	Stretch
Calves	Tight	Wearing high heels	Stretch
Shin	Weak	Not enough use in daily activities	Strengthen

Reprinted by permission from C. Kennedy-Armbruster and M.M. Yoke, *Methods of Group Exercise Instruction*, 3rd ed. (Champaign, IL: Human Kinetics, 2014), 45.

to complete. To gain muscular strength and mass, and to a limited degree muscular endurance, an appropriate resistance is one that allows you to complete 8 to 12 reps per set—to muscle fatigue with good form and control. To integrate this concept with the intensity guidelines, this is 60 to 80 percent of a person's 1RM. Typically, muscle fatigue occurs on a lower rep—by the last set of 12 reps, fatigue will usually occur around rep 8. Beginners can improve muscular fitness with one set but will realize additional gains as progression occurs. The SAID principle (specific adaptation to imposed demands) reminds us that the body will adapt to the specific challenges imposed as long as the program progressively overloads the system being trained (American Council on Exercise 2011).

> By manipulating reps, sets, and rest intervals between sets, you can target muscular strength, endurance, or hypertrophy. Make your program work for your goals!

If muscular endurance is your goal, perform a higher number of reps (15 to 25) for each set with a shorter rest interval and fewer sets (one or two per muscle group). Of course, this change will require an alteration in intensity—typically 50 percent of 1RM or less. Deconditioned or novice resistance trainers should begin with 10 to 15 reps at a very light intensity (5 or 6 on a scale of 1 to 10) if they can manage this with good technique.

Pattern

The 48-hour recovery rule is important for fitness gains and injury prevention. Remember that more is not always better. You should rest for at least 48 hours between sessions for *any single muscle group* (Garber et al. 2011). In fact, according to Schoenfeld and colleagues (2016), young strength-trained men benefitted more from longer periods of rest between sets (1 minute versus 3 minutes), even while performing their lifting routines. When you are strength training, you are actually tearing muscle down. When you rest, the muscle builds up again to be able to handle the next strength episode. People get injured when they do not rest long enough to allow the body to recovery. Also, within a given session, rest intervals of two to three minutes between each set of reps are most effective. Rest time can be reduced for a muscular endurance program.

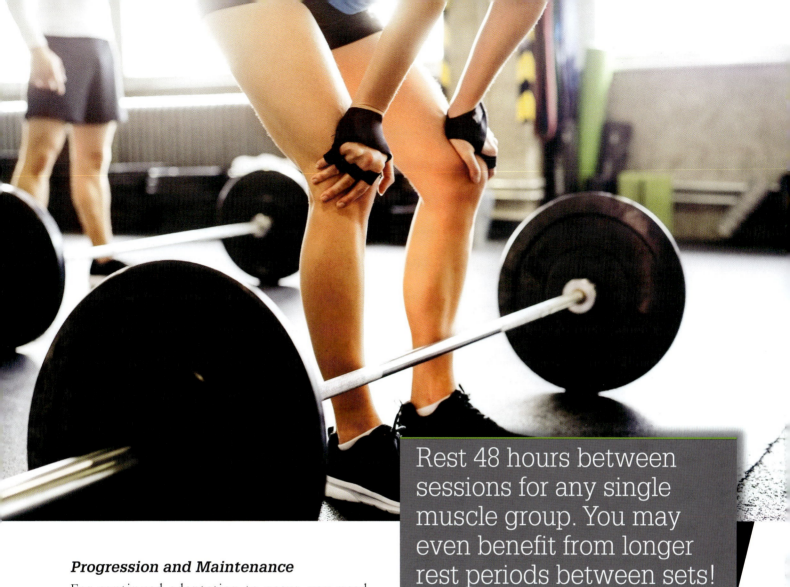

Rest 48 hours between sessions for any single muscle group. You may even benefit from longer rest periods between sets!

Progression and Maintenance

For continued adaptation to occur, you need progressive overload. As soon as you can do more than 12 reps easily, you need to increase the weight you are lifting. By increasing the weight, you will naturally fall back into the range of 8 to 12 reps. Other options for progressive overload are to increase the number of sets for each exercise or the number of days of training per week. Lack of time is the main reason people give for quitting.

If you have reached your muscular fitness goals and now want to focus on maintenance, you do not need to progressively increase the training stimulus. This means that that you can keep the same reps, sets, and weekly sessions. You can maintain muscle strength by training one day per week if you hold the training intensity or the resistance constant (Garber et al. 2011).

Finally, the FITT-VPP guidelines provided in this chapter target a general muscular fitness program for a relatively healthy adult. If you are training for a sport or event (like a marathon), you should find a coach who can help you meet these goals.

Analyzing Your Fitness Choices

"Do your quads hurt after climbing several flights of stairs to get to a class?" Then you will want to strengthen your quadriceps. "Do you have difficulty carrying heavy groceries or a pile of books?" Strengthening your biceps and deltoids will help with that. "Do you want to be able to tuck in your shirt and be satisfied that you look and feel good?" Working on your abdominals and obliques might be your priority. Think about what activities in your daily life you would like to have more strength to do and what matters to you. Then, identify which muscle group you want to

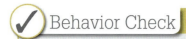

✓ Behavior Check

Incorporating Muscular Fitness Movements Into Daily Life

In addition to designing a formal muscular fitness training program, use these ideas to add muscular strength and endurance movements to your daily life:

- Choose a large backpack, load it down, and carry it (on both shoulders!) when you use active transportation.
- When carrying groceries and supplies into your room or apartment, try to lift as many as you can to transport your goods in as few trips as possible.
- Try to find a part-time job that works your muscles, such as with a lawn care service, a moving company, or a farm.
- Break up your computer screen time with sets of planks or push-ups in your room.
- Take the stairs instead of the elevator whenever you can.

strengthen. In other words, have a purpose for what you are doing outside of just "working out." Beginning strength trainers can find the FITT-VPP framework to get and keep muscular fitness complicated. Let's make sense out of how you might think about strength training before you design your own program. Understanding your choices will help you adhere to a regular program and gradually work up to the scientific guidelines outlined previously.

See the Functional Movement Training section after chapter 6. In it, you will find a practical method for choosing which exercises to include in your program. You'll start by thinking about which muscles you use more in daily living. Then you'll use a progression model—moving from functional movement to resistance exercise choices to a relevant stretch—that will be especially helpful if you are new to strength and endurance training.

The major muscle groups included in the Fundamental Movement Training section are the muscles of the calves, quads, hams and glutes, abdominals, lower back, hip abductors, hip adductors, chest and front of shoulder, upper back and shoulders, lats and middle back, front

> A general rule for safe weight training is the following: If you cannot control it, don't lift it!

of upper arm, and back of upper arm. It is useful to think of your major muscle groups as those that occur in pairs with nearly equal and opposite actions. For example, the chest muscles push away from the body, whereas the upper back muscles pull toward the body. Similarly, the quadriceps of the legs extend the knee joint and the hamstrings flex the knee joint. Nearly all muscle actions that occur in sports or during daily campus life use a combination of the major muscle groups. The special section on functional movement training will help you put this concept into perspective as you perform daily living activities and incorporate practical suggestions for muscular strength, endurance, and flexibility movements.

Safety Issues

Resistance training for strength, endurance, and power can provide many benefits. However, you should perform physical training safely in order to avoid injury and adverse consequences. In this section, we look at safety precautions to take while you train and briefly discuss supplements and drugs.

Safety While You Train

Follow these special considerations for strength training to avoid injury:

- *Don't skip the warm-up*. Cold muscles and tendons do not respond well to stress. Warming up may reduce the risk of injury, and you will feel better!
- *Mind the joints*. Proper form and technique are very important for injury prevention. Avoid bending while twisting.

- *Range of motion*. Unless you are performing a static exercise (e.g., plank), complete all exercises through the full range of motion for a given joint.
- *Don't forget to breathe*. Holding your breath can elevate your blood pressure and make you light-headed. Inhale when you are in the concentric or up phase (lifting) and exhale during the eccentric or down phase (lowering).
- *Eccentric training*. Avoid high-intensity eccentric training (unless you are a highly trained athlete under proper supervision), since it poses a significant risk for muscle soreness, joint injury, and muscle damage.
- *Use spotters and collars*. When using free weights, use appropriate collars and spotters at all times to prevent injury to yourself and your fellow exercisers.
- *Progress slowly*. Training too hard and too early is a primary reason for injuries. Start slow and progress appropriately so you can keep up your muscular fitness for a lifetime.

Friends don't let friends use steroids! If you suspect use and abuse, be a true friend—confront the situation and assist your friend get professional help.

Caution: Dietary Protein, Supplements, and Drugs

Dietary protein and supplements are addressed in chapter 8. It is fitting, though, to provide a brief mention of supplements. Resorting to extreme tactics with little regard for the potential health risks can be dangerous. Although some substances improve performance, the great majority are not regulated by the government (Food and Drug Administration [FDA]). They are ineffective and illegal and can be very dangerous.

Of special importance is the use and abuse of **anabolic-androgenic steroids (AAS)**, which are **ergogenic** but can be extremely dangerous and have long-lasting health effects. They are rarely prescribed for healthy young people and are not regulated by the FDA. These drugs, marketed as designer steroids, are considered recreational (i.e., illegal). Obtaining a prescription from a physician but using the drugs incorrectly also counts as illegal use. The National Athletic Training Association provides a detailed scientific position statement regarding AAS (www.nata.org/news-publications/pressroom/statements/position). Another great resource is WebMD (search "anabolic steroids"), which provides an extensive overview of steroids, as they are commonly called, and the health risks associated with their use and abuse.

Just like you wouldn't want friends to hurt themselves with other types of drug use and abuse, watch for signs and symptoms of steroid use. In addition to a regular well-designed resistance program, good health behaviors, including adequate nutrition, hydration, and sleep, are the key strategies to enjoying muscular fitness for a lifetime.

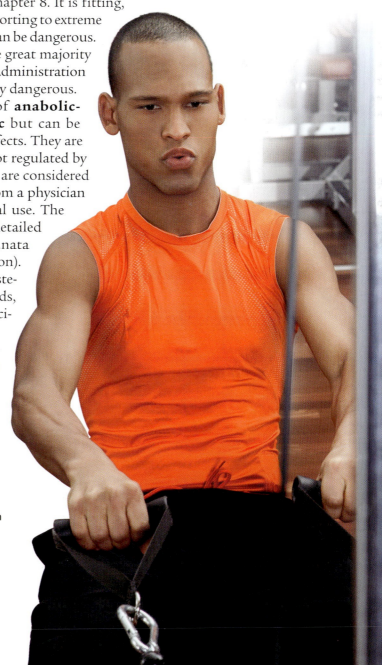

Building muscle through strength training is always better for your body than trying to use a pill a substance to gain muscle.

Summary

Muscular fitness, which includes muscular strength, endurance, power, and neuromotor movement, is a key component of health-related fitness. Your body's energy systems provide energy bucks to your contracting muscles, which pull on your bones to act like a leverage system. These contractions allow countless types of human movement actions, large and small. When you challenge the muscles with progressive overload using variable resistance machines, free weights, your body weight, or neuromotor capacity, muscles gain fitness due to both neural and muscle-fiber adaptations. Muscular fitness is very important for many sport and recreational activities. It can also enhance your daily campus life, especially if you tote a large backpack and sit and stand up with good posture. Good muscular fitness is also important for preventing injuries of your muscles and joints during work and play activities. Use the Functional Movement Training section—found after chapter 6—to help you design a regular muscular fitness program that you will be motivated to stay with for life. Lab 5.3 in the web study guide provides options for assessing your muscular strength. This will help you feel better, look better, reduce your risk for injury and pain, and increase your chance of living a long, independent life.

WEB STUDY GUIDE

Remember to complete all of the web study guide activities to further facilitate your learning, including the following lab activities:

Lab 5.1 Muscular Endurance: Push-Up Test

Lab 5.2 Muscular Endurance: Squat Test

Lab 5.3 Muscular Strength: %1RM Test

REVIEW QUESTIONS

1. Our muscles contain different types of muscle fibers that allow us to move freely throughout our day. What type of muscle fiber helps us run long distances without being tired? What type of muscle fiber allows us to run sprints? Which type of muscle fibers do you think you use more throughout the day and why?

2. List two positive and two negative consequences of using variable resistance machines, free weights, and your body weight to overload for muscular strength and endurance training.

3. Understanding muscle imbalances from daily living helps you choose a resistance training routine that will enhance your daily life. What are the opposing muscle groups to the following muscles: calves, quadriceps, abdominals, biceps, latissimus dorsi, and rhomboids?

4. How might you use the FITT (frequency, intensity, time, and type) model to outline a muscular strength and conditioning program?

5. Muscular strength and endurance training uses a particular volume of weight each session. Consider your workout plan. Calculate your total volume of weight lifted based on the sets and reps you do for your current workout. How might you use this total volume number to help you train and measure your progress?

6. List five ways you can incorporate muscular strength and endurance training into your daily life.

7. Outline three or four safety issues that are important to consider when using strength and conditioning equipment.

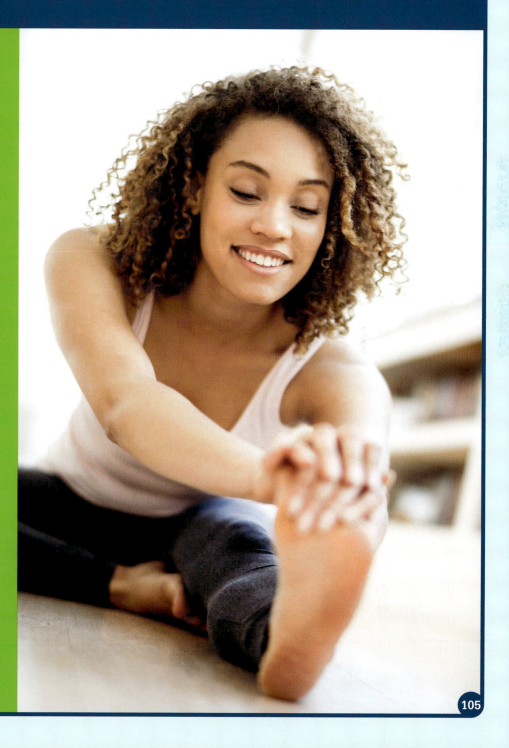

6

Flexibility, Neuromotor Fitness, and Posture

OBJECTIVES

❯ Understand the health benefits of flexibility and neuromotor fitness.

❯ Recognize that good posture makes you look good and feel good.

❯ Learn the evidence-based guidelines for flexibility and neuromotor exercise.

❯ Understand how to prevent low back pain through movement and proper posture.

❯ Develop a safe plan for enhancing your neuromotor fitness and flexibility that meets your needs.

❯ Incorporate strategies into your daily movement routine to enhance flexibility, neuromotor fitness, and posture.

KEY TERMS

connective tissue

dynamic stretching

flexibility

functional fitness

low back pain

neuromotor exercise

posture

proprioceptors

static stretching

stretch reflex

Chapter 5 explains how muscles work and provides principles to help you accomplish your personal goals for muscular fitness. We hope you took time to practice some functional strength and conditioning exercises. The Functional Movement Training section that appears after this chapter will help you gain perspective on strength, flexibility, and neuromotor training combined. These ideas for strengthening major muscle groups use different types of equipment and your own body weight. They are followed by examples of stretching exercises and neuromotor movements that will lend perspective on how these exercises fit into training for everyday living. The suggested stretch for each major muscle group is meant to enhance your flexibility.

Before finalizing your strengthening and stretching plan, review the guidelines for flexibility and see where else you could apply them in your life. Long and strong muscles are necessary for balance, which supports your overall health by reducing the risk of physical injury and helping you feel better after training for muscular strength and endurance training. After all, the purpose of performing most movements is to look and feel better. Leaving out stretching makes the muscles unhappy, since they shorten during muscle contractions and need to be lengthened at the end of a workout.

> Leaving a strength and conditioning workout without stretching is like forgetting to change the oil in your car. After going for a while without an oil change, your car will not work too well.

Neuromotor exercise (ACSM 2018) can be thought of as exercise training that involves the intersection between muscle capacity and flexibility. It is very important for functional fitness in your work, play, and daily movement. This chapter focuses on the evidence-based guidelines for flexibility and neuromotor exercise, as well as how you can apply them to your movement routine. The chapter ends with an important discussion on proper posture and its relationship to preventing low back pain.

All About Flexibility

Flexibility is the amount of movement that can be accomplished at a joint. Flexibility is described as range of motion (ROM) of a joint or set of joints. We do not have as much evidence-based knowledge of flexibility as we do of cardiorespiratory exercise and muscular strength and endurance. As the population ages, though, it is increasingly important to understand flexibility and apply it to daily living practices.

What Determines Flexibility?

Have you ever noticed that some people can bend themselves into a pretzel (and hold it!), while others can barely get out of a chair after sitting for a while? Flexibility, sometimes referred to as limberness, is about how freely your joints move, including the lengthening ability of the muscles that cross a given joint. Recall from the previous chapter that muscles often work in pairs. This means that many different muscle groups can influence the ROM of a joint. Here are a few primary factors related to flexibility training:

- *Joint structure*. There are many different types of joints in the body, and this affects joint ROM. For example, the ball-and-socket joint in the shoulder has the greatest range of motion of all the joints. The elbow is a hinge joint with much more limited movement (e.g., picking up and putting down objects).

- *Age and sex*. Flexibility is reduced with age, in part because of changes in the muscle fibers themselves. Women are more flexible than men throughout the life span due to their different bone structure and hormones.

- *Connective tissue*. The deep **connective tissues** of the body, including the fascia and tendons, can affect ROM. Fascia is a band of connective tissue below the skin that attaches, stabilizes, and separates muscles and other internal organs. Tendons attach muscle to bone. Ligaments are not elastic but do respond to regular stretching. They attach bone to bone. Age affects all the connective tissues listed previously, making them thicker and less flexible.

- *Muscle size*. Sometimes, typically in men, when muscles get big, ROM is reduced. For example, having large chest muscles can limit how far you can lift your arms overhead.

- *Proprioceptors*. These tiny sensors are located inside muscle fibers and provide information about joint angle, muscle length, and muscle tension. They can cause reflexes that prevent ROM. The stretch reflex (described in the section Mind the Stretch Reflex!) is an example of **proprioceptors** in the body.

- *Joint injury or repair*. Major injuries to joints that cause scar tissue often reduce ROM. Similarly, joint replacement can make a person less flexible. This typically occurs with knee replacements.

As you can see from the preceding list, many structures and principles are involved in a flexibility movement. For example, the triceps stretch shown in figure 6.1 also involves the posterior deltoid, rotator cuff muscles (teres minor and major), and the latissimus dorsi. The joint being stretched is the shoulder joint, a ball-and-socket joint that involves several muscles that stabilize the shoulder joint. Although this stretch is considered a triceps stretch, we know from the principles just described that there is much more going on with this simple stretch due to the connectedness of our muscles, joints, bones, and connective tissue structures.

Strength and Flexibility Can Interact!

A relative balance exists between the strength of a particular muscle group and the flexibility of both the muscle

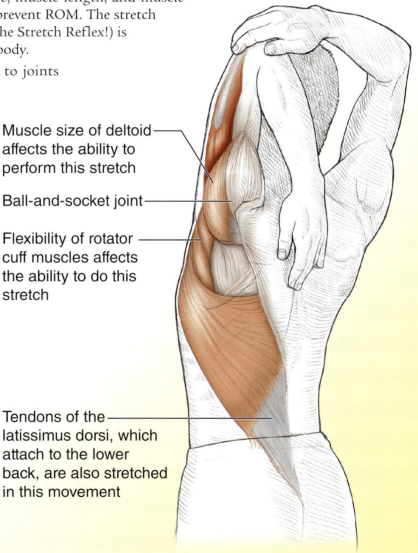

Muscle size of deltoid affects the ability to perform this stretch

Ball-and-socket joint

Flexibility of rotator cuff muscles affects the ability to do this stretch

Tendons of the latissimus dorsi, which attach to the lower back, are also stretched in this movement

Figure 6.1   Notice all of the muscles that are involved in the triceps stretch.

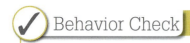

Stretching Feels Good!

People who adhere to regular stretching routines often incorporate stretching into daily living activities much like animals do—because it feels good to stretch. The next time you are not feeling good, try a few of the following stretches.

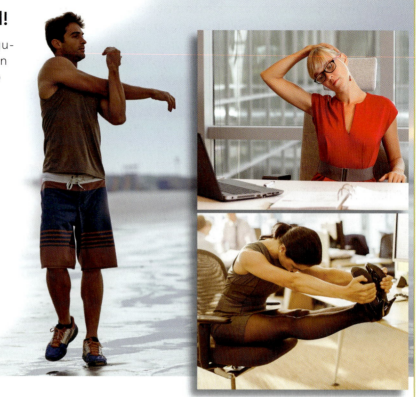

Stretch your arms while out on a walk, stretch your neck while sitting at your desk, or stretch your glutes and hamstrings at your desk or while standing.

Some people find that stretching in the morning starts the day off right, decreasing morning stiffness and increasing blood flow.

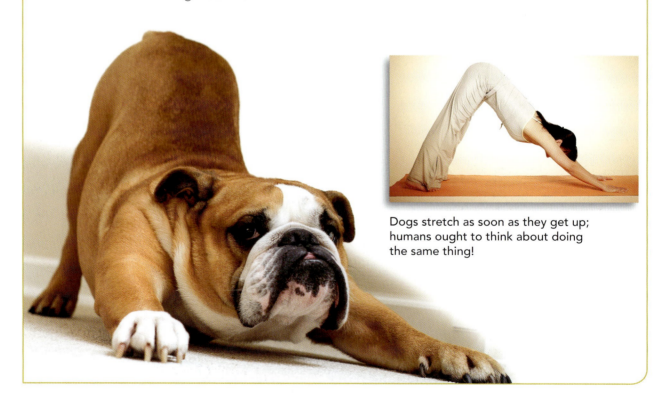

Dogs stretch as soon as they get up; humans ought to think about doing the same thing!

and the joint it crosses. If you have a great deal of flexibility in a specific muscle group, you may need to emphasize strength movements rather than stretching to avoid injury to joint structures and ligaments. On the other hand, if you are very strong but lack flexibility, then stretching is important. For example, gymnasts are often very flexible and can overstretch the spinal ligaments with their training, causing back pain and hyperflexible joint structures. Thus, to prevent joint pain, they should focus on core strengthening to counteract their flexibility. Most of us do not have issues with being overflexible; we are usually too tight in our muscles and joints from lack of movement and sitting. We also generally work in a forward-flexed position in front of a screen. In order to find that healthy balance between being flexible and strong, you will need to understand the evidence-based guidelines for flexibility.

Flexibility FITT: Frequency, Intensity, Time, and Type

As you might recognize by now, the FITT approach will also work for your flexibility plan. The best flexibility plan for you depends on your goals and interests. Choosing activities that you enjoy and that have minimum resource needs will help you stretch regularly. Figure 6.2 shows how you can fit the guidelines for flexibility training into your weekly schedule. If you cannot maintain your flexibility plan on a weekly basis, you might think about incorporating stretching into daily living. Much like the dog stretch or the suggested stretches at your desk featured in the sidebar Stretching Feels Good!, think about incorporating stretching movements that feel good throughout the day.

The special section on Functional Movement Training that appears after this chapter outlines ideas for stretching specific muscle groups. Think about incorporating stretching into your daily activities as well. When you sit on a bench or couch, turn and put one leg up on the bench to stretch your hamstrings, which get tight from so much sitting. When you get up from working at a computer, raise your hands above your head and take a moment to stretch the joints in your lower and upper back and shoulders. Sit back in your chair with arms extended to stretch your neck and upper-back muscles. Stretches like these fit well with daily living practices and allow you to meet the guidelines for stretching without going to a fitness facility.

To do this week

1. Wear backpack over both shoulders to strengthen lower back.
2. Establish weekend plans with friends.
3. Walk to class and don't forget umbrella and comfortable walking shoes.
4. **Follow the FITT principles for flexibility.**
   - **Frequency:** Stretch major muscle groups 2 to 3 times a week.
   - **Intensity:** Stretch to the point of slight tension and not pain, not bounce while stretching.
   - **Time:** Hold static stretches 10 to 30 seconds and do
   - **Type:** Perform 60 total seconds for each flexibility exercise remember to stretch between muscle strengthening exercises.
5. Watch one episode of my favorite Netflix series after dinner for a break.
6. Do homework for 2 hours.
7. Go to bed by 10:30 pm.

Figure 6.2 Make a weekly to-do list that includes the recommended parameters for flexibility training.

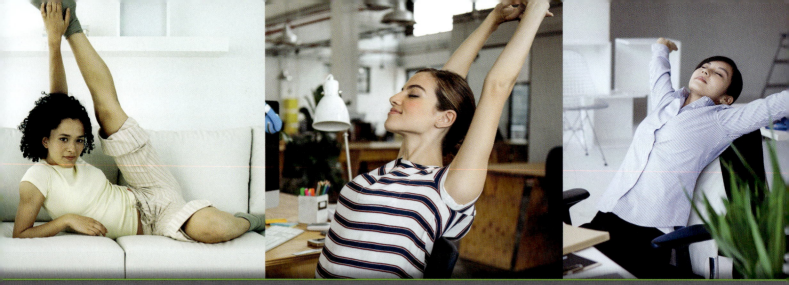

Try stretching your hamstrings on a park bench or couch, your latissimus dorsi when sitting or standing, or your upper back and chest muscles while sitting at your desk. Include stretching in your day to meet the FITT guidelines.

Frequency

Everyone, regardless of age or other demographics, can improve joint ROM. It is never too late to become more flexible. The other great news is that the ROM of a joint is improved immediately after performing targeted exercises, giving instant gratification. You can gain more permanent improvements in flexibility after doing a regular stretching program for three to four weeks if you perform flexibility exercises two or three times per week.

Intensity

Determining intensity for flexibility training is less complicated compared to what is needed to gain cardiorespiratory or muscular fitness. Stretch to the point of feeling tightness or slight discomfort but never pain. If you feel your muscle shaking, then reduce the range of motion slightly. Relaxing the muscle is important when thinking of intensity. Getting the mind and body to work together helps you see positive stretching outcomes.

Time

Although several types of flexibility exercises exist, the most common type for nonathletes is static stretching. The time recommendation is to hold each position for 10 to 30 seconds. Another time consideration is when to incorporate stretching into your day. Some research suggests that holding a stretch for more than 45 seconds can negatively affect muscular strength and power or sport performance. Thus, stretching before these types of activities is likely not great planning. Plus, given the fact that a stretching routine is more effective when the body is warm, it makes sense to stretch after cardiorespiratory or muscular fitness training. Passive warming can also be effective—consider stretching after a hot bath.

Type

Exercises that improve flexibility target the muscle–tendon units linked to major muscle groups. For more information, see chapter 5 and the Functional Movement Training section following this chapter. The Functional Movement Training section contains stretches for the calves, quads, hams and glutes, abdominals, lower back, hip abductors, hip adductors, chest and front of shoulder, upper back and shoulders, lats and middle back, front of upper arm, and back of upper arm. We suggest that you include these major muscle groups in your stretching practices. You may need to pay more attention to joints that are out of alignment due to work tasks, particularly muscles on the posterior (back) side of the body. Labs 6.1 and 6.2 in the web study guide will help you measure your flexibility so you have an understanding of which muscles you need to stretch regularly. The main types of stretching exercises include the following:

- *Static*. This is what most people think of when they picture stretching. **Static**

stretching involves slowly moving into a position and holding it for 10 to 30 seconds. Passive static stretching involves holding the limb or body part, with or without the assistance of a prop (e.g., bar, band, or partner). Active static stretching requires the muscle to be stretched to contract while the opposite muscle group is relaxed and stretched, which often occurs when performing yoga.

- *Slow dynamic*. This method involves a slow transition from one position to another with a progressive increase in the reach or ROM as the movement is repeated. Examples of **dynamic stretching** are lifting the knees high or stretching the inner and outer thigh muscles by slowly lunging side to side to dynamically increase the muscular range of motion.

- *Ballistic or bouncing*. Ballistic stretching is not recommended for the average person because the stretch reflex is often initiated (see the section Mind the Stretch Reflex!), which can lead to injury. With ballistic stretching, momentum produces the stretch and may cause the muscle to contract if it does not feel safe. If you continue to try to stretch the contracted muscle, it can cramp up or tear.

- *Proprioceptive neuromotor facilitation* (**PNF**). Although many different variations of the PNF method exist, it typically involves an isometric contraction (no joint movement and 3 to 6 seconds of a light to moderate intensity) of a selected muscle–tendon group followed by static stretching (10 to 30 seconds) of the same group. This is often termed contract–relax stretching.

All of the preceding methods can improve ROM. The best choice depends on your personal goals. For example, if your physical activities require you to perform ballistic movements (e.g., movements in basketball or dance), ballistic stretching might be a good choice but only after you have warmed up your muscles! If you find the complexities of PNF overwhelming, that technique is not a good choice for you. Generally speaking, static stretching is the safest and easiest to perform, particularly when warmed up. When stretching, choose any type you will do and enjoy on a regular basis.

Slow dynamic stretch option for the glutes and hamstrings.

Benefits of Being Flexible

Enhance, improve, or increase the following:
- Performance of daily activities
- Relaxation
- Mind–body connection
- Posture

Decrease or reduce the following:
- Muscle tension that can lead to pain and headaches
- Risk of low back and hip pain
- Risk of muscle or joint injury

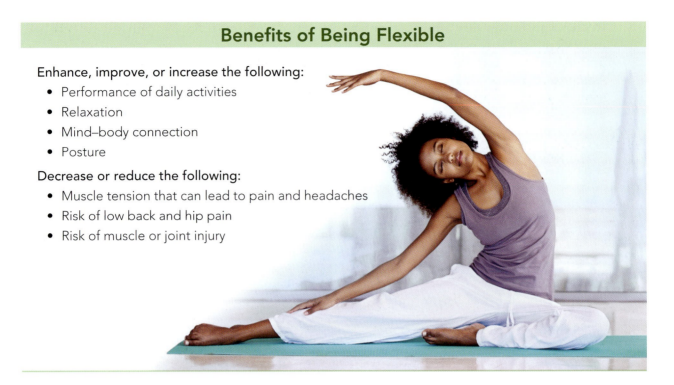

VPP: Volume, Pattern, and Progression

As with other components of fitness, volume, pattern, and progression (VPP) are probably important in flexibility training, but little research has been done in these areas. Although the optimal progression is not known, a good target is to perform two to four repetitions of each exercise, which results in about 60 seconds of total stretching time for each flexibility exercise. As with other fitness components, if you don't use it, you will lose it! Similar to cardiorespiratory and muscular fitness, it is much easier to maintain your flexibility than gain it.

Mind the Stretch Reflex!

The body has amazing protective capabilities, and the muscle system is no exception. A basic understanding of the myotatic stretch reflex, commonly called the **stretch reflex**, will help you design a safe and effective flexibility program.

Physiology

You may have heard the rule that the brain is in charge of how and if we move; reflexes are the exception. The stretch reflex is the most important reflex related to muscle movement. You might be familiar with reflexes from when your doctor performed the knee-jerk test by tapping your patellar tendon with a small hammer. This stretched your tendon and the quadriceps muscle and immediately resulted in a spontaneous muscle contraction, causing your foot to move. Essentially, a stretch reflex is your body's preprogrammed protection mechanism that autoregulates muscle length to prevent muscle tearing. This system is called a reflex because it does not involve the brain but rather operates directly through spinal cord control. This means that this process is rather quick and cannot be mentally overridden.

In brief, here's the physiology of the stretch reflex. Whenever your muscle experiences a sudden or excessive stretch, special receptors called muscle spindles or the Golgi tendon organ detect the action and immediately send an impulse for two simultaneous muscle actions:

- *Golgi tendon organ*. Contraction of the muscle, protecting it from being pulled too hard or beyond a normal range. Synergistic muscles are innervated so that they strengthen the contraction and help prevent injury.
- *Muscle spindles*. Relaxation of the antagonist muscles (the opposite muscle groups).

Without this inhibitory action, as soon as the stretched muscle began to contract, the antagonist muscle would be stretched, causing a stretch reflex. Both muscles would contract together if it were not for the stretch reflex process.

What Does the Stretch Reflex Mean for You?

The take-home point for the stretch reflex is that it needs to be respected in order to both prevent injury and maximize your flexibility exercises. For the full benefit when stretching muscles to enhance flexibility, focus on static stretching and stretching to the point of tension, not pain. If you overstretch or bounce and stretch, then the muscle shortens to protect itself. If you keep pulling on a shortened muscle, it might cramp up or, under extreme conditions, tear. When stretching, remember to relax and be patient. Use gentle, smooth, and pain-free movements to maximize benefits! See figure 6.3 for an illustration of the stretch reflex process.

> To experience a neuromotor exercise, try standing on one leg, and then close your eyes.

Neuromotor Exercise and Functional Fitness

Defining neuromotor fitness, sometimes called **functional fitness**, is more challenging than defining the other fitness components of cardiorespiratory fitness, muscular fitness, and flexibility. Did you know that the ACSM initially referred to neuromotor exercise as neuromuscular training (Bushman, 2012)? According to the American College of Sports Medicine (2018), neuromotor exercise involves motor skills, including balance, coordination, gait, and agility, and proprioceptive training. Yoga and tai chi are examples of physical activities that incorporate neuromotor exercise while also combining strength and flexibility. You use neuromotor exercise when you're carrying your laundry up or down a flight of stairs or when you jump over a puddle and land on one foot while carrying a backpack filled with books.

The benefits of functional fitness are well established for older adults because it enhances performance of daily tasks and prevents falling. Many sports training regimens involve various forms of balance and agility training. However, the science regarding the importance of neuromotor exercise for younger people is not well established. In labs 6.3 and 6.4 in the web study guide, you will test your balance, which is one aspect of neuromotor fitness.

The best way to enhance neuromotor fitness is not well known. Several body systems are involved in balance and other neuromotor activities. These systems include the sensory system (e.g., visual, auditory), the motor system, cognitive system, the somatosensory system (e.g., senses, touch, movement, body position, pain), and the vestibular system (located in the inner ear). Ideally, all of

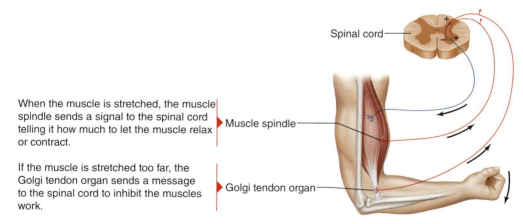

When the muscle is stretched, the muscle spindle sends a signal to the spinal cord telling it how much to let the muscle relax or contract.

If the muscle is stretched too far, the Golgi tendon organ sends a message to the spinal cord to inhibit the muscles work.

Figure 6.3   The myotatic stretch reflex. Special receptors (Golgi tendon organ and muscle spindles) are active during a strong contraction or stretch. They inhibit or facilitate muscle contraction in order to protect the muscle. These receptors are connected to the spinal cord, not the brain.

these systems work together to promote optimal balance in movement situations. We have a lot to learn about how integrated movements make us well. Expect more scientific information to emerge about this form of training.

Neuromotor Exercise FITT: Frequency, Intensity, Time, and Type

The American College of Sports Medicine (2018) recommends participating in functional fitness on two or three days for 20 to 30 minutes per day. The optimal intensity, volume, pattern, and progression for neuromotor exercise are not established. However, these guidelines serve as a gentle reminder that in order to improve your daily living status, enhance your health, and assist your functional fitness for life, your movement training should include movements you perform throughout the day or within your sport routine. If a recreation, leisure, or sport activity you enjoy requires better motor fitness, then your training program should prepare you to perform these motor movements well so you can avoid injury.

Physiological Teamwork for Flexibility and Neuromotor Fitness

Your muscles, tendons, ligaments, and sensory and nervous systems all work together to determine your flexibility and neuromotor fitness and—more importantly for your life—your *daily physical function*. We do many movements on one leg or off balance while playing sports. Think of a tennis player running after a

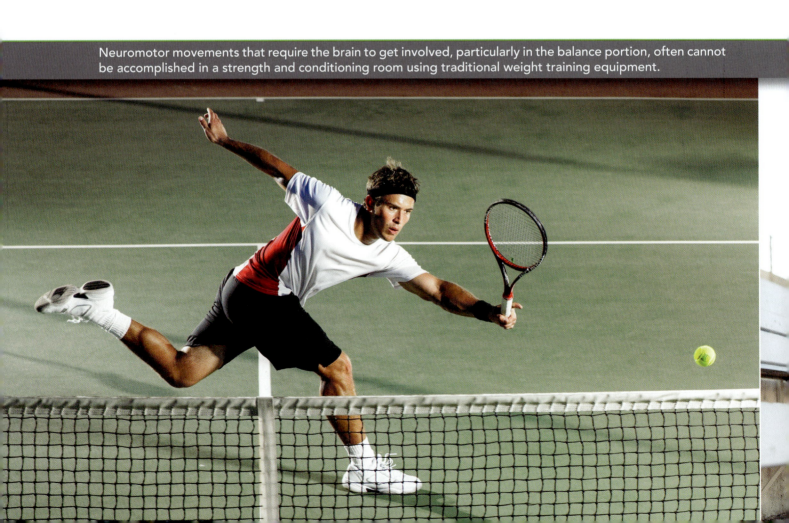

Neuromotor movements that require the brain to get involved, particularly in the balance portion, often cannot be accomplished in a strength and conditioning room using traditional weight training equipment.

ball and hitting it while off balance and on one leg. On a smaller level, we also have times in our daily lives where we are moving in a complex manner. During these moments, we need neuromotor control. This type of movement requires strength, flexibility, and a lot of communication from the brain related to balance and proprioception. It's hard to tell which muscle group to work in a strength and conditioning room to improve this kind of functional fitness. As with so many other things in life, practice the movement to move better daily.

Neuromotor Training Requires Destabilization

The guidelines for how to train neuromotor movements to gain neuromotor fitness are not easy to quantify. From a combined strength, flexibility, and neuromotor perspective, how might a person practice to become a better tennis player? Part of the answer is to play more tennis in order to practice more off-balance movements. Another option might be to practice bending over on one leg, lifting various weights in many directions. When we were little, we could easily pick up items on the ground, partially because we were lower to the ground, our knees were more flexible, and we did not weigh as much. As we get older, it becomes harder to bend over and pick things up, especially when standing on one leg. Functional fitness and fall prevention programs for older adults target many of these factors (base of support, eyesight, center of gravity, flooring surface) to safely challenge our movement systems to handle activities of daily living. Incorporating movements that will enhance neuromotor fitness into your daily life will require you to think about how to be destabilized. The next time you load the dishwasher or transfer clothes from the washing machine to the dryer, try to bend at the waist and do it on one leg!

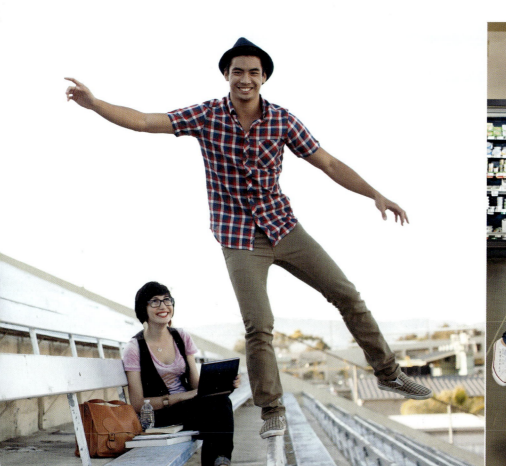

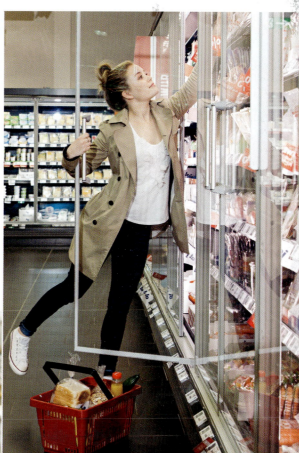

Creativity + Time = Fitness for Health

What tasks do you do that require your brain and body to work together in a complex manner? Think about it for a while and consider incorporating these movements (not just exercises) into your personal fitness plan. Your personal plan to develop flexibility and neuromotor fitness will be easier to formulate than the ones for cardiorespiratory and muscular fitness because you typically need fewer resources to regularly perform destabilization movements—just a little space and creativity. Even though there are many exercise toys on the market, you can do an awesome flexibility and neuromotor fitness program without equipment while working on your computer at a standing desk.

Preventing Low Back Pain

A conversation regarding flexibility and neuromotor fitness would not be complete without a discussion about low back pain. Low back pain, or relatedly neck or hip pain, is one of the most common health problems that bring a person to the doctor's office. It also creates a huge personal, social, and financial strain (Anderson 1998; Deyo et al. 1991; Katz 2006; Rapoport et al. 2004). The CDC (2001) defines **low back pain** as discomfort that limits activities and lasts for at least one day. Many people have a compromised quality of life because of low back pain. It is the second most common cause of disability for U.S. adults. An estimated 149 million days of work per year are lost due to back pain (Clarke et al. 2016). According to the National Institutes of Neurological Disorders and Strokes (2014), 80 percent of people will suffer from low back pain in their lifetime due to how they live and work (see figure 6.4). Low back pain is not just a problem for older adults. It is also one of

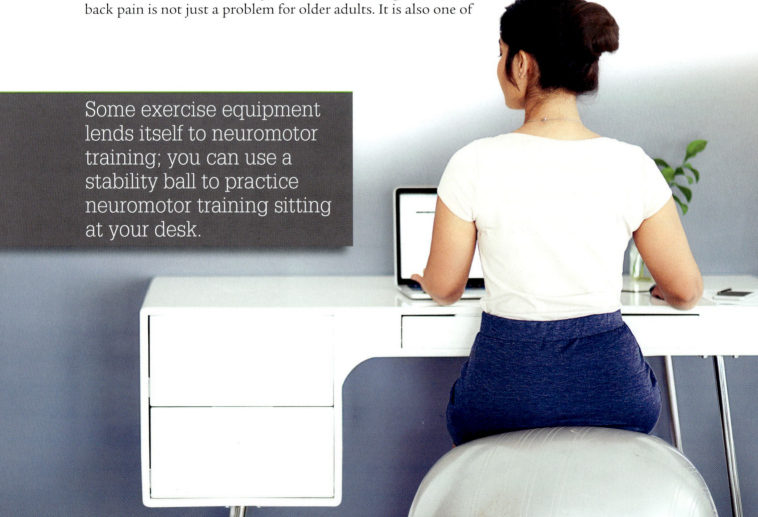

Some exercise equipment lends itself to neuromotor training; you can use a stability ball to practice neuromotor training sitting at your desk.

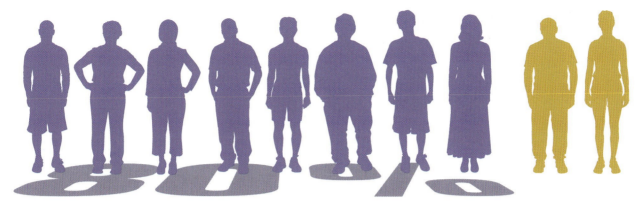

Figure 6.4 Eighty percent of adults will experience back pain at some point in their lifetimes.

the main causes of disability in people under 45 years old (Rubin 2007). Assessing flexibility and neuromotor fitness may give you an idea of your risk for low back pain and help you formulate a plan for preventing low back pain and other musculoskeletal aches and pains.

Causes of Low Back Pain

Low back pain can range from mild to extreme. It can arrive quickly or be a constant companion. Chronic back pain can be caused by diseases of the disc, various types of arthritis, sport injuries (e.g., a bad tackle in football), or an accident (e.g., car or bike accident). The majority of cases of low back pain, especially in young adults, are due to how we live our lives. Common factors due to lifestyle choices that are linked to back pain are being overweight, lifting heavy objects (without

being conditioned to do so), smoking, wearing poor footwear (especially high heels that alter the posture!), and being sedentary (Ricci et al. 2006). Mental states and emotions, including stress, anxiety, and depression, can also influence low back pain. If you suffer from chronic low back pain, visit your personal physician to rule out any major health issues before making any changes in lifestyle.

Stand Up Straight

How many times did a parent or grandparent tell you to stand up straight? Having good sitting and standing **posture** is critical for preventing back, shoulder, and neck pain. Good posture is also an important social signal that indicates engagement, energy, self-confidence, and self-respect. One key reason that it is so challenging

 Behavior Check

Essentials of a Functional Movement

As you decide which functional movements to practice on a regular basis, use this list to make sure you have incorporated all of their elements. Functional movements have the following characteristics:

- Incorporate multiple joints
- Use multiple muscles
- Are multiplanar (performed moving forward, sideways, or with rotation)
- Are done in a functional position (needed for activities of daily living)
- Incorporate balance
- Require core stability

> Good posture = more job opportunities. Many employers use posture as a way to evaluate confidence and maturity in an applicant.

to keep good posture as we go about our days is that we were not designed to be sitting in chairs. Many of us have muscle imbalances due to regular movement patterns that reinforce bad posture. How can you work on your posture in order to prevent back pain issues? A well-designed stretching and strengthening program can greatly enhance posture by improving muscular endurance of postural muscles, poor body mechanics, and muscle imbalances experienced from too much sitting. See the muscle group sections on lats and middle back, lower back, and abdominal muscles in the Functional Movement Training

section for specific information on stretching and strengthening exercises for postural muscles.

Good Muscle Balance + Daily Functional Movement = Back Pain Prevention

Although we all have different daily tasks, college students generally wear heavy backpacks to and from classes. If you wear your backpack over both shoulders as you walk to class, you are essentially strengthening your core muscles; this activity can be as useful as doing planks for your spinal joints and torso muscles. As your muscles become fit, you will have less fatigue from a given physical challenge, even if the challenge is transporting your backpack all around campus or carrying groceries into your apartment. It's important to connect the work you do to prevent back pain

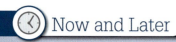 Now and Later

Have a Sense of Purpose

Now

Think about your exercise or movement routine now: Do you think it will benefit you later in your life? Which movements that you perform regularly and enjoy will make a difference in your body over the long term?

Later

A study published in the British Medical Journal (Cooper, Hardy, and Patel 2014) gives a wonderful overview of how important physical activity is for a life well lived. The study explains how 53-year-old subjects who performed well on grip strength, chair rise speed, and standing balance tests had lower disability and mortality rates than those who performed poorly. The study found that even light physical activity was beneficial: The more time people spent in light physical activity, the less subsequent disability they experienced. What do you strive to be like when you are 53 years old in terms of your functional fitness? What have the lives of your grandparents and parents been like after age 50? Consider this as you determine how to spend your time.

Take Home

As you prepare your movement plan for life, expand your goals beyond aesthetics. Keep in mind that a long-term health plan incorporates more than physical activity. The book *The Longevity Project* (Friedman and Martin 2012) suggests the following five items as ways to live longer. Number three is clearly focused on physical activity, and numbers two, four, and five could also be related to physical activity. These suggestions might enhance your chances of continuing a daily movement plan if you connect them to another important life task, such as socializing, doing functional movement that helps others, or embarking on a new physical challenge.

1. Reduce TV and screen time.
2. Improve social relations—spend time with friends.
3. Increase levels of physical activity—go for a long walk.
4. Help others and express gratitude to those who have helped you.
5. Take on new challenges to remain fresh and in the moment.

through strengthening and stretching movements with daily tasks so you can appreciate how your efforts help you function in your life. The ability to complete essential daily tasks will take on new meaning as you age. Muscular fitness, or lack thereof, is a key risk factor for physical disability.

Summary

Flexibility is a key component of health-related fitness. Neuromotor exercises integrate skill-related physical fitness components, including agility, coordination, balance, and reaction time. Flexibility is determined by age and health for a given joint. It is mainly affected by your muscles, which adapt very well to a stretching routine. Neuromotor fitness is how well your senses, brain and nervous system, and muscles work together to coordinate movement, especially under conditions that make you destabilized. These systems, and how well they collaborate, help you respond to life challenges. Good flexibility and neuromotor fitness are very important for many sport and recreational activities, but they can also enhance your daily campus life, especially while toting a large backpack and sitting and standing up tall and proud. Similar to how you'll improve and maintain cardiorespiratory fitness and muscular fitness, you'll want to design a regular flexibility and neuromotor training program that you can adapt throughout your life. Doing so will help you feel better, look better, reduce your risk for injury and pain (especially low back pain!), and increase your chance of living a long, independent life.

www WEB STUDY GUIDE

Remember to complete all of the web study guide activities to further facilitate your learning, including the following lab activities:

Lab 6.1   Lower-Body Flexibility: Sit-and-Reach Test

Lab 6.2   Upper-Body Flexibility: Shoulder Flexibility Test

Lab 6.3   Neuromotor Capacity: Sharpened Romberg Test

Lab 6.4   Neuromotor Capacity: Stork-Stand Balance Test

STUDY QUESTIONS

1. What are six primary factors that determine a person's flexibility?
2. Explain how training for flexibility and strength complement one another.
3. Using the FITT guidelines for training for flexibility, outline how flexibility might fit into your daily life.
4. List two or three benefits of being flexible.
5. Explain why the stretch reflex is an important concept to understand in order to enhance your flexibility training.
6. Define neuromotor training (functional training) and outline a few ways you might incorporate this type of training into your workout or movement plan.
7. List three or four elements of functional (neuromotor) training and give two examples of exercises or movements you might incorporate into your functional fitness training plan.
8. Define low back pain and explain two or three ways you can prevent low back pain using flexibility and neuromotor training.

Functional Movement Training

This special section on functional movement training contains over 90 exercises with photos. The web study guide also has narrated video of almost all of the exercises. Use the exercises in this section to design a program that fits your needs.

The exercises included here strengthen 12 major muscle groups. For each major muscle group, you'll find an anatomical illustration showing what part of the body is affected as well as the types of activities that involve those muscles.

Four types of exercises are included for each selected muscle group:

- Body weight
- Variable resistance machine
- Free weights
- Stretch

Neuromotor training options are included when possible to help you incorporate balance and stability.

Why Functional Movement Training?

This section suggests movement choices for strengthening and stretching major muscle groups to help you look and feel good. The movements in the exercises connect to activities you do every day. Functional movement training can start with muscle isolation movements that strengthen specific muscle groups in preparation for training multiple muscle groups. Both isolation and functional movements can prepare you for the various stages of life needs. A total-body functional workout will help you build and strengthen your body so you can be your best you, both inside and out.

This book emphasizes the importance of connecting your training choices with *why* you ought to train the musculoskeletal system in the first place. One reason could be that energetic people with good posture fare better when interviewing for jobs. Fitness and wellness also affect health care costs.

Because your "why" will change as you age, this section presents different options for movement using various types of equipment as well as body weight. If you want to get big biceps, you might use a variable resistance biceps machines for isolation training. If you want to focus on posture and lean abdominal muscles, planks and body weight curl-ups might work best. Alternatively, walking lunges with handheld weights allow you to work on balance and stability along with core training and save time. There are so many reasons and ways to improve the look and feel of your body. Make decisions that work best for you and your goals. Find what you like and what matters to you. The best exercise choices for strength and flexibility training are the ones you will perform regularly.

Always Warm Up Before Stretching and Strengthening

Remember to warm up thoroughly before performing strengthening and stretching movements. Break a sweat before you start working out. You might walk, jog, do your first set of strengthening exercises with a light weight, or mix cardio and strengthening movements.

Introducing Neuromotor Movements

Neuromotor movements generally incorporate balance and stability training into strength and conditioning movements. This section provides exercises for strengthening and stretching muscle groups that can be done throughout the life span. We hope you will find a sense of purpose in these movement options and the information you need to effectively perform the movements. Start training early for preventing falls so you can minimize your need for assisted care later in life. The habits you create in your 20s related to movement and exercise will follow you throughout your lifetime.

How Many Sets and Repetitions?

How do you select an appropriate load for strength training? **If you are a beginner, consider selecting a weight that allows you to perform one**

set of 12 to 15 repetitions comfortably. You will know that a weight is too much if you cannot complete 6 to 8 repetitions. If you can easily perform 12 to 15 repetitions, then you need to add more weight. How much weight should you use? Although there isn't an easy answer, think about the total volume you are lifting. For example, if you perform 10 repetitions of a biceps curl with two 10-pound (4.5 kg) weights, you have lifted 200 pounds (91 kg) total. For the same workload, you can increase the load and lift 20 pounds (9 kg) for 5 repetitions. Experiment with what works for you and which choices fit your goals. Muscles adapt best through progressive, incremental overload.

Remember that strength training is about breaking muscle down. Rest for 24 to 48 hours between workouts to allow the muscles to recover before you overload them again.

How Long Should I Hold Stretches?

Hold stretches for 20 to 30 seconds and perform each stretch two or three times. We recommend stretching in between strengthening movements or at the end of the workout. Remember not to bounce when you are stretching, since this can initiate the stretch reflex. Stretch to the point of tension, not pain, and hold stretches without allowing the muscle to shake. Focus on relaxing and elongating the muscle to improve flexibility.

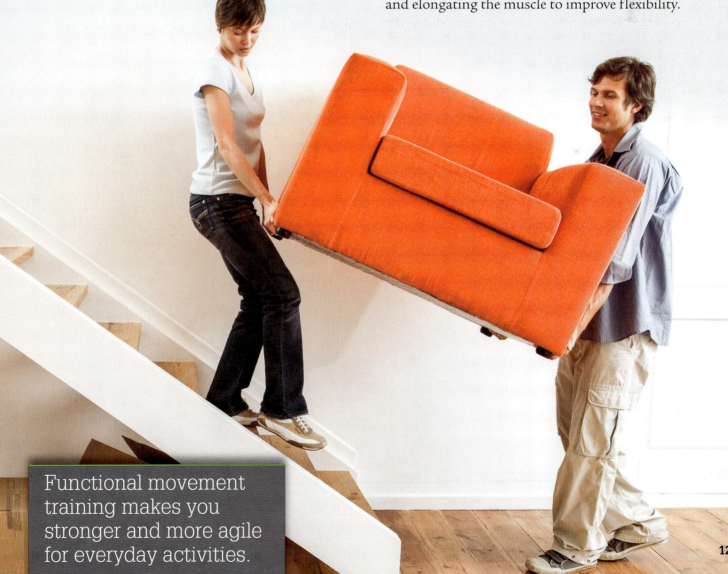

Functional movement training makes you stronger and more agile for everyday activities.

Calves

Gastrocnemius and Soleus

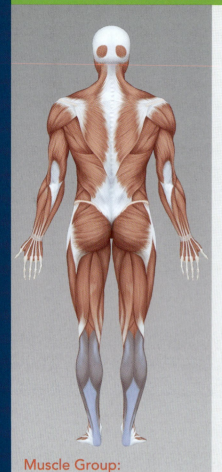

Daily activity use includes reaching up on toes, walking, running, and jumping

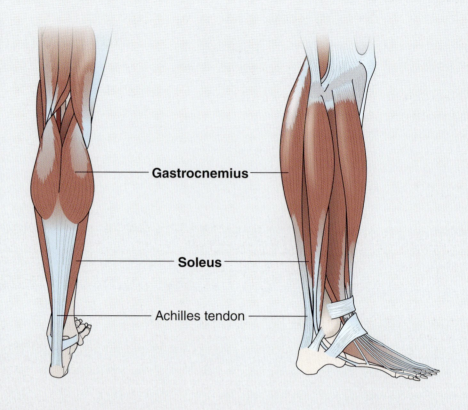

Gastrocnemius

Soleus

Achilles tendon

Muscle Group:
Gastrocnemius and soleus

Muscle Action:
Plantar flex ankles
30 to 50 degrees

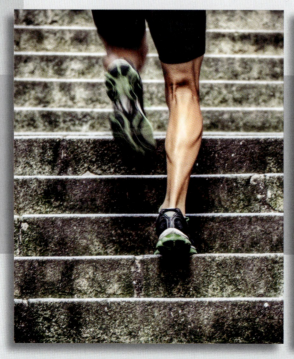

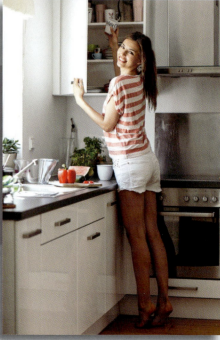

FUNCTIONAL MOVEMENT TRAINING

Calves Strengthening and Stretching

▶ Body Weight

Stand and lift both your heels 30 to 50 degrees off the ground. *More advanced:* Use a wall or a bar for support and lift one heel at a time or hold a dumbbell in each hand while lifting both heels off the ground.

Neuromotor training: Without using wall support, raise one heel at a time.

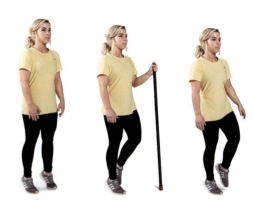

▶ Variable Resistance Machine

Use a heel raise machine or a leg press machine. A leg press machine is typically used to strengthen the quadriceps, the gluteus maximus, and the hamstrings. To engage your calves, lower your feet so that the balls of your feet are on the bottom edge of the platform. Then, raise your heels during the first phase of the exercise so that you are pressing with your toes. You can often use the same weight that you would for the leg press. However, you will want to increase your reps significantly.

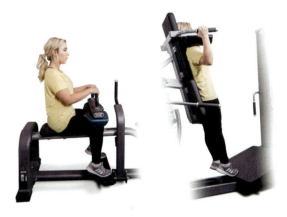

▶ Free Weights

Hold a dumbbell in each hand and raise your heels 30 to 50 degrees.

Neuromotor training: Hold a dumbbell in each hand, stand on one leg, and raise the heel of the support leg.

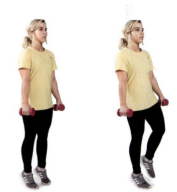

▶ Stretch

Step one foot forward and bend the front knee. Press your back heel toward the ground. This stretches the gastrocnemius of the back leg. Hold for 20 to 30 seconds. Then bend your back knee to stretch the soleus, keeping the front knee bent and the back heel down. Hold for 20 to 30 seconds. For both positions, the back toe is forward, heel is on the floor, and weight is shifted forward.

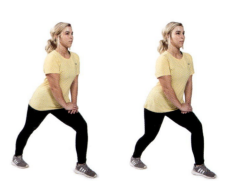

Quads

Quadriceps

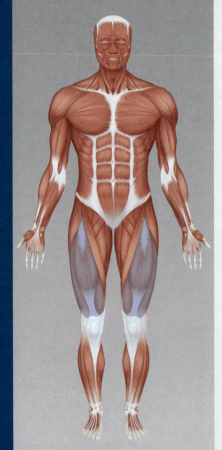

Daily activity use includes getting out of chairs, jumping, walking, and running

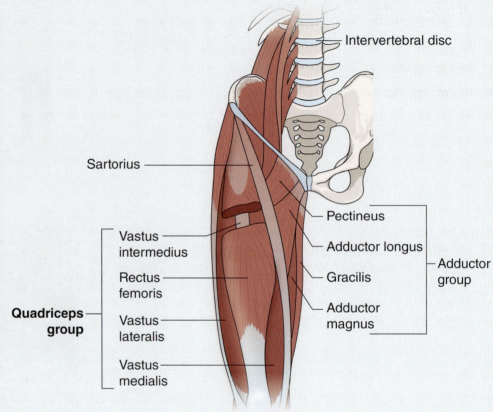

Intervertebral disc

Sartorius

Pectineus

Adductor longus

Gracilis

Adductor group

Adductor magnus

Quadriceps group

Vastus intermedius

Rectus femoris

Vastus lateralis

Vastus medialis

Muscle Group:
Quadriceps (rectus femoris, vastus intermedius, vastus lateralis, vastus medialis)

Muscle Action:
Hip flexion 90 to135 degrees and knee extension 5 to 10 degrees

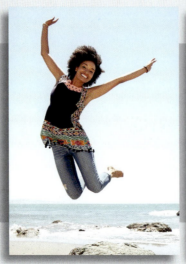

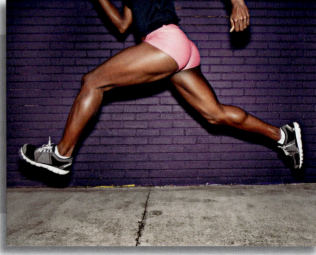

FUNCTIONAL MOVEMENT TRAINING

Quads Strengthening and Stretching

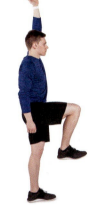
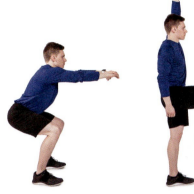

▶ Body Weight

Lower the hips as if to sit and lift the chest; extend your arms in front for balance; flex at the hips 45 degrees; keep your heels on the ground.

Neuromotor training: Raise one knee up, keeping the shoulders over the hips and balancing on one leg. Simultaneously, raise the arm on the same side of the standing leg straight up by your ear to maintain good posture and help with balance.

▶ Variable Resistance Machine

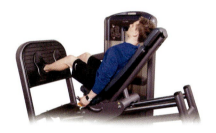
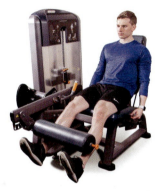

To strengthen your quadriceps, you can use a leg press or leg extension machine. Regardless of which machine you choose, be sure that you create a 90-degree angle with your legs to complete the exercises safely and effectively.

▶ Free Weights

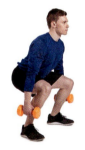
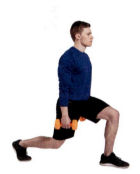

Squat with dumbbells in hands. Keep your head up and make sure your knees do not go over your toes.

Neuromotor training: Do alternating lunges, holding a dumbbell in each hand.

▶ Stretch

Lie on your side. Keeping the hips aligned, flex one knee and hold the top of one shoe or your toe; relax your head on your arm and relax the foot you are holding.

Neuromotor training: Perform the stretch while standing; do not hold on to a wall.

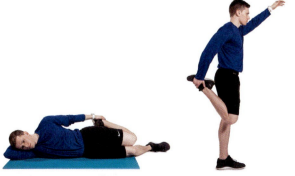

Hams and Glutes

Hamstrings and Gluteus Maximus

Daily activity use includes walking or running backward up a hill, stepping backward, and lowering items from a shelf

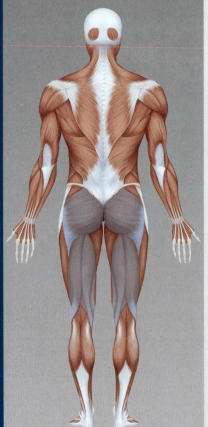

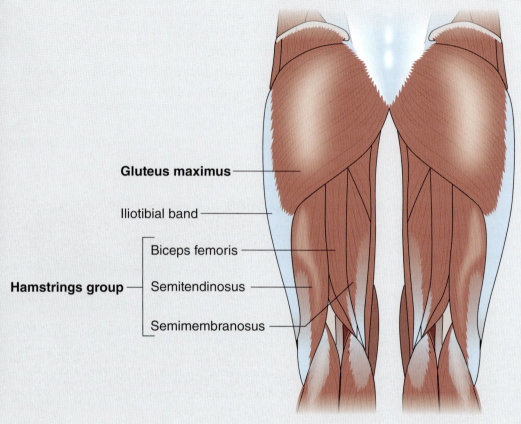

Gluteus maximus

Iliotibial band

Hamstrings group
- Biceps femoris
- Semitendinosus
- Semimembranosus

Muscle Group:
Hamstrings (biceps femoris, semitendinosus, semimembranosus) and gluteus maximus

Muscle Action:
Hip extension 10 to 30 degrees and knee flexion 130 to 140 degrees

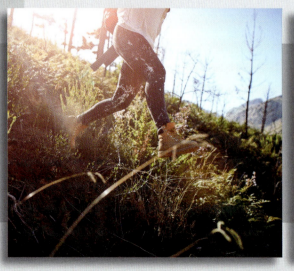

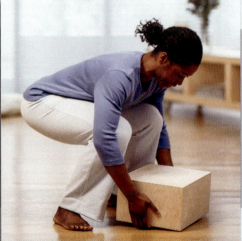

FUNCTIONAL MOVEMENT TRAINING

Hams and Glutes Strengthening and Stretching

▶ Body Weight

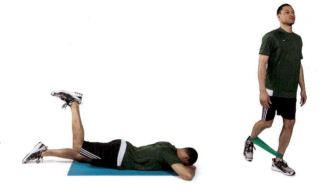

Lie on your belly and extend the hip 10 to 30 degrees, keeping the hip bone on the ground, and then flex the knee 90 degrees to maximize strengthening.

Neuromotor training: Stand on one leg, extend the hip, and flex the knee; add a band around the ankle for increased resistance.

▶ Variable Resistance Machine

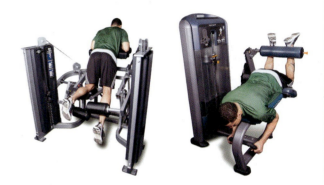

Options are standing hamstring curl and prone hamstring curl machines. Read placards carefully since there are many adjustments to make on both of these machines.

▶ Free Weights

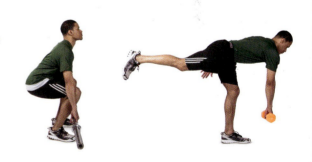

Perform a squat lifting a barbell while simultaneously extending at the hips and knees. Maintain a neutral spine throughout the entire movement and lift the bar using the hamstrings and glutes.

Neuromotor training: Hold a dumbbell or kettlebell in one hand and extend the opposite leg behind you; slightly bend the standing knee and raise the weight back up. Progress to using the arm on the same side as the extending leg.

▶ Stretch

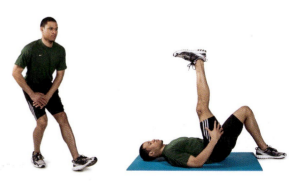

For the standing hamstring stretch, bend one knee and extend the other leg in front of you. Put all your weight on the bent knee, relaxing the straight leg. Tilt your hips backward to lengthen the hamstring muscle and keep the spine in line.

For the hamstring and gluteus maximus stretch, lie on your back and grasp the thigh of the raised leg with both hands. Keeping the knee of the opposite leg flexed, relax both the leg in your hands and your head on the ground.

Abdominals

Rectus and Transversus Abdominis and Obliques

Daily activity use includes maintaining posture, getting up out of bed, carrying items, and rotating the torso with weight in your hands (golfing)

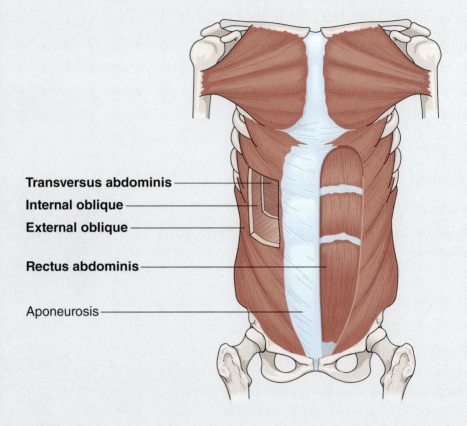

Transversus abdominis

Internal oblique

External oblique

Rectus abdominis

Aponeurosis

Muscle Group:
Rectus abdominis, transversus abdominis, internal oblique, and external oblique

Muscle Action:
Flex the spine 30 to 45 degrees, rotate the torso 20 to 45 degrees, and compress abdominal contents

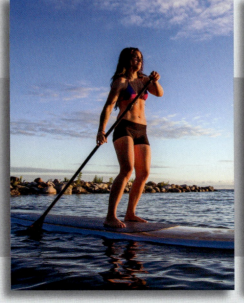

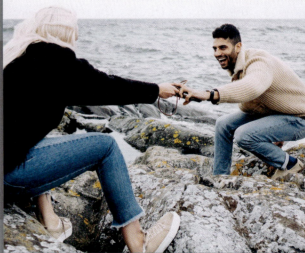

FUNCTIONAL MOVEMENT TRAINING

Abdominals Strengthening and Stretching

▶ Body Weight

Lie on your back with both hands behind the head and elbows out to the side (you should not be able to see your elbows), relax your head in your hands, and flex your spine 30 to 45 degrees.

Lie on your back; rotate your shoulder and point it toward the opposite knee, keeping the other shoulder on the floor. Continue by alternating the rotation to every other knee.

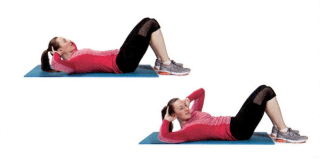

▶ Variable Resistance Machine

Use the abdominal flexion machine. Keep in mind that spine flexion is 30 to 45 degrees forward. Stay within appropriate range of motion.

Neuromotor training: Set the functional training machine for standing spinal rotation by placing elbows at your sides and biceps flexed; with knees slightly bent, rotate the spine side to side 20 to 45 degrees. Keep the abdominals tight and knees slightly bent as you rotate.

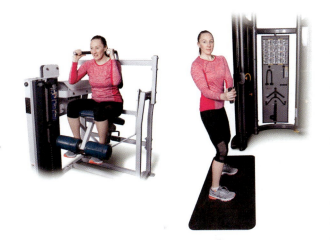

▶ Free Weights

Lie on your back on a stability ball with feet flat on the ground and knees bent at 90 degrees. Holding a weighted ball on your chest or over your head, flex the spine 30 to 45 degrees. Holding the ball overhead is more difficult because it creates a longer lever.

Neuromotor training: Sit on the ground and recline 35 to 45 degrees (flexing the spine), balancing with the heels on the ground, take a weighted ball and rotate side to side 20 to 45 degrees. Keep the abdominals tight as you rotate.

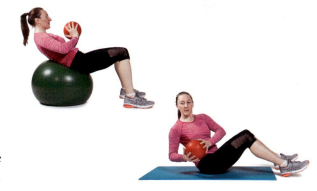

▶ Stretch

Lie on your back, point your toes, and slightly arch your back while extending your arms overhead to stretch your abdominals.

Lie on your belly and prop yourself up on your elbows; hold this position, keeping the spine in line and the hips on the ground at all times.

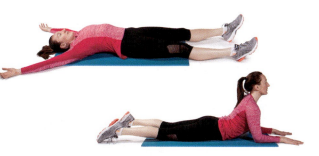

Lower Back

Erector Spinae

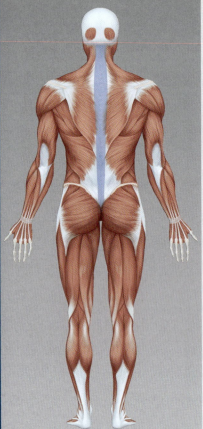

Daily activity use includes picking up a box from the floor and carrying a backpack over both shoulders throughout the day

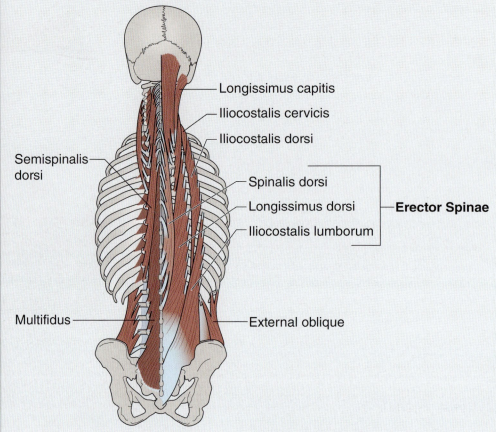

- Longissimus capitis
- Iliocostalis cervicis
- Iliocostalis dorsi
- Semispinalis dorsi
- Spinalis dorsi
- Longissimus dorsi } Erector Spinae
- Iliocostalis lumborum
- Multifidus
- External oblique

Muscle Group:
Erector spinae (iliocostalis lumborum, longissimus dorsi, and spinalis dorsi)

Muscle Action:
Extends the spine 20 to 45 degrees

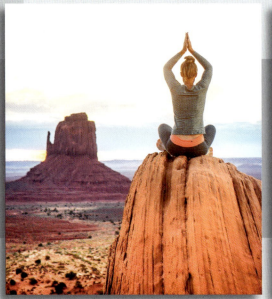

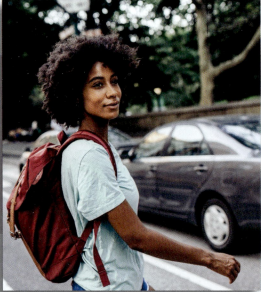

▶ **VIDEO AVAILABLE**

FUNCTIONAL MOVEMENT TRAINING

Lower Back Strengthening and Stretching

▶ ### Body Weight

Lie on your belly on the ground. With your arm fully extended (like Superman), simultaneously lift the right arm and the left leg and keep the hip bone on the ground. Repeat with the left arm and the right leg.

Neuromotor training: Lie on your belly on a stability ball with toes on the ground and extend the spine 20 to 45 degrees. For additional difficulty, raise the opposite hand and foot.

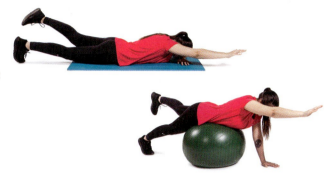

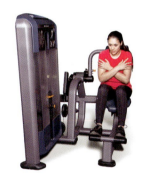

▶ ### Variable Resistance Machine

Use the lower back extension machine. Sit back into the seat before starting. Be careful to stay within the recommended range of motion for a back extension (20 to 45 degrees).

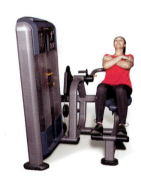

▶ ### Free Weights

Using a back-extension bench, flex the spine 20 to 45 degrees and then extend the lower back into an upright posture.

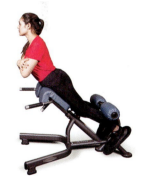

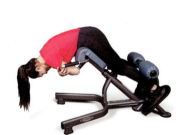

▶ ### Stretch

Lie on your back with knees bent and feet flat on the floor. Gently pull one knee toward your chest until you feel a stretch in your lower back. If you are comfortable, you can put your hands behind both knees, pull them to your chest, and hold.

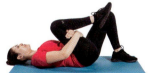

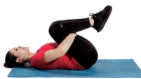

Hip Abductors

Gluteus Medius and Gluteus Minimus

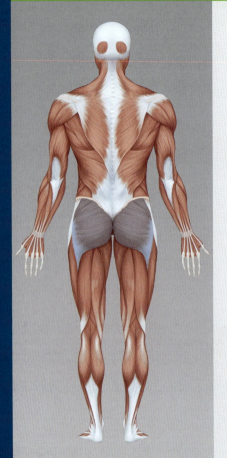

Daily activity use includes getting out of a car, keeping the hips in line when brisk walking, and stepping sideways

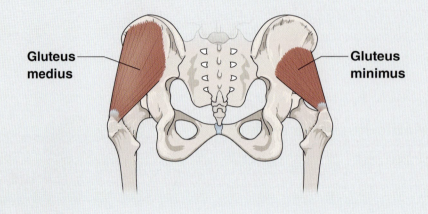

Gluteus medius

Gluteus minimus

Muscle Group:
Gluteus medius and gluteus minimus

Muscle Action:
Abducts the hip 30 to 50 degrees

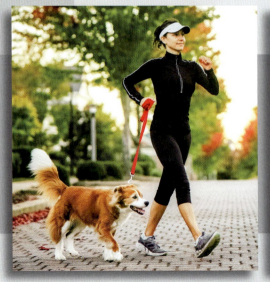

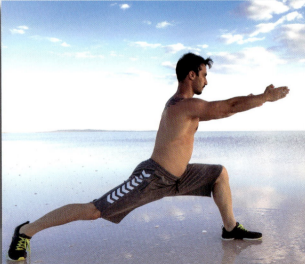

Hip Abductors

Gluteus Medius and Gluteus Minimus

FUNCTIONAL MOVEMENT TRAINING

Hip Abductors Strengthening and Stretching

Body Weight

Lie on your side with your head relaxed on your arm and your bottom leg bent, stacking the hips on top of each other to improve your base of support. Abduct (raise) your leg 30 to 50 degrees and then lower it, leading with the heel.

Neuromotor training: Perform the same 30- to 50-degree hip abduction movement in a standing position.

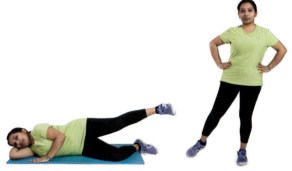

Variable Resistance Machine

Sit in a variable resistance hip abduction machine. Perform a bilateral hip abduction movement to 30- to 50 degrees.

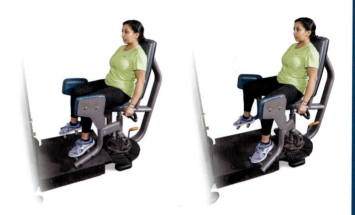

Free Weights

Place a resistance band around both legs above the knee. Side step in each direction 30 to 50 degrees.

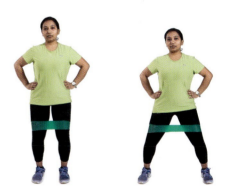

Stretch

For this stretch, sit on a mat, and place your right foot to the outside of your left knee. Place your left hand outside of your right knee and turn your head to look back. At the same time, rotate your right thigh inward. To modify this exercise if you have less flexibility, hold your leg with your hand rather than placing your arm on the opposite side of your leg. Repeat on the other side.

For a variation, stand up tall and place one foot behind the front leg. Lean the outside hip slightly outward to feel a stretch in the hip abductor. Repeat the movement on the other side.

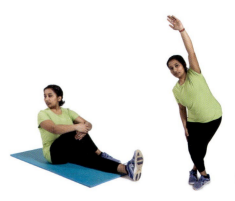

133

Hip Adductors

Adductor Longus, Brevis, and Magnus and Gracilis

Daily activity use includes stabilizing the body laterally on a bike and picking up heavy objects from the ground

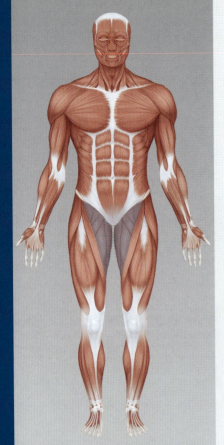

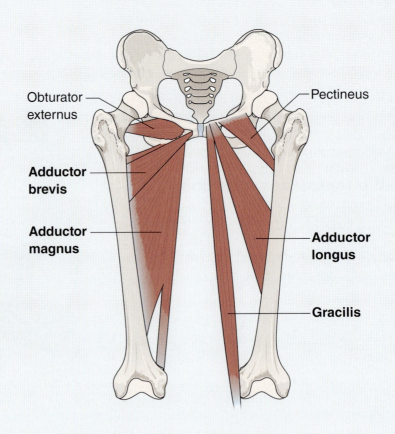

Obturator externus

Pectineus

Adductor brevis

Adductor magnus

Adductor longus

Gracilis

Muscle Group:
Adductor longus, adductor brevis, adductor magnus, and gracilis

Muscle Action:
Adducts the hip 10 to 30 degrees

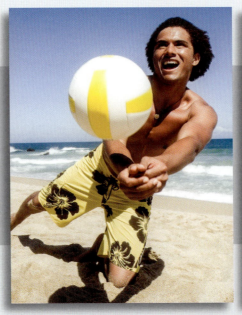

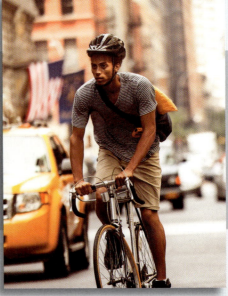

Hip Adductors

Adductor Longus, Brevis, and Magnus and Gracilis

FUNCTIONAL MOVEMENT TRAINING

Hip Adductors Strengthening and Stretching

▶ Body Weight

Lie on your side with your head relaxed on your arm. Line the hips up, bend the knee of the top leg, and place the foot on the ground to create a good base of support. Next, lift the bottom leg, adducting it 10 to 30 degrees.

Neuromotor training: Place a resistance band around one ankle and anchor the band to a chair. Stand with your shoulders over your hips, adduct one leg by crossing it in front of your body, adducting the hip 10 to 30 degrees. Alternate sides. Keep your spine in line and the range of motion to 30 degrees maximum. Lead with the heel and keep the toe forward.

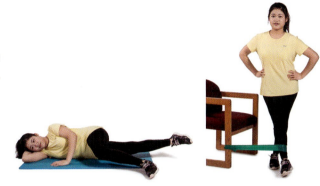

▶ Variable Resistance Machine

Use the hip adductor machine to perform hip adduction in a seated position.

Neuromotor training: Use a cable with a strap around the ankle. Leading with the heel, move the hip 10 to 30 degrees past the midline. You may choose to rest your hand on the machine for stability.

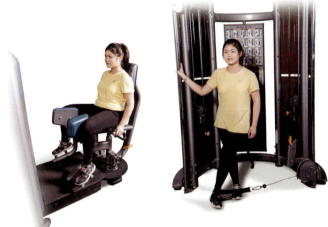

▶ Free Weights

Hold a dumbbell "goblet style" and perform a squat with the toes turned out slightly to engage the adductors. Allow the weight to stabilize in the center of the body.

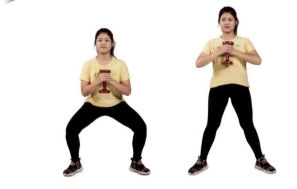

▶ Stretch

Put the soles of your feet together and let your knees relax to the sides, relax the elbows on your thighs, and keep your head up for proper posture. If your knees pop up, press them down slightly with your elbows.

For another option, move your legs to the straddle position and put your hands behind the buttocks; keep your head up. Lean your torso slightly forward and hold the position without bouncing.

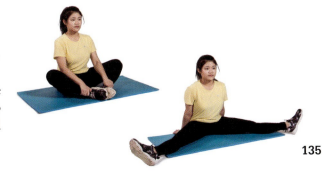

Chest and Front of Shoulder

Pectorals and Anterior Deltoids

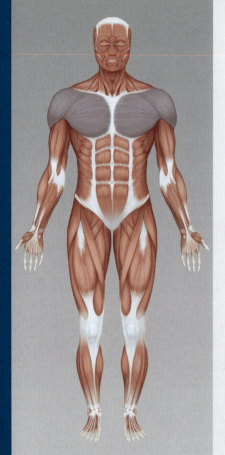

Daily activity use includes putting something heavy on a high shelf, carrying and lifting items in front of you, and lifting yourself up off the floor

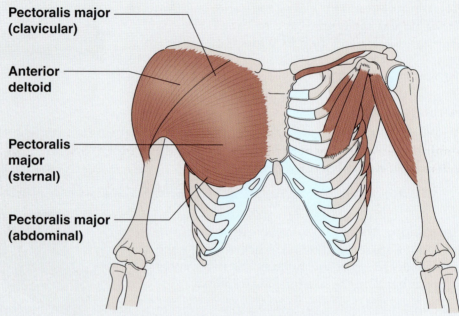

Pectoralis major (clavicular)

Anterior deltoid

Pectoralis major (sternal)

Pectoralis major (abdominal)

Muscle Group:
Pectoralis major and anterior deltoids

Muscle Action:
Anterior deltoid flexes the shoulder joint while pectorals horizontally adduct shoulders 90 to 135 degrees

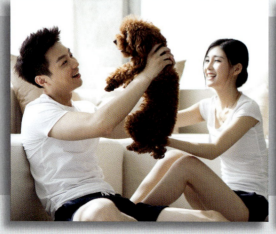

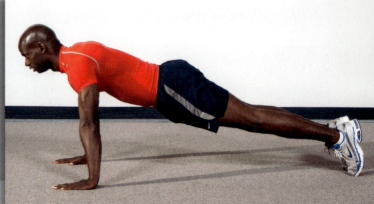

Chest and Front of Shoulder

FUNCTIONAL MOVEMENT TRAINING

Chest and Front of Shoulder Strengthening and Stretching

▶ Body Weight

Stand in front of a wall and step back a few feet. Lift your elbows so they are level with your shoulders. Maintain that distance between the hands as you position them on the wall in front of you. Slowly bend your elbows and perform a push-up.

Neuromotor training: Extend one leg behind you and balance while performing the same movement.

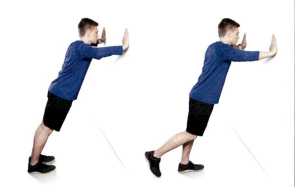

▶ Variable Resistance Machine

To perform a chest fly movement, adduct both arms simultaneously, keeping both feet on the ground and the chin and chest up.

For the seated bench press machine, simultaneously press both arms forward, keeping the feet on the floor.

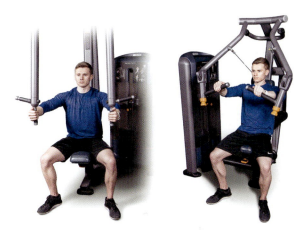

▶ Free Weights

Sit on a weight bench and, holding a dumbbell in each hand, keep the dumbbells close to your body as you lie back on your lower back. Simultaneously press the dumbbells straight up and return slowly. Make sure you do not let your elbows drop more than 10 to 15 degrees past a basic push-up position.

Neuromotor training: Hold a dumbbell in each hand and let your arms hang at your sides with the thumbs up. Flex one shoulder in front of you to 90 degrees while at the same time extending the opposite hip 10 to 30 degrees.

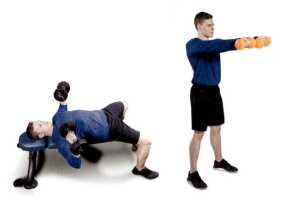

▶ Stretch

Stand and stretch both arms behind you. Clasp your fingers to stretch the pectoral and anterior deltoid muscles.

Standing in front of a doorway with knees relaxed, put one arm out to the side to hold onto the doorframe and lean slightly forward.

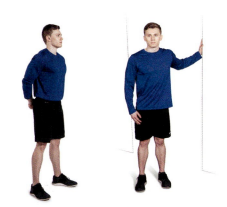

Upper Back and Shoulders

Rhomboids and Posterior Deltoids

Daily activity use includes rowing activities such as sweeping or vacuuming the floor, sitting up tall at a desk, or tucking your shirt in your pants

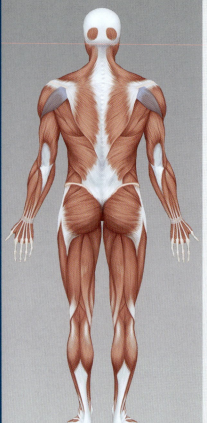

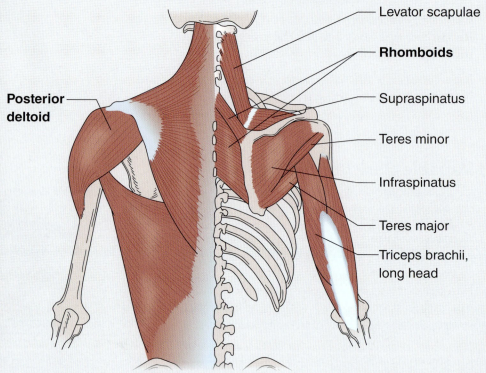

Levator scapulae

Rhomboids

Supraspinatus

Teres minor

Infraspinatus

Teres major

Triceps brachii, long head

Posterior deltoid

Muscle Group:
Rhomboids (rhomboid major, rhomboid minor) and posterior deltoids

Muscle Action:
Scapular retraction 15 to 20 degrees

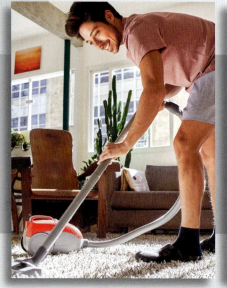

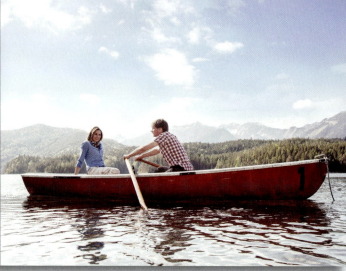

FUNCTIONAL MOVEMENT TRAINING

Upper Back and Shoulders Strengthening and Stretching

▶ Body Weight

Lie on your belly on a mat or a pillow, relax your feet, and stretch both arms in a *T* position. Relax the lower body and lift the arms and torso off the ground, keeping the head facing down, hips on the ground, and the feet relaxed.

Neuromotor training: Perform this same movement on a stability ball.

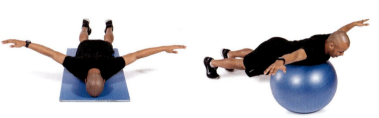

▶ Variable Resistance Machine

For the reverse fly variable resistance machine, lock your lower body in and put your feet flat on the floor. Reach up and grab the handles, then retract your scapulae at the same time, squeezing the shoulder blades together.

For the seated cable high row, be sure not to lean back on the second part of the movement but rather start and end with good posture, letting the bar touch your chest as you squeeze the shoulder blades together. Be sure to come back to an upright posture.

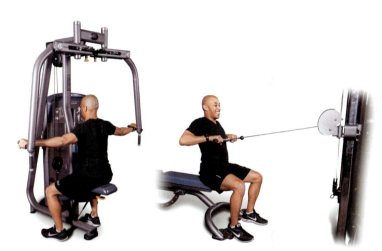

▶ Free Weights

Perform this exercise holding dumbbells in each hand. Keeping the spine in neutral, hinge at the hips, bending forward 45 degrees, bring arms out into a *T* position and squeeze the shoulder blades together.

Neuromotor training: Perform the same movement, but slightly lift one leg off the floor.

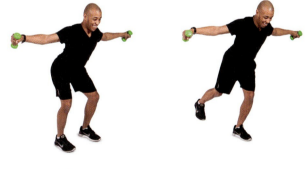

▶ Stretch

Stand and clasp both hands straight out in front of you. Round the middle back while slightly dropping the chin.

For the cat stretch on the floor, round the middle back. Inhale on the effort and exhale on the relaxation portion.

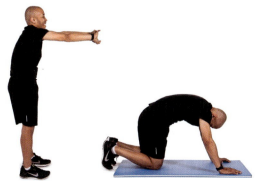

139

Lats and Middle Back

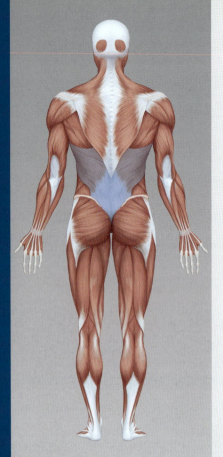

Daily activity use includes lifting up an object from the ground with one hand, performing a pull-up, and swimming

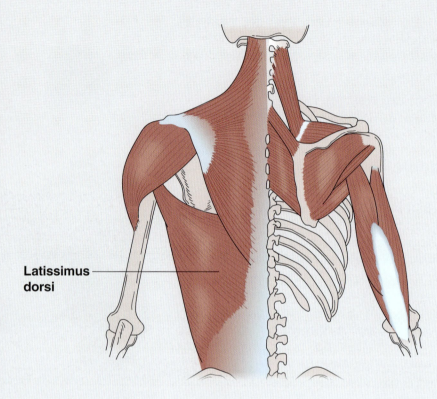

Latissimus dorsi

Muscle Group:
Latissimus dorsi

Muscle Action:
Shoulder adduction 80 to 100 degrees and shoulder extension 20 to 60 degrees

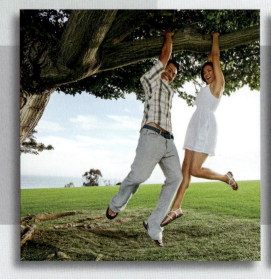

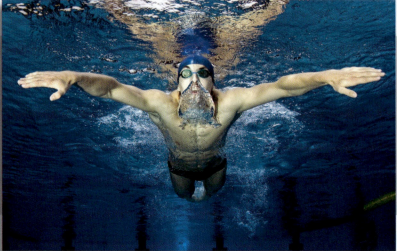

FUNCTIONAL MOVEMENT TRAINING

Lats and Middle Back Strengthening and Stretching

▶ Body Weight

Stand, holding a band in each hand overhead with approximately 6 to 8 inches of band between your hands. Anchor one arm overhead and adduct the other arm, bringing the elbow down to your side. Then alternate, bending one arm and then the other, bringing your elbow down to your side each time.

Neuromotor training: Perform this upper back exercise using TRX straps anchored to a rack or pull-up bar. Begin leaning back with your arms extended. Pull up toward the anchor using your upper back muscles. Slowly return to the starting position, keeping the back muscles activated.

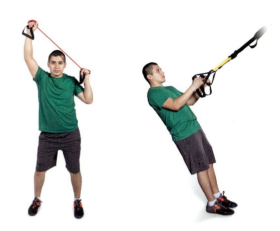

▶ Variable Resistance Machine

You can use a seated row machine or a lat pulldown machine. Using a seated row machine, perform a seated low row movement using a v-bar. Bend the knees slightly and row the arms, squeezing the middle back and lats while sitting upright. Using a lat pulldown variable resistance machine with either a bar or handles, lock the lower body in and simultaneously adduct the arms to the sides. Try not to let the handles drop below chin level.

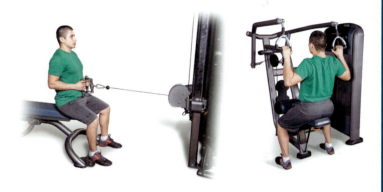

▶ Free Weights

Holding a dumbbell in each hand, lie on your back on a stability ball. Extend arms overhead to 180 degrees (arms by ears), then bilaterally flex arms with weights as if you are closing a hatchback on a car; stop the movement when the weights are at eye level.

Neuromotor training: Put a resistance band under one foot and hold the band with one arm. Pull the band up as if you are starting a lawnmower.

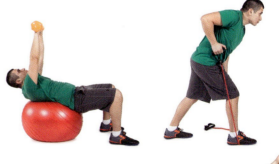

▶ Stretch

Kneel on the ground and extend both arms out in front of you, relaxing your hands on the floor. Look down and relax.

   In a standing position, reach one arm over to the side and let one hip turn slightly inward.

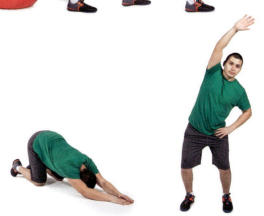

Front of Upper Arm

Biceps

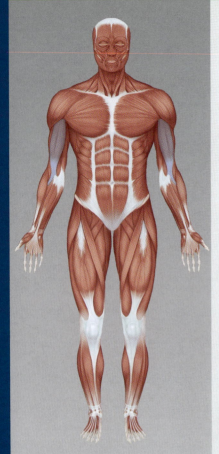

Daily activity use includes carrying groceries, picking up objects in front of you, and picking up objects from the floor and placing them on a table

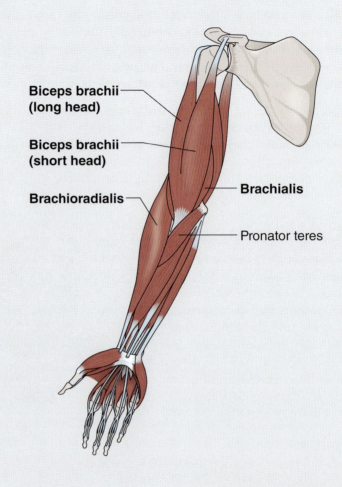

Biceps brachii (long head)

Biceps brachii (short head)

Brachioradialis

Brachialis

Pronator teres

Muscle Group:
Biceps (biceps brachii, brachialis, brachioradialis)

Muscle Action:
Elbow flexion, range of motion is 135 to 160 degrees

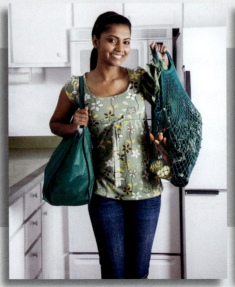

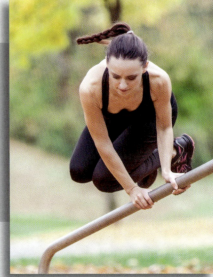

FUNCTIONAL MOVEMENT TRAINING

Front of Upper Arm Strengthening and Stretching

▶ Body Weight

Chin-ups and flexed-arm hangs from a bar are effective body weight exercises for the biceps. Because that equipment is not readily available, we show biceps curls here, which you can do with dumbbells or other heavy objects. Perform a bilateral biceps curl standing with feet shoulder width apart and holding light dumbbells.

Neuromotor training: Sit on a stability ball with your feet placed together and perform a bilateral biceps curl, using the 135- to 160-degree range of motion of elbow flexion.

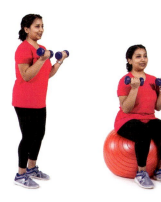

▶ Variable Resistance Machine

Using a straight bar and cable machine, or a biceps variable resistance machine, stabilize your shoulder joint on the pad and grab the handles to isolate the biceps. Curl your elbow 135 to 160 degrees and let the weight down slowly. Keep your abdominals tight and your knees slightly bent.

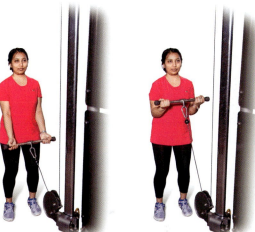

▶ Free Weights

Stand, holding dumbbells in each hand. With your palms facing up, flex the elbow, using a 135- to 160-degree range of motion. You can also perform this with the palms facing the sides of your body to work your brachioradialis.

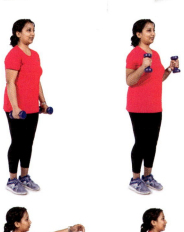

▶ Stretch

Extend arms straight out in front of you. Using one hand at a time, gently pull back the fingers of the other hand until a stretch is felt in the biceps.

Alternatively, clasp both hands behind the back to stretch both biceps at the same time. You can also stretch your biceps by reaching your arms behind the back without clasping your hands.

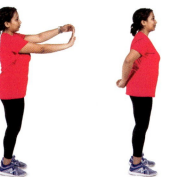

Back of Upper Arm

Triceps

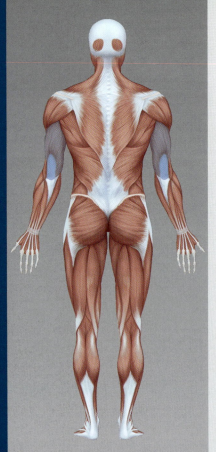

Daily activity use includes getting out of a chair, putting a box on a high shelf, and lowering a box from an overhead position

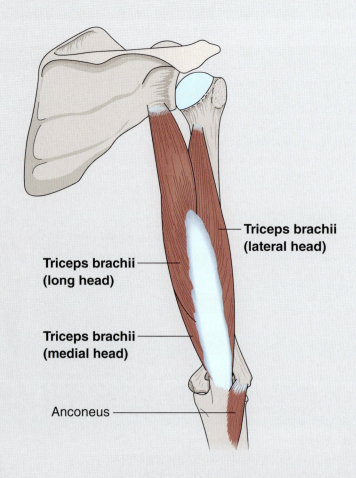

Triceps brachii (lateral head)

Triceps brachii (long head)

Triceps brachii (medial head)

Anconeus

Muscle Group:
Triceps (triceps brachii)

Muscle Action:
Elbow extension, range of motion is 135 to 160 degrees

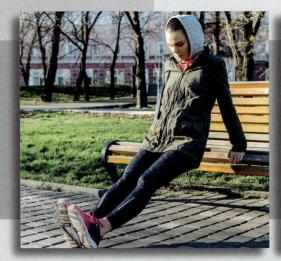

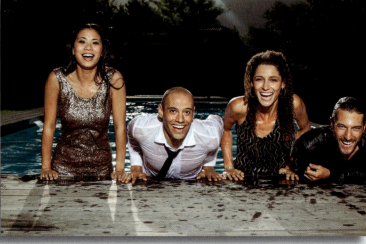

FUNCTIONAL MOVEMENT TRAINING

Back of Upper Arm Strengthening and Stretching

▶ Body Weight

Using a flat, stable bench, perform triceps dips. Flex and extend the elbows, keeping the knees bent and the head up.

Neuromotor training: Lift one leg as you perform the triceps dips on a bench.

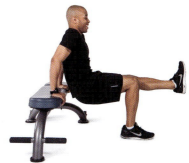

▶ Variable Resistance Machine

Adjust the handles on the triceps dip machine so you get the shoulders as close to the body as possible. Simultaneously extend the elbows and straighten the arms.

Neuromotor training: Stand close to a cable machine and extend both elbows 135 to 160 degrees, then let the bar up slowly.

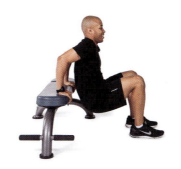
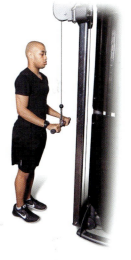

▶ Free Weights

Stand up tall with your knees slightly bent. Hold a weight overhead in both hands. Keeping the upper arms by the ears (perpendicular to the ground), bend the elbows, lowering the weight toward the neck until the elbows point straight up.

Perform the same movement while sitting on a stability ball.

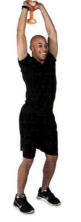
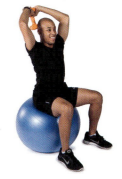

▶ Stretch

Point one elbow overhead, toward the ceiling. If the shoulder joint is not flexible, use a stretch band or a towel and slowly move the elbow upward. If you are more flexible, after pointing the elbow up, place the hand of that arm on your back. Using the other hand, slightly press the elbow down and point your fingers down your back.

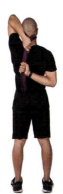
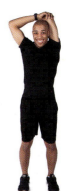

7

Body Composition

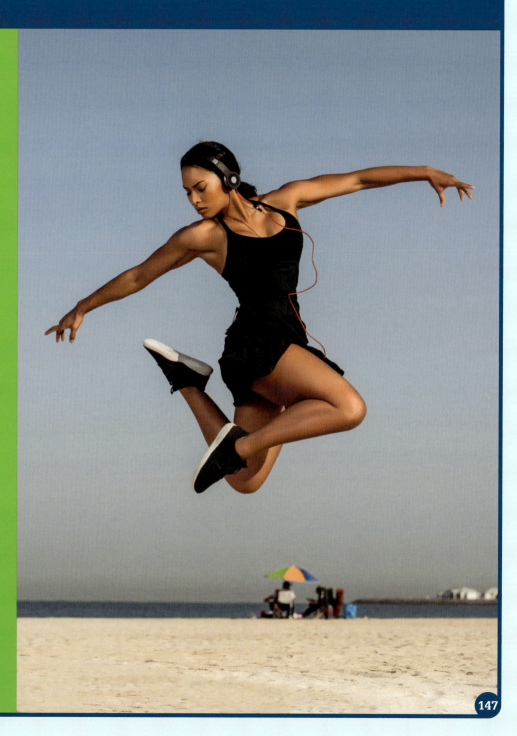

OBJECTIVES

❭ Understand that body composition includes muscle mass and bone mass in addition to fat.

❭ Learn the common ways to measure body composition in the research lab and for your personal assessment purposes.

❭ Recognize how fat, muscle, and bone mass relate to the primary diseases of obesity, sarcopenia, and osteoporosis.

❭ Use the "three-legged stool" of exercise and physical activity, nutrition, and hormones to manage your body composition to help you feel good and age well.

KEY TERMS

adiposity

air displacement plethysmography

bioelectrical impedance analysis (BIA)

body composition

body mass index (BMI)

bone density T-score

dual-energy X-ray absorptiometry (DEXA)

ectopic fat

essential fat

female athlete triad

hydrodensitometry (underwater weighing)

intermuscular adipose tissue

magnetic resonance imaging (MRI)

osteoporosis

percent body fat

sarcopenia

skinfold thickness

subcutaneous fat

visceral fat

Body composition is an important component of health-related physical fitness. A healthy body composition contributes to feeling well and being free of disease. As with the health-related physical fitness components discussed in previous chapters—cardiorespiratory fitness, muscular fitness, flexibility, and neuromotor fitness—body composition is important for functional fitness and sport performance. If you successfully manage your body composition, you will enhance how you look, feel, and move.

In this chapter, we'll look at the components of body composition, how to measure your body composition, and the benefits of a healthy body composition. You'll also get the opportunity to create a program to manage your body composition. You'll learn that healthy body composition is much more than body weight.

Body Composition Basics

Many people mistakenly think of **body composition** simply as body fat, but it is much more complex. Your weight can be divided into

> Body composition is much more than body fat. Your weight can be divided into three major components: fat mass, lean or muscle mass, and bone mass.

three major components: fat mass, lean or muscle mass, and bone mass. From an animal perspective, in earlier evolutionary times, fat was an efficient vehicle for energy storage. Life spans were so short that people did not contemplate diseases and conditions of old age. We now recognize that the three major components of body composition (fat, muscle, and bone) are all important health outcomes. However, in our modern times, body composition is often considered a social status symbol. A perspective of body composition that moves beyond body fat will help you design your personal program and successfully manage your body composition for a long, healthy life!

Measuring Body Composition

The measurement of body composition has evolved over the past several decades with technological advances and research that typically uses molecular models based on two, three, four, or six components (Heymsfield et al. 2005; 2015). Historically, the most common model used in clinical practice or for field applications was based on the two-component model, which divides the body into fat and fat-free components (Heymsfield et al. 2005, Pietrobelli et al. 2001). A recent gold standard in the research laboratory is a four-component model that divides the body into water, protein, fat, and water. Gold standards are highly accurate but require specialized equipment and trained personnel, which can be cost prohibitive and hard to locate. A three-component model of body composition, which divides the body into fat mass, lean soft tissue (including muscle), and bone mass, provides a useful conceptual model for body composition as it relates to health, especially for young adults. Therefore, this chapter uses the three-component model of body composition to frame important concepts for body composition.

Fat Facts

Although fat in the body is often thought of negatively in our society, it serves important functions. In addition to storing energy, fat cushions organs and helps regulate the body's temperature. Fat is also contained in all cell membranes. We all need a certain amount of fat for healthy body function. This is called **essential fat**. Women need a minimal amount of stored fat for reproductive purposes. The percentage of essential fat needed for health is ~3 to 5 percent for men and ~8 to 12 percent for women. Growing children and older adults need different levels of essential fat to remain healthy (Heymsfield et al. 2005).

Most of the fat available for stored energy purposes is located in adipocytes (i.e., fat cells).

When combined, these cells form adipose tissue. Hence, a common term to describe body fat is **adiposity**. The great majority of fat storage in the body is located either right beneath the skin (**subcutaneous fat**) or deep within the abdomen surrounding the organs (**visceral fat**). Visceral fat is often called intra-abdominal fat because it is located deep in your abdomen, underneath your abdominal muscles. Fat storage can also occur in less typical locations, such as within the liver, around the heart, or near bundles of muscle fibers. Minimal fat is stored in these locations, termed **ectopic fat**, in physically active normal-weight adults.

Figure 7.1 illustrates the main components of body composition of fat, protein, water, and bone

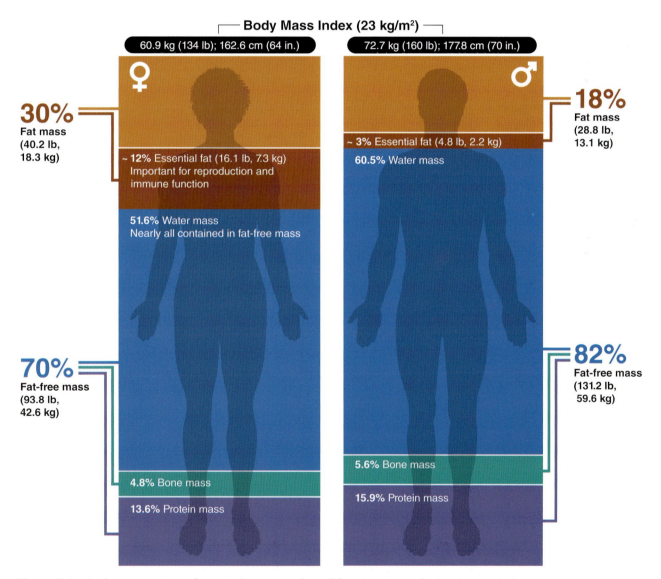

Body Mass Index (23 kg/m²)

60.9 kg (134 lb); 162.6 cm (64 in.) 72.7 kg (160 lb); 177.8 cm (70 in.)

30%
Fat mass
(40.2 lb,
18.3 kg)

18%
Fat mass
(28.8 lb,
13.1 kg)

~ **12%** Essential fat (16.1 lb, 7.3 kg)
Important for reproduction and
immune function

~ **3%** Essential fat (4.8 lb, 2.2 kg)

60.5% Water mass

51.6% Water mass
Nearly all contained in fat-free mass

70%
Fat-free mass
(93.8 lb,
42.6 kg)

82%
Fat-free mass
(131.2 lb,
59.6 kg)

5.6% Bone mass

4.8% Bone mass

13.6% Protein mass

15.9% Protein mass

Figure 7.1 Body composition of a typical young male and female with similar body mass indexes.

mass for an average healthy and normal-weight male and female college-aged students. In the figure, the percentage of fat mass, or **percent body fat**, for the average young adult means the percentage of the total body mass (or weight) that is fat mass.

Interactions Between Fat, Muscle, and Bone

Lean mass has a strong relationship to bone mass and density in adolescents and young adults (Weaver et al. 2016). This makes sense because muscles pull on bones whenever they contract, and this causes your bones to adapt. Also, as you gain or lose weight, not all of the weight change is due to increases or decreases in fat mass—you will also experience changes in lean mass and bone mass. The exact composition of the weight change is influenced by many factors, including your age and overall health, how much you exercise, and the quality of your diet, especially protein and bone nutrients like calcium and vitamin D (Shapses and Sukumar 2012).

Effects of Sex and Age on Body Composition

Both sex and the aging process influence body composition (Xiao et al. 2017). As depicted in figure 7.1, after puberty, the average man has greater muscle and bone mass and less fat mass than the average woman. These differences do not exist in prepubertal children and are primarily due to sex-specific differences in testosterone and estrogen for men and women, respectively.

Distinct changes also occur in fat, muscle, and bone mass with aging. Essentially, as a person moves beyond middle age, fat mass increases and muscle mass and bone mass decrease (Kohrt 2010; Looker et al. 2009). These body composition changes are a natural part of the aging process that are mostly caused by changes in hormones. However, the degree to which body composition changes with age is highly influenced by lifestyle choices, especially physical activity and dietary habits. Moving and eating well during your younger years helps you establish healthy habits.

> When trying to lose fat mass, make sure you include exercise, physical activity, and strength training in your weight-loss regimen to avoid losing muscle and bone mass!

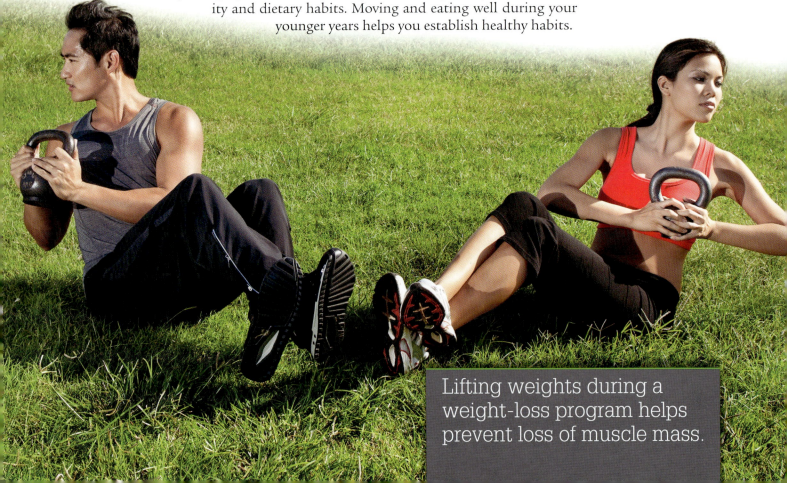

Lifting weights during a weight-loss program helps prevent loss of muscle mass.

Genetics Influence Your Body Type

Have you considered your family members' sizes and shapes? The question of nature versus nurture has been used to describe personalities, patterns of behavior, and body characteristics. Certainly, both factors play a role. One factor influenced by genetics is fat distribution (Bouchard and Perusse 1988). This is especially true for women, who vary in their fat patterning more than men do. For example, if you are female and most women in your family store extra weight in their midsection, you are likely genetically inclined to have an android (i.e., male) fat pattern, often called an apple shape. However, if your family members tend to store extra weight in the hips and thighs, they have a gynoid (i.e., female) fat pattern or a pear shape (figure 7.2). Some people are not an apple or a pear; their fat storage is more evenly distributed throughout their body regions and fat depots. Fat depots are not created equal with regard to their risk for health.

As with fat distribution, genetics often play a role in determining your body type. Researchers have seen a link between body composition and somatotype or body type (Slaughter and Lohman 1976). Three main body types exist:

- **Endomorph.** This is the roundest body type, with wider shoulders and hips. This type tends to be pear shaped, easily gain and regain weight, excel with strength activities such as weightlifting, and find weight-bearing exercise (e.g., distance running) more challenging.

- **Mesomorph.** The m in mesomorph is for muscle! These people typically have broad shoulders, are lean and muscular, and respond to exercise training with quick and very evident results. With their athletic build, they tend to excel at exercise and sport activities and manage their body composition very easily.

- **Ectomorph.** The ectomorph is thin and generally very linear, with narrow shoulders and hips. Regardless of their height, they have little fat or muscle, relatively speaking. These light-framed individuals excel at sports that require them to carry their weight, such as distance running.

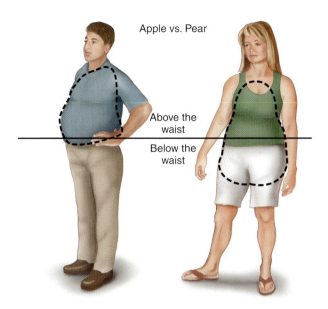

Figure 7.2 Do you have an apple or a pear body shape?

Reprinted by permission from K.E. McConnell, C.B. Corbin, D.E. Corbin, and T.D. Farrar, *Health for Life* (Champaign, IL: Human Kinetics, 2014), 70.

Most people have a blend of two different body types. Some bodies do not match any particular type. Both men and women can align with any of the three body types listed previously. Regardless of body type, everyone can benefit from meeting the guidelines for physical activity and exercise.

Assessing Body Composition

Body composition can be measured in many different ways. The greater the resources available, the more accurate the results. Methods commonly used in clinics and fitness facilities measure the whole body or regional parts of the body and are based on two-component and three-component models.

Body Composition in the Laboratory

The following sections provide an overview of some common laboratory methods for assessing body composition. This methodology and expertise might be used in research labs or in a hospital setting.

Body Density = Water Submersion

Hydrodensitometry, commonly called **underwater weighing**, is based on a two-component model of body composition that assumes the body is divided into fat and fat-free components. The density of the body determines the degree of body fatness and ranges from a theoretical .9 gm/dL for a purely fat body to 1.1 gm/dL for a purely fat-free body (i.e., lean) body (Pietrobelli et al. 2001; Heymsfield et al. 2005).

For example, if you were to put a pan that is greasy from frying a hamburger into a sink full of water, the fat droplets from the meat would rise to the top and any lean meat that had been left in the pan would go to the bottom. Fat floats because it is less dense than water and meat sinks because is it denser than water. The exact same principle applies for hydrodensitometry. In the swimming pool, people with higher levels of body fat float and tread water easily, whereas very lean, mesomorphic people have to work harder to stay afloat.

Density equals mass divided by volume. Humans cannot be put into a beaker to measure their volume; therefore, the difference between weight on land and weight underwater provides a calculation of body density. Underwater weighing requires a person to be completely submerged in a tank of water while their weight is obtained on a scale. Once body density is determined, a prediction equation is used to estimate relative adiposity, or percent body fat (i.e., %Fat).

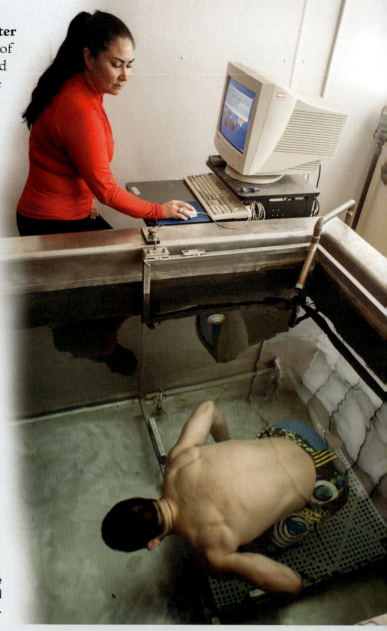

Underwater weighing, or the hydrodensitometry method, is used to measure body composition.

Body Density = Air Displacement

Air displacement plethysmography is very similar to underwater weighing. However, instead of using underwater weight, body density is determined from air displacement (Heymsfield et al. 2005; Lee and Gallagher 2008). This methodology uses a closed chamber called a BOD POD to acquire body density. When using the BOD POD, the person being measured should wear minimal clothing, remove air from their hair by wearing a swim cap, and sit very still. The BOD POD chamber measures the air volume changes with sophisticated computerized sensors. Once body density has been determined, similar to underwater weighing, the body density value is entered into an equation to estimate %Fat. The BOD POD offers many advantages compared to underwater weighing. It is safer and more comfortable for many populations, especially children, older adults, people with movement disabilities, and especially those who are afraid of water. The primary downside of the BOD POD is that it is expensive and requires a dedicated space that is free from rapid changes in temperature and air movement.

Dual-Energy X-Ray Absorptiometry

One of the best technological advances for body composition has been the **dual-energy X-ray absorptiometery** (**DEXA**). This equipment is available in many exercise science and nutrition departments at universities and in nearly all hospitals. This methodology is considered a three-component model since it measures fat mass, lean soft tissue (muscle), and bone mass (Heymsfield et al. 2005; Lee and Gallagher 2008). The DEXA works by exposing the body to low- and high-energy X-rays. The computer software then maps the body by pixel in terms of the composition of fat, lean tissue, or bone mass. DEXA provides both whole-body and regional (arms and legs) estimates of body composition. It also provides bone measures, including bone mass and bone density. DEXA is a very valid and reliable method for estimating body composition. It is very easy to undergo DEXA scanning; it just requires lying still on the back on a scanning table for a few minutes. In addition to the high cost and expertise needed, a small amount of radiation exposure occurs with DEXA scanning. The actual amount of radiation depends on the type and number of scans a person undergoes.

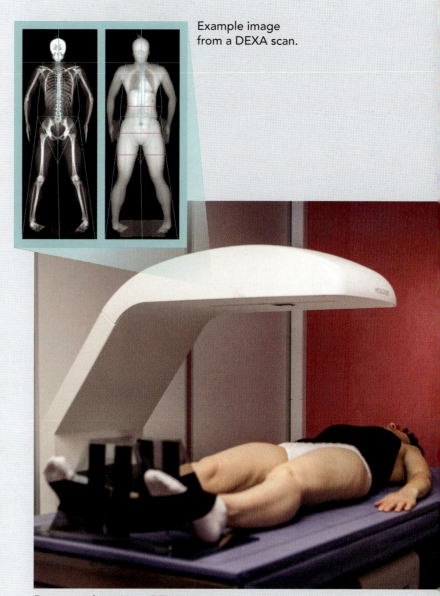

Example image from a DEXA scan.

Person undergoing a DEXA scan.

Magnetic Research Imaging (MRI)

Although it is not readily available, **magnetic resonance imaging** (**MRI**) is an important method for body composition assessment because it shows ectopic adipose depots (the presence of fat in places where only very small amounts of fat should be stored), including visceral fat (fat stored deep in the abdomen), which are a major health risk. MRI instruments are readily available in most hospitals and in many research centers. This technology can visually map the body by slices, or cross-sections. MRI is also used to assess fat infiltration into muscles, called **intermuscular adipose tissue**, which has been linked with a higher risk for metabolic diseases and poor muscle quality, the latter being associated with physical functional limitations and disability in older individuals (Addison et al. 2014).

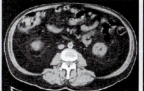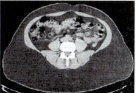

MRI images of visceral adipose tissue from a person with a large waist due to visceral fat and a person with a large waist due to subcutaneous abdominal fat.

Portable Options for Body Composition Assessment

To assess body composition on the sports field, at a health fair, or anywhere else that requires portable equipment, the two most common methods are bioelectrical impedance analysis and skinfold measurements. Both of these methods require some level of expertise to acquire quality estimates of body composition.

Bioelectrical Impedance Analysis

Bioelectrical impedance analysis (BIA) is considered suitable for laboratory, field, and personal use. This method is based on the fact that nearly all body water is contained within the fat-free mass of the body. Thus, if body water is measured, fat-free mass can be estimated. The difference in weight can be used to estimate fat mass and %Fat (Heymsfield et al. 2005; Lee and Gallagher 2008). A bioelectrical instrument sends a small electrical current through the body and measures the resistance to the current. Because water is a great conductor and fat is a good insulator, the balance between the two tissues determines the resistance to the current.

Based on previous research, the resistance and other factors such as height are used to estimate body water, which then can be used to estimate body composition based on research established equations. Because this methodology measures water, the person being tested must be properly hydrated. Testing when you are dehydrated or, less commonly, overhydrated can greatly affect the accuracy of this testing method. The quality of BIA instruments range greatly. High-level research-grade BIA instruments are multifrequency and more accurate and offer measures of where the body water is located (i.e., inside or outside the cell). Lower-cost BIA instruments offer a less accurate measure of total body water and %Fat.

Skinfolds

Skinfold thickness tests are often used in the field to assess body composition (Heymsfield et al. 2005). This method is based on the fact that a majority of stored fat is located just beneath the skin. Thus, once skinfold thicknesses have been obtained from several sites and summed, the total number reflects overall skinfold thickness, which represents %Fat. Experts recommend assessing sites from all body segments (Pollock and Jackson 1984). Because standardized measures can be taken on the legs, arms, back, and abdomen, this method can also give a quantitative measure of where you store your fat and the degree of change in various fat depots. However, this method cannot measure visceral adipose tissue, which is located underneath the muscle wall of your abdomen.

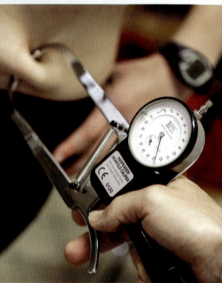

Acceptable measurements of skinfold thickness are a bit more challenging to get than BIA measures. First, an adequate caliper, the instrument needed to measure the skinfold, should be high quality. Research-grade calipers can cost several hundred dollars, and acceptable spring-loaded ones that are well calibrated are also expensive. Second, being able to obtain valid and reliable measurements requires much practice on many different body types. Finding a well-trained and experienced tester can be problematic. Third, having your skinfolds assessed requires a person to touch you on multiple parts of your body, which you may not find comfortable. Finally, when converting the sum of skinfolds into a %Fat estimate, the tester will need to choose from numerous prediction equations, which can influence the accuracy of the estimate. In summary, obtaining relatively accurate estimates from this method can be challenging, particularly when you want to use the method to assess change in %Fat.

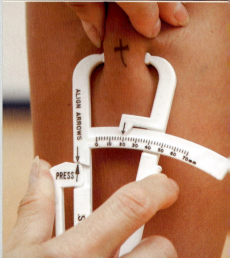

Research-quality calipers compared to low-quality calipers.

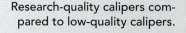

Personal Measurement of Weight Status and Body Composition

Whether you assess your body composition because you want to learn about your health risk or establish a baseline to track progress to help you make informed choices, your choice of method will depend on your purpose, the availability of equipment, testing expertise, and the amount of money you want to spend. At a minimum, you should monitor your weight and waistline if you do not have access to some of the more complex measurement devices outlined previously.

Weight Status

Weight status is evaluated primarily using **body mass index** (**BMI**), which is a ratio of weight to height. Although limitations exist for the personal assessment of body composition from BMI, the measure does provide a well-established index for health risk. Waist circumference is highly related to visceral fat. As lab 7.1 in the web study guide describes in more detail, proper measurement of height, weight, and waist is key to getting good baseline data and tracking changes over time. Therefore, investing in a good tape measure or consistently noticing your belt notch can help you understand your health status and keep your weight management on track. Be mindful of the four S's of monitoring your weight status:

- Same time of day
- Same day each week
- Same clothing (or none at all!)
- Same scale

Also, recognize that normal fluctuations in weight occur over the day and week, largely due to changes in body water that are influenced by your diet, especially salty and starchy foods. Other factors can affect your weight, such as the weather, stress, and hormonal changes, including those caused by the menstrual cycle if you are female.

Options for Personal Bioelectrical Impedance Analysis (BIA)

A number of personal BIAs can be purchased that range in price from $50 to 200, including handheld devices and stand-on scales. The latter are higher quality, and many of the more accurate personal devices are stand-on type scales that can

also measure weight. Remember to standardize your measurement protocol using the four S's mentioned previously, especially for factors that influence hydration. If you are using a scale at home, be sure to place it on an absolutely flat surface. Uneven bathroom tiles or plush carpeting can lead to an inaccurate reading. Finally, read the specific instructions for use, especially regarding equation selection, if this is an option. Similar to skinfold methodology, there are numerous prediction equations and selections that can affect quality. Although many companies provide personal BIA instruments, two manufacturers that have been in the BIA instrumentation business for many decades are RJL Systems for research-grade instruments and Tanita for personal instruments. You are encouraged to visit their websites for more information.

Quality Resources and Services

Beyond regularly monitoring your weight and waistline and perhaps considering the purchase of your own BIA device for home use, another great option is to pay for quality assessment services that use one of the techniques described earlier in this chapter. Many colleges and universities provide assessments of body composition through their health center or recreation center. In addition, many departments and medical centers have DEXA capabilities and offer testing services for a fee. Finally, higher-quality fitness facilities often have respectable BIA instruments and trained staff. It is highly recommended that you select conventional established methods for body composition testing as described in this chapter.

Be a Mindful Consumer of Body Composition Assessment

As a starting point, work on having a healthy perspective toward getting your body composition assessed. Ask yourself, do I have a healthy mindset whereby the process or results won't be counterproductive to my physical and mental health?

Purpose of Assessment

Before getting your body composition assessed, you should reflect on why you want the numbers. Do you want to know if you are in the healthy range? Are you trying to get a baseline so that you can track your progress in response to a new exercise or dietary program? Or are you comparing yourself to a friend and being competitive? Similarly, maybe you read the %Fat numbers of elite athletes or supermodels. These groups are not appropriate for comparison. Depending on your answer, perhaps you don't need to get your body composition assessed since the number will not help your health—physically or psychologically.

Body Composition Assessments Are Estimates!

You may have noticed when reading the preceding descriptions of body composition methods that they all provide *estimates* of %Fat. Another way to think of this is that the values they provide all have a degree of error. The only way to truly know what your body composition is would require you to be assessed as a cadaver (with chemical analysis), and we all agree that this would not be a good idea! With

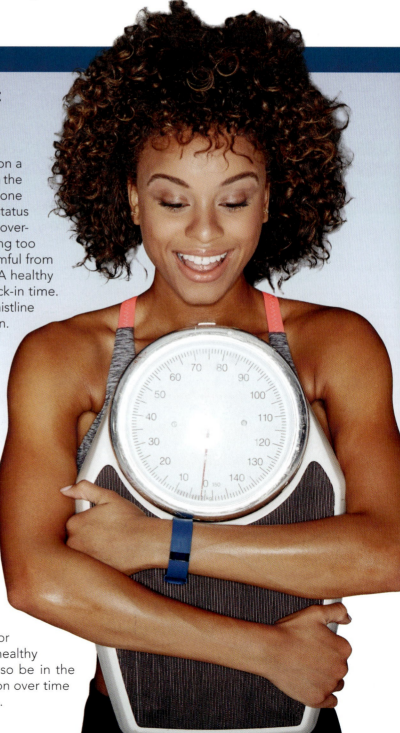

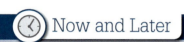 Now and Later

Find Your Assessment Sweet Spot For Life

Now

When was the last time you weighed yourself on a quality scale? Having a healthy relationship with the scale can be challenging in today's world. On one hand, we want to be mindful of our weight status and our body composition. On the other hand, over-monitoring, or being preoccupied with or giving too much importance to the numbers, can be harmful from an emotional and psychological perspective. A healthy strategy might be to determine a regular check-in time. The sweet spot for assessing your weight and waistline might be once a month or perhaps every season.

Later

The natural course for most people in today's society is a small, creeping gain in weight and fat mass every year after young adulthood. Although some of this change in weight is due to naturally occurring changes from the maturation and aging process, much of it is due to changes in lifestyle related to shifts in occupation, family structures, and our stress responses. Having a healthy mindset about your weight as you age will increase your chances of being both physically and psychologically healthy.

Take Home

The simple truth is that, from a health perspective, if you consistently meet the physical activity guidelines and the exercise recommendations put forth by the ACSM, especially for resistance training, and your waistline is in the healthy zone, your body composition naturally will also be in the healthy zone. Managing your body composition over time is a key strategy for staying healthy as you age.

methods for body composition assessment, you get what you pay for. This means that the more expensive equipment and sophisticated expertise will provide estimates that have lower levels of error. For example, DEXA can provide an estimate that has an error of only 1 to 2 percent. Alternatively, many BIA instruments on the market have an error rate of 4 to 5 percent (Heymsfield et al. 2005). Therefore, depending on your purpose for assessment, the availability of methods and expert testers, and your resources, the wiser choice might be not to get your body composition assessed since the level of error would be too great to inform you or your program plans.

Weight Status, Body Composition, and Your Risk of Chronic Disease

The three body composition components, fat mass, lean soft tissue (muscle), and bone, are directly linked to primary diseases. Having too much fat mass (a high %Fat), especially stored in certain places in the body, is defined as overweight or obesity. Overweight is linked to many chronic diseases and conditions that increasingly occur as a person enters middle age and beyond. However, having too little muscle mass and a low bone mass can also cause serious conditions and diseases that often arrive later in life.

Weight Status Classified

Table 7.1 lists the BMI classifications of underweight, normal weight, overweight, and obese, with subclassifications that are agreed on by the World Health Organization (WHO). Recall that BMI is a ratio of weight to height: It is calculated by dividing your weight in kilograms by height in meters squared. The calculation is more complicated if you would like to use the units of pounds and inches, so we recommend you use an online BMI calculator to determine your BMI. Because of the key link between waist size and visceral fat and the related risk for metabolic diseases, in addition to BMI, the table also includes risk based on waist circumference. This means that a person can have a normal or overweight BMI but be at an increased risk for disease due to an elevated waist size. The table lists subclasses of severity in both the underweight and obesity classifications.

BMI and Adiposity Relationships

A relatively strong relationship exists between BMI and %Fat across all age groups, which is why it is used to assess health status at the doctor's office. Additionally, much research supports the fact that for a typical adult, BMI levels in the overweight and obese categories are linked to increased risk of chronic disease and death. However, these predictions are not perfect. Many other factors, such as physical activity and exercise, diet quality, smoking, alcohol and drug habits, and stress, influence

Table 7.1 BMI and Waist Classifications

Weight status classification	Body mass index	Metabolic disease risk	Waist—Men	Waist—Women
Underweight, severe thinness	<16.0			
Underweight, moderate thinness	16.0-16.9			
Underweight, mild thinness	17.0-18.4			
Normal	18.5-24.9	Normal	≤94 cm (37 in.)	≤80 cm (31.5 in.)
Overweight	25.0-29.9	Increased	94-102 cm (37-40 in.)	80-88 cm (31.5-34.5 in.)
Obese, class I	30-34.9	Substantially increased	≥102 cm (40 in.)	≥88 cm (34.5 in.)
Obese, class II	35-39.9			
Obese, class III	≥40			

Data from WHO (2008).

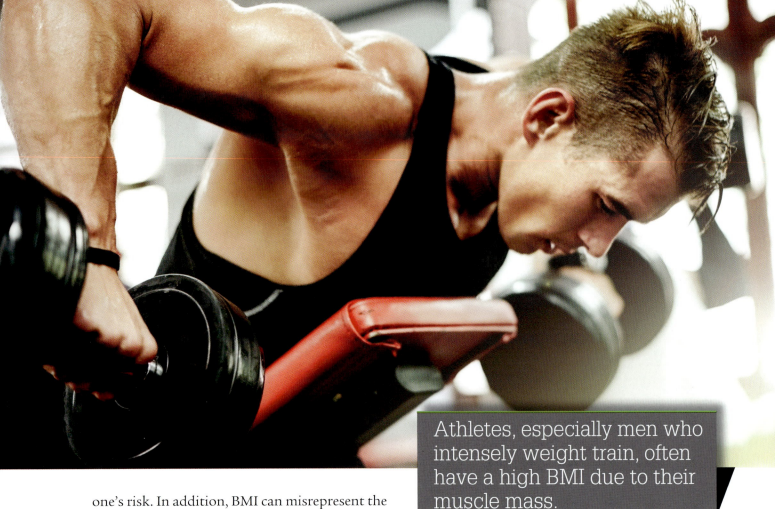

one's risk. In addition, BMI can misrepresent the body composition of a person. In the special cases that follow, interpret the BMI value with caution.

- *Heavily muscled athletes*. People who undergo a high intensity and volume of resistance training, typically men, often have a high BMI that is not due to increased fat mass. Their increased muscle mass increases their weight, thereby increasing their BMI as well.

- *Altered height*. Because height is in the equation to calculate BMI, any situation where height is altered will introduce error into the relationship between BMI and %Fat. For example, older adults lose several inches later in life. If their weight were stable, it would appear that BMI had increased.

- *Reduced physical activity*. In individuals who are bedridden or unable to walk due to illness, a spinal cord injury, or other health-related challenges, the relation between BMI and %Fat can also be greatly altered due to a reduced muscle mass. Even in people who can walk but choose to be very sedentary, reductions in muscle mass can cause the BMI to misrepresent %Fat.

%Fat Health and Fitness Categories

Unlike those established for BMI, no universally accepted norms for %Fat exist. However, the American College of Sports Medicine (2018) has determined a range of 10 to 22 %Fat and 20 to 32 %Fat as being satisfactory for health for men and women, respectively. Age, sex, and race may affect the level of %Fat that is in the healthy range (Gallagher et al. 2000). Table 7.2 highlights the %Fat ranges for men and women corresponding to the normal weight, overweight, and obese categories of BMI. Note that women have greater %Fat compared to men. A slight increase in %Fat (3 to 5 %Fat) is a normal part of the aging process.

The ACSM also supports using %Fat ranges to categorize body composition fitness for men and women into rankings of very lean, excellent, good, fair, poor, and very poor, with percentiles from 1 to 95 percent in 5 percent increments (American College of Sports Medicine 2018). Table 7.3 summarizes the main cut points within the categories for young men and women. Being excessively lean, which corresponds to a %Fat below 3 to 5 percent

Table 7.2   Percent Fat Classifications Based on BMI

	20-39 YEARS		40-59 YEARS		60-79 YEARS	
	Women	Men	Women	Men	Women	Men
BMI = 18.5 kg/m² (normal weight)	20%-25%	8%-13%	21%-25%	9%-13%	23%-26%	11%-14%
BMI = 25 kg/m² (overweight)	32%-35%	20%-23%	34%-36%	22%-24%	35%-38%	23%-25%
BMI = 30 kg/m² (obese)	38%-40%	26%-28%	39%-41%	27%-29%	41%-43%	29%-31%

Data from Gallagher et al. (2000).

Table 7.3   Fitness Categories for Body Composition Levels for Young Adults (20-29 Years Old)

		PERCENT FAT	
Percentile (%)	Category	Men	Women
95	Very lean	6.4	14.0
85	Excellent	10.5	16.1
60	Good	14.8	19.8
40	Fair	18.6	23.4
20	Poor	23.3	28.2
1	Very poor	33.4	38.6

Data from ACSM (2018).

for young men and 8 to 12 percent for young women, can be harmful to health.

Not All Fat Depots Are Equal

Where people store their fat influences their risk for many chronic conditions and diseases. Keep in mind that not all fat depots are created equal. Where you store fat as a healthy young adult depends on your genetics, sex hormones, and, to a lesser extent, your level of physical activity, diet quality, and your stress hormones.

As mentioned previously, changes in body composition occur with the aging process. The preferred storage depot shifts in women (somewhat in men, too) to store more fat centrally and less in the lower body. In addition, with higher levels of adiposity and a very sedentary lifestyle, you increase intermuscular adipose tissue. In simple terms, muscles get mushier with age. Remember that a mushy muscle is lower quality!

Another important site of ectopic storage is the liver. A small amount of fat in your liver is normal, but once it gets beyond 10 percent of the organ weight, you may be at high risk for fatty liver disease. There are two main types of fatty liver disease: alcoholic liver disease and nonalcoholic fatty liver disease. The latter type occurs mainly in middle-aged obese individuals. As expected, if this person also drinks heavily, the risk of fatty liver disease greatly increases. Remember to treat your liver right!

Preventing Sarcopenia: Keep Your Muscle Mass!

Relative healthy young adults have an adequate amount of muscle mass to meet the needs of their daily lives. However, during middle age (~45 to 65 years old), both men and women start to lose muscle mass at a greater rate. With advanced age, many older adults are at risk for **sarcopenia**, or age-related loss of muscle mass and strength. Sarcopenia is usually diagnosed in research or in the clinic using a DEXA scan to measure muscle mass of the arms and legs. Sarcopenia is one of the most important causes of functional decline and loss of independence in older adults.

Although this sounds like bad news for your life, the good news is that our muscles retain the ability to get stronger in response to resistance training well into our 90s. Much research documents that older adults of all ages with various chronic diseases can still safely strength train, which leads to physical functional benefits and

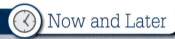

Now and Later

Mind the Muffin Top and Beer Belly!

Now

Although many healthy body shapes and sizes exist, if you are genetically inclined to store your excess calories in your abdomen, you need to be mindful of your waist size. A "muffin top" is a popular expression for a woman who is relatively thin but has a thick waistline, mainly because of subcutaneous fat storage in the abdomen due to poor dietary choices and a sedentary lifestyle. A similar label, often applied to men, is "beer belly," which can refer to storage of both visceral and subcutaneous fat in the abdomen. Poor core-muscle fitness and posture can also contribute to this condition.

Later

With the aging process, waistlines expand, especially in women who go through menopause. Having a larger-than-healthy waistline is a major risk factor for the Big Metabolic Three introduced earlier—cardiovascular disease, type 2 diabetes mellitus, and cancer—which often arrive in middle age. Similarly, having weak core muscles and poor posture predisposes you to low back pain and injury.

Take Home

By making healthy nutrition and physical activity choices on a regular basis, you can manage your waistline from the perspective of both fat storage and core strength and posture. This will pay major dividends later in life. You do not need have to have six-pack abs, but you should strive to stay within the healthy zone described in table 7.1.

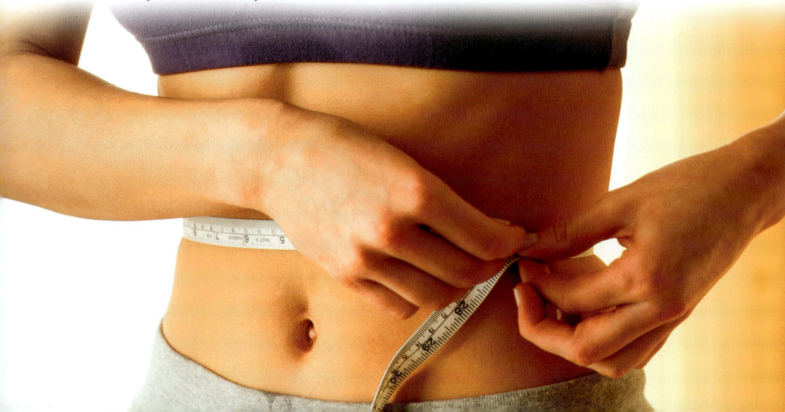

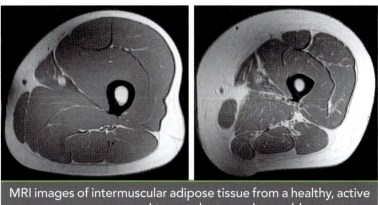

MRI images of intermuscular adipose tissue from a healthy, active young woman compared to a sedentary, obese older woman.

affords them the ability to live independently. For an awesome life as an older adult, build the habit of incorporating resistance training into your weekly movement routine. This single health behavior can pay great health dividends late in life!

Osteoporosis: Building the Bone Bank Early in Life Is Important

The term **osteoporosis** means "porous bone." Osteoporosis is a bone disease that occurs when the body loses too much bone, makes too little bone, or both. The bones become weak and are then at higher risk for breaking from nontraumatic injury such as a fall in the bathroom or on an icy sidewalk. Most people think of osteoporosis as a disease for little old ladies. In fact, osteoporosis affects all types of people. It is very serious and costly to our health care system. Osteoporosis is also silent, which means you can be completely unaware of having it until you suffer a fracture. More important to you as a young adult, the risk for osteoporosis starts early in life! The good news is that it is largely preventable with good health behaviors.

How Is Osteoporosis Diagnosed and Who Gets It?

Typically, screening for osteoporosis occurs based on a person's age and health history. In addition to measuring fat mass and lean soft tissue (mainly muscle), the DEXA instrument also measures bone mass and bone density. The **bone density T-score** value is the tool primarily used to diagnose osteoporosis. A T-score is simply the standard deviation below peak bone density of a young healthy person. Figure 7.3 summarizes the World Health Organization's definition of osteoporosis: a T-score below or equal to −2.5. This is equal to being 2.5 standard deviations below the peak bone density of a young healthy person of the same sex.

Age is the primary risk factor for osteoporosis because loss of bone is a normal part of the aging process. The following list presents other primary risk factors for this disease. Compare these factors to your personal demographics and health history.

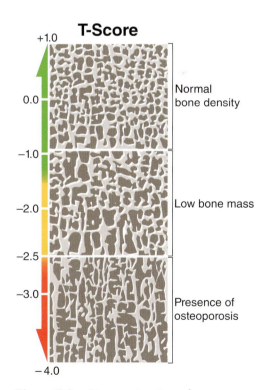

Figure 7.3. Diagnostic criteria for osteoporosis based on a DEXA T-score.

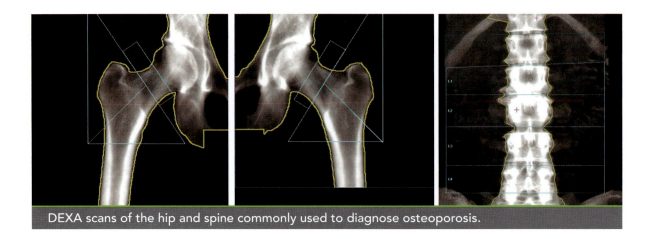

DEXA scans of the hip and spine commonly used to diagnose osteoporosis.

For more information, visit the National Osteoporosis Foundation website at www.NOF.org.

- *Sex*. Women have a greater risk of osteoporosis than men due to bone size and differing sex hormone profiles.
- *Race or ethnic group*. White and Asian people have greater risk of osteoporosis than African American people.
- *Diseases, conditions, and medical procedures*. Cancer, endocrine or hormonal disorders, autoimmune disorders such as lupus, and digestive disorders such as celiac disease are just a few health challenges that can increase risk for osteoporosis.
- *Medications*. Many medications (e.g., steroids) can compromise bones.
- *Nutrition*. Poor intake of calcium and vitamin D has a direct effect on bone health.
- *Physical activity and exercise*. Being sedentary, especially bedridden, greatly affects bone health.

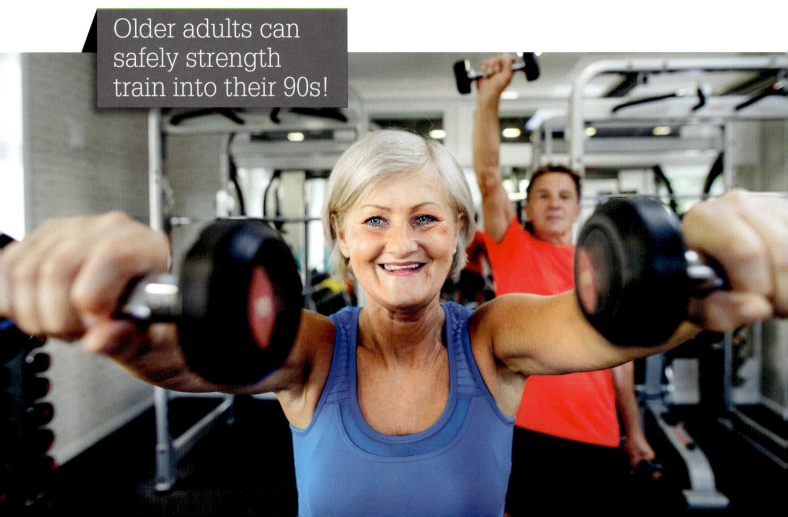

Older adults can safely strength train into their 90s!

The Bone Bank: Deposits and Withdrawals

With the aging process, all people lose bone mass and density. If you stay alive long enough, it is very likely that you will develop osteoporosis. When planning for retirement, the goal is to put money in the bank during your greatest earning years for the day when you retire and need to withdraw funds. If you planned correctly, you will not outlive your money. In this same way, the goal with bone health is to maximize your deposits in the bone bank, because sometime around middle age, especially for women who undergo menopause, you will begin to withdraw your bone mass and reduce your bone density. Therefore, the goal for your bone bank is to deposit as much bone as genetically possible and maximize your peak bone mass, and then flatten the withdrawal curve as you age (figure 7.4). This two-part strategy will help ensure that your bone density stays out of the fracture zone and that you do not suffer a bone fracture later in life due to osteoporosis, even if you live to be 90 years old or older!

> Maximizing your peak bone mass while you're young can reduce your fracture risk as an older adult. It pays to deposit in your bone bank early in life!

A Healthy Body Composition Benefits You—Today and in the Future!

A regular physical activity and exercise program and a healthy diet are important for having a healthy body composition. A healthy body composition means maintaining an appropriate level of fat mass, adequate muscle mass, and optimal bone mass and density for your stage of life. Although you won't be able to notice or feel your bone health status, having a good ratio between your muscle mass and fat mass will give you many benefits. You may notice that many of the benefits in the following list are very similar to those you read about in chapters 4 and 5. If you are dedicated to a regular fitness program and have good dietary habits, you will successfully manage your body composition!

Here are the many ways you will feel better and function better with a healthy body composition:

- *Energetic physical function*. Carrying around extra pounds of weight is like toting around an extra heavy backpack.
- *Enhanced work, recreation, or sport performance*. An unhealthy body composition can reduce your physical function, which can negatively affect your work, recreation, and sport performance.

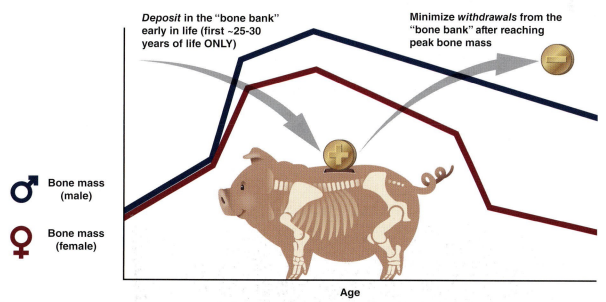

Figure 7.4 To keep your bones healthy for life, deposit more bone mass early in life and minimize withdrawals later in life.

- *Healthier self-esteem and self-image.* Obesity can affect psychological health. Being labeled as overweight or obese can hurt emotionally, which can lead to social anxiety and depression and negatively affect self-esteem. Many people live daily with body discontent.
- *Prevention of the Big Metabolic Three and physical function diseases and conditions.* Although the diseases and conditions of cardiovascular disease, diabetes, cancer, sarcopenia, and osteoporosis typically occur later in life, it bears repeating that these health challenges begin in early adulthood, often silently. Invest in your future best self by successfully managing your body composition.

Your Program for Managing Body Composition

Body composition is much more than body fat. Hopefully you are now thinking of your body as being made up of three components: fat mass, lean soft tissue (mainly muscle), and bone mass. Although weight management is discussed in chapter 9, the following information can remind you of key program components.

The Plan Depends on the Goal

Your plan to have a healthy body composition is highly dependent on your goal. Your personal goals may be functional in that when you work or play, you want to perform well. Or you may be more concerned with looking good and feeling good about the way you look. We all recognize that a healthy body composition is considered attractive in our society. We hope your goals will be about both your current and future self. Depositing in your "bone bank now" and throughout life can reduce your risk of osteoporosis. Plus, committing to a weekly routine of cardiorespiratory and muscle-strengthening exercises can reduce your risk for many diseases and conditions over your life span.

The Three-Legged Stool for Body Composition Management

An excellent conceptual model for a healthy body composition is the three-legged stool (figure 7.5). Unless all three legs of the stool are optimal, the stool will not function well. Regardless of the component—fat, lean soft tissue (muscle), or bone—optimal health depends on the three primary factors of exercise and physical activity, adequate nutrition, and appropriate hormones.

Physical Activity and Exercise: Movement Mode Matters

Hopefully, the previous chapters have convinced you of the importance of habitual movement and provided information to guide you in developing a personalized program that keeps you safely moving on a regular basis. With regard to body composition, mode really does matter! Consider these aspects of body composition management.

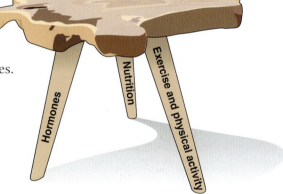

Figure 7.5   The three-legged stool for a healthy body composition: exercise and physical activity, nutrition, and hormones.

- *Fat mass*. Because cardiorespiratory endurance activities expend lots of calories and energy balance is very important for maintaining a healthy level of fat mass, choose activities that use lots of energy. The higher the intensity and the longer the duration of the activity, the greater the amount of energy expenditure.

- *Lean soft tissue* (*mainly muscle*). Any movement is better than none when working the muscles, but relatively high-intensity strength training is the most effective mode for gaining and keeping muscle mass.

- *Bone mass and density*. Bones must be loaded to adapt. The best loading for bone health comes from ground reaction forces (e.g., jumping, running), joint reaction forces (e.g., strength training), and novel forces. Many sport activities offer a combination of loading forces. Your young adult years are a prime time for building bone since your skill level allows you to play sports and safely weight train. Also, most young adults have healthy joints and bones that can tolerate overload.

Nutrition

Optimal nutrition is essential for a healthy body composition and, of course, calories do count for weight management. However, other nutrients are very important for body composition. For example, adequate protein intake is important for muscle maintenance and bone health, especially later in life. Micronutrients that are critical for bone health are calcium and vitamin D. Unfortunately, poor dietary habits and physical inactivity are major reasons for the rising rates of obesity, sarcopenia, and osteoporosis in our contemporary society.

✓ Behavior Check

Think of Bone Loading the Next Time You Move

Think about how you currently move. Have you ever thought about your bones when exercising or enjoying recreational activities? Jumping and lifting and carrying heavy things—weights in a strength and conditioning room, bales of hay, or a camping backpack—are great ways to load safely. Because many young adults do not meet the recommended physical activity guidelines for strength training, especially women, you might not be reaching the genetic potential of your "bone bank." Be creative to load your bones on a regular basis!

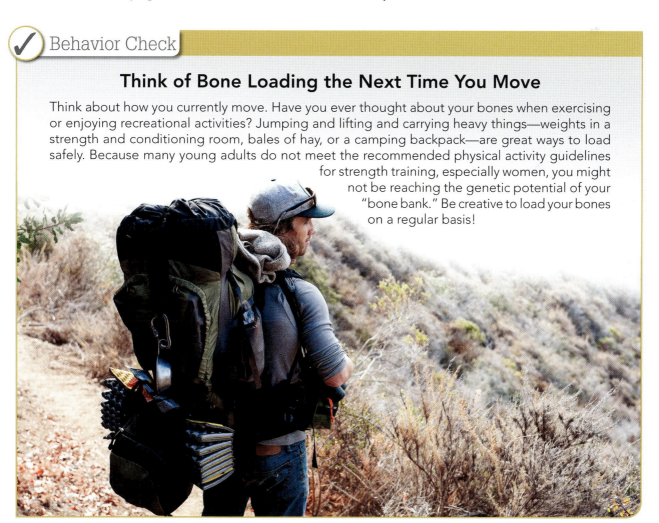

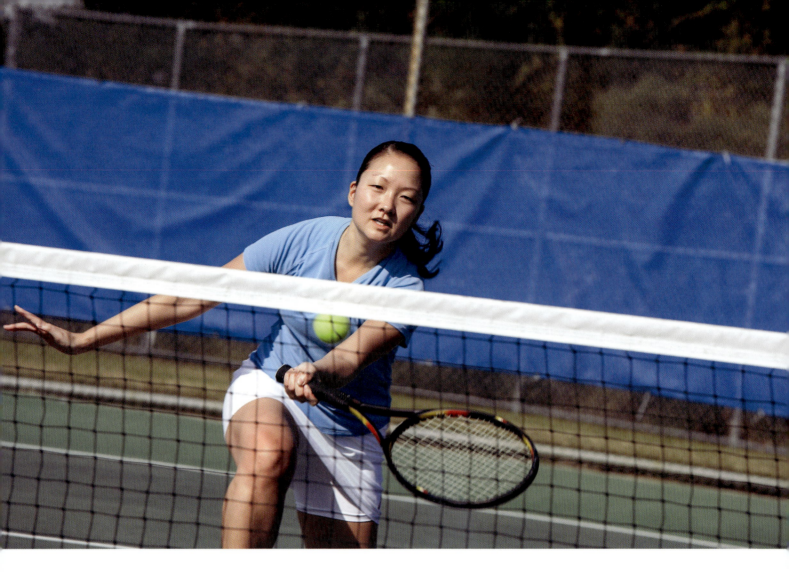

Hormones

Hormones also play a primary role in a healthy body composition. Sex hormones, testosterone and estrogen, and other growth hormones and factors play major roles in the differences in fat, muscle, and bone mass seen in men and women during and after puberty. Natural declines in these hormones that occur with aging are a key reason for changes in body composition, which include increases in fat mass and decreases in muscle and bone mass.

However, abnormal levels of hormones for a given life stage are also problematic for a healthy body composition. For example, many young women, for a variety of medical reasons, do not have a regular monthly menstrual cycle. If a young woman does not start to menstruate by age 16, misses three consecutive periods, or has a cycle longer than 35 days, bone loss could be occurring. This reduced estrogen state can lead to bone loss similar to what occurs in a menopausal woman.

Highly active women should be aware of the **female athlete triad**, which involves three distinct and interrelated conditions: disordered eating (with a range of poor nutritional behaviors), amenorrhea (irregular or absent menstrual cycles), and osteoporosis (low bone mass and poor bone quality leading to weak bones and risk of fracture) (Joy et al. 2014). The triad occurs most often in highly trained, very lean female athletes who excel in their sport by being very thin or lean (e.g., dancer, gymnast, distance runner). Although most common in women, men who aim to compete in weight class sports (e.g., wrestling, rowing, martial arts) can also be afflicted with a form of the triad. This provides a great example of the

> If you are female whose cycle is unexplainably irregular or absent (and you are not pregnant), see your physician. You might be compromising your bone health.

three-legged stool. The athlete greatly overloads her skeleton, but poor or inadequate nutritional intake disrupts her menstrual cycle and causes her estrogen levels to be much lower than what is normal. Her stool now has only one optimal leg: exercise. The triad, or any other reason for menstrual cycle disturbances, reduce the chance of reaching peak bone mass. For more information, see www.femaleathletetriad.org/athletes.

Summary

Body composition is the final component of health-related physical fitness, joining cardio-respiratory endurance, muscular strength and endurance, and flexibility. Although body composition is generally thought of as body fat, muscle mass and bone mass are also primary components. Accurate and adequate measurement of body composition can occur in both the research laboratory and the privacy of your home. Having optimal nutrition and participating in regular physical activity and resistance training can go a long way to successfully managing your body composition. The benefits of your efforts will pay off today with better physical function in your daily life, including in sports and active leisure activities. You will also look and feel great. However, the bigger payoff will occur in your future when you will have a much lower risk for chronic diseases and conditions and a greater chance of feeling and functioning better as you age. Make the commitment to manage your body composition today!

WEB STUDY GUIDE

Remember to complete all of the web study guide activities to further facilitate your learning, including **Lab 7.1 Body Composition: Weight Status and Waist Measurement**.

REVIEW QUESTIONS

1. Using a three-component model as a frame, list and describe the primary body composition components that can affect your health.

2. Describe the primary ways that body composition can be measured in the laboratory, in the field, and in the privacy of your home. Which method is the most accurate?

3. Body mass index (BMI) is a useful health index, but it does have limitations. When does caution need to be used when interpreting BMI to classify weight status?

4. Although chronic diseases often don't present until middle age, they often begin in young adulthood. Describe how the three body composition components relate to primary diseases that occur later in life.

5. List and describe the primary ways that a healthy body composition will make you both function better and feel better during your campus life.

6. What are the three legs of the body composition stool? What specific behaviors or factors do you need to address to apply these to your life as a young adult?

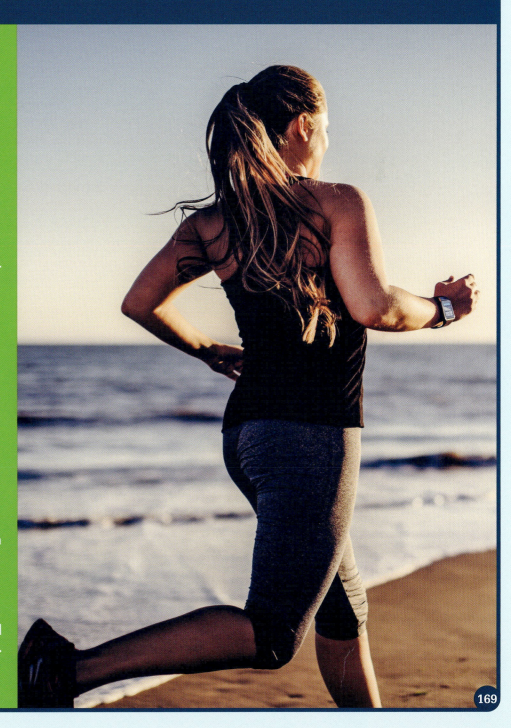

8

Fundamentals of Healthy Eating

OBJECTIVES

》 Understand the primary dietary components of macronutrients, micronutrients, and fiber and identify sources of each one.

》 Understand why each dietary component is important for health.

》 Realize that diet is much more than energy intake and that diet quality is important for health.

》 Find high-quality resources, including endorsed government and agency guidelines, to assist you in designing a healthy eating plan that fits your lifestyle, budget, and tastes.

》 Appreciate the key role that hydration plays in managing environmental stress and daily function.

》 Gain strategies to be a smart consumer.

KEY TERMS

antioxidants

complete protein

complex carbohydrates

free radicals

hydrogenated oils

incomplete protein

kilocalorie (calorie)

licensed dietitian (LD)

macronutrients

micronutrients

minerals

phytochemicals

refined carbohydrates

registered dietitian nutritionist (RDN)

saturated fatty acids

simple carbohydrates

trans fatty acids

unsaturated fatty acids

vitamins

whole grains

This chapter explores how to consistently eat a balanced and varied diet in a society that often provides unhealthy choices. Unlike doing physical activity, which is almost optional in our contemporary society, you must eat and drink to survive. Therefore, you'll need different skills for managing your eating behaviors than for your physical activity. Every time you have an opportunity to eat or drink, you have to make decisions about your diet. When it comes to a healthy diet, it may seem as though the advice is ever changing. To some extent, as more research emerges, this may be true, but the fundamentals of nutrition are not as confusing as you might think. A primary key to making consistent healthy choices is to find the time to plan so you have healthy foods that you enjoy readily available to you, helping you to stave off unhealthy temptations.

Eating Well: Balanced and Clean

While the expression "eating clean" doesn't have an official definition, this is a common and popular term used to describe eating foods that are as close to their natural state as possible. The term *processed* has taken on a negative connotation. Many people associate processed foods with those that are high in added sugar, salt, fat, and preservatives, but this is not always the case. Processing is simply altering a food product before consumption. Methods include freezing, pasteurizing, cooking, canning, preserving, baking, and fortifying with vitamins and minerals. Thanks to processing, we can enjoy a variety of foods throughout the year, safer foods, and foods that help prevent nutrient deficiencies. Although the idea to eat clean is good, being too rigid in this practice is often impractical and sometimes unsafe.

Beyond Calories to Fuel Quality

Many people reduce nutrition down to the energy content of food, or calories. However, the quality of your food also matters. If you put low-quality fuel into your car, it won't run very well. The same is true for your body—if you don't consistently provide it with high-quality fuel, you won't run very well. Running in this case goes beyond exercise to include your daily function on campus, such as mental concentration, motivational energy, and mood management. Running well in the long term includes reducing the risk for the Big Metabolic Three (cardiovascular disease, diabetes mellitus, and cancer) introduced in chapter 4, osteoporosis and sarcopenia introduced in chapter 7, and other chronic health conditions.

Essential Nutrients

A useful frame for your healthy diet is to start thinking beyond the good taste and pleasure of foods and drinks to the nutrients they can provide. Your diet should provide about 45 essential nutrients. These are deemed essential because your body cannot provide them, at least not without causing other conditions or diseases. The six main classes of essential nutrients include **macronutrients** (carbohydrates, fats, proteins), **micronutrients** (vitamins and minerals), and water.

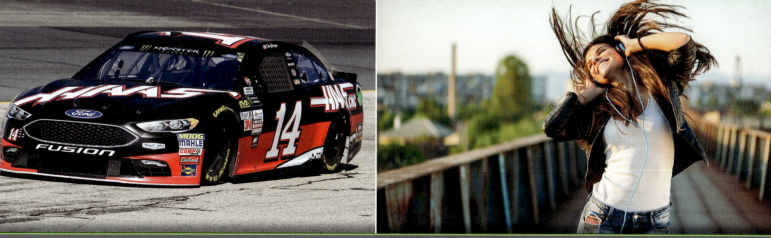

Just as race cars require high-quality fuel to run properly, your body needs high-quality food and drink to give you optimal energy.

Calories

A calorie is a unit of energy used to describe many scientific processes. When the word *calorie* is mentioned, what comes to mind? Something to be feared that can lead to unwanted weight gain? Something you require for energy to make it through the day? Do you think of this term when reading food labels? A **calorie** (or, more correctly, a **kilocalorie**) is the way that energy from foods is expressed. Since most people are familiar with the term *calorie*, which is also used on all food labeling, we will use it in this book rather than *kilocalorie*. Figure 8.1 lists the three primary macronutrients in order of energy density. Note that although alcohol is neither a macronutrient nor considered essential, it does contribute calories to daily energy intake if consumed.

Energy Needs

Energy needs are influenced by age, sex, height, weight, exercise or physical activity, and health conditions (e.g., pregnancy, diseases). In addition, a need or desire to lose, gain, or maintain weight can affect how many calories you need. The dietary guidelines in this chapter provide an estimate of energy needs based on age and sex, as well as physical activity levels. Chapter 9 explores energy needs more fully.

Carbohydrates: Great Energy Sources

During digestive processes, carbohydrates are broken down into glucose for use and are stored in the liver and muscles as glycogen. They are the body's main source of energy, and glucose is the

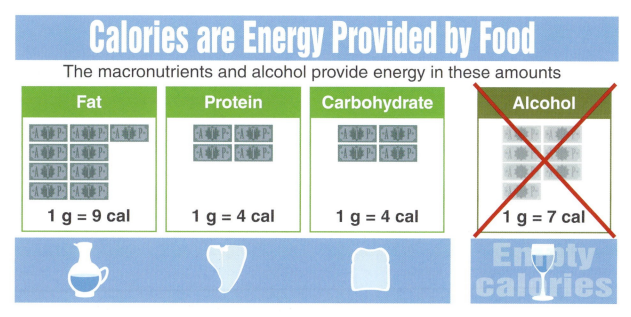

Figure 8.1 Macronutrients and alcohol vary in the number of calories, or "energy bucks," they provide per gram.

sole energy source for the brain. Carbohydrates provide working muscles with a readily available energy source, especially during high-intensity exercise. From an energy-storage perspective, compared to fat and protein, carbohydrate is stored in very small amounts in the body.

What foods can you think of that contain carbohydrates? If you think of bread, potatoes, pasta, and cookies, you are certainly correct, but carbohydrates are actually found in most of the foods we consume. Compared with the other macronutrients, carbohydrates contribute the most energy in terms of daily caloric intake. Table 8.1 summarizes the types of carbohydrates that are classified as **simple carbohydrates** or **complex carbohydrates**, which are further divided into **refined carbohydrates** and **whole grains** (Institute of Medicine 2005).

Simple Carbohydrates

Your taste buds identify simple carbohydrates because they add sweetness to our foods. Although they are found naturally in fruits and milk, simple carbohydrates are also added to soft drinks, fruit drinks, candy, desserts, yogurt, condiments, and plant-based milks such as soy milk.

Beware of Added Sugars

Added sugars are those that do not occur organically in foods. They are added by the consumer or food manufacturers. If you put brown sugar in your oatmeal or honey in your tea, you have added sugars to your diet. Sugars that naturally occur in fruits or milk are not considered added. Many foods that are high in added sugars are low-quality fuel, providing unneeded calories and minimal nutrients. In addition to increasing your risk for obesity and other metabolic diseases, added dietary sugars are also linked with tooth decay, or cavities.

Added sugars in the American diet are a major public health concern. On average, in the United States, added sugars account for 270 calories, or 13 percent of calories per day. The largest sources of added sugars are sugar-sweetened beverages, sweet snacks, and desserts. It is recommended that added sugars of the diet contribute 10 percent or less of your daily caloric intake (U.S. Department of Health and Human Services and U.S. Department of Agriculture 2015). Although we often recognize intentional additions of sugar (i.e., a scoop of sugar in your morning coffee), hidden sources in packaged foods are more challenging to identify. These may include yogurt and peanut butter, processed fruit blends or punches, and snacks. Reading the ingredient list or food label to determine how much added sugar a food contains can greatly inform your food selections.

> Starting in 2020, if not earlier, it will be easier than ever to detect added sugars in food because food labels will clearly state "Added Sugars" in grams.

Complex Carbohydrates: Refined Carbohydrates and Whole Grains

Whole grains are complex carbohydrate sources that include the germ, endosperm, and bran of

Table 8.1 Types of Carbohydrates

Simple carbohydrates (sugars): Lack vitamins, minerals, and fiber	Complex carbohydrates: Provide vitamins, minerals, and fiber
Monosaccharides: single-sugar molecules • Glucose • Fructose • Galactose	Starches: long, complex chains of sugar molecules • Grains (wheat, rice, oats) • Legumes (beans, peas, lentils) • Tubers and vegetables (potatoes, yams, corn)
Disaccharides: double-sugar molecules • Sucrose or table sugar (fructose + glucose) • Maltose or malt sugar (glucose + glucose) • Lactose or milk sugar (galactose + glucose)	Fiber (nondigestible carbohydrates) • Soluble (oats, barley, legumes, some fruits and vegetables) • Insoluble (wheat bran, vegetables, whole grains)

Data from Institute of Medicine (2005).

the grain (figure 8.2). Compared to processed carbohydrates, whole grains are often more energy dense and contain more nutrients, including fiber, B vitamins, and minerals (Whole Grains Council n.d.). When whole grains are refined, the germ and bran are often removed, mainly leaving behind the starchy endosperm. This processing is how brown rice becomes white rice and whole wheat flour becomes white flour. Foods made from refined grains are often enriched and fortified with vitamins and minerals, but not all nutrients lost during the refinement process are replaced. Refined carbohydrates are thought of as less nutritious than whole grains. For this reason, the U.S. Department of Agriculture (USDA) recommends that consumers choose half of their grain sources from whole grains. Some examples include brown rice, whole wheat or whole grain bread, whole wheat pasta, quinoa, and popcorn. Whole grains play an important role in weight management and gastrointestinal health due to their fiber content (U.S. Department of Health and Human Services [USDHHS] and U.S. Department of Agriculture 2015).

Fiber: Beyond Bathroom Business

If the discussion of fiber makes you snicker due to its well-known link to essential bathroom business, you are not alone, but the benefits of fiber are no laughing matter. Fiber, unlike the starchy component of plant carbohydrate that is digested, is the nondigestible carbohydrate in plants. A noncarbohydrate substance called lignin that is found in plants such as grains, fruits, legumes, and vegetables also contribute to dietary fiber intake. As fiber moves through the intestinal tract, it provides bulk for fecal matter in the large intestine, which ultimately assists in elimination. Depending on the type of fiber you consume, the bacteria processing in the large intestine results in gas, which is why too much fiber, especially when not regularly consumed, results in intestinal gas (Institute of Medicine 2005).

Two types of dietary fiber exist, both of which are important for health. The first, soluble or viscous fiber, delays stomach emptying, slows glucose uptake into the blood after eating, and reduces absorption of cholesterol. Good sources of this type of fiber are oat bran and some fruits and legumes. The second, insoluble fiber, increases fecal matter bulk and prevents constipation, hemorrhoids, and other digestive disorders. This type of fiber is found in wheat bran or psyllium seed. Psyllium is found in some cereals and fiber supplements and laxatives to aid digestion. Even though humans

> Keep your bathroom business in order by meeting the recommendation for fiber intake: 25 grams per day for women and 38 grams per day for men (USDHHS and USDA 2015).

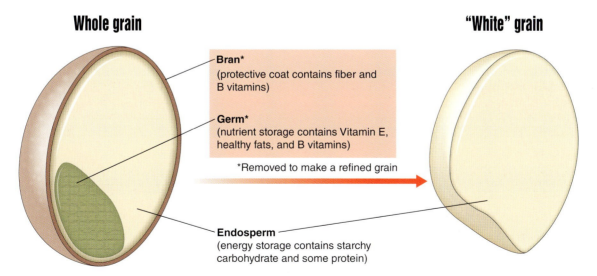

Whole grain

Bran*
(protective coat contains fiber and B vitamins)

Germ*
(nutrient storage contains Vitamin E, healthy fats, and B vitamins)

*Removed to make a refined grain

"White" grain

Endosperm
(energy storage contains starchy carbohydrate and some protein)

Figure 8.2 Whole grains include the germ, endosperm, and bran of the grain, while refined grains have only the endosperm.

cannot digest fiber, it is critical to aid digestion of other foods. See table 8.1 for food choices that provide good sources of both soluble and insoluble fiber (Institute of Medicine 2005; U.S. Department of Health and Human Services and U.S. Department of Agriculture 2015).

Fats: Unsaturated, Saturated, and Trans Fats

Dietary fats also have a bad reputation. In fact, you might think of them as the good (unsaturated), the bad (saturated), and the ugly (trans fats). High levels of certain fats in the diet can increase risk for cardiovascular disease. Fats also pack the most calories per gram, so people usually limit their intake if they want to lose or maintain weight. However, as explained in chapter 4, dietary fats can help with energy balance, especially under conditions of intense physical exertion or labor. Dietary fats assist your body in absorbing fat-soluble vitamins and add flavor and texture to foods. If you have ever eaten a very-low-fat cookie, you probably have noticed how dry it is compared to a conventional higher-fat option.

As illustrated in figure 8.3, the current recommendation for dietary fat is 20 to 35 percent of your total daily caloric intake. Similar to carbohydrates, there are several different types of dietary fats based on sources (e.g., animal versus plant). A few fats, linoleic acid and alpha linoleic acid for example, are essential fatty acids, so they must be consumed in the diet (Institute of Medicine 2005; U.S. Department of Health and Human Services and U.S. Department of Agriculture 2015). Food processing alters dietary fat properties. Thus, not all dietary fats are equal with regard to their effect on health.

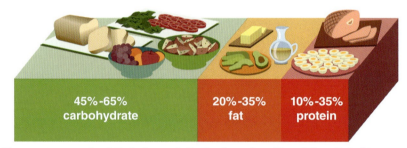

Recommended Intake of Calories for Healthy Adults

45%-65% carbohydrate | 20%-35% fat | 10%-35% protein

Figure 8.3   Recommended macronutrient distribution for adults.

Dietary Fat Types

Table 8.2 summarizes the types of fatty acids and gives examples of foods that contain them. Although many foods contain a combination of **saturated fatty acids** and **unsaturated fatty acids**, you can typically tell the main source by the characteristics of the food. Saturated fats are primarily contained in animal products, such as fatty meats and butter; however, they are also contained in oils from tropical plants, including coconut and palm oils. They are easy to identify because they are solid at room temperature. Alternatively, unsaturated fats most often come from plant sources. Fatty fish, such as salmon, also provide unsaturated fats. These sources are typically liquid at room temperature. Unsaturated fats are often further described by their chemical structure as monounsaturated fats (MUFAs) and polyunsaturated fats (PUFAs). PUFAs are classified by their chemical structure into omega-3 and omega-6 sources (Institute of Medicine 2005; U.S. Department of Health and Human Services and U.S. Department of Agriculture 2015).

Dietary Fat Processing: Hydrogenation

Because the food industry is on a quest to bring products to the marketplace that offer taste at a lower price with a longer shelf life, food scientists have discovered

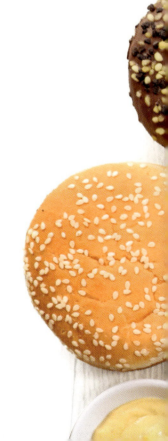

Table 8.2 Types of Fatty Acids

Type of fatty acids	Common example foods
Saturated • Keep to 10% or less of daily caloric intake	• Animal fats, especially fatty meats (e.g., beef steaks) and poultry fat and skin • Butter, cheese, and other high-fat dairy products • Palm and coconut oils
Trans • Avoid, if at all possible	• Small amount occurs naturally in animal fats such as beef and dairy • Convenience foods, including cookies, crackers, and some popcorn • Deep-fried fast foods that contain partially hydrogenated oils
Monounsaturated	• Olive, canola, and safflower oils • Avocados and olives • Peanut butter (without added fats!) • Many nuts such as almonds, cashews, and pecans
Polyunsaturated: omega-3	• Fatty fish: salmon, white albacore tuna, anchovies, and sardines • Walnuts, flaxseed, soybean oils, dark-green leafy vegetables
Polyunsaturated: omega-6	• Corn, soybean, cottonseed oils (used in margarines and salad dressings)

Data from Institute of Medicine (2005); U.S. Department of Health and Human Services and U.S. Department of Agriculture (2015).

processes to change naturally occurring fats. One common process is hydrogenation, which takes an unsaturated vegetable oil and converts it to a mixture of saturated fatty acids that creates a more solid fat from a liquid fat. What is the benefit of **hydrogenated oils**? Hydrogenation increases stability of oils so that they can be reused for deep-frying, which is often used in restaurant businesses. Hydrogenation also improves the texture of many foods, for example, making pie crusts flakier. Finally, hydrogenation is the critical process that makes a margarine or vegetable shortening from a liquid oil.

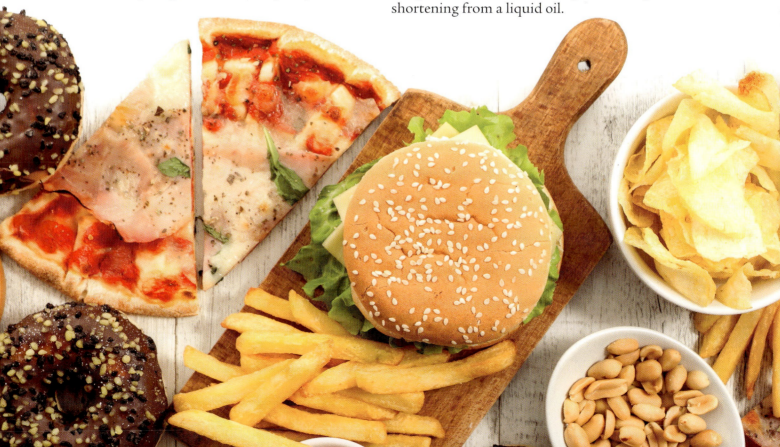

Trans Fats Banned From Processed Foods

The hydrogenation process also changes some unsaturated fatty acids into **trans fatty acids** (trans fats), which changes their chemical structure for many of the reasons described previously. Although very small amounts of trans fats occur naturally in animal fats, including beef and dairy products, the great majority of trans fats consumed in the American diet come from packaged and commercially available foods (i.e., fast foods) that contain partially hydrogenated oils. Nearly all baked and fried foods contain high levels of saturated and trans fats. Unfortunately, the consumption of trans fats has been linked to a significant increase in coronary heart disease. In response to this discovery, in 2015, the U.S. Food and Drug Administration (FDA) required all food manufacturers to stop putting trans fats into our food supply. By 2018, all food manufacturing companies should be in compliance and trans fats will be eliminated from our food supply; however, it will still be very important to check food labels for partially hydrogenated oils (U.S. Food and Drug Administration 2018).

Dietary Fats as Part of a Healthy Eating Pattern

The role that dietary fat plays in chronic diseases, especially cardiovascular diseases, is complicated. Although the negative role that trans fats play in chronic diseases is pretty clear, the role that saturated and unsaturated fats play is a source of ongoing scientific investigation. Certainly, diets higher in fat pose a challenge for weight management given their high caloric density. Subsequently, obesity is linked with the Big Metabolic Three. However, the risk of developing any of these diseases is multifactorial, with other dietary factors such as added sugars and both genetics and physical activity playing key roles.

So, how should you eat with regard to dietary fats? The primary strategy is to think of eating as a daily and weekly pattern and not in terms of one food or food group. The available evidence suggests that the majority of Americans would benefit from reducing their total fat intake. The USDA recommends that saturated fat intake make up no more than 10 percent of daily calorie intake (U.S. Department of Health and Human Services and U.S. Department of Agriculture 2015). Strat-

---

✔ Behavior Check

Going Nuts for Coconut Oil?

When was the last time you drastically changed your diet because you read about a new trendy food? Coconut and coconut oil are trendy foods that some people believe will make you healthier and happier. Many people fall for the claims that certain superfoods will change their lives. If you stay grounded in basic nutrition knowledge, you will be able to resist the urge to follow each new trend and instead stay with the fundamentals of eating a balanced and variable diet. For the record, coconuts and the oil from them are high in saturated fat and ought to have a small place in your diet.

What inaccurate nutrition trends have you fallen for?

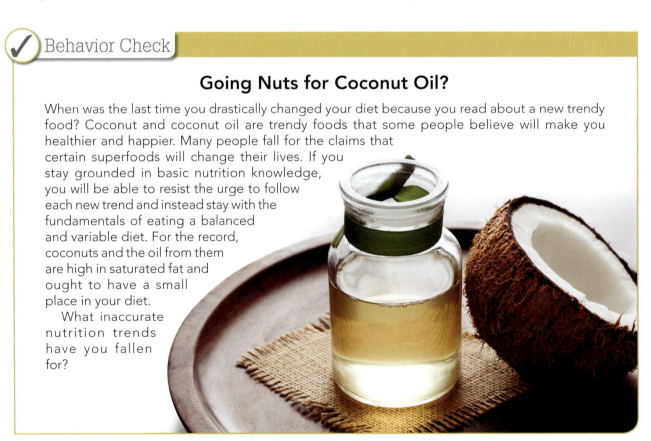

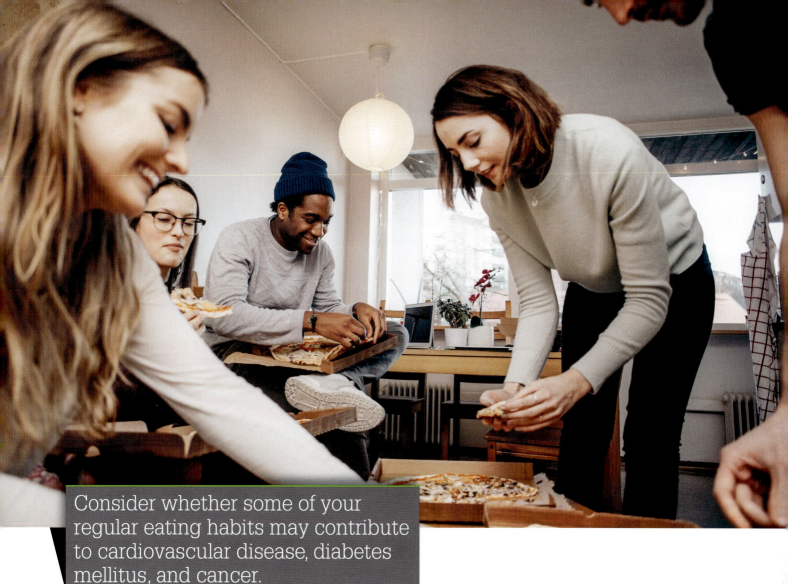

Consider whether some of your regular eating habits may contribute to cardiovascular disease, diabetes mellitus, and cancer.

egies to achieve this include limiting fatty meats, cheeses, and milks, using oils such as canola or olive to prepare foods rather than coconut oil or butter, and snacking on fruits and vegetables instead of prepackaged snacks such as cookies and potato chips.

Protein: Building Blocks of Muscle and Tissue

Of the macronutrients, protein is a popular dietary topic. However, for most Americans, protein contributes the least amount to their daily calories. Most people think about muscles when they think about protein. However, protein is also important for bones, blood, enzymes, cell membranes, some hormones, and optimal immune function. Thus, being protein deficient can be harmful to many systems within the body. The building blocks of proteins are amino acids. Twenty amino acids

exist in food and nine of these are essential, which means they cannot be synthesized by the human body and must be consumed. The remaining 11 amino acids can be created through various metabolic processes (Institute of Medicine 2005). Having adequate protein intake in your diet is clearly important for health. Similar to carbohydrates and fats, there are different sources of dietary protein. Understanding the quality of dietary protein sources will help you design your personal nutrition program.

Protein Quality: Complete and Incomplete

Many foods contain protein, but high-quality protein comes from animal foods such as meats, eggs, dairy products, poultry, seafood, and soy. Lower-quality protein foods, sometimes referred to as **incomplete proteins**, primarily come from plant sources. If you are a vegetarian or you limit your meat intake for health, taste, or financial reasons, you should be able to meet your protein requirements by eating a variety of protein-rich plant foods in your daily diet. Experts used to think that incomplete protein foods had to be consumed together to gain the benefits of a complete protein. For example, grains are low in the amino acid lysine, while beans and nuts (legumes) are low in the amino acid methionine; therefore, when eaten together (e.g., rice and beans, peanut butter on whole wheat bread), they form a **complete protein** (Palmer 2014). However, research now shows that these foods can be consumed over the course of a day for the same benefits.

How Much Protein Is Enough?

Because protein is good for muscles, we often think that eating more is better. Adequate intake is considered .8 to 1.2 grams per kilogram (or .4 to .6 grams per pound) of body weight for most healthy adults, even if they are recreationally active (Palmer 2014). As depicted earlier in figure 8.3, the recommended range for protein is 10 to 25 percent of total daily calories (U.S. Department of Health and Human Services and U.S. Department of Agriculture 2015). Nearly all Americans consume adequate levels of protein in their diets. Consuming above the recommended amounts of protein is typically not harmful except potentially in the following situations:

- *Kidneys and dehydration*. The metabolic processing of dietary protein challenges kidney function and produces more urine excretion, which is not a problem if you have healthy kidneys and you don't consume too much protein. However, if your kidneys are compromised, which often happens with age, or protein intakes are excessive, you could be damaging your kidneys and causing dehydration.

- *Calories*. Excessive protein, if not incorporated into muscle or tissue growth or repair, will be stored as excessive energy in the form of adipose (fat) tissue. Many dietary protein sources are high in fat and can provide unneeded energy.

- *Financial considerations*. High-quality protein sources can also tax your budget. Protein powders and bars and other packaged foods can be expensive.

- *Disordered eating*. Being very rigid with eating routines, including with protein foods and supplements, can be a sign of disordered eating. Having quality protein in your diet is important, but if this aspect of

Dietary protein is provided by both animal and plant sources, including meats, dairy, legumes, soy foods, grains, seeds, and nuts.

your diet is starting to compromise your social relationships and ability to enjoy a variety of foods in a variety of settings, take care to explore your relationship with dietary protein.

Are Protein Supplements Needed?

Many people on the quest for bigger muscles resort to protein supplements in the form of protein powders, bars, or drinks. Adequate protein can be obtained in the diet through whole foods, and supplements are typically not needed. Furthermore, using protein supplements can lead to excessive protein intake that can be dangerous to your health. Plus, dietary supplements are not regulated like food products in the market. Alternatively, as you can see in table 8.3, many protein sources are not very portable and require refrigeration. Protein powders, bars, and drinks are a great option for a quick snack, so some supplements may have a place in your dietary plan.

Table 8.3 Protein Content of Foods Commonly Selected for Protein Content

Food	Serving size	Energy (calories)	Grams of protein
Meat, poultry, and seafood			
Ground beef (cooked; 90% lean)	3 oz (85 g)	184	22
Pork chop (boneless, broiled)	3 oz	144	22
Chicken breast (grilled)	3 oz	128	26
Salmon	3 oz	156	23
Tuna (canned in water)	1 oz (30 g)	24	5.5
Egg (cooked, poached)	1	72	6
Dairy			
Milk (nonfat or skim)	1 cup	83	8
Yogurt (plain skim milk)	6 oz (170 g)	95	9.8
Yogurt (Greek, plain nonfat)	6 oz	100	17
Cheese (cheddar)	2/3 oz (20 g); 1 slice	78	4.6
Cottage cheese (1% milk fat)	4 oz (110 g)	81	14
Legumes and peas			
Lentils	1 cup	230	18
Black beans (boiled)	1 cup	227	15
Chickpeas (boiled)	1 cup	269	14.5
Peas (boiled)	1 cup	230	16.4
Soy foods			
Tofu*	1/2 cup	190	20
Soy milk* (light, plain)	1 cup	70	6
Seeds and nuts			
Pumpkin seeds (dried)	1/4 cup	180	9.75
Peanut butter* (smooth)	2 tbsp	191	7
Almonds (dried)	1/4 cup	206	7.25
Walnuts (black, dried)	1/4 cup	194	7.5

*Varies by manufacturer.

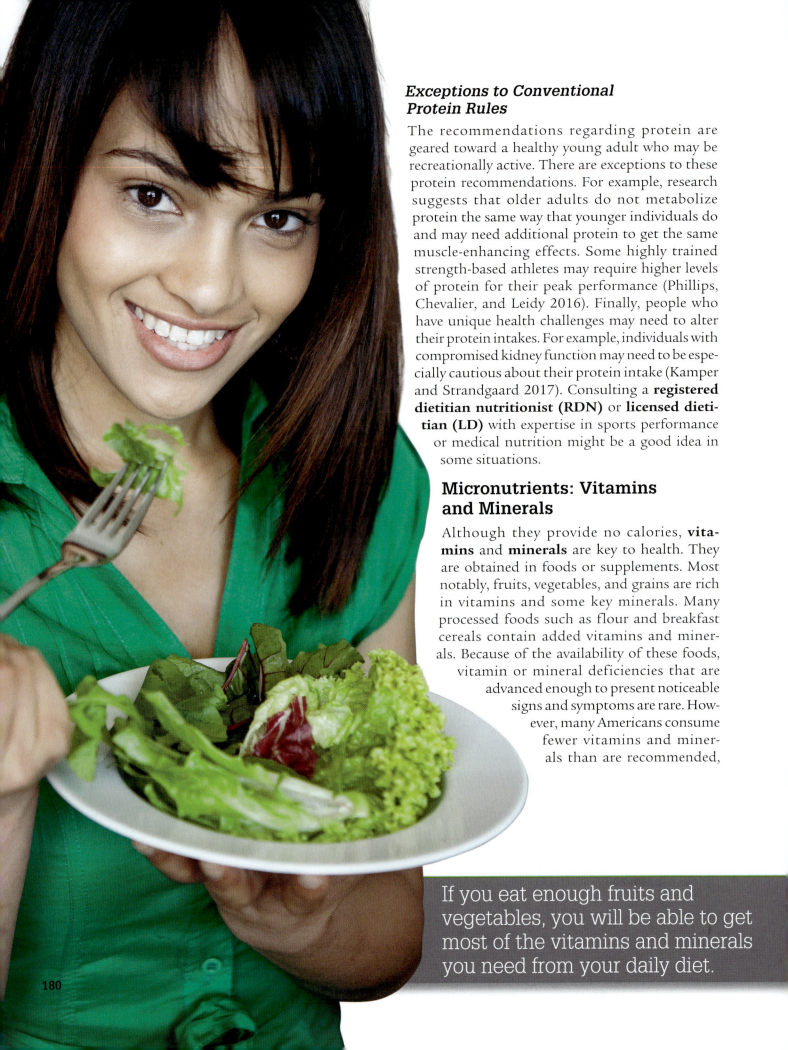

Exceptions to Conventional Protein Rules

The recommendations regarding protein are geared toward a healthy young adult who may be recreationally active. There are exceptions to these protein recommendations. For example, research suggests that older adults do not metabolize protein the same way that younger individuals do and may need additional protein to get the same muscle-enhancing effects. Some highly trained strength-based athletes may require higher levels of protein for their peak performance (Phillips, Chevalier, and Leidy 2016). Finally, people who have unique health challenges may need to alter their protein intakes. For example, individuals with compromised kidney function may need to be especially cautious about their protein intake (Kamper and Strandgaard 2017). Consulting a **registered dietitian nutritionist (RDN)** or **licensed dietitian (LD)** with expertise in sports performance or medical nutrition might be a good idea in some situations.

Micronutrients: Vitamins and Minerals

Although they provide no calories, **vitamins** and **minerals** are key to health. They are obtained in foods or supplements. Most notably, fruits, vegetables, and grains are rich in vitamins and some key minerals. Many processed foods such as flour and breakfast cereals contain added vitamins and minerals. Because of the availability of these foods, vitamin or mineral deficiencies that are advanced enough to present noticeable signs and symptoms are rare. However, many Americans consume fewer vitamins and minerals than are recommended,

> If you eat enough fruits and vegetables, you will be able to get most of the vitamins and minerals you need from your daily diet.

which can predispose them to chronic conditions later in life. Visit sources such as www.webmd.com, www.eatright.org, and the interactive website for dietary reference intake (U.S. Department of Agriculture n.d.a) to determine the specific intakes based on your age, sex, and other important factors.

Vitamins

Vitamins are organic substances required in small amounts to assist with the chemical reactions within the body. They are essential for the production of red blood cells and maintenance of key systems, including the nervous, skeletal, and immune systems. Vitamins E and C and the precursor to vitamin A (beta-carotene) are also considered **antioxidants**, which are known to block the formation and action of **free radicals**, substances produced during regular metabolic processes that are known to promote aging and cancer. Antioxidants are part of a broader class called **phytochemicals**, located in plant foods, that prevent chronic diseases. In addition to the vitamins that are contained in food and supplements, a few vitamins are made in the body, including vitamin D in response to sunlight and vitamin K from intestinal bacteria processes, although consumption of vitamins D and K is still needed for optimal health (Institute of Medicine 2005; U.S. Department of Agriculture n.d.b).

The 13 vitamins required for human health are divided into fat- or water-soluble categories based on how they are absorbed, transported, and stored in the body. The four fat-soluble vitamins (A, D, E, and K) are carried by special protein carriers in the blood and stored in the liver and adipose tissues (hence, the name *fat-soluble*). The nine water-soluble vitamins (B_6, B_{12}, biotin, C, folate, niacin, riboflavin, thiamin, and pantothenic acid) are absorbed directly into the bloodstream, where they travel freely. Water-soluble vitamins are removed by the kidneys and excreted in urine. Because of these differences, it is more difficult to have excessive water-soluble vitamins in your system compared to fat-soluble vitamins (Institute of Medicine 2005; U.S. Department of Agriculture n.d.b).

Minerals

Minerals are nonorganic elements that are required for human health, primarily to regulate body processes, grow and maintain bodily tissues, and produce energy (see table 8.4). Of the 17 essential minerals, the key minerals that are needed in amounts greater than 100 milligrams per day are calcium, chloride, phosphorous, magnesium, potassium, and sodium. The essential trace minerals needed in very small amounts are copper, fluoride, iodine, iron, selenium, and zinc (Institute of Medicine 2005; U.S. Department of Agriculture n.d.b).

Too Much and Too Little

Unless an individual has very abnormal eating patterns, perhaps due to an eating disorder, or is oversupplementing with vitamins and minerals in pill or power form, excessive intake of vitamins and minerals is rare. Fat-soluble vitamins are of greatest concern because they are stored in the body, which can increase the risk of toxicity. Inadequate intake of vitamins and minerals is very common, especially of those highlighted in table 8.4. Chronically poor nutritional habits are more common than nutritional deficiencies. Poor habits can result in an increased risk for chronic diseases later in life, including heart disease and osteoporosis. The majority of Americans, if they eat a varied nutritionally balanced diet on most days, do not need to take supplements to obtain adequate amounts of vitamins and minerals. Relying on supplements to gain the majority of your vitamins or minerals also makes you miss other important substances contained in food, such as fiber.

> Colorful fruits and vegetables provide many key vitamins and minerals as well as fiber and energy!

The Importance of Hydration

Hydration is an underappreciated health behavior. Water makes up 50 to 60 percent of our body weight. Compared to other nutrients, water is by far the most important. The human body can live several months (depending on body size and composition) without food but only a few days without water. Water is essential because it is the medium for chemical reactions and temperature regulation and the main component of blood. We lose water on a continual basis through urine and feces, evaporation from breathing processes, and, of course, from sweat.

Table 8.4 Key Vitamins and Minerals Commonly Lacking or Excessive in Young Adults

	Common dietary source	Major function
Vitamin A	• Milk and cheese • Carrots, spinach, and other deep green and orange vegetables	• Maintenance of vision • Skin health • Health of linings of mouth, nose, and digestive tracks • Function of immune system
Vitamin C	• Citrus fruits • Peppers, broccoli, brussels sprouts, tomatoes, and strawberries	• Maintenance and repair of connective tissue, bones, teeth, and cartilage • Promotion of healing • Aids iron absorption
Vitamin D	• Fortified milk and butter • Fish oils • Egg yolks	• Development and maintenance of bones and teeth • Promotes calcium absorption
Folate	• Green leafy vegetables and oranges • Whole grains and legumes	• Metabolism of amino acids • Synthesis of RNA and DNA • New cell synthesis
Calcium[a]	• Milk and milk products • Tofu • Fortified products (orange juice, bread) • Green leafy vegetables	• Formation of bones and teeth • Control of nerve impulses • Muscle contraction • Blood clotting
Iron[a]	• Meat and poultry • Fortified grain products • Dark green vegetables • Dried fruit (raisins)	• Contributes to hemoglobin and myoglobin • Enzymes • Immune function
Magnesium[a]	• Grains and legumes • Nuts and seeds • Green vegetables • Milk • In water supply (except soft water)	• Nerve impulses • Energy systems • Enzyme activation
Sodium[b]	• Table salt • Soy sauce • Fast and processed foods, especially lunch meats, canned soups, and vegetables	• Body water balance • Acid–base balance • Nerve function
Potassium[a]	• Meats and milk • Fruits and vegetables • Grains and legumes	• Body water balance • Nerve function

[a]Indicates that many young adults do not obtain enough iron, calcium, magnesium, or potassium in their diets.

[b]Indicates that most Americans have too much sodium in their diets.

Data from U.S. Department of Agriculture (n.d.); U.S. Food and Drug Administration (n.d.).

Fluid recommendations for a young adult woman is approximately 2.7 liters per day, with 2.2 liters (9 cups or 72 ounces) coming from beverages. For an adult man, the recommended intake is around 3.7 liters per day, with 3.0 liters (13 cups or 104 ounces) coming from beverages (Institute of Medicine 2004). All fluids, including coffee and tea, count toward total daily amounts. Your need for fluids is highly dependent on exercise and sweating, which is greatly affected by temperature, humidity, and exercise intensity (American College of Sports Medicine 2011). For example, a runner who runs several hours in a hot, humid outdoor environment in direct sun will lose much more water from sweat compared to someone working out in an air-conditioned facility. A good rule of thumb is to replace each pound of weight lost due to sweat with 16 fluid ounces of water. To do this accurately, you need to weigh yourself before and after an intense sweat-producing workout.

Severe dehydration causes weakness and can lead to death. Fortunately, most people do not get dehydrated except in emergency situations or in response to a major illness such as the flu; however, many people are chronically slightly dehydrated, which does not often lead to thirst. In addition to the color of your urine (see figure 8.4), other signs of mild dehydration are headaches, tiredness, lack of mental focus, and dizziness when standing up rapidly. Get in the habit of drinking a large glass of water when you get up in the morning, with each of your meals, and right before you go to bed.

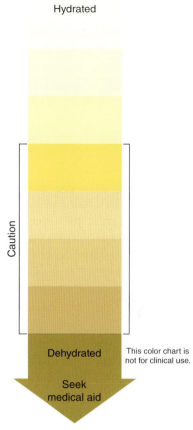

Urine Color Chart

Hydrated

Caution

Dehydrated

This color chart is not for clinical use.

Seek medical aid

Figure 8.4 An easy way to determine if you are hydrated is to check the color of your urine.

Nonessential Components: Alcohol and Caffeine

Alcohol and caffeine are not nutrients; however, both are often dietary components (U.S. Department of Health and Human Services and U.S. Department of Agriculture 2015). If you choose to consume alcohol and caffeine, similar to other aspects of your diet, you should strive to make wise choices.

Alcohol

Alcohol is a drug and must be respected for its many body-altering effects and the risk for addiction. However, the role that it plays in terms for energy balance and chronic disease is also important. Although it provides 7 calories per gram, alcohol is not considered a nutrient because it is not needed by the body. If alcohol is mixed with fruit or a sugar-sweetened beverage, the caloric content is increased. Chronic overconsumption of alcohol is a risk factor for many chronic diseases, including breast and stomach cancers, cardiovascular diseases, obesity, and fatty liver disease.

If you choose to consume alcohol, think about your alcohol consumption as a potential risk to your metabolic health and consider the recommendation of one drink or less per day for women and two drinks or less per day for men. (See figure 11.11 for what qualifies as one drink.) Remember that alcohol is a diuretic, which means it will dehydrate you. Finally, alcohol use and physical activity are not a good combination. Although many activities provide entertainment centered around the interaction between alcohol and sports, the risk of injury potentially increases due to slowed reaction times and impaired judgment. If these events take place out in the hot sun, the dehydration effects of the alcohol and the environment can be interactive and result in heat illness. Just don't do it.

Caffeine

Similar to alcohol, caffeine is also a part of our social and cultural fabric. Most of us choose caffeine to start our day and aid in performance, both mentally and physically. Caffeine is not a nutrient and does not contribute to your caloric intake; however, it is the most widely used drug worldwide. Do you consume your caffeine in sugary energy drinks, heavily sweetened coffee, or black tea? Be aware of the calorie content and added sugar in many tea and coffee drinks served at coffee shops, not to mention caffeinated sodas. More caffeine is not necessarily better for energy or mental focus; depending on your tolerance, excessive caffeine intake can actually make you less able to focus. Caffeine abuse is also related to anxiety. In moderation, which can be defined as three to five cups per day (up to 400 milligrams), caffeine can be part of a healthy diet (U.S. Department of Health and Human Services and U.S. Department of Agriculture 2015).

Common caffeinated coffee beverages include drip or brewed coffee (12 milligrams per fluid ounce [mg/fl oz]), instant coffee (8 mg/fl oz), espresso (64 mg/fl oz), and specialty beverages made from coffee or espresso (e.g., lattes). Other common sources include brewed black tea (6 mg/fl oz), brewed green tea (2 to 5 mg/fl oz), and caffeinated soda (1 to 4 mg/fl oz). Beverages within the energy drinks category have the greatest variability (3 to 35 mg/fl oz). If caffeine is added to a food, it must be included in the listed ingredients on the food label. Caffeinated beverages can vary widely in their caffeine content, so read labels carefully (U.S. Department of Health and Human Services and U.S. Department of Agriculture 2015).

The Many Benefits of a Healthy Diet

Now that you have been introduced to the primary considerations on your quest to have a balanced and clean diet, let's discuss motivational reasons for managing your behavior. Why is eating healthy important to you? Contemplate what affects your food choices, from your family traditions to your college friends, your mood and stress, or even your budget. Whatever your reasons, there are many benefits to consuming a healthy diet that can benefit you now so you can be a healthier version of yourself in the future.

Weight Management

Energy balance can be a challenge. Without understanding calorie counting and recognizing where calories are hidden in your diet, you may struggle to manage your weight. For example, many people do not recognize how many calories in their daily diet come from their drinks in the form of sweetened sodas, sport beverages, coffees, and teas. Learning about macronutrients and their associated calorie counts will help you understand the energy-in side of the energy balance equation, as explored in chapter 9.

Feeling and Performing Better

Fuel quality and hydration matter when it comes to performance, whether it is physical, mental, or social. Feeling sluggish because you are dehydrated can reduce the quality of your day. Skipping breakfast can give you a case of low blood sugar midmorning during primetime morning classes, which can make you shaky or perhaps give you a headache. Recall that your nervous system, especially your brain, uses glucose as its primary fuel source. Thus, mismanaging your blood sugar can compromise your ability to concentrate. Too much caffeine can also increase your anxiety. How you eat and drink can directly influence how you feel and how you perform.

Investment in a Healthier Future Version of Yourself

Over and above the link between dietary intake and weight management, diet has major implications for your risk of many chronic diseases, including the Big Metabolic Three and diseases related to body composition (osteoporosis, sarcopenia). Although these chronic diseases and conditions do not typically arrive until you are middle aged or an older adult, healthy eating has direct implications for the risk factors.

Nutrition Recommendations and Resources

Many types of diets can be healthy and balanced. You have many different options to accommodate your food preferences and budget. The food choices available to us on a daily basis can make it challenging to consistently make healthy choices. How do we know what and how to eat and drink to be healthy? Scientists and governmental agencies have collaborated to provide recommendations and resources to aid the design of your personal nutrition program. You can also use apps to track your efforts. Finally, in addition to making sure that you are accessing quality food sources, you are encouraged to consult a registered dietitian,

especially if you have unique dietary challenges such as food allergies.

Dietary Reference Intakes

Issued by the Food and Nutrition Board of the Institute of Medicine, the dietary reference intakes (DRI) are standards for nutrient intake that help prevent nutritional deficiencies and reduce the risk of chronic diseases (Institute of Medicine 2006).

Four specific reference values exist for recommended intakes and optimal safety:

1. *Estimated average requirements*. The intake levels for nutrients estimated to meet the needs of half of healthy individuals in a particular group.

2. *Recommended dietary allowance* **(RDA)**. The average daily level of intake sufficient to meet the nutrient requirements of nearly all healthy people (97 to 98 percent).

3. *Adequate intake*. Established when evidence is insufficient to develop an RDA and is set at a level assumed to ensure nutritional adequacy.

4. *Tolerable upper intake level*. The maximum daily allowance unlikely to cause adverse health effects.

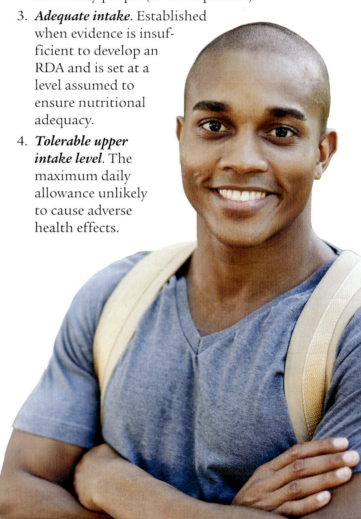

Typically lower than recommended nutrients occur; however, more is not always better and can actually be dangerous. You are encouraged to access the free interactive DRI website to determine your personal daily nutrient recommendations (https://fnic.nal.usda.gov/fnic/dri-calculator/).

Dietary Guidelines for Americans

The DRIs are very specific recommendations regarding macronutrient and micronutrient intakes. In contrast, the Dietary Guidelines for Americans (DGs) are general principles for good nutrition practices (U.S. Department of Health and Human Services and U.S. Department of Agriculture 2015). The DGs are jointly issued by the USDA and the U.S. Department of Health and Human Services (USDHHS). These guidelines are updated and revised every five years. Similar to the DRIs, the DGs are supported by extensive research and are designed to prevent chronic diseases.

Can MyPlate Be Your Plate?

Even though you may completely understand the recommendations for healthy eating, it still can feel overwhelming to put your knowledge into practice. A picture is worth a thousand words. MyPlate is the USDA's visual teaching tool for helping Americans meet their recommended intake of food groups (figure 8.5). This online source provides a wealth of information on how to make the healthy choice the easy choice. A major theme of this tool is personalization—you can customize the recommendations to fit your goals, health needs, tastes, and other factors. Some of the key messages of MyPlate are that selecting a variety of nutrient-dense foods and consuming all foods and beverages in moderation will provide a strong framework for your balanced dietary plan. Lab 8.1 will provide an opportunity to determine your basic knowledge of nutritional practices using the interactive ChooseMyPlate website.

Dietary Patterns

Several dietary patterns can provide optimal nutrition. No one dietary pattern is best for all people, but several common and complete diets are options. A key point of the DGs is that several eating patterns can be a healthy choice as long as they have (1) many nutrient-dense foods that are rich in vitamins, minerals, and other nutrients but are relatively lower in calories and (2) minimal empty-calorie foods that are high in added sugars and saturated fats. The USDA advocates that diets have balance,

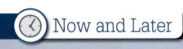

Now and Later

Calcium Intake

Now

Because of the quality of many diets, few people meet their recommended calcium intake. Some of the best calcium sources are low-fat dairy products such as milk and yogurt. If you do not like milk or are lactose intolerant, try to get calcium from other sources in your diet such broccoli or fortified orange juice. The intake recommended for young adults is 1,000 milligrams per day; this includes food and supplements (U.S. Department of Health and Human Services and U.S. Department of Agriculture 2015).

Later

The calcium recommendation increases to 1,200 milligrams per day for older men and women. Because of the loss of estrogen for women and changes in hormones that occur with the aging process for all people, bone loss rapidly increases after middle age. People with low calcium intake have accelerated bone loss.

Take Home

To reduce your risk of bone fracture later in life, build your bone bank by getting an adequate amount of calcium in your diet. If you do not like dairy or other foods that contain calcium, consider a supplement.

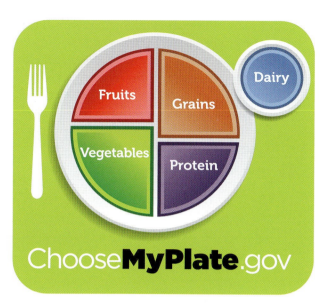

Figure 8.5 Go to ChooseMyPlate.gov to learn more about how to balance the five food groups.
USDA's Center for Nutrition Policy and Promotion.

moderation, and variety. USDA-recommended options in addition to the MyPlate model include the Healthy Mediterranean-Style Eating Pattern and the Healthy Vegetarian Eating Pattern (U.S. Department of Health and Human Services and U.S. Department of Agriculture 2015).

Mediterranean-Style Eating Pattern. This diet is characterized by patterns common in cultures of the Mediterranean region and includes frequent consumption of unsaturated fatty sources, such as seafood and olive oil, and plenty of fruits and vegetables, but not quite as much dairy as the typical American diet. The Mediterranean diet has been associated with positive health outcomes.

Healthy Vegetarian Eating Pattern. A vegetarian dietary plan has an essential difference from all other diets in that foods of animal origin are restricted (meats, poultry, fish, eggs, milk; U.S. Department of Health and Human Services and

U.S. Department of Agriculture 2015). People select vegetarian diets for health reasons, religious preferences, ethical reasons, or out of concern for the environment. These diets tend to be lower in calories, saturated fats, and cholesterol and higher in legumes, soy products, nuts and seeds, whole grains, fruits, vegetables, and fiber.

Various vegetarian diets exist. Adherents may eat only plants (vegans); plants and dairy products (lacto-vegetarians); plants, dairy products, and eggs (lacto-ovo vegetarians); or plants, dairy products, eggs, and fish or seafood (pescatarian). Some people deviate from their plan for special social occasions, due to circumstances (e.g., travel), or for occasional variety (partial or semivegetarians).

Depending on how restrictive the vegetarian plan is, there may be challenges to having a nutritionally adequate diet, especially with regard to protein, calcium, vitamin D, iron, and B vitamins, depending on whether dairy or eggs are included in the diet. Vitamin and mineral supplementation may be necessary. Consultation with a RDN may be a good idea, especially for growing children and teens, pregnant and lactating women, or people with a chronic health condition (Melina, Craig, and Levin 2016).

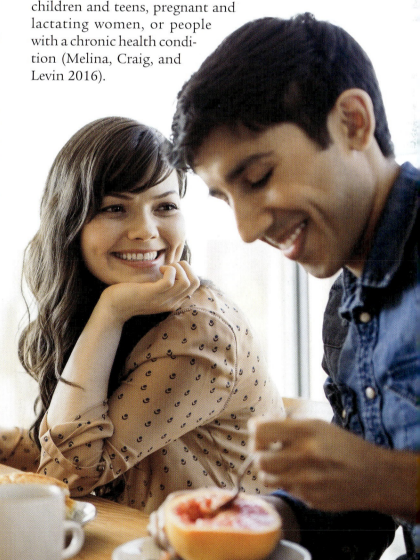

Selected Nutrients of Concern

In addition to patterns, the DGs also identify a few nutrients that are of concern given their intakes and links to chronic diseases (U.S. Department of Health and Human Services and U.S. Department of Agriculture 2015). You are advised to limit intake of the following:

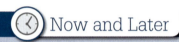 **Added sugars**. Reduce added sugars to no more than 10 percent of daily calories, or about 4 and 6 tablespoons of sugar for women and men, respectively. Americans currently consume at least double this amount.

! **Fats**. These guidelines target a reduction in saturated fats and trans fats. Given the recent food processing laws, reducing trans fats should not be a major challenge in the future. Saturated fats should be limited to less than 10 percent of daily calories. Americans obtain their saturated fats mainly from full-fat dairy products (e.g., whole milk), fast foods such as pizza and hamburgers, baked goods like cookies and cakes, as well as meat and eggs.

! **Sodium**. Adults should consume no more than 2,300 milligrams of sodium on a daily basis. Packaged or convenience foods are the main source of sodium, in addition to what is that added during cooking or at the table with the saltshaker.

Replacing foods that are high in added sugars, fats, and sodium with more fruits, vegetables,

---

Now and Later

Sustaining You and the Earth

Now

Choosing to consume a diet closer to a vegetarian and Mediterranean diet can save you saturated fat calories and money, if you prepare your food at home. For example, a large pot of bean soup can be relatively inexpensive to make in your Crock-Pot compared to a similar amount of a beef stew.

Later

Small choices add up over time for your waistline, arteries, and your pocketbook. These small choices also add up for our environment. For example, Americans could reduce their diet's environmental footprint just by eating less meat and dairy. Beef and dairy cattle and the food products that end up on your dinner table are very environmentally expensive in terms of land use, water use, greenhouse gas emissions, and, ultimately, ecosystem disruption.

Take Home

On your way to being a healthier you, remember to think socially when acting personally. Food choices affect your health, but they also have major long-term effects on our planet. This does not mean that everyone should be a vegetarian; however, by making small changes, you can be healthier and help our planet, too. For example, try meatless Mondays or eat only plant-based foods for one day per week. This could not only increase your fruit and vegetable intake but help you discover some new favorite dishes as well.

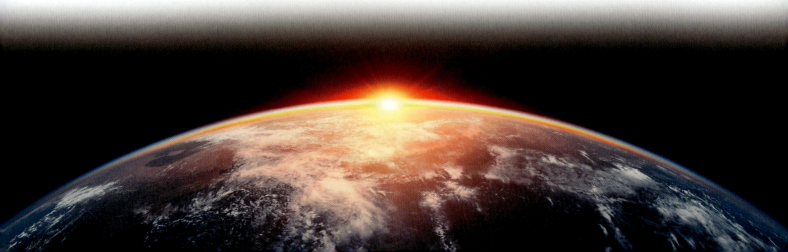

whole grains, and low-fat dairy foods will go a long way toward improving your diet quality. Try to find opportunities to practice subbing in healthy foods.

Reading Food Labels

The FDA requires labeling for all packaged foods. Food labels are not required on fresh meat, poultry, fish, fruits, and vegetables, although you can find nutrient information for these foods on the USDA website. One way to meet the recommendations highlighted in MyPlate is to select unprocessed foods. Dried beans and nuts, fresh or frozen fruits and vegetables, low-fat dairy, whole grains such as brown rice and oatmeal, and lean, fresh meats are all examples of nutrient-dense foods that likely do not have extensive food-label ingredient lists.

Food Labels Provide Nutrient Facts

In the next few years, all food manufacturers will need to comply with a new rule passed in 2016 by the FDA, which will require an updated food-label format (see figure 8.6; U.S. Food and Drug Administration 2017a). The five mandatory requirements for all food labels are statement of identity (what is the product), net contents of package, nutrition information, list of ingredients in order of largest to smallest percentage, and manufacturer information. Based on recommendations by experts, the following changes were made:

- Calories and serving size fonts are enlarged.
- Calories from fat were removed.
- Added sugars are now clearly listed.
- Vitamins C and A are no longer required.
- Vitamin D and potassium have been added to iron and calcium, and the micronutrient amounts are listed.

Lab 8.2 in the web study guide will give you an opportunity to practice your food label reading skills.

The translation of the DRIs and DGs are further accomplished for the consumer by FDA laws that govern communicated dietary standards to the public, most recognizable in the form of daily values. This is most evident on food labels where the daily values represent appropriate intakes for a 2,000-calorie diet, expressed as a percentage.

Food Package Nutrient and Health Claims

Knowing food label language can also greatly assist you on your trip to the grocery store.

Food-labeling regulations by the FDA require that products meet very distinct definitions before they can make the following types of food-packaging claims.

- *Health claim and a qualified health claim*. These indicate that a food or ingredient helps to reduce the risk of a disease or health-related condition (e.g., "Adequate calcium throughout life may reduce the risk of osteoporosis.").
- *Structure or function claim*. This indicates that a nutrient has an effect on the normal structure or function of the body (e.g., "Calcium builds strong bones.").
- *Nutrient content claim*. This makes a statement about the level of a nutrient in a product (e.g., "Excellent source of calcium."). The majority of claims on food packages are nutrient content claims.

Nutrient content claims can be very confusing. Commonly used terms include *free*, *low*, *reduced* or *less*, *healthy*, *light*, *high*, *good source*, *more*, *lean* or *extra lean*, *high potency*, *modified*, *fiber source*, and *antioxidants*. Many of these terms can be applied to different products or foods targeting calories, fat, cholesterol, or sodium. For current information, go to the FDA website and review the Nutrition Labeling and Education Act (U.S. Food and Drug Administration 2014).

Common Dietary Limitations: Allergies and Intolerances

Having allergies or intolerances to various food sources is common. Food allergies often start early in life and may be outgrown, while others can develop in adulthood. They occur when your body's immune system reacts to a substance, most often a protein within a food. Signs of a food allergy are similar to other allergies, ranging from a runny nose or itchy eyes to a major life-threatening anaphylactic event (i.e., cannot breathe; Wolfram 2017).

A food intolerance is not the same as a food allergy. The symptoms are not comfortable (generally

Nutrition Facts

Serving Size 1 cup (228g)
Servings Per Container about 2

Amount Per Serving

Calories 250	Calories from Fat 110

	% Daily Value*
Total Fat 12g	18%
Saturated Fat 3g	15%
Trans Fat 3g	
Cholesterol 30mg	10%
Sodium 470mg	20%
Total Carbohydrate 31g	10%
Dietary Fiber 0g	0%
Sugars 5g	
Proteins 5g	
Vitamin A	4%
Vitamin C	2%
Calcium	20%
Iron	4%

* Percent Daily Values are based on a 2,000 calorie diet. Your Daily Values may be higher or lower depending on your calorie needs:

	Calories:	2,000	2,500
Total Fat	Less than	65g	80g
Saturated Fat		Less than	20g 25g
Cholesterol	Less than	300mg	300mg
Sodium	Less than	2,400mg	2,400mg
Total Carbohydrate		300g	375g

For educational purposes only. This label does not meet the labeling requirements described in 21 CFR 101.9.

① Serving size

This section is the basis for determining number of calories, amount of each nutrient, and %DVs of a food. Use it to compare a serving size to how much you actually eat. Serving sizes are given in familiar units, such as cups or pieces, followed by the metric amount, e.g., number of grams.

② Amount of calories

If you want to manage your weight (lose, gain, or maintain), this section is especially helpful. The amount of calories is listed on the left side. The right side shows how many calories in one serving come from fat. In this example, there are 250 calories, 110 of which come from fat. The key is to balance how many calories you eat with how many calories your body uses. *Tip: Remember that a product that's fat-free isn't necessarily calorie-free.*

③ Limit these nutrients

Eating too much total fat (including saturated fat and trans fat), cholesterol, or sodium may increase your risk of certain chronic diseases, such as heart disease, some cancers, or high blood pressure. The goal is to stay below 100%DV for each of these nutrients per day.

④ Get enough of these nutrients

Americans often don't get enough dietary fiber, vitamin A, vitamin C, calcium, and iron in their diets. Eating enough of these nutrients may improve your health and help reduce the risk of some diseases and conditions.

⑤ Percent (%) daily values (DVs)

This section tells you whether the nutrients (total fat, sodium, dietary fiber, etc.) in one serving of food contribute a little or a lot to your total daily diet.

The %DVs are based on a 2,000-calorie diet. Each listed nutrient is based on 100% of the recommended amounts for that nutrient. For example, 18% for total fat means that one serving furnishes 18% of the total amount of fat that you could eat in a day and stay within public health recommendations. Use the Quick Guide to Percent DV (%DV): 5%DV or less is low and 20%DV or more is high.

⑥ Footnote with daily values (DVs)

The footnote provides information about the DVs for important nutrients, including fats, sodium, and fiber. The DVs are listed for people who eat 2,000 or 2,500 calories each day.

– The amounts for total fat, saturated fat, cholesterol, and sodium are maximum amounts. That means you should try to stay below the amounts listed.

Figure 8.6 Everything you need to know about the new FDA nutrition label.
Reprinted from U.S. Food and Drug Administration (2018).

include abdominal cramping and diarrhea), but they are not life-threatening, although they could lead to dietary deficiencies if left untreated (Wolfram 2017).

Although many types of food allergies are known, nearly 90 percent are related to what are commonly thought of as the Big Eight:

- Milk and eggs
- Shellfish (shrimp, lobster, crab) and fish (pollock, salmon, cod, tuna, snapper, eel, tilapia)
- Peanuts and tree nuts (walnuts, cashews)
- Wheat and soy

Gluten deserves a special mention given the recent interest in it and the range of conditions associated with it. The gluten-sensitivity spectrum ranges from an allergy to an intolerance to celiac disease. Gluten is a protein found in common cereal grains, mainly wheat, barley, rye, and spelt. Symptoms depend on the degree of sensitivity, ranging from mild allergy symptoms and diarrhea to more intensive digestive distress to headaches, muscle and joint pain, fatigue, and an increased risk for small-intestine destruction and cancer. Increased research and public attention to gluten sensitivity has created greater awareness, and many gluten-free products may be found in the marketplace. If you suspect you have an intolerance, consult your physician and consider a screening for diagnosis. Although a gluten-free diet is currently very popular, it is neither intended for weight loss nor is it nutritionally superior.

If you suspect or know you have a food allergy or intolerance, several steps can improve your quality of life:

- *Meet with a registered dietitian nutritionist.* An RDN can assist you with designing an eating plan that is nutritionally adequate and meets your lifestyle.

- *Learn about ingredients in your food.* Navigating menu items and dishes, especially when foods include a combination of ingredients, can be challenging. Ask questions and do your research.

- *Read labels carefully.* The FDA has mandated that food companies specify on product labels if foods contain any of the Big Eight allergens.

- *Inform friends and family.* Explain your food allergy so that your friends and family can accommodate your food requirements during social gatherings. This is especially critical if your allergy causes a life-threatening reaction.

Although you may choose a gluten-free diet for a variety of reasons, it is not necessarily nutritionally superior.

Dietary Supplements

Supplement sales are a big business. Dietary supplements include vitamins, minerals, herbals and botanicals, amino acids, enzymes, and many other products. They can also come in a variety of forms: traditional tablets, capsules, and powders, as well as drinks and energy bars. Before supplementing, think carefully and check with your physician or an RDN. Remember that some supplements can cause damage to your health.

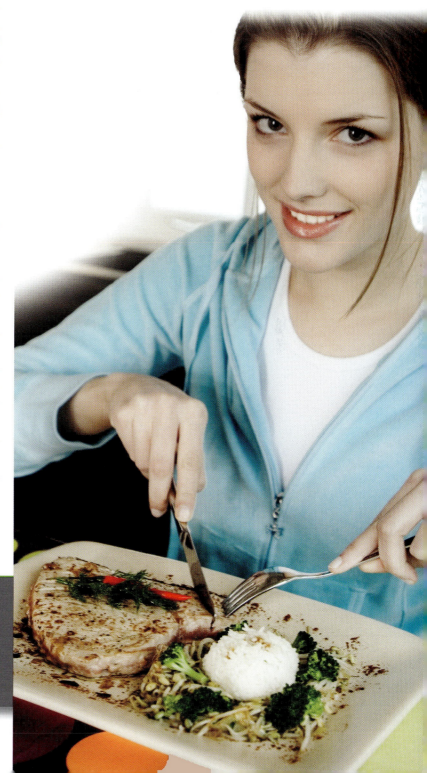

When Is a Supplement Needed?

Although a balanced dietary plan is the best way to meet your optimal vitamin and mineral needs, a supplement is needed in certain situations:

- Women of childbearing age who are planning to become pregnant should consume adequate amounts of folate or folic acid (synthetic form) to prevent neural tube defects in the baby.
- People who are older than 50 often have a reduced ability to absorb B12. In addition to eating foods that supply this important vitamin, they may need supplements.
- Women with heavy menstrual cycles may need additional iron to prevent anemia.
- Older people, those with dark skin, or people who remain indoors most of their days may need vitamin D supplementation.
- Vegans may need B_{12}, calcium, and iron supplementation.

Supplements Are Not Regulated by the FDA

The FDA does not regulate dietary supplements (U.S. Food and Drug Administration 2017b). In fact, manufacturers do not have to prove a supplement is safe or effective before selling it. The FDA can take action to remove or restrict the sale of a supplement after it has been on the market and has been proven unsafe. For this reason, consumers should exercise caution when choosing to use any supplements.

Manufacturers of supplements can voluntarily test their products for quality control. Those that meet the USP Dietary Supplement Verification Services are awarded the USP verified mark, which assists

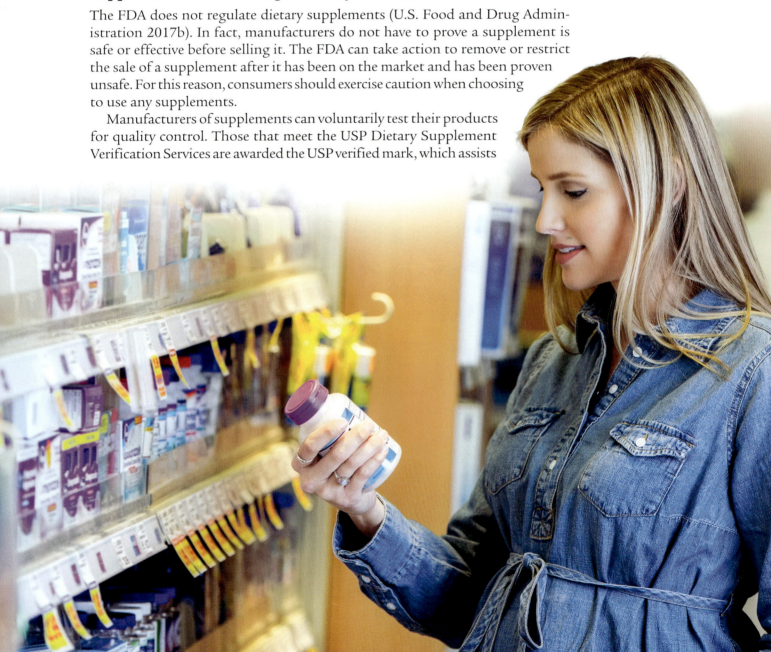

suppliers and consumers in determining quality. However, if a company does not pay for these services, this does not necessarily mean that their product is inferior. For more information, see www.usp.org/about.

Protein Supplements

Although young, healthy, recreationally active adults with good dietary habits do not need protein supplements, these products are popular. Protein supplements are typically delivered in bars or powders and come from either soy or whey protein. Soy protein powder contains protein isolated from the soybean and made from the soybean meal. Whey is obtained from dairy milk processing. There are also differences between protein isolates and concentrates in terms of the grams of protein, and often of the carbohydrate and fat, they contain. For example, for people who are lactose intolerant or struggle to digest dairy products, whey isolate may provide benefits because it is low in lactose. Remember, too much protein can be hazardous to your health. If you decide to use protein supplements, do your research and read labels carefully, since many protein bars on the market have a lot of added sugar.

Food Safety Basics

Food allergies and intolerances are a concern for some people, but food safety is everyone's concern. If you have ever suffered from food poisoning, you understand how sick you can get from contaminated food. The federal government provides excellent resources to help keep you safe with regard to food practices. They advocate these four simple steps for food safety (see www.foodsafety.gov for more information):

1. *Clean*. Wash your hands and surfaces often! Illness-causing bacteria can survive in many places around the kitchen. Unless you wash your hands, utensils, and surfaces the correct way, you could spread these bacteria.

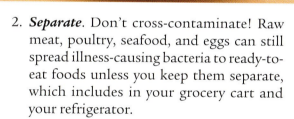

2. *Separate*. Don't cross-contaminate! Raw meat, poultry, seafood, and eggs can still spread illness-causing bacteria to ready-to-eat foods unless you keep them separate, which includes in your grocery cart and your refrigerator.

3. *Cook*. Cook to the right temperature! The danger zone for bacteria that cause food poisoning is between 40 and 140 degrees Fahrenheit (4 to 60 degrees Celsius). Bacteria multiply quickly, so knowing the right temperatures for various foods and cooking methods is essential.

4. *Chill*. Refrigerate promptly! Illness-causing bacteria can grow in foods within two hours, especially in a warm environment. Therefore, cooling foods promptly is critical. Keep meat and dairy consistently cool by placing them near the back of fridge.

See figure 8.7 for tips on planning wisely and choosing carefully in order to keep you on the right path as you design your personal diet plan.

Healthy Choices Require Planning

The more you plan ahead in terms of will power, food purchasing, and preparation, the more you will be able to stick to a healthy diet. Making the healthy choice on a routine basis while managing a complicated daily schedule will require you to invest some thought and action into your nutritional plan.

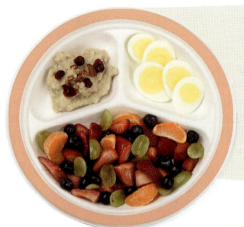

Start With Breakfast

Healthy fueling should be part of your planning. An important fuel of the day is typically breakfast. Know yourself. If you need a good breakfast to feel and perform well, plan the time to invest in this behavior.

Plan Your Fuel To-Do List

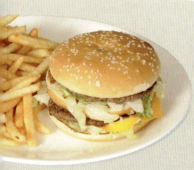

Stressful week of exams coming up! My main goals:

• Eat out only once this week. Eat homemade meals or at the dining hall the rest of the time.

• Plan all my meals so I don't overeat or overspend.

• Stay in budget at the grocery store.

• Pack healthy snacks and water in my backpack.

Plan for Healthy Eating at the Dining Hall

• Plan ahead of time what you will eat and make up your mind to stick with that plan.
• If you know you will be spending a long time at the dining hall, make a plan for how much you will eat and at what times. This will help you avoid mindless eating.
• Apply the knowledge you have gained from this chapter to your choices of food in the dining hall.

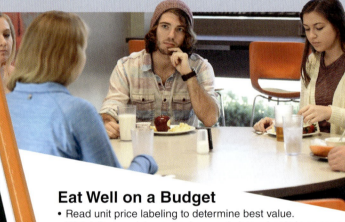

Eat Well on a Budget

• Read unit price labeling to determine best value.
• Watch for specials on produce and shop what is in season.
• Try frozen vegetables: They are just as nutritious as fresh and decrease likelihood of spoiling if they are not consumed right away.
• If storage is available, purchase frequently consumed foods in bulk.
• Make a grocery list and avoid shopping when you are hungry
• Share spices, condiments, and other pantry staples with roommates and alternate preparing meals.
• Invest in a slow cooker so you can make large batches of food to refrigerator freeze for later meals.
• If you notice that some fruits are not getting used, wash and dry them thoroughly and freeze for later use in smoothies, pancakes, breads, or oatmeal.
• Buy meat in bulk and freeze what you won't be able to use right away.
• Choose water instead of soda, sweet tea, or fruit-flavored beverages.

Avoid Fast-Food Foibles

Fast food is generally not a healthy choice, but we turn to that option when we haven't planned ahead. In addition, fast food can cost two or three times more than eating at home. Plan ahead by buying ingredients to make quick and easy food. For example:

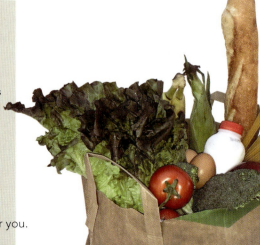

• Tortillas, shredded cheese, and sausage to make breakfast burritos
• Fresh vegetables put into containers for grab and go with hummus or cottage cheese dip
• Baked potatoes stuffed with salsa, broccoli, and low-fat cheese or cottage cheese
• Canned black or red beans heated and eaten over rice with low-fat cheese sprinkled on top

Eating out has a place in your life, but it should be the treat for the week, not a daily occurrence.

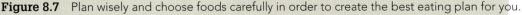

Figure 8.7 Plan wisely and choose foods carefully in order to create the best eating plan for you.

Consult sources endorsed by scientific and government agencies for the highest quality information.

Be Informed to Make the Best Food Decisions

No one diet is best. Most of the time, eating well really means making high-quality fuel choices. This starts with accessing quality information. The food marketplace can be overwhelming with the choices and marketing strategies. Be a smart consumer by consulting trusted and reliable sources and knowing the difference between trends and facts.

- United States Department of Agriculture (USDA)
- Food and Drug Administration (FDA)
- The Food and Nutrition Board
- The Academy of Nutrition and Dietetics

Who Should I Trust to Advise Me?

It is important to know the difference between a "nutritionist" and a Registered dietitian (RD) or Licensed dietitian (LD), which are sometimes abbreviated as a registered dietitian nutritionist (RDN).

Registered Dietitian	Nutritionist
Education and training established by the Accreditation Council for Education in Nutrition and Dietetics	
Bachelor's degree with a specifically designed curriculum	Anyone can call themselves a nutritionist
Must complete an extensive internship	
Must pass a rigorous registration examination	

Are Whole Foods Better?

It depends. Some food processing is healthy because it increases shelf life. However, packaged or processed foods often give you more of the bad stuff and less of the good stuff.

Read food labels. Compared to a processed food, eating the whole food version typically provides more vitamins and minerals, fiber, and healthy fats and less sodium, added sugars, and preservatives. If the ingredient list is long, chances are there are healthier alternatives.

Should I Choose Organic and Non-GMO Foods?

Before you spend the extra money on an organic and non-GMO product, are these foods healthier than conventional foods?

Organics

Although it is intuitive that organic foods might be healthier and prevent chronic diseases, at this time research does not support organic foods as being more nutritionally healthful than conventional foods. However, a consumer may choose to purchase organic foods due to other perceived benefits such as supporting small farms and decreasing overall pesticide use in the environment.

GMOs

Non-GMO foods have recently become a major consumer demand. Genetic modification techniques allow for introduction of new traits or greater control of other traits to increase the efficient use of natural resources, resistance to diseases, or nutrient profiles. There is no scientific consensus that currently available GMO crops pose any health risk compared to conventional food. However, public concerns are ongoing. The longer term effects have not been studied as GMO foods have only been on the market for a few decades.

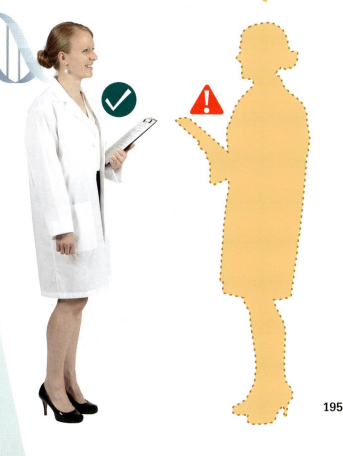

195

Summary

Having a high-quality diet on most days of your college life will require you to have a fundamental understanding of your personal macronutrient (protein, carbohydrate, and fat), micronutrient (vitamins and minerals), fiber, and hydration needs. Although many people think of diet as calories or energy intake, eating a high-quality diet can greatly influence how you feel and perform, academically and socially, as well as prevent many chronic diseases and conditions later in life. The government and other scientific organizations provide many guidelines and quality resources to assist you in planning a healthy diet. Being able to determine quality foods, supplements, and resources as a smart and informed consumer will be essential to maintaining your health. Finally, beyond physiological needs, food is meant to be enjoyed as a source of pleasure and is an important part of our social lives. Practice the primary principles of moderation, variety, and balance to ensure a healthy diet.

www WEB STUDY GUIDE

Remember to complete all of the web study guide activities to further facilitate your learning, including the following lab activities:

Lab 8.1   ChooseMyPlate Quiz

Lab 8.2   Practicing Reading Food Labels

REVIEW QUESTIONS

1. List the three macronutrients along with the recommended amount of each in the daily diet in terms of percent of caloric intake (as a range). List three food sources that best represent each macronutrient group.

2. Explain why fiber is so important for health, the two primary types of fiber, and two food sources of each type.

3. List several factors that influence daily water intake needs. Describe three strategies that can enhance your daily hydration levels. What is an easy test to determine if you are adequately hydrated?

4. Do you need a vitamin or mineral supplement to be healthy? Describe a few situations where a supplement might be needed to enhance health.

5. List and describe key resources that you might access to obtain quality information based on scientific evidence to inform your dietary selections.

6. Being a smart consumer spans health and budget concerns. Describe five key strategies for eating clean and well that will also allow you to stay on budget.

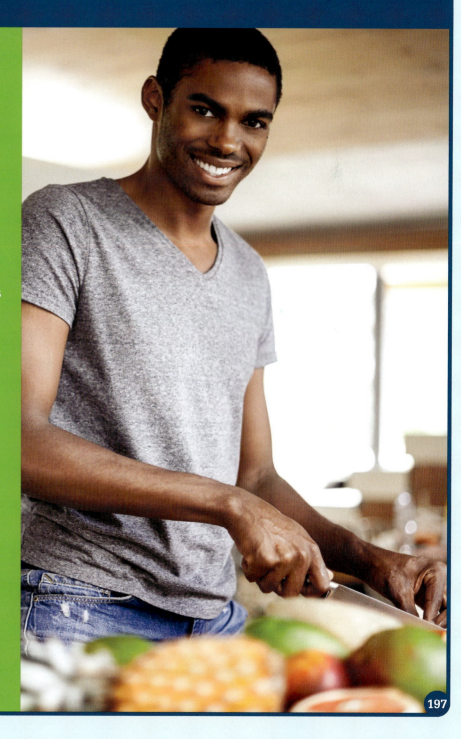

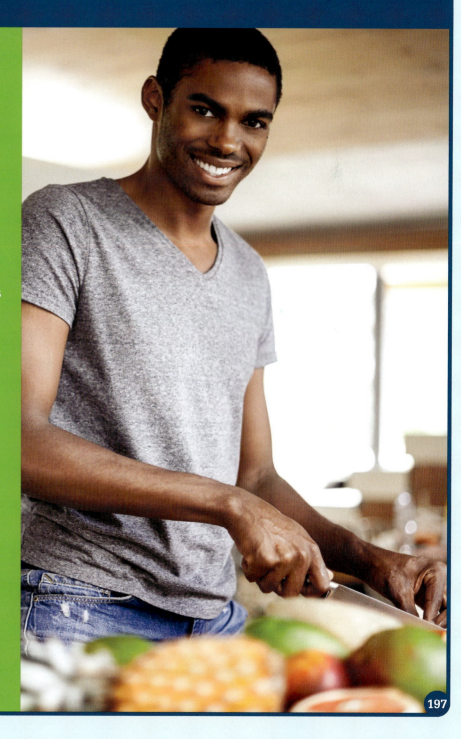

Weight Management

OBJECTIVES

❱ Recognize that obesity is the greatest health challenge of our modern times and understand how it affects health.

❱ Know the primary factors that contribute to weight status.

❱ Learn energy balance principles that influence weight status on a short-term and long-term basis.

❱ Become familiar with weight-management strategies that are useful for all weight statuses and life stages.

❱ Respect that regular exercise and physical activity are critical for weight management for most people.

❱ Understand that weight management can cause psychological distress and that a healthy body image is important for long-term physical and mental health.

❱ Recognize when professional help may be needed for weight-management issues and learn the resources that are available.

KEY TERMS

anorexia

binge-eating disorder

body dysmorphic disorder

body image

bulimia nervosa

energy balance

energy density

exercise addiction

glycemic index

muscle dysmorphia

obesity

obesogenic environment

overweight

resting metabolic rate (RMR)

satiety

thermic effect of activity (TEA)

thermic effect of meals (TEM)

We think about healthy weight management a lot. Weight management is not only a critical public health issue, but it can also cause a significant amount of psychological distress. Whether you are trying to prevent weight gain, lose weight, or maintain weight loss, managing both sides of the **energy balance** equation can be a struggle. Weight management means far more than looking good or feeling good about the way you look. Being overweight or obese links to a long list of physical and mental conditions and diseases. This chapter provides a social–cultural perspective of weight management that can be applied to your life. It also discusses weight-management strategies to help you balance your personal energy balance equation, with a special highlight on the importance of energy expenditure. Our final focus is on psychological concerns regarding weight management. Specific information about how to get help for yourself or a friend is included.

Weight Management: Our Greatest Modern Health Challenge

Current prevalence data for **overweight** and **obesity** indicate that approximately 70 percent of American adults are overweight and 38 percent are obese (Centers for Disease Control and Prevention 2016). Figure 9.1 shows the prevalence of obesity in the United States by sex and age. Importantly, obesity affects all sectors of the population, including children, all over the world. On average, people gain weight as they age until becoming an older adult,

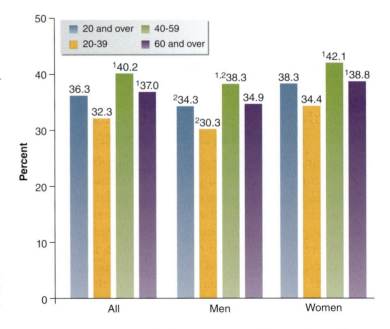

Figure 9.1 Prevalence of obesity among adults aged 20 and over, by sex and age, United States, 2011 to 2014.

[1]Significantly different from those aged 20 to 39.

[2]Significantly different from women of the same age group.

NOTES: Totals were age adjusted by the direct method to the 2000 U.S. census population using the age groups 20 to 39, 40 to 59, and 60 and over. Crude estimates are 36.5 percent for all, 34.5 percent for men, and 38.5 percent for women.

Reprinted from C.L. Ogden et al., "Prevalence of Obesity Among Adults and Youth: United States, 2011-2014," NCHS Data Brief 207 (2015): 1-8.

If about 70 percent of the population is overweight or obese, why is 30 percent able to maintain a normal weight? Beyond inheriting good genes, most people who are successful in managing their weight eat a clean and balanced diet and regularly spend energy by being active (Hill and Wyatt 2013).

when late in life they typically lose weight. Thus, when people become overweight or obese early in life, they will likely struggle to manage their weight their entire lifetime, although a sustained change in lifestyle can alter this course. The energy balance equation, which is explained further later, is very simple in concept: Energy in – energy out = weight status. However, the factors that influence our eating and moving habits and patterns are very complicated. The causes of obesity are multifactorial. What causes one person to be overweight compared to another is unique and personal. This chapter reviews some strong themes related to weight management to help you make better decisions.

Obesity: A Disease Linked to Many Other Diseases and Conditions

Obesity has been defined as a disease by the American Medical Association. Although overweight and obesity are diagnosed using body mass index (BMI) and waist circumference (see table 7.1), the state of being obese is strongly associated with being "overfat." As chapter 7 explains, the storage of too much fat, especially in the abdominal region, is strongly linked to many other conditions. Therefore, the behaviors that lead to the state of overweight or obese—poor nutrition and a sedentary lifestyle, in addition to the excess fat storage in the body—are linked to many diseases and conditions spanning both physical and psychosocial domains (Centers for Disease Control and Prevention 2017), as shown in figure 9.2.

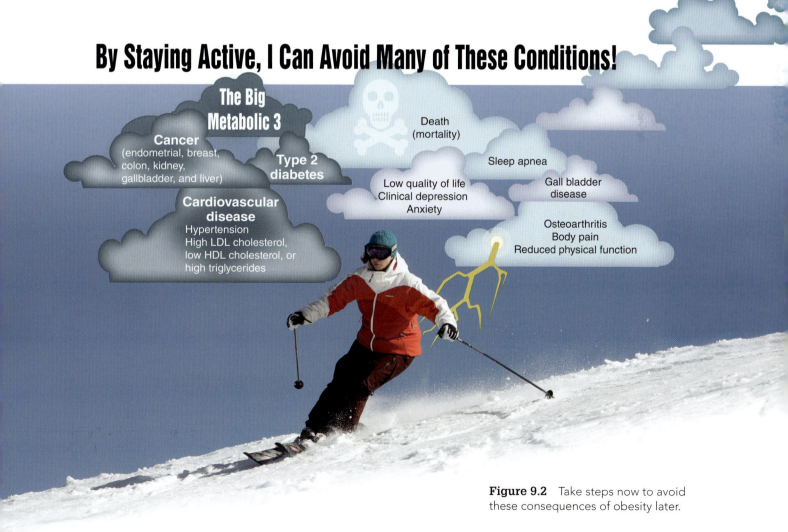

Figure 9.2 Take steps now to avoid these consequences of obesity later.

Think Socially, Act Personally

The struggle to manage weight causes a great deal of emotional distress and human suffering. How do we think socially and act personally? Inadequate weight management is often due to a mismatch between our genetics and our ability to adapt to societal changes. With all of its comorbidities, obesity is currently challenging health care costs and will continue to have major effects in the future. From a social perspective, two major demographic shifts in our modern society will influence our health care system.

1. Because more people are obese at a younger age, chronic diseases and conditions arrive earlier in life. For example, hypertension and type 2 diabetes mellitus used to be very rare in young adults but now are more common.

2. Older adults are predicted to outnumber young adults in the decades to come. This demographic shift, coupled with people becoming obese younger, will lead to a significant percentage of the population living with chronic conditions.

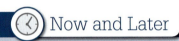 Now and Later

Obesity, Functional Fitness, and Quality of Life

Now

Have you thought about what it means to be functional? The concept of functional fitness applies to various aspects of life. Functional fitness spans from mental (cognitive) to psychosocial to physical abilities. Just as physical activity and exercise play key roles in functional fitness, obesity affects your ability to function daily with zest and joy.

Later

Obesity at any age is problematic for health. However, for older adults, obesity has major implications for physical function, especially of the lower body, which leads to reductions in walking function and increases risk for physical disability. Obesity in older adults is a major risk factor for admission to an assisted care facility. Do you have a grandparent who is in an assisted care facility? Why did they end up there? Was it due to diseases of the heart or their joint conditions? Did they get arthritis or have uncontrolled diabetes? Did they simply lack the strength to be able to move their own body weight?

Take Home

Although it can be very challenging to think about your weight, you will go a long way toward preventing physical disability throughout your life span if you pay attention to weight management early in life. From a practical perspective, later in life, you may be able to retain your independence longer if you manage your weight.

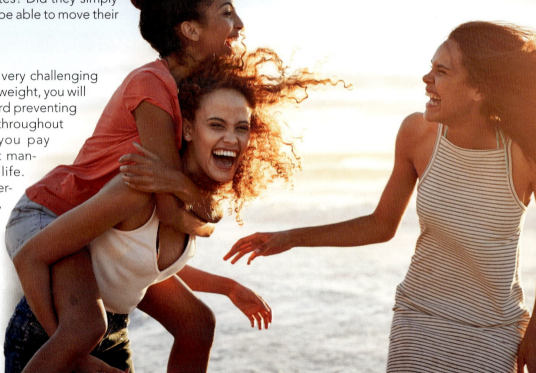

Poor lifestyle choices that result in obesity, when coupled with our aging society, will greatly strain our health care system in terms of quality, low-cost delivery. As you work to manage your weight, think of the benefits to yourself as well as the world (figure 9.3). We are all in this weight management struggle together.

Genetics + Modern Society = Energy Imbalance

Obesity scholars believe we are challenged to manage our weight because we are living in an obesogenic environment (Bouchard and Katzmarzyk 2010). This means that we have a mismatch between our genetics and our technologically advanced society. Long ago, we lived in a society where our food supply was unpredictable and sometimes scarce. Because of this, we were required to be physically active, mainly to seek food and shelter and avoid being someone else's lunch. However, our environment has undergone enormous changes since those very early days. We now have a very complicated social structure and a built environment. These changes have produced what is termed an **obesogenic environment**, where it is very easy (behaviorally speaking) to overeat high-calorie, tasty food, have minimal physical activity, and sit too much. Our biological predisposition to engage in these behaviors creates a positive energy balance, so keeping our weight in a healthy range can be a constant challenge.

If you struggle with weight management, think of your challenge as a universal problem as well as a personal challenge. This does not mean you should not take personal responsibility for your weight-management behaviors, but recognize that you are not alone in your struggles. There are very valid evolutionary reasons for your current situation. Alternatively, if you are a person who rarely struggles to manage your weight, resist the urge to be smug about your normal weight state. Although you live in the same social and built environment as your overweight and obese friends, chances are that you do not have the biological predisposition to overeat or remain inactive, or maybe you learned behavior-management techniques at an earlier age, which are now just a normal part of your behavioral patterns.

Your Family Tree: Nature and Nurture

The heritability of BMI is estimated to be 40 to 70 percent, which means that about half of your weight status and body composition can be attributed to your genes and the other half to environmental influences. (Bray et al. 2016). Links between your family tree and the chance that you will be obese have been discovered for body size, body-fat storage depot (Are you an apple or a pear?), resting metabolic rate, and how challenging it is to gain or lose weight, plus many other factors. However, you probably know families where the parents are obese and the children are not, or vice versa, which suggests that although some of the risk of obesity is inherited, it can be altered through lifestyle choices.

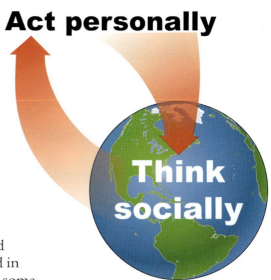

Figure 9.3   As you work to manage your weight, consider how your personal actions affect those around you.

We have engineered physical movement out of our daily lives by creating a built environment that includes more buildings, less green space, and automobile transportation.

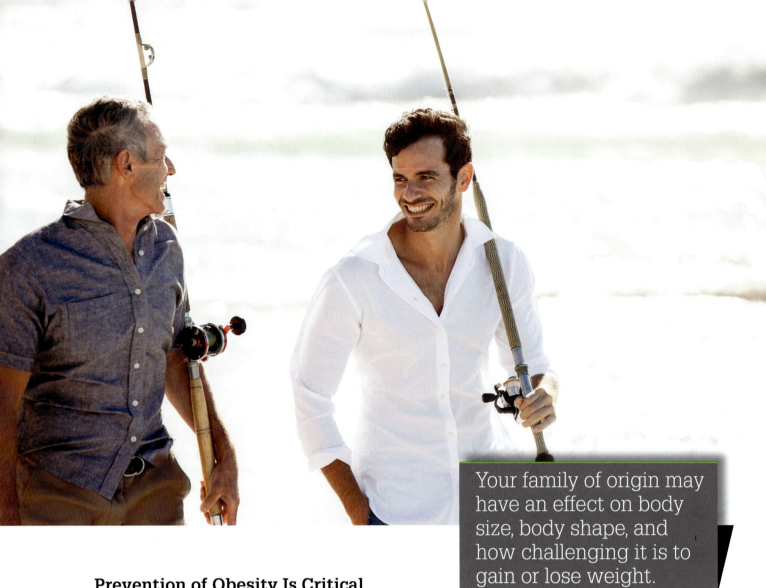

Your family of origin may have an effect on body size, body shape, and how challenging it is to gain or lose weight.

Prevention of Obesity Is Critical

Much research and public health efforts have targeted obesity prevention in younger people. This helps to reduce the risk of associated comorbidities occurring at an earlier age and prevent various social issues such as low self-esteem. However, another important reason to prevent obesity in adolescents is because once a person is obese, it becomes very challenging to ever obtain normal weight status. Also, the longer a person is obese, the lower the chance he or she could ever obtain a normal weight, so a person who has been obese since childhood will likely still be challenged by weight management as a middle-aged or older adult (Reinehr 2017).

The normal trajectory for weight change is to gain a small amount of weight each year after young adulthood (see figure 9.4). Greater than 90% of both men and women gain weight every year moving into a higher BMI category (e.g., normal weight to overweight or overweight to

obese) by middle-age (Malhotra et al. 2013) These weight changes can be larger or smaller due to many life events that affect hormones (e.g., pregnancy, menopause), health status (e.g., cancer), or psychosocial well-being (e.g., grief, stress). Any major weight change (gain or loss) that cannot be explained by behavior such as a new exercise program or dietary program should be checked by a physician to rule out other diseases or conditions.

A sweet spot exists in weight and weight behavior monitoring that needs to be acknowledged. Because weight gain is the normal pattern in our obesogenic society, it is important to intentionally monitor your weight status, as described in chapter 7. However, being hypervigilant about your weight and related behaviors suggests an eating disorder or exercise addiction, which can compromise your physical and mental health. Try to stay in the sweet spot of weight monitoring where you

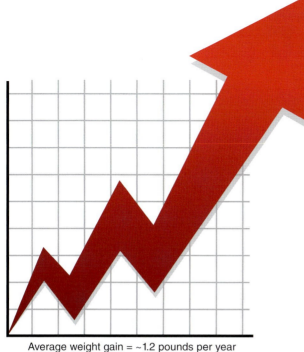

Average weight gain = ~1.2 pounds per year

Figure 9.4   Weight-gain trajectory.

are aware of your weight-management behaviors but are not obsessive about them. That way, when you get off track, you can notice it in a relatively short period of time and make corrections to get back in energy balance.

Energy Balance Math

Trying to remain in energy balance (see figure 9.5) is challenging without a firm understanding of the fundamentals that influence the equation. Most people understand the energy-in side of the equation, at least conceptually. The energy-out part is a bit more complicated. Remember as you start to assess the math of your personal energy balance equation that it is highly variable. Losing weight requires a disruption of the energy balance equation; more energy needs to be going out than coming in. Alternatively, gaining weight requires a greater amount of energy coming in than going out. Keep in mind that how you unbalance the energy balance equation can have a major effect on your body composition, including your muscles and bones.

Energy In

As discussed in chapter 8, the macronutrients vary in their energy content on a gram basis. Carbohydrate, protein, alcohol (not considered an essential nutrient), and fat provide 4 to 9 calories per gram. On your quest to balance calories in with energy spent, don't forget about diet quality, especially macronutrient balance. For example, diets that are higher in fiber, have a higher protein content, or have a lower **glycemic index** are linked to **satiety**, which theoretically should help align your energy intake with your energy expenditure (Tremblay and Bellisle 2015). Certain carbohydrates are higher on the glycemic index, which means they raise your blood sugar more quickly than other carbohydrate foods. In general, refined sugars and breads have a higher glycemic index than vegetables and whole grains. Relatedly, carbohydrate foods that are found in nature have a much lower glycemic index than those of refined and packaged foods.

Energy density is also a main factor to consider. Regularly consuming foods with a greater energy density makes weight management more challenging. Energy density refers to the number of calories per gram of food. If you choose foods relatively low in calories, you can have larger portions and more of them. Foods with a low energy density have a high water content, such as soups or foods that absorb water during cooking like rice. Foods with a high energy density are typically high in fat and sugar and have a low water content. Examples include cheese, peanuts, and sweets.

As chapter 8 describes, fuel quality matters. Eating clean (on most days) is very important for long-term weight management. Because most foods and beverages are mixed in their macronutrient content, detecting calories can be challenging. It requires education, attention, discipline, and maybe even a really great app! Reducing energy intake is a key strategy for weight loss. Compared to energy expenditure, most people find it easier to reduce their dietary intake than to spend the same amount of energy engaging in exercise or physical activity.

Energy Out

Energy expenditure can be categorized into the three components of resting metabolic rate, thermic effect of activity (TEA), which requires skeletal muscle contraction and movement, and food processing costs. Excluding highly trained endurance athletes, most people spend the most energy on a daily basis through resting metabolic

Energy Balance

Weight management is really an issue of energy balance:

Energy In – Energy Out = Weight Status

FUEL QUALITY MATTERS

Eating "clean" on most days—that is, eating whole foods, or foods that are minimally processed or refined that contain little added sugar or sodium—is very important for long-term weight management.

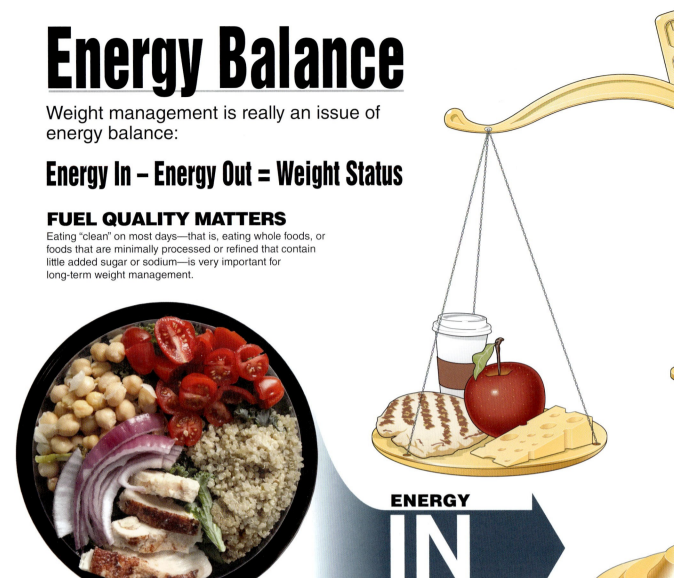

ENERGY

IN

GLYCEMIC INDEX

High glycemic index foods are those that raise blood sugar more quickly, like refined sugars and breads. It's better to choose foods with a lower glycemic index, like vegetables and whole grains. Foods with a lower glycemic index help you balance your blood sugar better and avoid low blood sugar, which typically triggers eating.

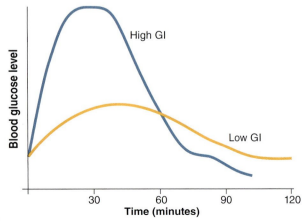

High GI

Low GI

Blood glucose level

30 60 90 120
Time (minutes)

Soup

Cheese

LOW

HIGH

Rice

Sweets

Nuts

ENERGY DENSITY

Energy density refers to the number of calories per gram of food. Consuming lower energy density foods means you can have higher portions with a relatively low calorie content.

Figure 9.5 Weight management involves finding the balance between energy in and energy out.

Energy expenditure has three components

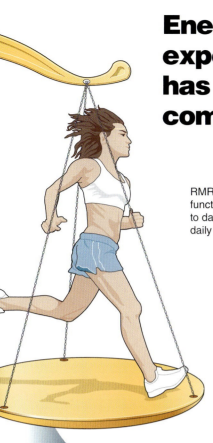

Age

Hormones

Environment

Exercise/physical activity

Weight change

RMR (resting metabolic rate)

RMR is the energy expended to maintain all vital functions in the body at rest. It is the largest contributor to daily energy expenditure, using ~60%-75% of daily calories. Many factors influence RMR...

TEA
(thermic effect of activity)

TEA is any and all muscle contractions that expend energy over and above RMR. This includes sitting, typing at a keyboard, walking for active transportation or intentionally exercising, etc. TEA is the factor that is most adjustable on a daily basis with regards to the energy expenditure side of the equation. Body size, especially lean mass, also impacts the amount of energy expended during a given session. For example, a large male will expend more energy than a small female doing the same activity. Components of FITT greatly influence exercise energy expenditure.

**FITT:
Frequency
Intensity
Time
Type**

ENERGY
OUT

TEM (thermic effect of meals)

The energy cost to process and digest food can be altered by food choices but is so small in its contribution to energy OUT that it is not typically considered an important player in energy balance.

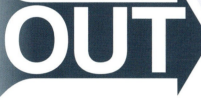

DO THE ENERGY BALANCE MATH

	RMR	TEM	TEA	Comments
Young male (20 yr) 5'10; 160 lb BMI: 23 kg/m²	1900	300	800	😊 Active
Young female (20 yr) 5'4; 134 lb BMI: 23 kg/m²	1470	230	600	😊 Active
Middle-aged male (55 yr) 5'10; 188 lb BMI: 27 kg/m²	1760	240	400	☹ Sedentary
Middle-aged female (55 yr) 5'4; 157 lb BMI: 27 kg/m²	1320	180	300	☹ Sedentary

rate. However, we have the most control over muscle contraction and movement, so this area is a key target for balance on the energy-out side. The energy cost of processing and digesting food can be altered by food choices, but this component contributes so little to energy out that it is not typically considered an important player in energy balance.

Resting Metabolic Rate

Resting metabolic rate (RMR) is the largest contributor to daily energy expenditure, using 60 to 75 percent of daily calories. Simply put, maintaining vital functions when the body is at rest takes a lot of energy—your body has to keep the heart beating and the lungs inflating, maintain body temperature and blood pressure, and so on. The higher your RMR, the more energy your body is using while at rest. Many factors influence RMR from person to person, including genetics. RMR can also change on a daily basis for an individual. The main factor consistently influencing RMR is muscle mass. Muscle mass is highly metabolically active compared to fat or bone mass. This is one reason that the average man can eat more calories than the average woman without gaining weight. Other factors that influence RMR include the following:

- *Hormones*. Several hormones influence RMR; those connected with the thyroid are primary. Sex hormones also influence RMR (e.g., RMR changes throughout the menstrual cycle).
- *Age*. Due to many factors, including hormones, RMR decreases with age.
- *Environment*. Very cold or very hot environments can influence RMR.
- *Exercise and physical activity*. Exercise can influence RMR. Intense sessions elevate RMR for many hours. RMR is consistently elevated in highly active people due primarily to their increased lean body mass.
- *Weight change*. RMR decreases with weight loss. This is one reason it is more challenging to keep losing weight without continuing to adjust energy balance by reducing energy intake or expending energy through exercise or physical activity.

Thermic Effect of Activity (Muscle Movement)

The **thermic effect of activity (TEA)** refers to any and all muscle contractions that use energy over and above RMR, including sitting, typing at a keyboard, walking for active transportation, or intentionally exercising. TEA is the factor that is the most adjustable on a daily basis with regard to the energy expenditure side of the equation. Body size, especially lean mass, also affects the amount of energy used during a given session. For example, a large man with more lean mass will spend more energy for weight-bearing activities. If he runs the same miles at a given intensity compared to a smaller woman, he will spend more energy. Components of FITT, introduced in earlier chapters also greatly influence exercise energy expenditure.

- *Frequency*. The more you move, the more energy you use.
- *Intensity*. The higher the intensity, the greater the caloric expenditure during the session and after the session due to elevations in RMR.
- *Time*. The longer the activity is performed, the more energy is used. This is why energy expenditure charts typically express energy as calories used per minute.
- *Type*. This factor is critical because aerobic endurance activities use more energy than strength, flexibility, and neuromotor types of movement.

Table 9.1 provides examples of common exercise modes for an average man and woman, illustrating how different energy expenditure can be depending on mode, intensity, and body size. Remember also that some activities are not constant. For example, weightlifting uses a similar rate of kilocalories per minute compared to cycling at 10 miles (16 km) per hour; however, the exertion portion of the weightlifting session does not last very long.

Thermic Effect of a Meal

The **thermic effect of meals (TEM)** represents the small energy cost of food processing, that is, chewing, digesting, transporting, metabolizing, and storing ingested calories. The exact cost depends on the amount of food and its caloric and

Table 9.1   Average Values for Energy Expenditure During Various Physical Activities

Activity	Men (kcal/min)	Women (kcal/min)	Relative to body mass (kcal/kg/min)
Basketball	8.6	6.8	.123
Cycling			
• 11.3 km/h (7.0 mph)	5.0	3.9	.071
• 16.1 km/h (10.0 mph)	7.5	5.9	.107
Handball	11.0	8.6	.157
Running			
• 12.1 km/h (7.5 mph)	14.0	11.0	.200
• 16.1 km/h (10.0 mph)	18.2	14.3	.260
Sitting	1.7	1.3	.024
Sleeping	1.2	0.9	.017
Standing	1.8	1.4	.026
Swimming (crawl), 4.8 km/h (3.0 mph)	20.0	15.7	.285
Tennis	7.1	5.5	.101
Walking, 5.6 km/h (3.5 mph)	5.0	3.9	.071
Weightlifting	8.2	6.4	.117
Wrestling	13.1	10.3	.187

Note. The values presented are for a 70-kilogram (154 lb) man and a 55-kilogram (121 lb) woman. These values will vary depending on individual differences.

Reprinted by permission from W.L Kenney, J.H. Wilmore, and David L. Costill, *Physiology of Sport and Exercise*, 6th ed. (Champaign, IL: Human Kinetics), 133.

macronutrient content. Protein is the most expensive to digest and process, meaning it requires more energy than other foods. In spite of the many factors that influence thermic effect of feeding energy costs, the total amount of energy used is minimal—only ~10 percent of energy intake.

Weight Management Strategies

Although most people think of weight management as reducing weight, energy balance principles also apply when wanting to gain weight. However, since most people are trying to be leaner and lighter than they currently are, the focus in this section is on applying the energy balance equation to weight loss. It is useful to think of weight management in phases: weight-gain prevention, weight

loss, and weight-loss maintenance. For most people, it is easier to prevent weight gain than to lose weight. Relatedly, maintaining weight loss is the most challenging phase of all due to many factors, including alterations to RMR and the permanent changes in lifestyle that must occur.

If you are currently at a normal weight, it is in your best interest to try to remain this way (using healthy practices!), especially as you age. If you are interested in losing weight and motivated to do it, don't think that it is impossible to lose weight and keep it off, but know that it might prove to be challenging. Small choices over many days, months, and years really do add up. Most people have a slow, steady weight gain throughout their life. To successfully manage your weight in our obesogenic environment, you will need to create a lifestyle that respects energy balance principles most days.

Healthy Strategies for Tipping the Energy Balance Scale

To change your weight status, you need to unbalance your energy balance equation over a given period. Three general principles should always be respected for healthy weight management:

1. Try not to lose more than 2 pounds (1 kg) per week. Rapid weight loss is harder to maintain long term because it can potentially disrupt your RMR and often causes greater muscle and bone mass loss.

2. Include both sides of the energy balance equation. By reducing both your energy intake and increasing your energy expenditure, the total energy deficit will be more manageable in both the short and longer term. For example, if your goal is to cause a daily deficit of 500 calories, you could reduce energy intake by 300 calories and spend an additional 200 calories in physical activity.

3. Small changes in weight pay big health benefits. Although the path to weight loss can be long, challenging, and frustrating, small reductions in weight (around 3 to 5 percent of body weight) can reduce your risk for several chronic diseases if accomplished by improving your diet quality and moving on a regular basis (Jensen et al. 2014).

Reducing Energy Intake

In our society, *diet* is both a noun and a verb. Everyone has a diet but not everyone is dieting. Managing caloric intake can be challenging because we live in a world of good and plenty. Several key strategies exist for reducing calories in without making you feel deprived; however, to make it work well, you will probably need to mix and match these strategies depending on your social situation. A word of caution is in order. Your precise caloric needs depend on your body size, activity level, age, and other factors. On your quest to unbalance your energy balance equation, be careful not to take in fewer than 800 calories per day unless you are under medical supervision. You will feel unwell (low energy, difficulty concentrating) and you probably won't be getting your required nutrients (as described in chapter 8). Your body requires a certain amount of high-quality fuel to perform well. Very-low-calorie diets are unsustainable; you are setting yourself up for failure. Table 9.2 highlights a few key strategies for reducing energy intake and how you might apply them to daily living.

> One primary key to sustained weight loss is to crank up your fat-burning metabolic machinery. This is best accomplished through a high level of physical activity and exercise and good dietary choices.

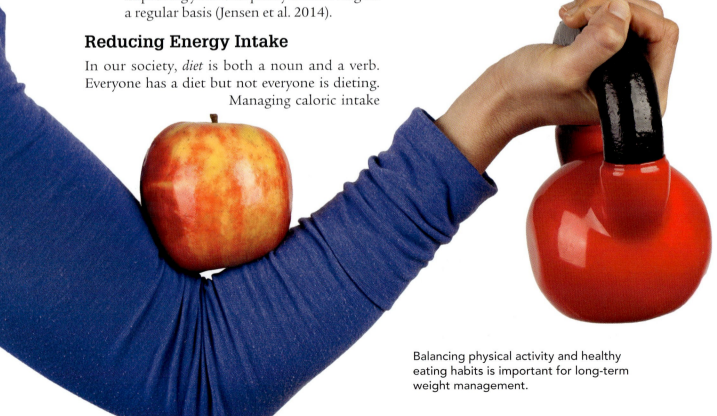

Balancing physical activity and healthy eating habits is important for long-term weight management.

Table 9.2   Strategies for Reducing Energy Intake by Altering Dietary Intake

Energy intake reduction strategy	Implementation of strategy
Portion sizes	Overconsumption of total calories is linked to portion sizes. • Order the smaller meal, split a meal, use smaller plates and bowls.
Energy density	Weight or bulk of food helps with feeling of fullness. • Substitute fruits and vegetables for chips and crackers because they have a lower energy density (i.e., fewer calories per gram).
Fiber	High-fiber foods make you feel fuller. • Add or substitute fruits and vegetables for many options at meals, including your dessert or appetizers.
Macronutrient balance	Having a protein and healthy fat source at each meal or snack might assist with satiety. • Add nuts or Greek yogurt to your cereal; avoid pure carbohydrate meals such as orange juice and banana for breakfast.
Meal timing	Skipping meals can make it hard to manage your blood sugar and sabotage your efforts to make good choices and manage your portion sizes. • Try to eat smaller meals or snacks throughout the day.
Dietary fat	At 9 kcal/g, fat provides many calories, often hidden in foods such as salad dressings. • Select low-fat options when available; avoid fried foods as much as possible.
Added sugars and sweets	Added sugars over the day can really add up. • Reduce intentionally adding sugar (e.g., sugar in coffee) and minimize sweets, saving them for a special treat after a long week or for an event such as a celebration.
Processed foods	Processed foods have many hidden calories in terms of added fat and sugar. • Eat processed foods sparingly in your diet and select those that have minimal processing and additives; know how to accurately and confidently read food labels.
Move to earn "indulgence energy bucks"	If you regularly move and spend energy, you can afford a few indulgence energy bucks. • Try to move at least 30 minutes per day at a moderate intensity to keep your metabolism healthy (Hill and Wyatt 2013).

Move More: Expend More Energy

Previous chapters provide details about how to move more and sit less. All modes of exercise and types of physical activity play a role in health; however, two modes are key to managing the energy balance equation. First, as indicated previously, aerobic endurance activities not only improve the health of your cardiorespiratory systems but also use up a lot of energy. The higher the intensity and the longer the duration of the activity, the more energy that is spent and the greater the influence on RMR. Remember that cardiorespiratory activities can be very intentional (e.g., going out for a run) or they can be woven into your daily life in the form of active transportation.

Second, resistance training is critical for keeping your muscle mass as metabolically active as possible. This is important during all phases of weight management (preventing weight gain, weight loss, and maintenance), but it may be especially critical during the active weight loss phase due to the link to your RMR described previously. From the perspective of your future healthiest self, regular strength training is the key to preserving your muscle mass and RMR as you age, especially through middle age and beyond.

Think about incorporating these daily strategies into your life:

- Ban the bus and any other step-saving device, such as elevators, escalators, and moving sidewalks. Don't let anyone steal your steps. Start to think of them as ways to spend your energy bucks.
- Load your backpack as much as possible. This will increase the intensity of your transportation walk. Be sure to have good posture in order to avoid back or shoulder pain or injuries.
- When planning your cardiorespiratory exercise, try to work hard for longer periods to really stimulate your metabolism.

- Stand when possible and fidget (if socially acceptable) to spend calories throughout the day.
- Take planned breaks from sitting. For example, if one of your buildings has stairs, try to get up and walk the stairs for a few minutes every hour. Think of these breaks as energy-buck spenders even if they spend just a few cents per break.
- Consistently do resistance training overloading beyond your body weight. This is especially important for women, who often focus exclusively on cardiorespiratory activities for weight management. Don't underestimate the key role that muscle mass can play in energy balance.

Buyer Beware: Be a Smart Consumer

The weight management business is a booming industry. Because so many people struggle to manage their weight, the marketplace has responded with many plans, programs, pills, supplements, and aids. This is very concerning because when the struggle for weight management gets very frustrating and subsequently emotional, many people get desperate. This feeling of desperation often leads people to make bad decisions. Most products on the market target either dietary

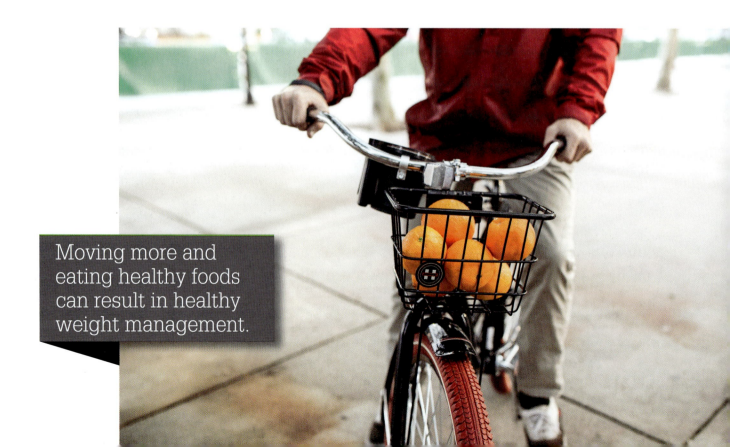

Moving more and eating healthy foods can result in healthy weight management.

> **Weight management is a lifestyle choice. A product that is advertised as a quick fix is likely too good to be true.**

intake (products to curb your appetite) or RMR, with the latter idea being to increase your RMR so that you use more energy while at rest. The majority of products are ineffective and can be dangerous. The FDA does not regulate dietary supplements. A good source to check is the FDA public notification site, which informs the public of products that have hidden active ingredients that are potentially harmful. (Go to www.fda.gov and click on the Food tab.) If a product sounds too good to be true, it likely is. To safely manage your weight, you need to keep your energy equation in balance by following the principles described in this chapter, which can be implemented over a lifetime.

Prescription Drugs and Surgery

Medical options are available for weight management. Prescription drugs have been developed over the years that influence energy consumption and energy expenditure or interfere with energy absorption. A more complete review is beyond the scope of this book. Recognize that all prescription drugs on the market have a limited effect on weight status in the long term (i.e., they lose their effectiveness; some are approved only for short-term use) and many have numerous side effects. Also, many people regain any weight lost when stopping the medication. All medications work best in conjunction with a behavioral modification program reinforcing the importance of managing lifestyle, typically both sides of the energy balance equation, for long-term weight management success.

Surgical treatment of obesity, known as bariatric surgery, is often considered a last resort. As such, it is typically recommended only for people who have morbid obesity (BMI > 40 kg/m², or 35 kg/m² with other major risks due to obesity). Bariatric surgery is growing in prevalence worldwide. Essentially, bariatric surgery involves reducing the size of the stomach to reduce the amount of food a person can eat. Although it is very effective, the risks associated with this procedure are not minimal, including nutritional deficiencies, chronic nausea and vomiting, and serious postoperative complications that can result in death. For long-term success, behavioral modification strategies are essential. For more information, see www.webmd.com (search gastric bypass surgery) or https://asmbs.org/patients.

Potential Interactive Implications of Stress, Sleep, and Alcohol

Alcohol, stress, and sleep have important implications for weight management. Many people have good intentions to adhere to healthy weight-management behaviors but fail to do so for a variety of reasons. A common theme often expressed is that stressful lifestyle issues can work against energy-balance practices. Lab 9.1 will help you utilize SMART goal planning to set effective long and short term goals for healthy eating practices.

1. *Stress*. Emotional and psychosocial stressors play major roles in the health of our society. Our 24/7 go-go-go world alters our cardiovascular and neuroendocrine systems and often challenges our psychosocial well-being.
   - Energy in: Stress has been shown to increase the selection of starchy, sweet foods (junk food). Feeling pressed for time can lead you to select more fast food and processed food.
   - Energy out: High levels of stress can cause fatigue, which then can reduce your motivation to move, resulting in more sitting.

2. *Sleep*. Many people are chronically sleep deprived, which can also lead to many behavioral changes.
   - Energy in: Fatigue may reduce your motivation to stick with healthy food choices. It might also increase your intake of caffeine, which increases your energy intake if taken as sweet drinks (e.g., soda, sweetened coffees).
   - Energy out: As with stress, fatigue reduces your interest in moving.

3. *Alcohol*. Drinking alcohol can have implications beyond the substance abuse concerns discussed in chapter 11.
   - Energy in: At 7 calories per gram, alcohol can affect your weight-management plan. Depending on how much and often you

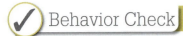
Do You Spiral Up or Down?

Your behavior choices can help you spiral either up or down in terms of your overall health. Have an honest conversation with yourself about how you manage pressure and stress. For example, when you are tired from your hectic schedule and stressed due to a major exam, do you eat lower-quality foods such as fast foods, snack foods, sweets, or candy? Do you reach for sugary sodas or sweet coffees to give you energy to power through? Alcohol may also play a role in your stress management. Alternatively, do you make sure to adhere to your exercise routine because you know it will help you manage your stress? Try to recognize and manage your triggers.

Make a plan to replace behaviors that will have a negative effect on your health with positive behaviors. For example, if you binge on chocolate when you are stressed, plan for a healthier replacement: You might plan to go for a walk, take a hot bath or shower, or listen to relaxing music. Find a plan that will work for you so that when life issues arise, you are prepared to deal with them.

indulge, especially if you drink heavy beer or sweet mixed drinks, the calorie intake can be substantial.

- Energy out: Consuming too much alcohol can cause fatigue and reduce your interest in adhering to your exercise plan or engaging in active transportation or recreation. Recall that alcohol is a diuretic, so it can also dehydrate you, which influences your movement performance. Finally, the metabolism of alcohol, if consumed excessively, will reduce the use of fat as a fuel source.

Daily Movement Is Essential for Weight Management

Regular exercise and physical activity are essential for all three phases of weight management. However, how much exercise you will need to perform and why you need to do it might change.

Prevention of Weight Gain

The role of energy expenditure in preventing weight gain is not well established because of challenges with study designs. However, we can assume that the role that energy expenditure plays would be important, especially with advancing

age when RMR begins to decline. High levels of activity, especially resistance training, lessen the RMR decline that occurs after middle age by maintaining muscle mass and keeping existing muscle mass metabolically active.

Weight Loss and Healthy Body-Composition Change

Incorporating both cardiorespiratory and resistance training into your weight-loss program is essential. First, it will allow you to eat more (i.e., restrict energy less) to meet the same energy deficit goals, which will help you stick with your program. Second, it will promote the healthiest body-composition change. When we try to lose weight by restricting calories alone, more of the weight loss comes from lean tissue (muscle mass) compared to when exercise and physical activity are included in the program. Loading your bones when undergoing weight loss will help reduce bone loss, which typically occurs with caloric restriction and weight loss. Finally, moving, especially with higher-intensity cardiorespiratory and strength training, will help protect against reductions in RMR that occur with weight loss. With specific attention to FITT guidelines for weight loss, the ACSM suggests performing moderate- to vigorous-intensity (as tolerated) aerobic activities that use large muscle groups for a minimum of

30 minutes per day, progressing to 60 minutes per day, on at least five days per week (American College of Sports Medicine 2018).

Weight Loss Maintenance

If exercise and physical activity are important during weight loss, they are even more important for weight-loss maintenance. Research suggests and the ACSM endorses that an increased amount of cardiorespiratory activity is needed for weight-loss maintenance (American College of Sports Medicine 2018). With specific attention to the FITT guidelines, weight-loss maintenance has been linked to performing moderate- to vigorous-intensity (as tolerated) activities using large muscle groups on at least five and closer to seven days per week, progressing to 250 minutes per week. You can do these four hours per week of cardiorespiratory activity with intentional exercise and lifestyle activities such as active transportation as long as they are of a moderate intensity. Some of the best evidence for the importance of energy expenditure for weight-loss maintenance comes from the National Weight Control Registry, which is a longitudinal study of successful weight losers and maintainers that also offers an online weight-management program. The primary successful strategies include using a macronutrient balance approach to eating (see table 9.2) and a high level of physical activity, or exercise, of 60 minutes per day (Hill and Wyatt 2013).

Psychological Concerns Regarding Weight Management

We live in an environment that makes it challenging to manage weight using healthy behaviors. On top of that, our society values being thin and fit. Many people live in a constant state of psychological distress related to **body image** issues. Nearly all body image issues stem from a lack of congruence between what people look like (or think they look like) and what they feel they should look like based on cultural messages, family pressures, and individual belief systems. A continuum exists with healthy body image on one end and

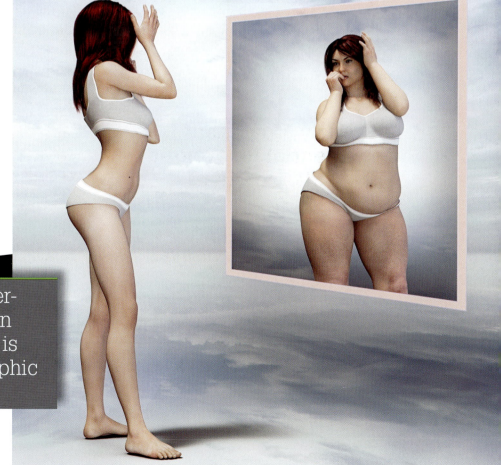

Seeing yourself differently in a mirror than how others see you is called body dysmorphic disorder.

life-threatening eating disorders on the other end. Unfortunately, it is becoming increasingly rare to find a person, male or female, who is content with their body shape, size, and appearance. Although an in-depth review of these issues is beyond our scope, you are encouraged to seek professional resources if you or someone you care about struggles with these issues. Weight management should take place in a positive and supportive atmosphere, including the attitudes you create within yourself. With few exceptions, most people can be relatively healthy at any weight. Moreover, being content in one's own skin—regardless of appearance—and being self-confident is an attractive feature.

Developing and Maintaining a Healthy Body Image

Body image is the perceptions, images, evaluations, and emotional feelings regarding one's appearance that may span the entire body or target a certain body part. Developing a positive body image is essential to psychosocial well-being and successful weight management. A negative body image can cause great mental anguish, damage self-esteem, interfere with healthy relationships and social activities, and lead to depression. When extreme, it is often termed **body dysmorphic disorder**. Lab 9.2 in the web study guide will help you explore your personal body image.

Reducing Body Size and Fatness: Anorexia, Bulimia, and Exercise Addiction

Negative body image and unhappiness with weight status can lead to more serious issues such as eating disorders and other unhealthy weight-management behaviors. Unfortunately, eating disorders are becoming increasingly common for both men and women of all ages. The most common disorders related to a negative body image are **anorexia**, **bulimia nervosa**, **binge-eating disorder**, and **exercise addiction**:

- *Anorexia*. Although often expressing interest in food, people who suffer from anorexia do not eat enough to maintain a normal weight and often have a very low BMI. This condition mainly afflicts young women but is getting more common in older women and men. Even more sadly,

sometimes this starvation condition results in death.

- *Bulimia nervosa*. A person with bulimia nervosa engages in recurrent episodes of binge eating followed by purging, typically through vomiting or using laxatives and diuretics. Bulimia is more challenging to identify because these behaviors are performed in private and people often have a normal weight. However, fluctuations in weight can be a sign. The binge–purge cycle greatly stresses many systems of the body, including the teeth and esophagus, liver and kidneys, and the heart.

- *Binge-eating disorder*. People who binge eat often do so uncontrollably in response to stress, strong emotions, or conflict. The uncontrolled eating episode is followed by shame and depression and ramped-up efforts in weight management. These people are almost always obese and compromise their health. In addition, they also live with higher rates of anxiety and depression.

- *Exercise addiction*. Note that although most behaviors center on energy intake, obsessive or excessive exercise may also be used to achieve weight control.

Increasing Body Size and Muscle Mass: Muscle Dysmorphia

Although eating disorders often bring to mind young women on a quest to be very thin, men can also be prone to a **muscle dysmorphia** disorder where they struggle with their eating and exercise behaviors. In this situation, people (typically men, but also women) do not see themselves as muscular and fit despite being very well conditioned, with good muscle mass and tone. In the case of men who strive to be larger, this condition is often referred to as "bigorexia." Even though the goal of people who struggle with this condition is the opposite of that of people with conventional eating disorders (i.e., trying to be bigger with more muscle as opposed to smaller), the root cause is often the same—a poor body image that results in unhealthy eating and exercise behaviors. The mental anguish can be just as serious and lead to life-endangering behaviors, including steroid use.

When Professional Help Is Needed

Sometimes the best course of action in life is to recognize you need help and wisely secure quality resources for yourself. Weight management is no exception to this rule.

Psychologist or Therapist

Although you or someone you know may not suffer from a diagnosed eating disorder, many people have symptoms of an eating disorder or a body image disturbance severe enough to compromise their quality of life. Having an honest conversation is the start to increasing your well-being. However, sometimes professionals are needed. Most college campuses have counselors who can provide quality assistance with these issues or a referral to a professional in the community. Working with a professional counselor can help address both problematic eating disorders and the misuse of food and activity to manage stress and emotions. Anxiety or depression are often key underlying issues that cause further problems with weight-management behaviors.

If you are worried about yourself or a friend, a great resource for eating disorders is the National Eating Disorders Association (www.national eatingdisorders.org).

Registered Dietitian Nutritionist (RDN)

As mentioned in chapter 8, an RDN can help with personal dietary plans. This is especially important if you have special dietary needs due to chronic illness or a food allergy. A few sessions may be all you need to understand some key principles and get on your way to healthier fueling.

Working With a Certified Fitness Trainer

Although the fundamentals of how to move in terms of the established guidelines have been discussed extensively, sometimes you need additional assistance to set up a program or improve your adherence as you get started. When selecting a professional fitness trainer,

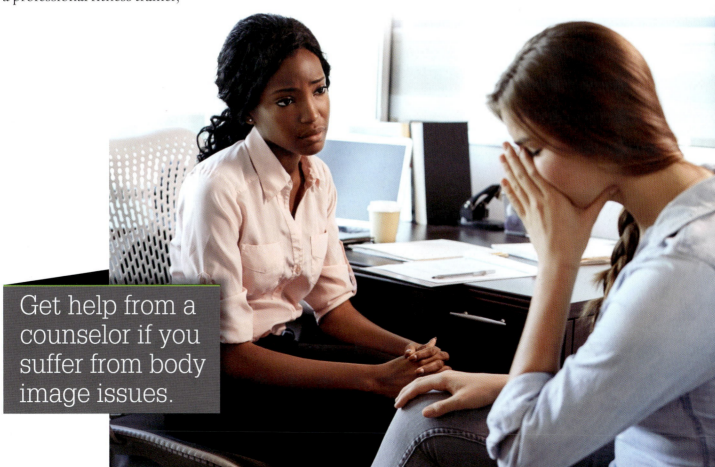

Get help from a counselor if you suffer from body image issues.

look for someone who is certified by the NCCA (National Commission for Certifying Agencies, www.credentialingexcellence.org/ncca) and who aligns with your goals and personality. These standards were put in place to protect the health, welfare, and safety of the public. Just as you would not go to a doctor who has not passed a medical board examination, you would be wise to select a fitness trainer who has been nationally certified by an organization that has gone through the NCCA accreditation process.

Medical Evaluation

Finally, if your weight changes for no apparent reason or does not change in response to your intentional manipulation of energy intake or expenditure, you are encouraged to see a physician. Unexplained weight change is always cause for concern. Although you are young and the risk is minimal, conditions such as hyper- or hypothyroidism or cancer can alter your weight.

Summary

Weight management is a challenge in our obesogenic society, where we have so much accessible, highly palatable food and minimal need to use energy to survive. To manage weight, we need to pay constant attention to the energy balance equation, especially energy intake and energy expenditure through physical activity and exercise. Movement, especially cardiorespiratory and resistance training, can enhance your weight-management success. Movement and exercise maintain or enhance your resting metabolic rate and spend energy to keep you closer to energy balance. You can gain many strategies for remaining in energy balance by educating yourself and paying attention to your daily behaviors. Managing weight can be very emotionally challenging, and disturbed eating and exercise behaviors can greatly damage mental and physical health. Knowing when to seek professional assistance may be a key part of your weight-management program.

www WEB STUDY GUIDE

Remember to complete all of the web study guide activities to further facilitate your learning, including the following lab activities:

Lab 9.1   Healthy and SMART Weight Management Plan

Lab 9.2   Stepping Toward a Positive Body Image

REVIEW QUESTIONS

1. How do relatively recent changes in our social and built environments contribute to our ongoing public health challenge with weight management?

2. List the four primary components of the energy balance equation. On the side of energy out, which factor explains the greatest amount of daily energy expenditure for most people? Which factors can be manipulated in the short term to cause an energy deficit to lose weight?

3. Describe three strategies you could use to manage energy intake without feeling greatly deprived.

4. Which primary modes of exercise should be incorporated into your weight-loss program? Justify their use from a mechanistic perspective.

5. Briefly explain the major eating disorders with regard to signs and symptoms.

6. List and explain how various professionals might be able to help you with your goals related to a healthy and sustainable weight-management program.

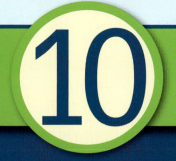

Stress Management

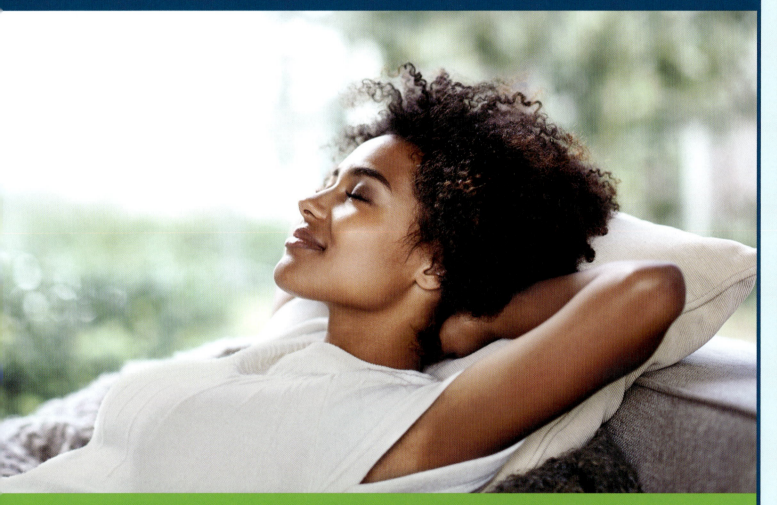

OBJECTIVES

❭ Define *stress* and *stressor* and recognize that perception of both is personal.

❭ Recognize that stress is not always bad and spans from eustress to distress.

❭ Explain the acute physiological and psychological stress response.

❭ Understand how chronic stress, if unmanaged, can cause physical and emotional health problems.

❭ Recognize the primary stressors for college students.

❭ Describe key strategies, especially sleep and physical activity, that can help manage stress.

KEY TERMS

adrenal glands

adrenocorticotropic hormone (ACTH)

allostatic balance (allostasis)

allostatic load

autonomic nervous system (ANS)

corticotropin-releasing hormone (CRH)

cortisol

depression

endocrine system

epinephrine (adrenalin)

fight-or-flight response

generalized anxiety disorder

hypothalamus

hypothalamus-pituitary-adrenal axis (HPA axis)

mantra

mindfulness meditation

norepinephrine (noradrenaline)

panic disorder

parasympathetic nervous system

personality

pituitary gland

social anxiety disorder

stress

stressor

sympathetic nervous system

time management

Transcendental Meditation

Do you ever feel overwhelmed by your to-do list? Are many of your days full of constant hassles? Stress is a natural part of our lives, but how you react to it can have major implications for your health and well-being. This chapter targets stress management, beginning with an overview of the stress response. Importantly, it emphasizes the implications of mismanagement of stress for health, now and in your future. Common sources of stress for the college student are highlighted, including academic performance, finances, and social and intimate relationships. Finally, this chapter explores key strategies for managing stress, especially physical activity and quality sleep.

The Contemporary Stress Experience

The primary sources of stress for most people are related to social and psychological challenges, including our relationships and occupational performance. For college students, performing well academically is equivalent to full-time employment and has many of the same stressors. Regardless of the source of stress, it is important to recognize when you are stressed, the sources of the stress, and how to manage these stressors. Can you manage your stress so that it

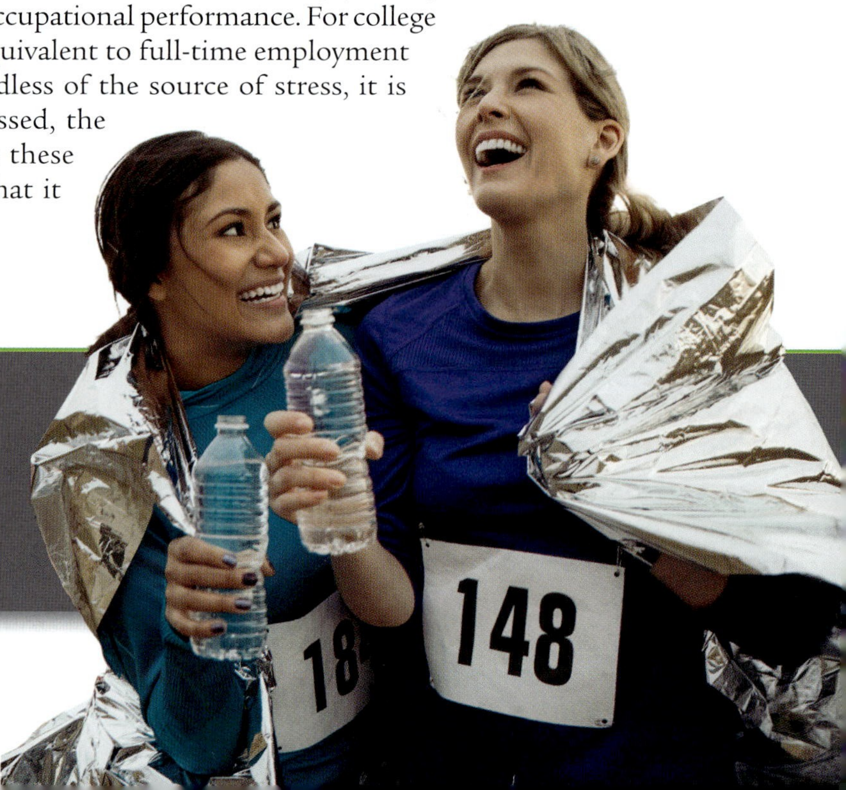

Being stressed and not having coping techniques can be like running a marathon and never crossing the finish line.

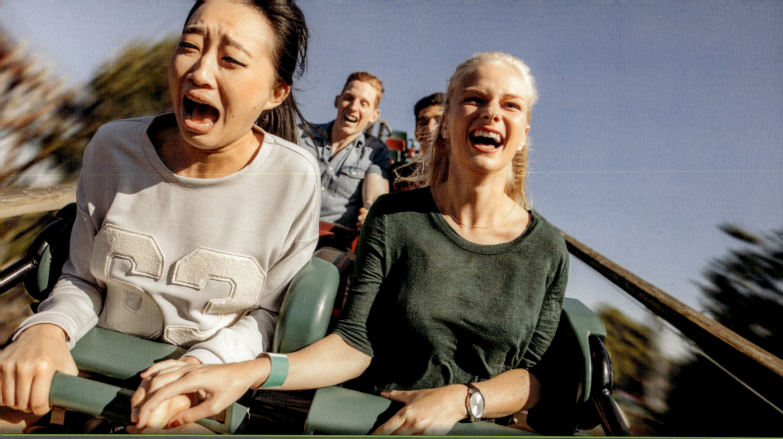

How an event or situation is viewed is highly individual; one person's awful stressor is another person's adventure.

does not negatively affect your health and life? The answer is yes, but, as with most health habits, it will take intentional strategies and effort.

Stress Defined for Better or Worse

Most people view **stress** as some unpleasant threat. Most dictionaries define it along the lines of a "strain or tension of a physical, mental, or emotional type" or "feelings or conditions that occur when a person perceives that a demand exceeds their personal or social resources." Thus, stress is generally considered a negative experience and something to be avoided. A few major myths are that stress is the same for everyone and it is always bad for you (American Psychological Association n.d.b). However, if there is no healthy tension, most people become bored and lose motivation to engage in life. Therefore, stress can be helpful because it motivates us to be productive, try new things, and engage in our social world.

This brings us to another important stress concept. It is very useful to differentiate the stimulus from the response. The stress stimulus is considered the **stressor**. You probably know from your life experience that not all stressors produce the same response in different people (see figure 10.1). A given stressor may be very distressing only if it occurs under specific conditions—for example, a stressor may result in a higher stress response when you

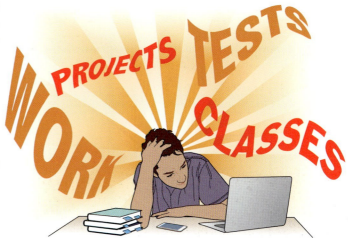

Figure 10.1 College students have many stressors related to their academic courses and employment obligations. Develop a personal stress-management plan to prevent adverse health outcomes.

219

are short on sleep, hungry, or very pressed for time. An important concept discussed in this chapter is that you cannot always control the stressors in your life (e.g., your midterms all landing on the same day), but you can alter the way you *perceive* and *react to* the stressors, which will greatly alter your experience of stress from both a physiological and emotional perspective.

Eustress Versus Distress

Stress can be thought of as being on a continuum from good to neutral to bad. The good stress, eustress, occurs when you are looking forward to a planned event and you anticipate that it will be a positive experience. Examples of eustress might include going on a long-awaited vacation, learning how to drive, or going to college. It is also being excited to experience something new or different. Distress is when you are exposed to negative circumstances that are often out of your control. Examples of distress include failing a major exam, especially after you invested a lot of time in your preparation, enduring an unanticipated physical injury, or breaking up with your romantic partner. Distress, especially if it is ongoing, is the type of stress that negatively affects your health and well-being. Figure 10.2 depicts a conceptual model of how eustress and distress interact on a continuum.

The Stress Response

How do you feel when you are stressed? How does your body know how to react when faced with a stressor? The body responds to stressors, both physiologically and psychologically. Understanding these different responses will help you develop stress-management skills. Allostasis is the process of achieving stability or balance, or homeostasis, through physical or behavioral changes. Therefore, a stressor is anything that throws your body out of **allostatic balance (allostasis)**, and the stress response is your body's attempt to return to homeostasis. No matter whether the stressor is physical, psychological, or social, or even an anticipation of a challenge, the body responds with the same physiological cascade. Thus, being too hot or too cold, hungry, or worried about an important exam can all activate the stress response.

Physiological Response: Two Systems Work Together

When the body is exposed to a stressor, two systems within the body are responsible for your nearly immediate physical response to the stressor: the **fight-or-flight response**. Earlier in our evolution, this response was completely appropriate because without it, many humans would have been killed by predators. Nowadays we rarely have to run away or physically fight a predator, but this same response system gets set in motion with psychological or social challenges or even by the anticipation of these challenges. The stress-response teamwork of the nervous and the endocrine systems causes the fight-or-flight response.

The **parasympathetic nervous system**, a primary arm of the **autonomic nervous system (ANS)**, is in control during relaxed states. The **sympathetic nervous system**, the other primary

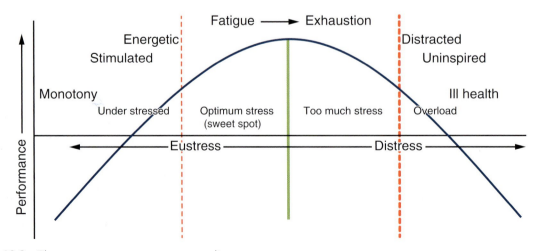

Figure 10.2   The stress curve: eustress versus distress.

arm of the autonomic nervous system, is a key player in the stress response. Its nerves release **norepinephrine (noradrenaline)** to signal nearly every organ, sweat gland, blood vessel, and muscle to prepare your body to move in the fastest, most efficient manner possible (to run or prepare to fight!). The **endocrine system** is coordinated with the nervous system through the **hypothalamus**, which signals the **pituitary gland** with **corticotropin-releasing hormone (CRH)**. The pituitary gland then signals the **adrenal glands** with **adrenocorticotropic hormone (ACTH)**, which releases the key hormones **epinephrine (adrenalin)** and **cortisol** (the primary hormone). This cascade is often summarized as the HPA axis, which is short for **hypothalamus-pituitary-adrenal axis (HPA axis)**.

Activation of the HPA axis is like a short-term crisis in the body, shifting resources from any longer-term bodily functions, such as digestion, immune function, or reproduction (see figure 10.3). When the stressful situation is over, the parasympathetic nervous system returns the body to its resting prestress state, or into homeostatic balance (e.g., the heart rate returns to resting levels). Longer-term projects now begin to take priority again, including digestion, energy storage, and reproductive function. The immune system can now repair any injuries to prepare for the next threat. Changes in the shape and function of the HPA axis are involved in many mood disorders, including anxiety disorders and depression, and insomnia (Sapolsky 2004). Learning to manage your stress is critical for protecting the health of your HPA axis and keeping it appropriately sensitive to realistic stressors.

What Affects Your Stress Response?

Although we all experience both physiological and psychological stressors and exhibit the same cascade of bodily changes in response to them,

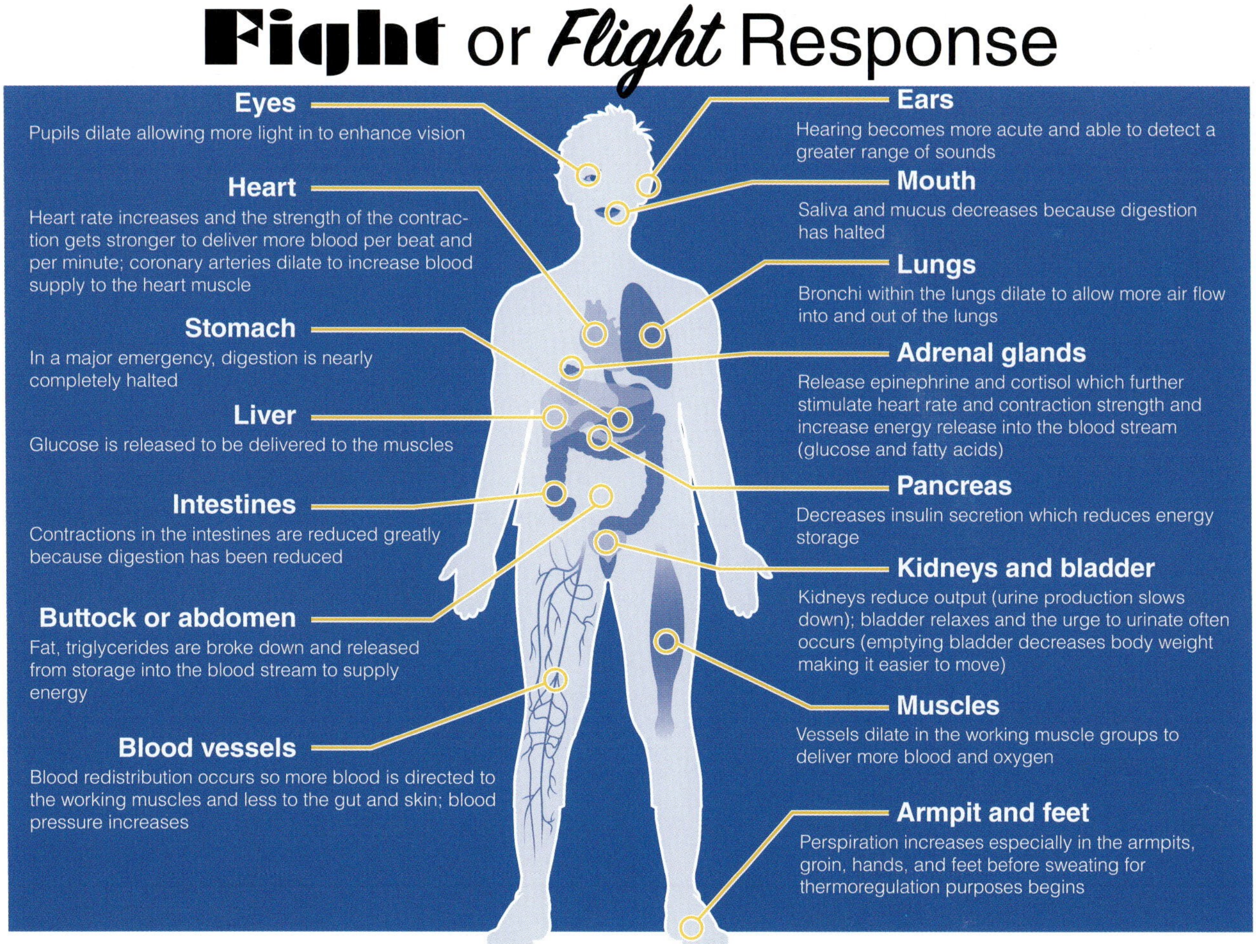

Figure 10.3   The physiological responses of your body to stress.

the magnitude of the stress response varies greatly from person to person and for an individual in different situations. A few of the primary factors that influence the stress response are your cognitive evaluation of the situation (how you think about it) and your emotional reaction to the challenge or the threat. Your personality might also influence your stress response in general and your specific reactions to a given stressor.

Cognitive Evaluation: Can I Cope?

When presented with a stressor, most people immediately process the threat cognitively to assess the situation—that is, you think it through. Although several well-established psychological theories exist, most align with the idea that the level of stress experienced is highly dependent on a few key questions you ask yourself (Lazarus and Folkman 1984):

1. Is there potential for harm or threat?
2. If yes, if anything can be done, will my resources be enough?
3. If my resources are not enough, can I cope with the resulting situation?

The cognitive evaluation of the threat and your ability to cope will be greatly influenced by your past experience with the situation and your perception of control. Having a bad experience with a situation or event will nearly always result in more stress in similar future situations (Sapolsky 2004). For example, having the course outline and knowing the date of the final exam, the structure of the exam, and the material to be covered will make the exam less stressful compared to unannounced exams or situations where you have been given no guidance on how to prepare. Also, if you have been successful with comprehensive exams in the past, given your academic abilities and your study habits, the next round of exams will be less stressful.

Emotional Responses: Does It Matter to Me?

Psychological stress is often thought of as the emotional response we have when we perceive an event or situation as a threat to our well-being. However, you have to care about the outcome of the situation in order for your stress response to be triggered. If you don't care much about the outcome, you won't perceive the event as a threat and therefore will have a minimal stress response. However, if the stakes are high, the situation will pose a significant threat or challenge, triggering a larger stress response (Sapolsky 2004). This is why you would probably perceive a minor quiz in an elective class as less stressful than a comprehensive final exam in a core class in your major, especially if the latter could influence your GPA enough to alter your chance of getting into a competitive graduate program. This is also why hearing the news of a stranger passing will not cause a stress response, whereas losing a loved one, especially someone who is in your daily life, can be a significant stressor.

Personality Influences the Stress Response

Think about the personalities of your family members and close friends. Some people seem very calm and able to handle anything that comes their way, while others are anxious about anything that disrupts their daily routine. These traits are aspects of **personality**. Personality can influence how you perceive and respond to stressors. There are many ways to characterize personality, and many researchers have attempted to classify personality into types.

With specific reference to the stress response, there are different personality types (American Psychological Association n.d.c). The most well-known type is a Type A personality. In general, people with Type A personalities are very competitive and impatient. They are hard-working overachievers who are highly concerned with time management. Type B personalities are in contrast to Type A personalities and are more relaxed, less competitive, and calm. Research has shown that being Type A can increase the risk for coronary artery disease, especially if it is linked to being hostile, time-pressured, and socially insecure (Sapolsky 2004). Other personality types, such as the worry wart who pessimistically sees danger and disaster everywhere and catastrophizes everything, also tend to have a chronically activated stress response and a higher risk for anxiety and depression (American Psychological Association n.d.c).

Although most people do not fit neatly into

> Learning to manage your stress is critical for protecting your health.

one personality type, the important point is that your personality can influence how you perceive stressors and your physiological (heart rate, blood pressure, hormone levels) and psychological responses to them (Sapolsky 2004). Some personalities chronically activate a stress response that is much higher than it should be for a given stressor.

Modern Life and the Stress Response Mismatch

A stressor is anything that knocks you out of homeostatic balance and the stress response is what your body does to reestablish homeostasis. If you are a lion chasing your lunch or a zebra trying not to become a lion's lunch, the physiological stress response is wonderfully adapted and appropriate for this short-term crisis situation. Unlike species that are less cognitively advanced, humans can turn on the stress response just by thinking about potential stressors. This worry can throw our systems out of homeostatic balance even if the event will occur (or maybe not even occur) far in the future (Sapolsky 2004). Humans get very stressed about many things that have no relevance to other mammals. For example, a major final exam or failing course grade, a text that ends a relationship with a romantic partner, or a low bank balance from too much debit card

 Now and Later

Personality and Stress

Now

By this stage of life, you are likely aware of your main personality traits. Without getting too caught up in the alphabet of the personality typing, you might be able to align yourself with one of the types described in the text. When you understand factors you cannot change—such as genetic contributions to your personality or aspects of your temperament formed in your childhood—you can better choose the strategies that might help you manage your stress.

Then

Many students assume that their stress level will go down after they graduate. This is not typically the case because life gets even more complicated, with multiple social roles and professional and family demands. Continual unmanaged stress has been linked to chronic conditions such as cardiovascular disease, anxiety disorders, and depression (Sapolsky 2004). Many of these stress-related diseases and conditions begin to show up during midlife.

Take Home

You may not be able to change your basic personality, but you can learn to manage your stress response by working on positive thinking, learning from the stressful experience, and practicing stress-management techniques. Stress management is a key health behavior that will help you feel better now and have a long, happy, and healthy life.

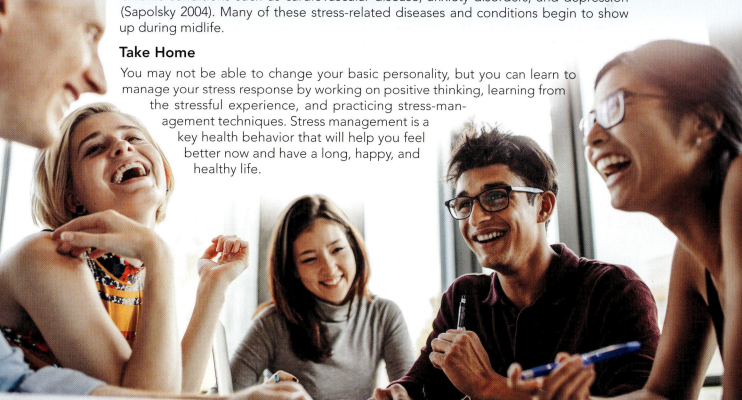

action over the weekend can cause great distress for many college students.

For the great majority of nonhuman animals on the planet, the physiological stress response is about managing a short-term crisis. The problem with humans is that, given our complicated social environment and technological advances, our stress response is not being turned on just every once in a while. Instead, the stress response is being set off for some people multiple times per day or even nearly all day long. This is the conceptual basis of stress-related disease. The physiological stress-response system evolved to assist us in short-term physical emergencies, but now we are turning it on for longer periods of time (months or years), worrying about issues such as our relationships, finances, employment, and social status.

Allostatic Load Leads to Chronic Conditions and Diseases

We experience similar responses from a variety of physical, psychological, and social stresses. We also know that if stressors go on for a long period of time, they can make a person sick. A contemporary theory of how chronic stress actually causes disease is the concept of **allostatic load**, which is defined as the wear and tear on the body that occurs due to chronic stress exposure and the neuroendocrine response to the stress. Another way to understand this concept is that repeated stress that causes a stress response can be managed, but

getting back into allostatic balance takes a great deal of effort and having to constantly rebalance eventually wears a person down.

In his book *Why Zebras Don't Get Ulcers*, Robert Sapolsky (2004) explains this concept well. He calls it the "two elephants on a seesaw" model of stress-related disease. Figure 10.4*a* shows two small children balancing on a seesaw, which is relatively easy to do. This illustrates allostatic balance, when nothing stressful is occurring in your life. The small children depict the low levels of stress hormones in your system. In contrast, Figure 10.4*b* shows two elephants trying to balance the seesaw. The size of the elephants represents the huge amount of stress hormones in your system in response to some real (or anticipated, or theoretical) stressor. As you can see, the elephants can balance, but costs and consequences are involved in achieving this, including the following effects:

- *Allocation of effort*. It takes an enormous amount of energy to balance two elephants on a seesaw. This means that energy must be diverted from longer-term investments like reproduction and repairing and rebuilding projects (i.e., immune system) to handle the chronic short-term emergencies.

- *Collateral damage*. Although the seesaw might be able to be balanced, other damage will occur because the large elephants cause a lot of wear and tear. Fixing an issue in the body that creates such a high load of stress hormones often causes damage somewhere

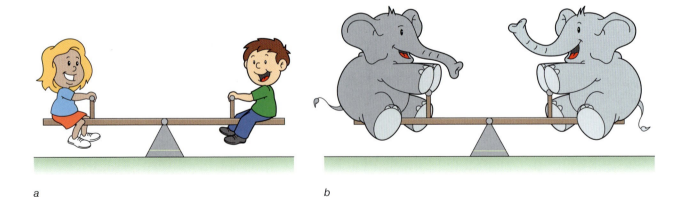

a   *b*

Figure 10.4   The "two elephants on a seesaw" model of stress-related disease (Sapolsky 2004). *(a)* Allostatic balance, with the children representing low levels of stress hormones. *(b)* Allostatic load, in response to chronic stress. The elephants represent the abundance of stress hormones in response to real or anticipated stress. The elephants can balance, but not without creating conditions for chronic diseases.

else in the body. You can get back into allostatic balance by using your elephants (huge levels of stress hormones), but using your elephants for extended periods of time will create a mess somewhere else in the body. This essentially is allostatic load.

- *Complicated dismount.* When these large elephants are no longer needed because the stress has been reduced, they will have a hard time getting off the seesaw gracefully. For example, if one jumps off, the other will crash to the ground due to its massive weight. This illustrates that sometimes stress-related disease can be caused by turning off the stress response too slowly or turning off the different components of the stress response at different speeds. Some hormones will be high while others are low, but they should generally run parallel. This effect also has negative health implications.

Conditions and Diseases Affected by the Stress Response

Repeatedly turning on the stress response can damage your health. It is not the stressor that makes us sick, it is the stress response itself (especially if it is purely psychological) that predisposes us to certain conditions and diseases, which then make us sick. Table 10.1 summarizes the main systems that are adversely affected by chronic activation of the stress response, along with a brief description of their mechanisms (Sapolsky 2004).

Common Stressors and Hassles of College Life

Activation of the stress response typically occurs in three situations. First, an acute physical crisis can occur (e.g., accidentally stepping off a curb in front of a speeding car). Second, a chronic physical challenge can occur, which might be a chronic health condition or a major extended illness, although modern medicine typically helps us avoid long-term pain and discomfort. Third, we encounter psychological and social disruptions, the primary causes of stress in our modern world that were described earlier in the chapter. Essentially, the basic health needs of humans are covered, but we create lots of stressful challenges

Table 10.1   Primary Systems Affected by Chronic Activation of the Stress Response

System	Primary mechanism	Symptoms or related diseases
Cardiovascular	• Increases in heart rate and blood pressure at rest • Chronic system inflammation	• Hypertension • Coronary artery disease
Metabolic	• Elevated levels of glucose and fat in the bloodstream	• Atherosclerosis • Type 2 diabetes
Digestion	• Change in appetite (1/3 of stressed people eat less and 2/3 eat more) • Changes in acid levels and blood flow in stomach	• Weight loss or obesity • Irritable bowel syndrome • Ulcers (stress makes some types worse)
Immune	• Mechanisms not well established	• Colds and flu • Cancer (potentially)
Sex/Reproductive	• Menstrual cycle irregularity • Erection difficulties • Loss of interest	• Infertility • Impotence
Brain	• Neuron networks altered • Less neurogenesis (fewer new neurons produced)	• Reduced concentration and memory performance • Dementia (potentially)

Stress and the Aging Process: Before and After Office

Take a look at some of the United States presidents when they were sworn into office and compare them to photos taken near the end of their terms. What do you notice? Chronic activation of the stress response is implicated in the aging process. The pictures of presidents when they were sworn in to office compared to when they departed office suggest that highly stressful positions accelerate aging.

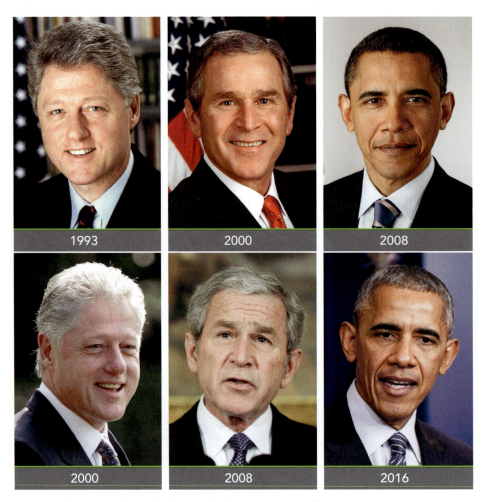

Photos of U.S. presidents before and after serving in office.

in our own minds! Some of these concerns are legitimate (e.g., deadlines or being worried about a loved one's health); however, our stressful challenges are often not grounded in reality or within our control, which suggests that we should not be activating our stress response to fight or flee from them.

Big Stressors and Little Stressors

Stress-response activators can be broken down into major life events and daily hassles. Major life events can be further divided into environmental

or natural events that are unforeseen and out of our control, such as living through a hurricane or witnessing a terrorist attack like the events at the World Trade Center in 2001. The second type of major life event is also not within our control and includes things such as death of a loved one, divorce (even more so if not your choice), disability, or a life-threatening illness (Lazarus and Folkman 1984).

Although we usually don't consider them as important as major life events, daily hassles are a significant contributor to our stress response.

These minor but common events lead to frustration, annoyance, anger, and distress. These can include things like being stuck in traffic, having an argument with someone, and worries about money and relationships. Daily hassles can occur all day long and are highly linked to psychological and physical symptoms of stress (Lazarus and Folkman 1984).

Signs and Symptoms of Excessive Stress

The numerous signs of excessive stress span physical, emotional, and behavioral categories (table 10.2). Not all people experience all of the symptoms all of the time, and a given symptom may show up in response to different stressors. Being able to recognize your personal stress symptoms will help you act quickly to make behavioral changes before your stress becomes an anxiety disorder or depression. Think of your personal stress signs as a glowing orange "check engine" light on your dashboard. In lab 10.1 in the web study guide, you will identify two main life stressors and develop a plan as

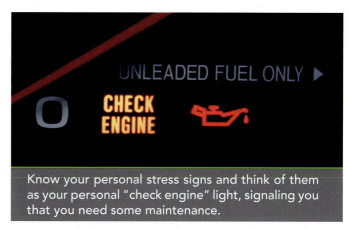

Know your personal stress signs and think of them as your personal "check engine" light, signaling you that you need some maintenance.

to how you will cope with and change the effects of these stressors in your life using the decisional balance behavioral tool discussed in chapter 3.

Specific Stressors of College Life

Over and above the general stressors of life, college, especially during your first year, can involve specific stressors. As you review the following categories, recall

Table 10.2   Potential Signs of Excessive Stress

Physical	Emotional	Behavioral
Headaches	Easily angered, short tempered	Difficulty falling or staying asleep
Muscle tension; neck or back pain	Feeling depressed or down	Increased alcohol and substance abuse
Upset stomach, including nausea, constipation, and diarrhea	Feeling jittery	Loss of appetite or overeating comfort foods
Dry mouth and difficulty swallowing	Crying	Changes in connections with friends and family
Chest pains and rapid heartbeat (at rest)	Becoming easily frustrated	Avoidance techniques with devices
Fatigue, low energy	Feeling overwhelmed	Reduced performance in job or school
Frequent colds and infections	Feeling bad about yourself (low self-esteem)	
Excessive sweating		
Clenched jaw and grinding teeth		

From Center for Diseases Control (2017); American Psychological Association (n.d.); Sapolsky (2004).

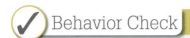

Behavior Check

What Are Your Top Stressors?

Recent representative data from college students indicated that within the past 12 months, approximately 57 percent of students reported their level of overall stress to be more than average or tremendous. Students identified the following parts of life as being traumatic or very difficult to handle: academics (50 percent), finances (33 percent), intimate relationships (31 percent), sleep difficulties (31 percent), and other social relationships (30 percent; American College Health Association 2017).

Take a few minutes to do a stressor inventory and determine your top five stressors. If you have minimal stressors, your life may be lacking challenge. If you have lots of stressors, you might be on overload. Remember that what constitutes a stressor is very personal. Try to determine if these top stressors are temporary or chronic. A temporary stressor might be a challenging course that will be finished at the end of the term. A chronic stressor might be having to balance a full academic load and a part-time job to pay for college for many years. At the end of the chapter, you will revisit these stressors and develop a stress-management plan to help you cope with and reduce the negative effects of stress in your life.

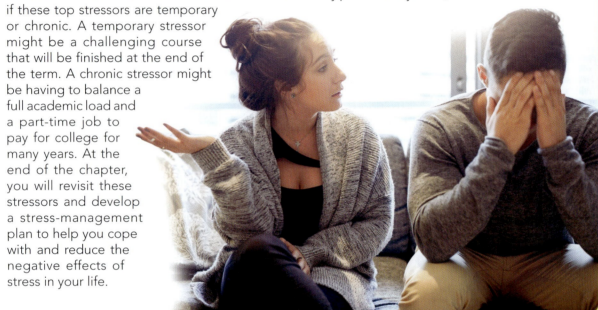

that one person's stress is another person's thrill. While you might dread the first day of class because you don't know anyone, your more extroverted roommate might bounce out the door looking forward to meeting new people.

Academic Challenges

The heavy workload in college can be a challenge. Many students who attend college were very good students in high school; however, they may find college more challenging with its increased academic rigor and expectations. The workload can be intense, and professors operate independently, which means they often don't know if their midterms land on the same day for you. There is also much less structure in college than in high school, with fewer homework assignments and more comprehensive final exams.

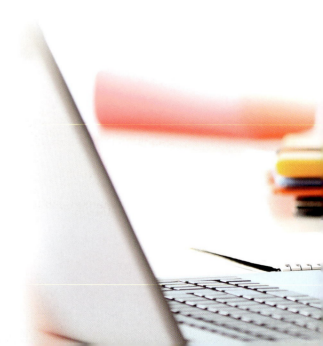

Changing Social Roles, Relationships, and Identity

The transition to independence can be stressful even if it is welcome. Many challenges are interrelated, including the following examples:

- **Family.** Moving away from home can cause relationships with your family to change. Moving away can be welcome or cause great homesickness if your family is one of your primary social supports.

- **New friends and relationships.** Meeting different people can be exciting but also a source of strain and even overwhelm you, depending on your personality. Navigating your new social dynamics on a daily basis can be stressful.

- **Roommates.** Sharing space with new living partners can be challenging, especially if you had your own room and bathroom at home.

- **Self-image.** As you leave high school, you will need to adjust your identity. Maybe you were the smart one or the talented athlete or captain of the cheerleading team. Transitioning to college life can be a struggle as you recognize that you are just one of many different types of students.

- **Larger social issues and choices.** College can also be a time where you are exposed to many lifestyle choices, including sexual activity, alcohol use, and other issues such as sexual orientation, religious beliefs, and political affiliations. Stress can arrive based on your tolerance of these lifestyle choices and differences. They could also make you question your own beliefs and choices.

Environment Changes

The transition to college will come with many changes in your physical environment, especially if you are living in the residence halls. You will sleep in a new bed in a new room with a new bathroom arrangement. You will eat in the dining halls rather than your own kitchen. Transportation on campus and around town will be different. Finding out where to go for classes and other requirements can be a source of stress. Noise stress may be different compared to your home, which may disrupt your sleep.

Academic challenges are the number one stressor for college students.

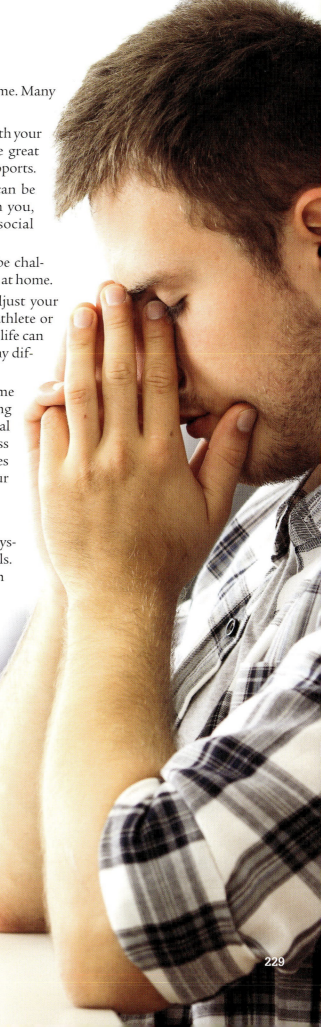

Financial Pressures and Future Worries

College costs continue to rise, which stresses both students and their families. There are also many hidden and unplanned costs in college, including course fees, textbooks, and fees to join organizations. Many students now work part-time to offset these rising costs, which can be stressful due to fatigue and time constraints. The student loan debt that accumulates can also be a source of chronic stress and worry.

Many students who struggle to find a major and settle into a career path are stressed because they know a good education is also supposed to prepare them for the workplace and put them on the path to financial independence. This decision-making process, combined with financial pressures, can be overwhelming. Managing your life, which includes managing your money, is an essential component of becoming an independent person.

Time Management

Many students struggle to manage their time and often complain that there is not enough time in the day. College can open up tremendous freedom in your daily schedule. However, this lack of structure can also be a source of stress because you will need to make yourself accountable and structured in order to simultaneously manage your academic, social, and, potentially, your work lives. Figure 10.5 shows how college students use their time, on average.

Key Stress-Management Strategies

Since we all have stressors in our lives, and there are times when these stressors are more significant and debilitating than others, it's important to learn how to put these life events into perspective and to have a coping plan in place. Like stressors, strategies for managing stress are personal. One tactic may help you more than your roommate and some strategies will work better for combatting certain stressors. This section describes the primary strategies that have been well researched.

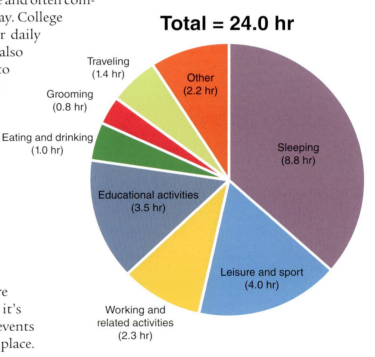

Total = 24.0 hr

Traveling (1.4 hr)
Grooming (0.8 hr)
Eating and drinking (1.0 hr)
Other (2.2 hr)
Sleeping (8.8 hr)
Educational activities (3.5 hr)
Leisure and sport (4.0 hr)
Working and related activities (2.3 hr)

Figure 10.5   Time use on an average weekday for full-time university and college students.

Note: Data include individuals aged 15 to 49 who were enrolled full time at a university or college. Data include nonholiday weekdays and are averages for 2011 to 2015.

From Bureau of Labor Statistics (2016).

Exercise and Physical Activity

As this textbook describes in great detail, exercise and physical activity have many benefits for your health, including your mental health. Exercise can help you manage stress and anxiety and is used to help prevent or treat mild depression (Office of Disease Prevention and Health 2008). Many modes are important, but the cardiorespiratory modes are the best researched. Regular daily movement of at least a moderate intensity can prevent stress from getting out of control (i.e., prevent the "check engine" light from going on). You can also temporarily increase the amount of exercise you do when you are facing a short-term stressor, such as during finals week.

Fuel Your Body

Stress has effects on dietary intake (Sapolsky 2004). Under stress, you may be tempted to overconsume calories or increase your intake of less healthy foods. Coping by eating for comfort is often termed *stress eating*. It typically involves selecting foods that are less healthy in terms of added sugars, saturated fats, and sodium. When pressured for time, you may take in excessive caffeine, which can increase stress and anxiety in both the short and long term. However, many people have a reduced appetite in response to stress, so making healthy fuel choices throughout the day is important. Being hungry with low blood sugar is a stressor. Stress hormones can cause your blood sugar to be less balanced, which can further contribute to stress levels. People most often skip breakfast due to stress, which can then cause low blood sugar during prime productive hours in the morning (American Psychological Association 2014). How should you eat to help manage stress? Essentially, the best advice is to eat a healthy and balanced diet (see chapter 8 for more information on nutrition).

Social Support

Social support is also a primary strategy for reducing your response to life's stressors. Being tended and befriended in times of stress and being a social support to others in times of need reduce the stress response, especially to psychological stressors (Sapolsky 2004). It is important to get social support from the right person, the right network of friends, and the right community. We all know people who would increase our stress response if we asked them for help.

Instead of placing the management of friendships, which take time, into the "fun" category, start thinking of these activities as a health behavior. Fostering new friendships, maintaining established relationships, and seeking to keep family connections healthy are all critical to your health. The college experience presents opportunities to join many different clubs and organizations, ranging from church, sports, political, and volunteer experiences. Many of these are run as registered student organizations at your institution. Finally, if you are struggling with relationship issues or are suffering from loneliness, most campuses have counseling services that offer many services either for free or at a reduced cost. Gaining good relationship skills is an important investment in your health. Invest in yourself.

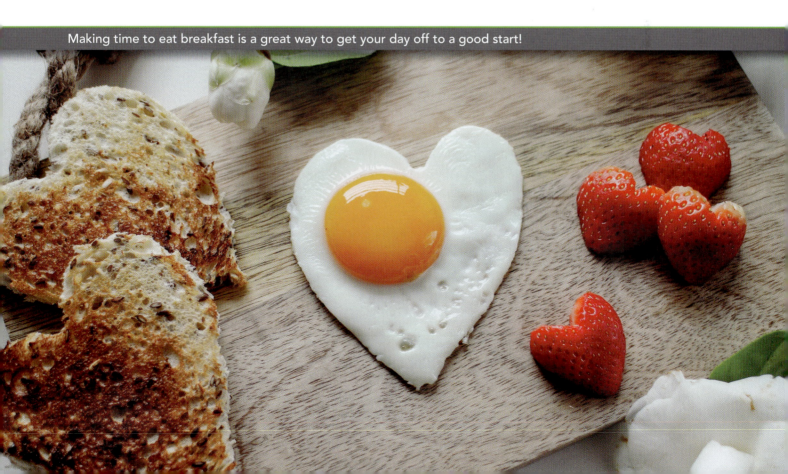

Making time to eat breakfast is a great way to get your day off to a good start!

Relaxation Techniques and Meditation: Quieting the Mind

Relaxation techniques often combine breathing and focusing on pleasing thoughts and images to calm the mind and the body. Common examples of relaxation response techniques are biofeedback, deep breathing, guided imagery, progressive relaxation, and self-hypnosis. Mind and body practices, such as meditation and yoga, are also sometimes considered relaxation techniques (National Institutes of Health 2017). When performed on a regular basis, meditation has been shown to reduce the negative effects of psychological stress (Goyal et al. 2014), and biological evidence includes reduction in stress hormones (Sapolsky 2004). Many different types of meditation exist, and most are focused on adopting thoughts and ideas that are positive and affirming. Two common methods are **mindfulness mediation** and **Transcendental Meditation**. Mindfulness meditation reduces psychological stress and the stress response through learning how to be mindful of the present moment, as opposed to thinking about the past or future. Transcendental Meditation emphasizes using a **mantra**, which is a word or phrase that is repeated to reach a point where your attention is no longer focused on the distressing thoughts.

Managing Your Life and To-Do List

Setting goals and priorities to keep you organized and prepared can help you manage your stress level. Oversleeping, running late for class, and rushing through your morning in a disorganized manner will almost certainly cause a stress response. Arriving to class and realizing that you forgot about the exam scheduled for that day will cause your cortisol levels to increase. Consciously thinking through what must get done and what can wait for another day as well as prioritizing your work *and* your rest is critical (University of South Florida n.d.).

Time management means successfully and efficiently prioritizing and scheduling one's time. There are only 24 hours in your day and 7 days in your week; therefore, choices are a constant challenge. Figure 10.6 illustrates steps that might offer some insights to increase your skills in managing your time, which is really about managing your life.

Managing Stress Through Sleep

Sleep is a stress-management technique because the stress response can cause sleep disturbances and lack of quality sleep greatly increases the stress response to life's challenges. For optimal health, learn how much you personally need to sleep to function properly and then use strategies to make sure you get this quantity and quality of sleep. In our society today, regular good sleep is becoming very rare and is often thought of as a luxury reserved for a few or for vacation times. Your sleep behaviors are just as important for your health and academic performance as eating well and exercising.

Sleep Quantity and Quality

As you will see figure 10.7, sleep is an important health behavior, and many people struggle to get enough quality sleep (Watson et al. 2015). College students need seven hours or more of sleep per night; however, the amount of sleep a person needs varies, especially with age. Infants, children, and adolescents need the most sleep. Most adults require seven to eight hours per night. Some people function well on 5 hours, whereas others need 10 hours of sleep to feel their best (American Sleep Association n.d.).

Learn to Manage Your Time

 Set goals and priorities: Write a "To Do List" to help you stay focused.

Make a plan: Determine the milestones you want to accomplish and by when.

 Divide big tasks into smaller tasks: Chip away at the bigger task by breaking it up into smaller, more manageable pieces.

Set a deadline: Determine realistic deadlines so you can see your accomplishments.

Take breaks: Determine a set time you will work on a project without any distractions (including your phone). Set a timer and work until the alarm goes off, and then reward yourself by taking a break.

Be organized: Have a place for all of your belongings so you don't have to take extra time in your day to search for them.

It's OK to say no!: Recognize your limitations and realize it is okay to say no and focus on your priorities.

Enlist the help of friends and colleagues: Ask others to help you.

Anticipate the unexpected: Allow extra time to complete your projects as problems may arise that are not under your control.

Record everything in a journal or calendar: Record all appointments, project due dates, and events in your calendar, and keep it updated.

Prioritize: Focus on what is most critical and needs your attention.

Determine when you are the most productive: Are you a morning person, night person, or middle of the day person? Notice when you have the most energy and complete your most demanding projects at this time of the day.

Figure 10.6   Use these tips to successfully manage your time and lower your stress.

Beyond quantity, uninterrupted (i.e., not fragmented) sleep is also very important for sleep quality so that each of the five stages of sleep can be experienced, especially stages 3 and 4 and REM (rapid eye movement) sleep. Typically, if uninterrupted, a healthy sleeper will pass through all five stages of sleep in a sleep cycle of 90 to 110 minutes, with the length spent in the stages changing through the night (American Sleep Association n.d.).

- Stage 1 sleep:
  - Light sleep occurs.
  - Drift in and out of sleep.
  - Can be awakened easily.
  - Eyes move slowly and muscle activity slows.
  - Often have a sense of falling or muscle spasms of jerks.
- Stage 2 sleep:
  - Eye movements stop.

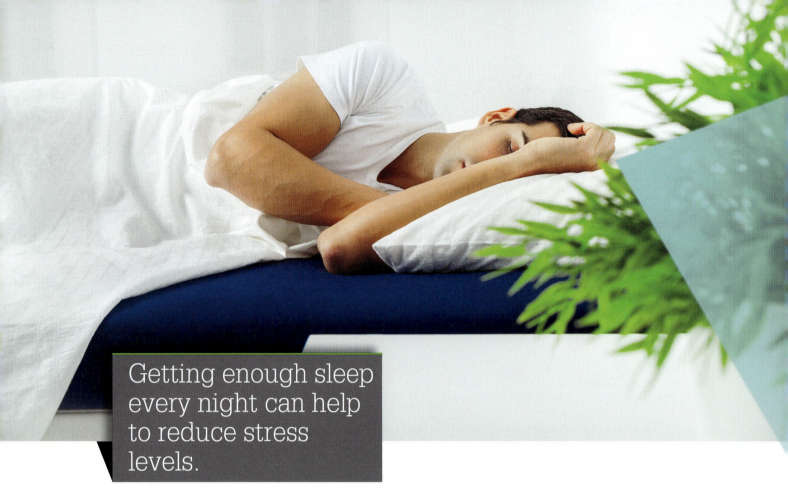

Getting enough sleep every night can help to reduce stress levels.

- ◦ Brain waves become slower.
- ◦ Rapid brain waves occur occasionally.
- • Stages 3 and 4 sleep:
  - ◦ In stage 3, slow brain waves appear called delta waves.
  - ◦ By stage 4, delta waves are the only brain waves.
  - ◦ Stages 3 and 4 are deep sleep with no eye or muscle activity.
  - ◦ If awakened, people are groggy and may be disoriented.
- • REM sleep:
  - ◦ Breathing becomes rapid, irregular, and shallow.
  - ◦ Eyes jerk rapidly in random directions.
  - ◦ Muscles in arms and legs become temporarily paralyzed.
  - ◦ Heart rate increases and blood pressure rises.
  - ◦ If awakened in this stage, many people recall bizarre or illogical dreams or thoughts.

If you feel drowsy during the day, you likely are not getting enough sleep. If you routinely fall asleep within five minutes of lying down, you likely have major sleep deprivation (American Sleep Association n.d.). Inability to get to sleep or stay asleep and sleep disorders such as excessive snoring or sleep apnea are also a concern (Centers for Disease Control and Prevention 2017b).

Therefore, it's important to get regular sleep with regular sleep cycles and stages instead of skipping sleep for many days and then planning to catch up on weekends or holiday breaks (figure 10.7). An excellent sleep resource is the American Sleep Association (www.sleepassociation.org). Speak with your personal physician if you are concerned about your sleep patterns.

Thirty-three percent of the U.S. population reports chronically not getting enough sleep, which is less than 7 hours of sleep in a 24-hour period (Centers for Disease Control and Prevention 2017c).

Health Risks Associated With Poor Sleep

Regular, good sleep is essential for optimal health and a high quality of life. Without it, we experience

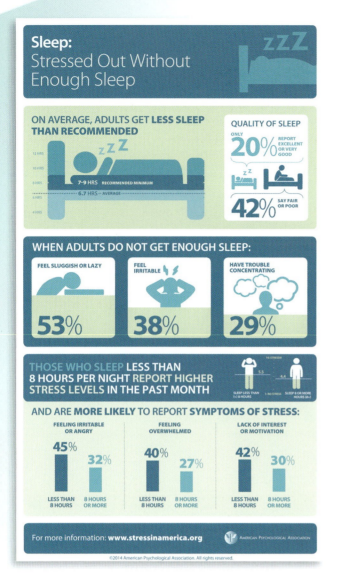

Figure 10.7   Where do you fall in this illustration? If you're not getting enough sleep, can you identify with some of the consequences?

Reprinted from American Psychological Association. www.apa.org/Images/2013-sia-Sleep-Infographic-1024_tcm7-166594.jpg

adverse physical and mental consequences. These include an increased risk of accidents, injuries, cardiovascular and metabolic diseases, and mental health afflictions such as depression. Lack of sleep also negatively affects mental alertness and focus and contributes to poor behavioral choices in general. Chronic sleep deprivation stimulates the stress systems, contributing to allostatic load. If you have poor sleep habits, you are at risk of developing numerous chronic health conditions that will negatively affect your life, now and in the future (Watson et al. 2015; American Sleep Association n.d.).

Strategies for Enhancing Sleep and Energy Levels

Like most health behaviors, sleep is a habit. Therefore, having good sleep habits can help you get a good night's sleep on a regular basis. Lab 10.2 in the web study guide will help you assess your sleep quantity and quality and craft a personal plan for getting the sleep you need. The following considerations will help you explore your sleep habits (Centers for Disease Control and Prevention 2016a):

- Be consistent: Get up and go to bed at the same time every day. This includes weekends and holiday or vacation breaks from school.

- Make sure your bedroom is cool (not too warm), peaceful, and quiet. Your mattress and pillows should be comfortable.

- Install dark curtains or blinds over your bedroom windows or wear an eye mask.

- Make your bedroom a screen-free zone. Do not share your bed with your computer and cell phone.

- Eat small meals before bedtime and resist the temptation to have pizza, tacos, and other spicy foods a few hours before bed. Some foods can cause indigestion, or acid reflux, which worsens when lying down.

- Limit your caffeine in the late afternoon or early evening (this includes chocolate and energy drinks) and limit alcohol and other fluids before bed to reduce the chances of having to use the bathroom during your sleep cycle.

- Being physically active during the day can help you fall asleep more easily at night.

- Talk to your health care provider about any medications you are taking and their effect on your sleep, since some may cause drowsiness. You may be able to take these types of medications before bed so you can stay awake for class and sleep at night.

Social, Stressed, and Sleepless

The college years, especially the early ones, can be stressful, which affects sleep quality. Also, due

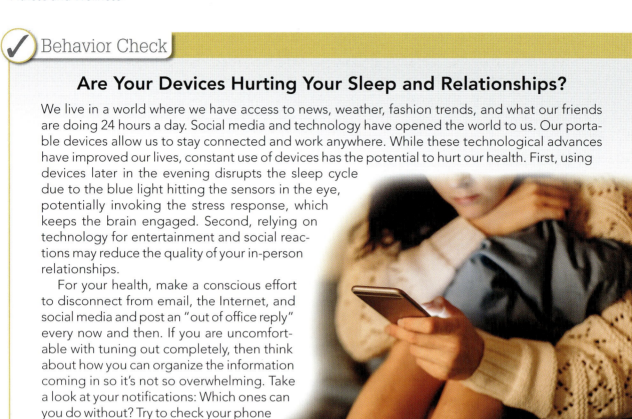

✓ Behavior Check

Are Your Devices Hurting Your Sleep and Relationships?

We live in a world where we have access to news, weather, fashion trends, and what our friends are doing 24 hours a day. Social media and technology have opened the world to us. Our portable devices allow us to stay connected and work anywhere. While these technological advances have improved our lives, constant use of devices has the potential to hurt our health. First, using devices later in the evening disrupts the sleep cycle due to the blue light hitting the sensors in the eye, potentially invoking the stress response, which keeps the brain engaged. Second, relying on technology for entertainment and social reactions may reduce the quality of your in-person relationships.

For your health, make a conscious effort to disconnect from email, the Internet, and social media and post an "out of office reply" every now and then. If you are uncomfortable with tuning out completely, then think about how you can organize the information coming in so it's not so overwhelming. Take a look at your notifications: Which ones can you do without? Try to check your phone for messages just once an hour while studying. Plan screen-free days, either once a week or during a holiday.

to the new relationships and environment of campus, your social life can gear up significantly. You may find that the three factors of social life, stress, and sleep are intertwined. Social lives can cause stress, but social support is also very important for stress management. If you give more hours to your social life, you will have less time for academic work and sleep. Being pressed for time and under-slept can also cause stress. Learning to balance the competing demands of all that you *have to do* and all that you *want to do* is a challenge that you will likely have for all of your working years. Learning this balance will serve you well, both now and in the future. Two important keys are keeping the positive energy and getting professional help if needed.

Keeping the Positive Energy: Habitual Movement is Key

Of all of the stress-management strategies outlined in this chapter, a relatively high level of exercise and physical activity is one of the most important. Being regularly physically active at a moderate to high intensity, especially the cardiorespiratory and resistance training modes, can help manage stress and reduce the risks for anxiety disorders and mild depression. This level of activity is also linked with improved sleep quality (Office of Disease Prevention and Health 2008). Finally, regular activity can also help you maintain mental and physical energy (Puetz, O'Connor, and Dishman 2006), which can help you accomplish the *have to do* and the *want to do* tasks on your list. In this way, your daily movement is the cornerstone of your plan to keep you spiraling up instead of down in your sleep behavior and stress responses.

Know When to Get Help

Triggering your stress response can be unpleasant, which is why most people define stress in a negative way. Triggering your stress response now and again is not a problem for most of us. But for some people, repeated or sustained stress-response activation can lead to more serious mental health challenges, including anxiety disorders and depression.

Anxiety Disorders

Chronic stress can progress to an anxiety disorder (National Institutes of Mental Health 2016a). For example, **generalized anxiety disorder** is a condition where a person displays excessive anxiety and worry for months, with several relatively intense symptoms that do not go away and can get worse with time. **Panic disorder** presents with recurrent unexpected panic attacks, which are sudden periods of intense fear that might include heart pounding (palpitations), sweating, trembling, sensations of choking, shortness of breath, and sometimes a feeling of impending doom. People with **social anxiety disorder** have a marked fear of social or performance situations in which they expect to be embarrassed, judged, or rejected, triggering a stress response. Anxiety disorders can greatly reduce quality of life, causing great distress, straining class or work performance, and hindering relationships.

Depression

Also related to stress and a close cousin to anxiety disorders is **depression**. Many different types of depression exist, and the most concerning type is major depressive disorder or clinical depression. Symptoms include persistent sadness, feelings of hopelessness, changes in sleep patterns (difficulty sleeping, early-morning awakening, or oversleeping), changes in appetite or

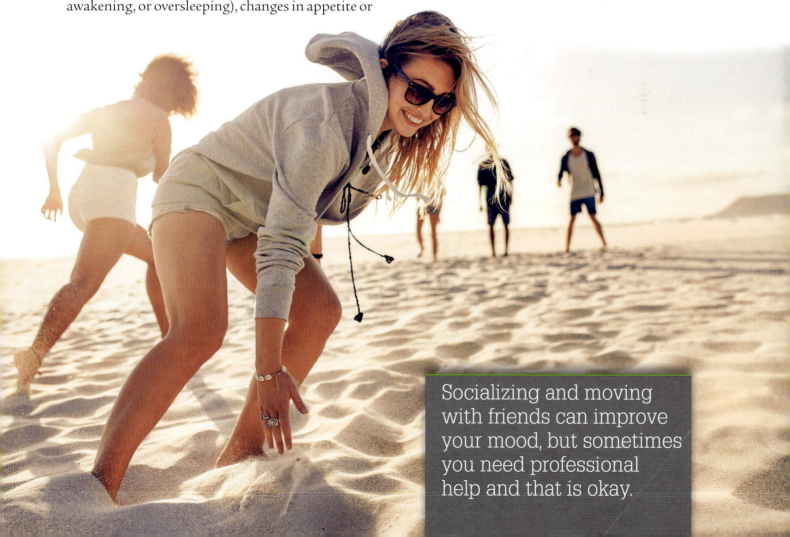

Socializing and moving with friends can improve your mood, but sometimes you need professional help and that is okay.

weight, decreased energy, and aches and pains that occur for at least two weeks (National Institutes of Mental Health 2016b). This is not a mild case of the blues in response to a temporary event. A defining feature of depression is loss of pleasure. Along with major depression, great grief and guilt also occur; these can be incapacitating. Unfortunately, depression is highly linked to suicide.

Professional Help

When you experience a "warning light" with respect to sustained stress symptoms, try to manage your stress response through the strategies described in this chapter. If you find that after a few weeks you are unable to do so, get some help to prevent longer-term health issues. Sometimes there are medical reasons for anxiety or depression. For example, some medications have side effects that can mimic anxiety disorders or depressive symptoms. Low blood sugar can also cause feelings of anxiety. Seeing a health care professional can help you sort through the various physiological, situational, or emotional reasons for your current struggle. Nearly all colleges and universities have a student health center that offers services for both medical and psychological challenges that students routinely face. Know your resources and get help sooner rather than later.

Summary

We all experience stressors, especially psychological and social challenges. Although many stressors are good because they keep you engaged and challenged, too much challenge, especially for an extended period of time, can be overwhelming. Managing your stress response is important for preventing longer-term negative health effects. Understanding your personal stressors, learning to read your "warning light," and practicing good stress-management strategies can help you cope and feel better. A regular physical activity and exercise program of a moderate to high intensity and healthy sleep practices are both foundational to managing your stress response and maintaining a high energy level to meet the demands of your busy schedule.

WEB STUDY GUIDE

Remember to complete all of the web study guide activities to further facilitate your learning, including the following lab activities:

Lab 10.1   Evaluating and Balancing Stress

Lab 10.2   Sleep as a Health Behavior

REVIEW QUESTIONS

1. Stress can be considered eustress or distress. Define each and provide typical examples for a college student.
2. What is the stress response and how do the neural and endocrine systems work together to cause it?
3. Define *allostatic load* and describe its importance as the link between chronic stress and health implications.
4. Describe three systems that are negatively influenced by chronic stress and the mechanisms and the common conditions and diseases related to the system.
5. Describe common stressors for college students.
6. Stress symptoms are a "check engine" light for your health. Describe five common symptoms of chronic stress.
7. List the six key stress-management strategies described in this chapter and provide an example of each that might be used by a college student.

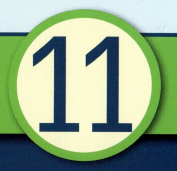

Remaining Free From Addiction

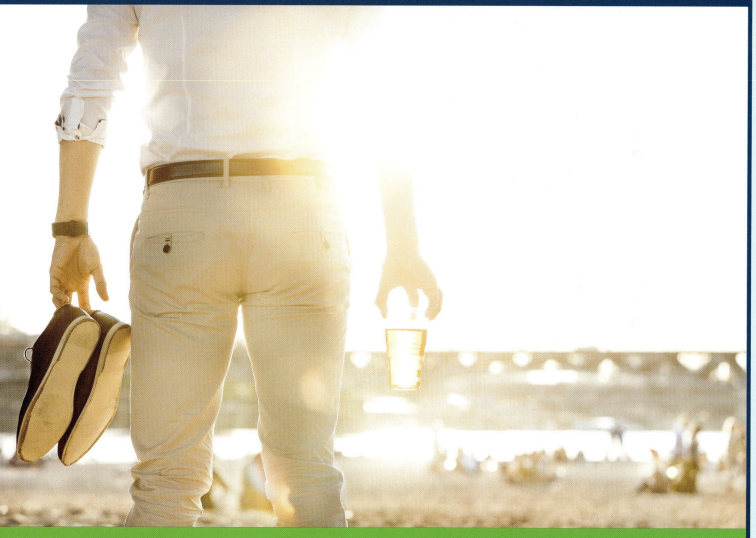

OBJECTIVES

❱ Define addiction.

❱ Explain why people develop substance and behavioral addictions.

❱ Differentiate between substance and behavioral addictions.

❱ Know the short- and long-term effects of addiction on the body and on relationships with others.

❱ Identify treatment options for addiction.

KEY TERMS

addiction

behavioral addiction

binge drinking

blood alcohol concentration

central nervous system (CNS)

club drugs

cocaine

dependence

depressants

drug abuse

drug misuse

heroin

illegal drugs

illicit drugs

marijuana

nicotine

opioids

psychoactive drugs

stimulants

substance abuse

Substance and behavioral addictions can take over one's life, often leading to debilitating disabilities and even death. You may know someone who is struggling with an addiction, so you know how serious the problem is. An estimated 27.4 million Americans aged 12 and older have a significant problem with drugs or alcohol (Substance Abuse and Mental Health Services Administration 2015). Addictions are most likely to begin during adolescence and young adulthood (Grant et al. 2010). Addicts end up in situations where they are not able to care for themselves and can become reliant on community resources for survival. Addiction

is a complex issue that is neither the result of a lack of willpower nor a sign of weakness. Research has shown that drugs have an effect on the brain that makes quitting difficult, even for those who have a great desire to do so. This chapter focuses on how and why people become addicted to drugs and certain behaviors. It also provides information about resources for treatment and prevention of the most commonly abused substances.

Drugs are either used as intended or prescribed or they are misused or abused. **Drug misuse** is when a drug is being taken for reasons other than what it is intended for, for example, taking an antihistamine to feel high rather than to relieve allergy symptoms. **Drug abuse** is when an individual takes a drug not as prescribed or intended consistently and over a long period of time.

Types of Addictions

Two primary types of **addictions** exist: substance addiction and behavioral addiction. Both types can lead to serious health and social outcomes, such as breaking the law, being arrested, poor decision making, increased risk of sexual assault

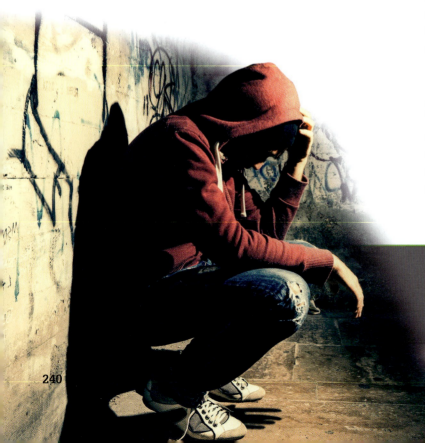

Addictions are complex and are not the result of a lack of willpower.

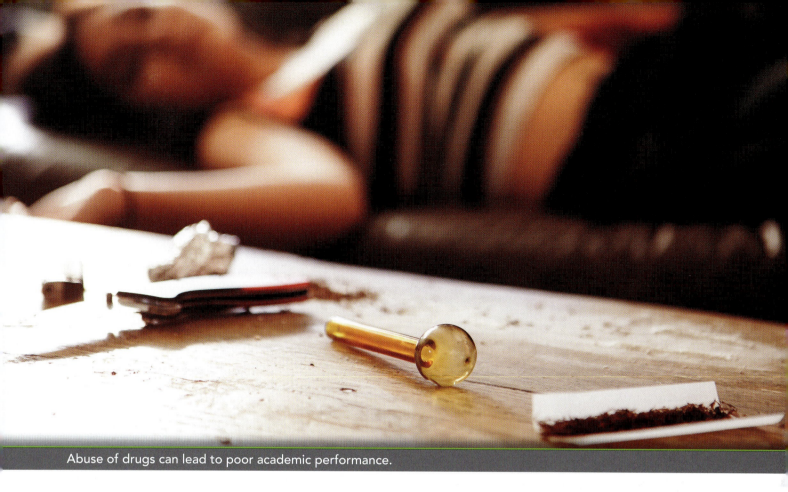

Abuse of drugs can lead to poor academic performance.

(as the victim or the perpetrator), memory loss, and unemployment. Addiction can have fatal consequences if treatment is not sought or is not successful.

Substance Abuse: Drug Addictions

Substance abuse is using drugs not as intended or prescribed but rather illegally or in doses that lead to harmful consequences. When drugs are taken repeatedly and not as prescribed, chemical changes to the brain occur that lead the individual to seek more of the drugs because of the euphoric and pleasurable effects. The primary chemical that causes these feelings is dopamine. The release of this chemical motivates an addicted person to continue taking these drugs over and over. After a long period of taking drugs, the brain produces less of the dopamine, and the addicted person develops a tolerance that diminishes the euphoric feelings. This results in the desire and need to take the drug in higher doses, which can lead to an addiction. Long-term use of drugs affects the brain's ability to process what are considered simple functions such as learning, judgment, decision making, adapting to and dealing with stressful situations, memory, and healthy behaviors (National Institute on Drug Abuse 2016b). Although many addicts are very aware of the negative effects of abusing drugs, this knowledge alone is not enough to help them stop—this is the reality of addiction.

Treatment of Substance Addictions

The good news is that, like many diseases and illnesses, addictions can be treated. However, in many cases, a cure is not achieved because there is always the possibility of relapse. Still, many people in recovery succeed at managing their addiction for the rest of their lives. Approximately 1.5 percent of the U.S. population sought treatment for a substance abuse problem in 2013. The majority of those sought help for alcohol abuse, followed by marijuana abuse (Substance Abuse and Mental Health Services Administration 2014). The most common type of treatments used by those seeking help were self-help groups (e.g., Alcoholics Anonymous, Narcotics Anonymous) and outpatient rehabilitation facilities. The best chance of success is a combination of addiction treatment medication with behavioral therapy that is specific to the needs of the patient. Unfortunately, the primary reason that people with substance abuse problems do not follow through is lack of resources to afford treatment or lack of health care coverage (37.3 percent; Substance Abuse and Mental Health

241

Services Administration 2014). The second most common reason is that the person is not ready to stop using the substance (24.5 percent).

Treating drug abuse and addictions may require the use of medications; however, all treatment options must include behavior therapies in order to have the best chance at success. FDA-approved medications exist to treat addictions to cocaine, heroin, and methamphetamines. Examples of behavioral treatment options include cognitive

behavioral therapy, community-based therapies, contingency management or motivational incentives, and 12-step facilitation therapy (National Institute on Drug Abuse 2017b).

Behavioral Addictions

People can get a high on other things besides drugs and alcohol (see figure 11.1); many have **behavioral addictions** that result in some of the same euphoric feelings and negative outcomes

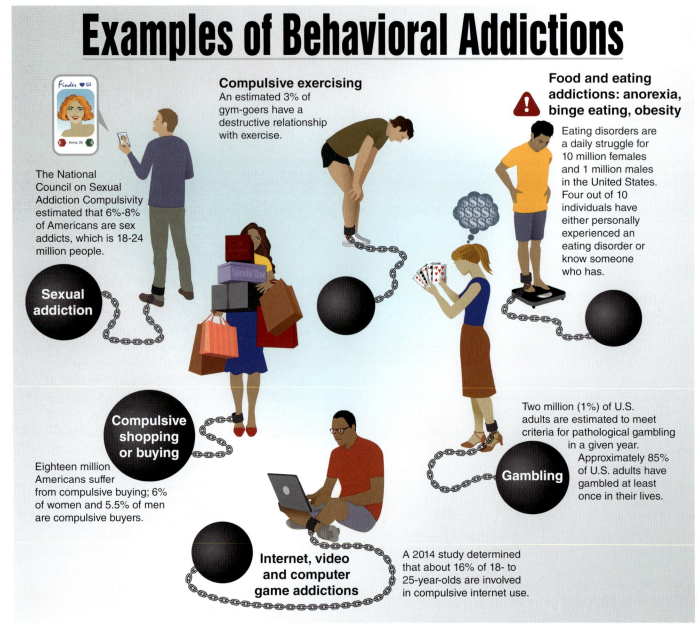

Examples of Behavioral Addictions

Compulsive exercising
An estimated 3% of gym-goers have a destructive relationship with exercise.

Food and eating addictions: anorexia, binge eating, obesity

Eating disorders are a daily struggle for 10 million females and 1 million males in the United States. Four out of 10 individuals have either personally experienced an eating disorder or know someone who has.

The National Council on Sexual Addiction Compulsivity estimated that 6%-8% of Americans are sex addicts, which is 18-24 million people.

Sexual addiction

Compulsive shopping or buying

Eighteen million Americans suffer from compulsive buying; 6% of women and 5.5% of men are compulsive buyers.

Internet, video and computer game addictions

A 2014 study determined that about 16% of 18- to 25-year-olds are involved in compulsive internet use.

Two million (1%) of U.S. adults are estimated to meet criteria for pathological gambling in a given year. Approximately 85% of U.S. adults have gambled at least once in their lives.

Gambling

Figure 11.1 Behavioral addictions occur when the desire to get a high through certain behaviors becomes chronic and out of control.

Data from Bragg (2009); Koran, et al (2006); National Council on Problem Gambling (2014); Addiction Hope (2017); BBC News (2014); Eating Disorder Hope (2017); National Eating Disorders (2016).

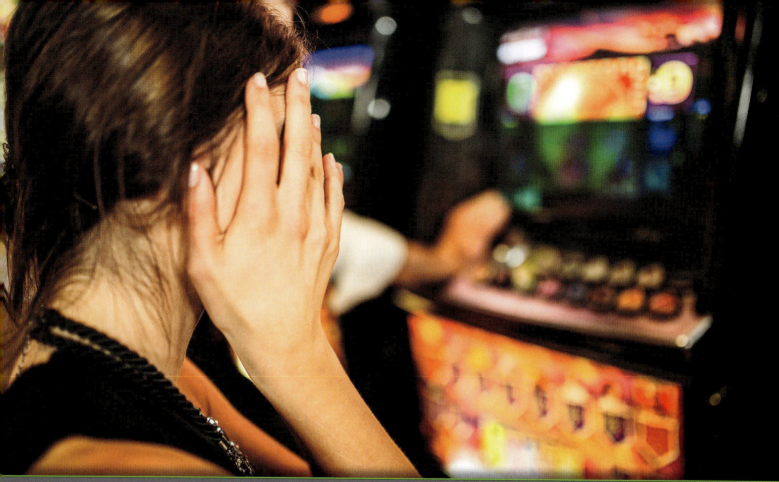

If a desire to get a high from any activity becomes chronic or out of control, it has become an addiction.

as experienced with substance abuse. Behavioral addiction is not often a topic of discussion because society tends to focus on substance addiction. The desire to feel good and get a high through certain behaviors is very common, and behavioral addiction can become chronic and out of control despite the negative consequences. People with behavioral addictions experience similar highs to people with substance abuse problems because the brain releases the same chemical during the addictive behavior as when taking drugs.

Examples of behavioral addictions include compulsive buying, gambling, internet addiction, video or computer game addiction, sexual addiction, excessive tanning, plastic surgery addiction, binge eating disorder (food addiction), excessive exercising, and risky behavior addiction (e.g., skydiving, rock climbing). See chapter 9 for information on addictions related to exercise and food.

People with behavioral addictions spend excess time in a day engaged in that behavior and are unable to reduce that time; they do not have control over this behavior. Eventually the addic-

tive behavior leads to the inability to carry out normal daily activities (e.g., going to work) and maintain positive relationships with others. A common characteristic of behavioral addictions is the inability to resist the temptation to behave in a way that is harmful to the individual or others. This is similar to the inability to resist the urge to drink alcohol or use cocaine. Many people with behavioral addictions report experiencing intense cravings prior to the behavior. Once they engage in the behavior, they feel a sense of relief, somewhat like the high that is experienced with drug or alcohol abuse. The pleasure and gratification that accompanies the addictive behavior prevents the individual from recognizing its destructive effects (Grant et al. 2010).

Treatment of Behavioral Addictions

Many people with behavioral addictions experience numerous relapses and have a difficult time stopping these behaviors without professional help. Treatment options for behavioral addictions are much like those for substance abuse, including psychosocial support and medication, along with the traditional 12-step self-help support groups, motivational enhancement, and cognitive behavioral therapies (Grant et al. 2010). These treatment methods focus on identifying the specific behaviors that led to the negative outcomes (e.g., financial ruin, loss of close relationships, loss of employment) for the individual. They also help the person cope with the need for feelings of euphoria experienced when engaging in these destructive behaviors. These therapies provide alternative coping mechanisms for when addicted individuals are in high-risk situations and help them develop a plan that specifically identifies healthier behaviors they can implement for life.

What Is Substance Abuse Addiction?

We will now turn to discussing substance abuse. Consider for a moment how you would define drug addiction. Would your definition include how frequently a person uses a substance, how much is used, or a combination of those factors? Would it include other aspects, such as not being able to stop or always wanting more? The *Diagnostic and Statistical Manual of Mental Disorders* (American Psychiatric Association 2000) defines people as being addicted to, dependent on, or abusing alcohol or **illicit drugs** if they meet three or more of the following six **dependence** criteria specifically related to the use of hallucinogens, inhalants, and tranquilizers:

1. Spent a great deal of time over a period of a month getting, using, or getting over the effects of the substance.
2. Used the substance more often than intended or were unable to keep set limits on the substance use.
3. Needed to use the substance more than before to get desired effects or noticed that the same amount of substance use had less effect than before.
4. Unable to cut down or stop using the substance every time they tried or wanted to.
5. Continued to use the substance even though it was causing problems with emotions, nerves, mental health, or physical problems.
6. Found that the substance use reduced or eliminated involvement or participation in important activities.

A seventh criterion related to the use of alcohol, cocaine, heroin, pain relievers, sedatives, and stimulants was recently added. This last criterion

 Behavior Check

Your Attitudes About Drug Use: Do You Agree or Disagree?

Think about whether you agree or disagree with each of these statements (Centers for Disease Control and Prevention 1988):

1. Drug dependence happens when using drugs every day.
2. Most people who use drugs have financial problems.
3. Smoking cigarettes helps people control their emotions.
4. Using illegal drugs prevents people from being responsible.
5. Marijuana helps people cope with life stressors.
6. Smoking can cause people to age prematurely.
7. Cocaine can help reduce sleeping problems.
8. Drugs help people to be more creative.
9. Using drugs can lead to the loss of self-control.
10. Alcohol use can negatively affect relationships with family and friends.
11. People can remain relatively healthy even if they use illegal drugs.

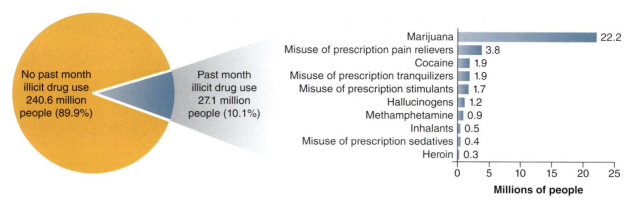

Figure 11.2 Number of past-month illicit drug users among people aged 12 or older, 2015.

Note: Estimated numbers of people refer to people aged 12 or older in the civilian, noninstitutionalized population in the United States. The numbers do not sum to the total population of the United States because the population for NSDUH does not include people aged 11 years old or younger, people with no fixed household address (e.g., homeless or transient people not in shelters), active-duty military personnel, and residents of institutional group quarters, such as correctional facilities, nursing homes, mental institutions, and long-term care hospitals.

Note: The estimated numbers of current users of different illicit drugs are not mutually exclusive because people could have used more than one type of illicit drug in the past month.

Reprinted from Center for Behavioral Health Statistics and Quality (2016).

is related to withdrawal symptoms that vary by the abused substance (e.g., having trouble sleeping, cramps, hands trembling). With this additional criterion, a respondent was defined as having dependence if three or more of seven dependence criteria were acknowledged related to these specific substances.

Addictions become a concern when a person is not able to attend to his or her daily responsibilities (e.g., not paying bills on time, neglecting relationships, arriving late to work, not attending school, or missing appointments). The addiction begins to consume the individual's life and prevents him or her from attending to daily responsibilities and obligations. This often leads to taking more of the drug and using it longer than intended. Additionally, addiction can be considered a dependence on a substance that when stopped or reduced leads to psychological and physiological tolerance and withdrawal symptoms. Figure 11.2 shows that in 2015, an estimated 27.1 million Americans aged 12 and older surveyed had used an illicit drug within the past month. The most commonly used drug was marijuana, followed by prescription pain relievers.

Risk Factors: Why Do Some People Become Addicted?

Many factors can lead to an addiction. It can be hard to predict whether someone has an addictive personality and will develop dependence on drugs or behaviors that are harmful to them or others. Drugs have an effect on the brain that hinders the ability to stop taking them, causing many people to have a very difficult time quitting despite their desire to end the addictions.

The more risk factors a person has, the more likely an addiction is to occur. The primary factors are as follows (National Institute on Drug Abuse 2017b):

- ***Biology***. Genetics account for about half of a person's risk for developing an addiction. In addition to genetics, sex (men are more at risk than women), ethnicity, and mental health issues increase the possibility. People of color experience an increased incidence of substance abuse due to lack of access to health care, inappropriate care, and higher social, environmental, and

Signs of addiction include the need to use a substance more than before to get desired effects and the inability to cut down or stop using it.

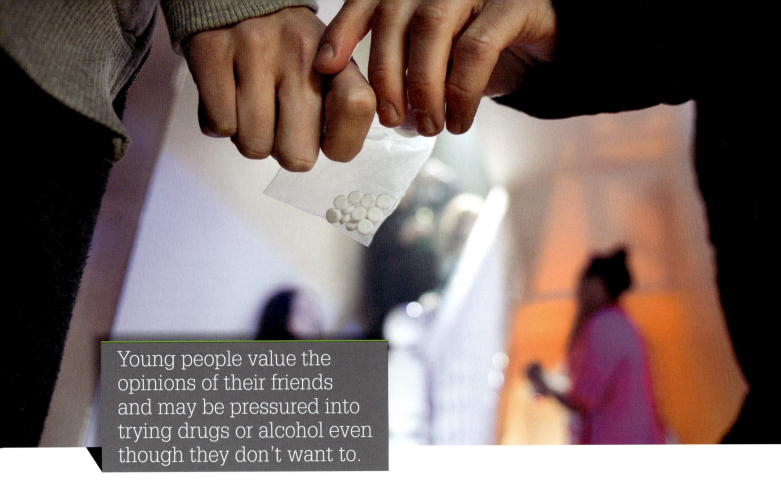

Young people value the opinions of their friends and may be pressured into trying drugs or alcohol even though they don't want to.

socioeconomic risk factors (Substance Abuse and Mental Health Services Administration 2016).

- **Environment**. Family, friends, peers, socioeconomic status, and quality of life affect addictions. Lower socioeconomic status, pressure from peers to use drugs or participate in risky behaviors, significant stress, early exposure to drugs, physical and sexual abuse, and parental guidance all influence the risk.

- **Development**. The earlier drugs are introduced or the risky behavior is initiated, the more likely an addiction to drugs or a behavior is to develop. The teenage years are when most addicts experiment with drugs and risky behaviors. These years are critical for brain development, so teens are less likely to demonstrate good judgment and exhibit self-control.

College Students and Addictions

The use of illicit drugs among college students has increased in recent years. Unfortunately, a change in this trend does not appear to be on the horizon. The prevalence of illicit drug use with college students increased from 34 percent in 2006 to 41 percent in 2015 (Johnston et al. 2016). In 2013, first use of illicit drugs among people aged 12 or older averaged 7,800 new users per day, and the average age at initiation was 19 years old. The first drug of choice for 70.3 percent of this population was marijuana, followed by nonmedical use of pain relievers (Substance Abuse and Mental Health Services Administration 2014).

The types of drugs most commonly used among college students include marijuana, amphetamines, heroin, inhalants, cocaine, and club drugs. Figure 11.3 shows the prevalence of drug use by college students. Johnston and colleagues (2016) reported results of a long-term survey on drug use among adults. At the turn of the century, the annual prevalence of marijuana use among young adults attending college was 36 percent. This declined in 2006 to 30 percent, but then increased in 2015 to an all-time record of 38 percent. Use of nonprescription amphetamines increased signifi-

Use of cocaine, heroin, and ecstasy is increasing among college students. Students also abuse prescription medications like Adderall and Ritalin (National Institute on Drug Abuse 2017b).

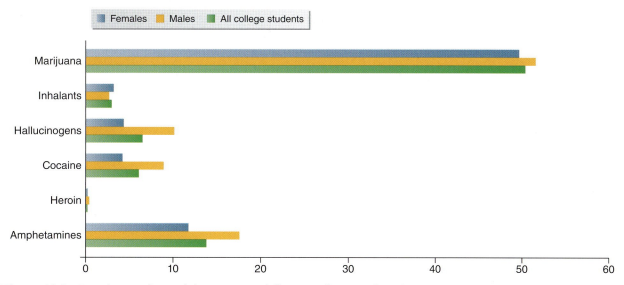

Figure 11.3   Prevalence of use of drugs among full-time college students by sex, 2015 (%).

Reprinted from L.D. Johnston et al., *Monitoring the Future: National Survey Results on Drug Use 1975-2015* (Ann Arbor MI: Institute for Social Research, The University of Michigan, 2016), 370. www.monitoringthefuture.org/pubs/monographs/mtf-vol2_2015.pdf

cantly among college students between 2008 and 2012 from 5.7 percent to 11.1 percent, respectively. However, use leveled off at 9.7 percent in 2015. College students reported using Adderall five times more often than Ritalin, very likely to help them improve academic performance. Figure 11.4 shows that while stimulant use among college students has decreased, cocaine use is increasing.

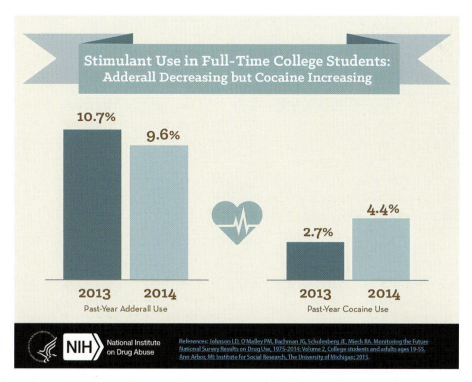

Figure 11.4   Stimulant use among college students in 2014: Adderall use is decreasing but cocaine use is increasing.

Reprinted from National Institute on Drug Abuse (2016a).

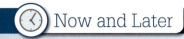
Substance Abuse and a Lifetime of Negative Consequences

Now

The best way to prevent substance abuse is to never try illicit drugs. There are many ways to prevent becoming addicted while in college (Kilpatrick 2016). Review the following information to stay drug free, now and for life:

- Become involved in extracurricular activities.
- Attend all classes and take advantage of assistance from professors to do well.
- Make a commitment to get at least eight hours of sleep a night, get some physical activity every day, and maintain a healthy weight.
- Hang around people who do not use illicit drugs or drink alcohol. Attend social events where these substances are not offered.
- Take courses or attend events to learn more about the dangers of drugs and alcohol, signs of addiction, and the connection between these substances and the prevention of sexual assault.
- Contribute to substance abuse prevention on your campus by volunteering to be part of alternative, responsible ways to have fun.

Later

Addictions to drugs and alcohol become chronic conditions that are very difficult to control despite the harmful and fatal outcomes. No single factor can predict whether or not a person will become

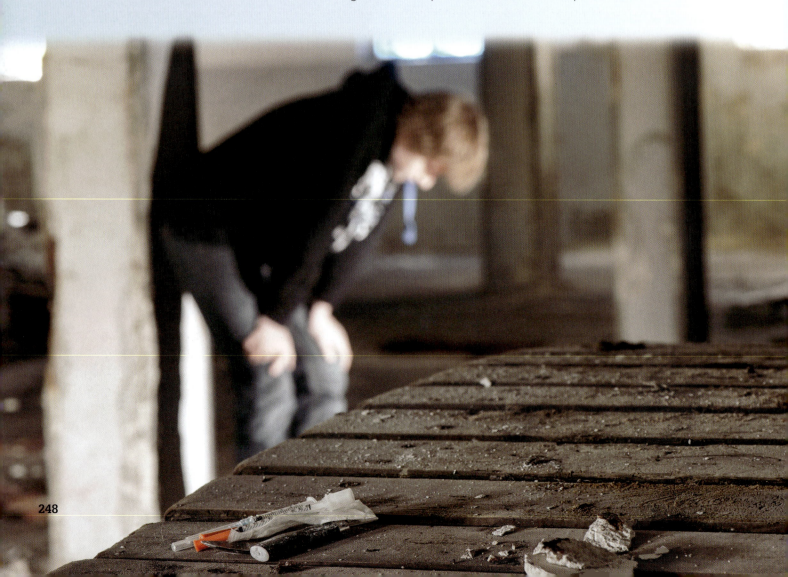

addicted to drugs because many reasons related to genetics, environment, and development can cause an addiction. Review these facts to understand the negative consequences that may happen later, should you develop an addiction:

- The changes in the brain occur over time, leading to an overstimulation of dopamine that creates the euphoric feeling and the need to take the drug more often and in higher doses.
- Alcoholics are more likely to get divorced (Cranford 2014), with a divorce rate of 50 percent when one spouse drinks heavily (Caba 2013).
- About 9,000 babies are born each year to narcotic-addicted women (Physicians Committee for Responsible Medicine n.d.), and about one baby born each hour is addicted to opiate drugs in the United States (Patrick et al. 2012).
- Staying on the job is more difficult. Addicts are 2.7 times more likely to have injury-related absences (National Council on Alcoholism and Drug Dependence 2015).
- Accidents can occur at work. Eleven percent of the victims who died while working had been drinking alcohol (National Council on Alcoholism and Drug Dependence 2015).
- Addiction makes it difficult to keep a job. Workers who had three or more jobs in the previous five years are about twice as likely to be current or past-year users of illegal drugs as people who have held a single job (National Council on Alcoholism and Drug Dependence 2015).
- Relapse can occur often. However, this does not mean an addicted individual cannot return to therapy and try again. He or she may require a different approach or therapy to successfully manage the addiction.

Take Home

The best way to prevent substance abuse is never to try illicit drugs. Lab 11.1 in the web study guide provides specific examples of situations that are common for many college students, which may involve the use of drugs and alcohol. Take a look at the situations and think about how you would respond. It's always good to have a plan in place to help you and your friends avoid using drugs and alcohol. Should you find yourself addicted to drugs or alcohol and want information to help you stop, contact your university's drug and alcohol center or call the national hotline at 800-662-HELP (4357). The Substance Abuse and Mental Health Services Administration's national helpline is a free, confidential, 24/7, 365-day-a-year treatment referral and information service (in English and Spanish) for individuals and families facing mental health or substance use disorders. You can also call the Drug and Alcohol Abuse Hotline: 888-328-2518.

Psychoactive Drugs

Psychoactive drugs include cannabinoids (marijuana), opioids (heroin and opium), **stimulants** (cocaine, amphetamine, and methamphetamine), **club drugs** (MDMA, Rohypnol, and GHB), dissociative drugs (ketamine and PCP), hallucinogens (LSD, mescaline, and psilocybin), anabolic steroids, inhalants, and prescription medications (CNS depressants, stimulants, and opioid pain relievers). This section presents facts about each of these drugs, including their alternate names, incidence of use, mechanism of action, and short- and long-term effects.

ILLEGAL DRUGS

Illegal drugs are limited in their production and use by governments. In the United States, commonly used illegal drugs include marijuana, heroin, inhalants, cocaine, and methamphetamine. Marijuana has become legal in some states; in some others, it is available with a prescription. Inhalants can be purchased legally as household substances, but the substance is considered illegal if used for getting high. Most states have penalties for selling or providing common inhalants to minors.

MARIJUANA

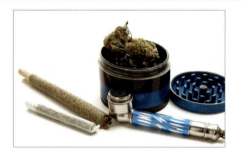

Marijuana is derived from the *Cannabis* plant. The active ingredient that causes changes in the brain is THC, or delta-9-tetrahydrocannabinol.

Alternate names: Blunt, dope, grass, herb, pot, skunk, weed.

Incidence of use: Marijuana is the most commonly used drug in the United States (Substance Abuse and Mental Health Services Administration 2015). There are approximately 6,600 new users every day (Substance Abuse and Mental Health Services Administration 2014). Figure 11.5 shows the increase of marijuana use among full-time college students.

Mechanism of action: Typically smoked in a rolled cigarette (joint) or with pipes or a bong (a device that uses water); can also be ingested in foods like brownies, cookies, or candy.

Short-term effects: Marijuana is quickly absorbed in the lungs and bloodstream, then travels to the brain and other organs in the body. It results in altered senses (for example, seeing brighter colors), a distorted sense of time, mood swings, inability to have normal body movements, difficulty with thinking and problem solving, and impaired memory (National Institute on Drug Abuse 2017f).

Long-term effects: Leads to impairments related to thinking, memory, learning, and how the brain makes connections between these cognitive functions. Impairments can be permanent (National Institute on Drug Abuse 2017f).

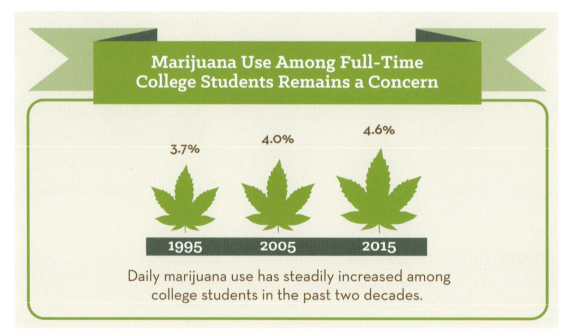

Figure 11.5 Marijuana use among full-time college students, 2015.

Reprinted from National Institute on Drug Abuse (2016a).

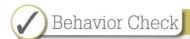
Behavior Check

Legalization of Marijuana

Marijuana is currently an illegal drug in the United States as a whole. However, it is legal for medical use in 29 states and the District of Columbia and for nonmedical (recreational) use in 8 states. One of the reasons given for why marijuana should be legalized is because of its medicinal uses in helping with pain and nausea; however, most physicians are not trained to prescribe marijuana and are unsure of the best method of administration for their patients: smoking, ingesting, or vaping. Those who support legalization claim that marijuana is less dangerous than alcohol and less harmful and addictive than tobacco. They believe that fewer dollars will be spent prosecuting minor offenses if using marijuana is no longer a crime.

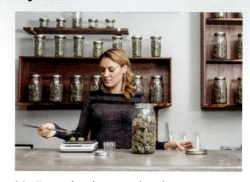

Marijuana has become legal in some states. These specialty stores are making marijuana more easily accessible.

- What do you think?
- What are your attitudes and values about the use of marijuana for recreational reasons?
- What are your attitudes and values about the use of marijuana for medical reasons?
- Does the legalization of marijuana lead to increased use?

HEROIN

Heroin is a drug classified as an opioid. It is made from morphine, which is extracted from the seed pod of the Asian poppy plant, and has no accepted medical use in the United States (Substance Abuse and Mental Health Services Administration 2015).

Alternate names: Smack, dope, mud, horse, junk, H, black tar, brown sugar.

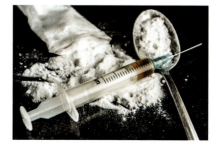

Incidence of use: In 2015, .3 percent of young adults aged 18 to 25 were current heroin users and .6 percent were past-year users, a total of 217,000 young people (Center for Behavioral Health Statistics and Quality 2016). Approximately 23 percent of people who use heroin become dependent on the drug (National Institute on Drug Abuse 2017d). In 2013, the average age at first use among recent heroin initiates aged 12 to 49 was 24.5 years (Substance Abuse and Mental Health Services Administration 2014).

Mechanism of action: Injected, inhaled by snorting or sniffing, or smoked.

Short-term effects: Alters areas in the brain that affect pain, arousal, blood pressure, and breathing (National Institute on Drug Abuse 2017d).

Long-term effects: Deterioration of sections of the brain that affect decision making and responses to stressful situations, severe pulmonary complications like pneumonia, infections of the heart lining and valves, abscesses, constipation and gastrointestinal cramping, and liver and kidney disease. Chronic use of heroin leads to physical dependence; the body has become accustomed to having the drug in its system. A chronic user will experience severe symptoms of withdrawal within a few hours of stopping; these include restlessness, muscle and bone pain, insomnia, diarrhea and vomiting, cold flashes with goose bumps, and kicking movements. During withdrawal, users also experience severe cravings for heroin that often lead to relapse (National Institute on Drug Abuse 2017d). Overdosing causes breathing complications that result in brain damage or a coma due to lower oxygen levels in the brain.

The risk is high: Almost one-fourth of people who use heroin become dependent on it.

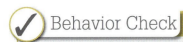

Behavior Check

Needle Exchange Programs

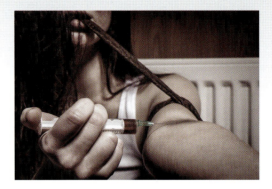

People who inject drugs are at high risk of contracting HIV and hepatitis C (HCV) because blood or other bodily fluids remain in the needle and syringe. Many injectable-drug users share their needles, thus increasing the risk of acquiring these fatal diseases. HCV is a common blood-borne infection, especially among injectable-drug users. Engaging in unprotected sex with an injectable-drug user may increase the risks of acquiring HIV and HCV (National Institute on Drug Abuse 2017d).

Due to this increased risk, many communities have initiated needle exchange or syringe services programs to help reduce the chances of injectable-drug users spreading these diseases. These programs provide free access to sterile needles, safe disposal of used needles and syringes, and counseling on risk reduction and safer sex practices (Centers for Disease Control and Prevention 2017d).

- What do you think about needle exchange programs? Are they effective? Why or why not?
- Does a needle exchange program contribute to the problem of addiction?
- Does a needle exchange program prevent the spread of fatal diseases like hepatitis B or HIV?
- Do you think needle exchange programs give the message that it is okay to use intravenous drugs?
- What are other ways communities can prevent the use of illegal intravenous drugs besides implementing needle exchange programs?

INHALANTS

Inhalants are chemical vapors that are breathed in and cause a mind-altering effect. These include the following:

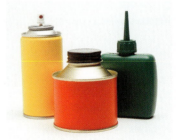

- *Volatile solvents:* Liquids from common household and industrial products that vaporize at room temperature.
- *Aerosols:* Sprays that contain propellants and solvents, such as those found in spray paints, deodorant, hair sprays, vegetable oil sprays for cooking, and fabric protector sprays.
- *Gases:* Vapors from medical anesthetics gases used in household or commercial products.
- *Nitrites:* Liquids from pain medications for heart conditions that are used primarily as sexual enhancers.

Alternate names: Laughing gas (nitrous oxide), snappers (amyl nitrite), poppers (amyl nitrite and butyl nitrite), whippets (fluorinated hydrocarbons), bold (nitrites), and rush (nitrites; National Institute on Drug Abuse for Teens 2017).

Incidence of use: Approximately 46.8 percent of initiates of inhalants in 2013 were younger than age 18; the average age at first use among recent initiates aged 12 to 49 was 19.2 years (Substance Abuse and Mental Health Services Administration 2014).

Mechanism of action: After being inhaled through the nose or mouth, chemicals quickly pass into the bloodstream and then travel to the lungs, brain, and other body organs. Users sniff or "snort" fumes from containers, spray aerosols directly into the nose or mouth, "bag" fumes by sniffing the inside of a plastic or paper bag where substances have been sprayed or deposited, "huff" from an inhalant-soaked rag stuffed in the mouth, or inhale from balloons filled with nitrous oxide (National Institute on Drug Abuse 2012b).

Short-term effects: Volatile solvents, aerosols, and gases affect the central nervous system (CNS). Nitrites dilate the blood vessels and relax the muscles. Inhalants alter one's mood by producing pleasurable effects; however, they can also result in dizziness, drowsiness, slurred speech, lethargy, depressed reflexes, general muscle weakness, and stupor (National Institute on Drug Abuse 2012b).

Long-term effects: Toxic chemicals can remain in the body for a long period of time. They are absorbed by the fatty tissues in the brain and central nervous system, causing muscle tremors and spasms that affect daily activities like walking, bending over, and talking. Users may experience difficulties having conversations with others and solving complex problems, as well as clumsiness (National Institute on Drug Abuse for Teens 2017).

COCAINE

Cocaine is a very powerful and addictive stimulant that is derived from coca leaves that grow in South America. Initially developed to treat illnesses and serve as a local anesthetic, it has detrimental effects on the brain when used repeatedly (National Institute on Drug Abuse 2016c).

Alternate names: Blow, candy, coke, crack, rock, snow (National Institute on Drug Abuse 2017a).

Incidence of use: In 2013, 601,000 people aged 12 or older had used cocaine for the first time within the past 12 months; this averages to approximately 1,600 initiates per day (Substance Abuse and Mental Health Services Administration 2014). Cocaine use among college students declined between 2006 and 2013 but increased between 2014 and 2015 (figure 11.6).

Mechanism of action: Inhaled, smoked, or mixed with heroin (speedball) and injected into a vein.

Short-term effects: Enlarged pupils, increased energy and alertness, violent behavior, heart attacks, strokes and seizures, euphoria, anxiety, paranoia, psychosis, and an increase in body temperature, heart rate, and blood pressure (National Institute on Drug Abuse 2017b).

Long-term effects: Permanent loss of sense of smell, nosebleeds, damage to the nose, difficulty swallowing, and a decreased appetite that leads to poor nutrition and significant weight loss (National Institute on Drug Abuse 2017b).

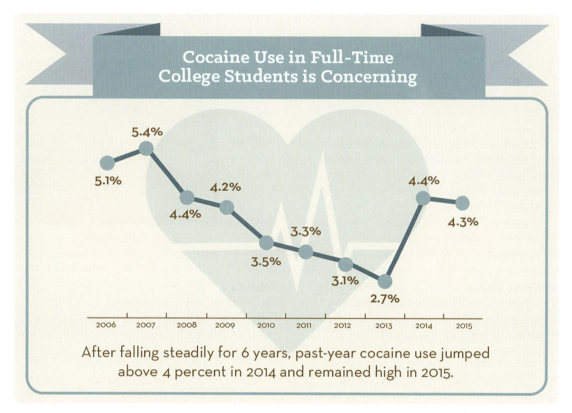

Figure 11.6   Cocaine use in full-time college students, 2006 to 2015.

Reprinted from National Institute on Drug Abuse (2016a).

METHAMPHETAMINE

Methamphetamine is an extremely addictive stimulant drug that is a white, odorless, bitter-tasting crystalline powder. The effects of the drug can last up to 24 hours, with an average duration of 6 to 8 hours (Foundation for a Drug-Free World n.d.).

Alternate names: Meth, crystal, chalk, ice.

Incidence of use: In 2012, approximately 1.2 million people reported using methamphetamine within the last year, and the average age of new users was 19.7 years old (Volkow 2013).

Mechanism to action: Taken orally, smoked, snorted, or dissolved in water or alcohol and injected. The drug gets to the brain the fastest when it is smoked or injected. It produces an immediate, intense euphoria. Due to the short-acting power of the stimulant, users quickly adopt a binge-and-crash pattern in order to sustain the high (National Institute on Drug Abuse 2017e).

Short-term effects: Anxiety, confusion, insomnia, mood disturbances, violent behaviors, psychosis (e.g., paranoia, hallucinations, and delusions), increased wakefulness, increased physical activity, decreased appetite, increased respiration, rapid heart rate, irregular heartbeat, increased blood pressure, and increased body temperature (National Institute on Drug Abuse 2017e).

Long-term effects: Reduced motor skills, impaired verbal learning, emotional and memory problems, extreme weight loss, severe dental problems ("meth mouth"), skin sores caused by scratching, increased risk of contracting infectious diseases like HIV and hepatitis B and C (National Institutes on Drug Abuse 2017e).

Other facts about meth: Methamphetamine has become a highly abused drug because it can be manufactured in concealed laboratories in homes with ingredients such as pseudoephedrine, a common ingredient in cold medicines. Pharmacies keep track of the number of products containing pseudoephedrine that individuals purchase in a day (National Institute on Drug Abuse 2017e). This is why you have to get these medicines from the pharmacy rather than an over-the-counter aisle.

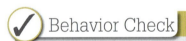 Behavior Check

Treatment for Drug Abuse and Addiction

Medications available to help addicts wean off of opioids include buprenorphine, methadone, and naltrexone. Buprenorphine and methadone work by binding to the same cell receptors that heroin does with less of an effect, helping reduce cravings so the user can wean off the drug. Naltrexone blocks opioid receptors and prevents the drug from having an effect. Some patients have trouble complying with naltrexone treatment, but a new long-acting version given by injection in a doctor's office may increase this treatment's efficacy.

Emergency medication is also available for overdoses (National Institute on Drug Abuse 2017d). Naloxone effectively reverses opioid and heroin overdoses. It is an inexpensive, quick-acting medication that restores breathing within minutes. Health care providers can administer naloxone and physicians can prescribe it to someone at risk of an overdose.

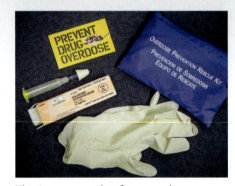

This is an example of an overdose rescue kit that can be used to assist someone who is experiencing an opiate overdose.

- What do you think about providing overdose rescue kits to addicted individuals or a family member or friend of the drug user?
- Would you want this kit if you had a friend or family member addicted to opioids or heroin? Why or why not?
- Do you think providing the kits to addicts keeps them from seeking treatment for their addiction because they know they have a safety net in case of an overdose?
- Does this medication save a life or enable an addiction?

Meth Labs and Future Life Plans

Now

Look at the number of meth labs across the United States (figure 11.7). The lifetime user rate is 3.3 percent among people aged 18 to 25, and meth use continues for many people into middle age (6.4 percent of lifetime users are age 26 and older; Center for Behavioral Health Statistics and Quality 2016).

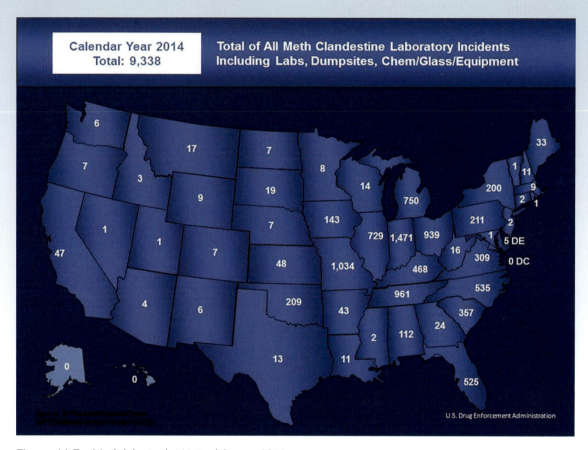

Figure 11.7 Meth labs in the United States, 2014.

Reprinted from Drug Enforcement Administration, *Methamphetamine Lab Indicants*, 2004-2014.

Later

How does this map influence where you would want to go to graduate school, look for employment, engage in recreational activities, raise a family, and eventually retire?

Take Home

The choices we make, such as geographic location or the friends we spend time with, can influence our ability to remain free from addiction.

PRESCRIPTION DRUGS

Prescription drugs are prescribed to treat common disorders, but when they are obtained without a prescription and consumed in higher doses than prescribed, they can become addictive. Commonly abused prescription medications are **opioids**, **central nervous system (CNS) depressants**, and stimulants. The most common prescription drugs that are abused by teens and college-age students include Adderall, Ritalin, cold medicine with codeine, and OxyContin.

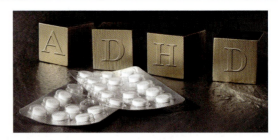

College students use prescription medications like Adderall illegally to help them focus on their academic responsibilities.

ADDERALL AND RITALIN (STIMULANTS)

Alternate names: Kiddy coke (or kiddy cocaine), poor man's cocaine, uppers, vitamin R, R-ball, skippy, smarties, Kibbles & Bits, Diet Coke, R pop, Coke Junior, Jif, study buddies (Ritalin Abuse Health n.d.).

Incidence of use: An estimated 6.4 percent of college students between the ages of 18 and 22 use Adderall in a recreational way (Substance Abuse and Mental Health Services Administration 2015). Young adults are most likely to abuse the prescribed stimulants Adderall (60 percent of users) and Ritalin (20 percent of users; Feliz 2014).

Mechanism of action: Swallowed, snorted, smoked, injected, or chewed.

Prescribed use: Prescribed to treat children, adolescents, or adults diagnosed with attention-deficit hyperactivity disorder (ADHD).

Short-term effects: Increased alertness, attention, and energy; increased blood pressure and heart rate; narrowed blood vessels; increased blood sugar; opened-up breathing passages.

Long-term effects: Heart problems, psychosis, anger, paranoia (National Institute on Drug Abuse 2014).

High doses: Dangerously high body temperature and irregular heartbeat; heart failure; seizures.

COLD MEDICINE WITH CODEINE (CNS DEPRESSANT)

Alternate names: C-C-C, triple C, Orange Crush, Dex, Drex, DXM, robo, robo-dosing, robo-fizzing, velvet, vitamin D, syrup head (Stop Medicine Abuse n.d.).

Incidence of use: One in 30 teens reports using over-the-counter (OTC) drugs to get high (Stop Medicine Abuse n.d.).

Mechanism of action: Orally via tablet, capsule, or syrup; sometimes mixed with alcohol or soda.

Prescribed use: Used to treat lower and upper respiratory congestion and symptoms associated with colds and flu.

Short-term effects: Hallucinations, sedation, euphoria, impaired motor functions, increased heart rate and blood pressure, extreme agitation.

Long-term effects: Addiction, liver damage, central nervous system depression, respiratory depression, lack of oxygen to the brain (National Institute on Drug Abuse 2017c).

OXYCONTIN (OPIOIDS)

Alternate names: Hillbilly heroin, blues, kickers, OC, Oxy.

Incidence of use: An estimated 2.1 million people in the United States abuse prescription opioid pain relievers (Substance Abuse and Mental Health Services Administration 2013).

Mechanism of action: Swallowed, snorted, injected.

Prescribed use: Treat moderate to severe pain.

Short-term effects: Pain relief, drowsiness, nausea, constipation, euphoria, confusion, slowed breathing, death.

Long-term effects: Unknown (National Institute on Drug Abuse 2017b).

OTHER COMMONLY ABUSED DRUGS

Table 11.1 outlines the most commonly abused club, dissociative, and hallucinogenic drugs. Club drugs tend to cause mild hallucinogenic effects and lowered inhibitions. Use of dissociative drugs can lead to the feeling of being separate from one's body and environment, impaired body movements, long-term feelings of anxiety, tremors, numbness in hands or feet, memory loss, and nausea. Hallucinogenic drugs cause altered states of perception and feeling, hallucinations, and nausea.

Table 11.1 Commonly Abused Club, Dissociative, and Hallucinogenic Drugs

Facts	MDMA (methylene-dioxymethamphetamine)	GHB (gamma-hydroxybutyrate)	Rohypnol (flunitrazepam)	Ketamine (ketalar SV)	LSD (lysergic acid diethylamide)	Mescaline
Category	Club drug	Club drug	Club drug	Dissociative drug	Hallucinogen	Hallucinogen
Street names	Ecstasy, Adam, Eve, lover's speed, uppers	Georgia home boy, liquid ecstasy	Forget-me pill, Mexican Valium, R2, roofies	Cat Valium, K, Special K, vitamin K	Acid, blotter, cubes, microdot	Buttons, cactus, mesc, peyote
How administered	Swallowed, injected, snorted	Swallowed	Swallowed, snorted	Injected, snorted, smoked	Swallowed, absorbed through mouth tissues	Swallowed, smoked
Short-term effects	Mild hallucinogenic effects, lowered inhibitions, anxiety, chills, muscle cramping	Drowsiness, nausea, headache, disorientation, loss of coordination, memory loss	Sedation, muscle relaxant, confusion, memory loss, dizziness, impaired coordination	Numbness, impaired memory, respiratory depression, cardiac arrest	Increased body temperature, heart rate, and blood pressure, loss of appetite, sweating, weakness, impulsive behavior	Increased body temperature, heart rate, and blood pressure, loss of appetite, sweating, weakness, impulsive behavior
Long-term effects	Sleep problems, depression, impaired memory, hyperthermia, addiction	Unconsciousness, seizures, coma	Addiction	Death	Flashbacks, hallucinogen persisting perception disorder	

Adapted from National Institute on Drug Abuse (2017b).

Alcohol

Alcohol is often used in social situations, to celebrate events and milestones, and to relax after a long day. It affects people differently depending on how much and how often alcohol is consumed, age, health status, and family history (National Institute on Drug Abuse 2017b). According to the Centers for Disease Control and Prevention (2017b), excessive drinking accounts for 88,000 deaths in the United States every year. Research has shown that children of alcoholics are close to four times more likely to develop a drinking problem, and the risk increases when a child has family experiences related to an alcoholic parent who is depressed, if both parents abuse drugs and alcohol, if the alcohol abuse by the parents is severe, or if there is aggression and violence (National Institute on Alcohol Abuse and Alcoholism 2012).

In general, consuming alcohol is not typically of great concern. However, it becomes a problem when one drinks too much and can no longer manage everyday activities such as attending classes, going to work, paying bills, and attending to family responsibilities. Alcohol becomes a problem when individuals become

> In the United States, 88,000 people die every year due to excessive drinking.

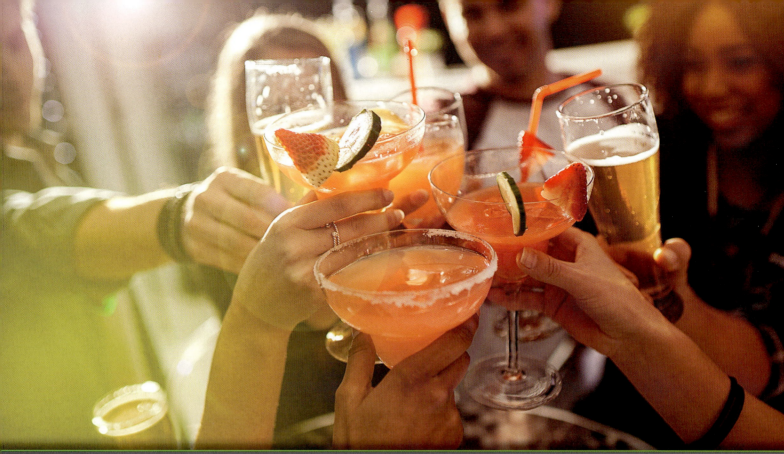

College students can drink responsibly by planning their activities with friends in advance, including knowing when to stop drinking to keep the blood alcohol levels within legal limits and developing a plan to keep each other safe (e.g., designated drivers, getting a taxi, making sure no one in the group is left alone).

dependent and cannot complete daily tasks. Additionally, the alcohol abuser experiences increased health care costs due to comorbidities (conditions or diseases caused by alcohol abuse), lost productivity and wages due to hangovers (cannot go to work), crime, relationship and family problems, and early deaths due to chronic health conditions.

Alcohol use and abuse on college campuses are common despite the number of alcohol-related illnesses, injuries, and deaths among college students. It is important to learn about the negative consequences of alcohol use as a moderate drinker, binge drinker, or heavy drinker. It is never too late to quit using alcohol or to learn how to drink responsibly and in moderation to make healthy decisions that influence the short- and long-term effects on the body. Figure 11.8 shows the rates of drinking among college students compared to others their age who are not students: Students attending college have higher rates of binge drinking and are more likely to drink until intoxication.

In the 2013 National Survey on Drug Use and Health (Substance Abuse and Mental Health Services Administration 2014), the prevalence of full-time college students aged 18 to 22 who drank alcohol in the past month was 59.4 percent. Thirty-nine percent of surveyed students reported binge drinking (consuming five or more alcoholic drinks on an occasion) in the past 30 days and 12.7 percent participated in heavy drinking (five or more drinks on an occasion at five or more occasions in a month) in the same time period. College students are more likely than their peers in the same age range who are not enrolled full time in college to drink alcohol, binge drink, and participate in heavy drinking; this trend has continued since 2002 (Substance Abuse and Mental Health Services Administration 2014). Excessive drinking is associated with health and social issues that include impaired driving, violence, risky sexual activity, and unintended pregnancies (Centers for Disease Control and Prevention 2017b). Figure 11.9 shows the pattern of binge drinking among college students and their peers not enrolled in college between 2002 and 2013. Figure 11.10 shows the rates of binge drinking from the same time period among college students by sex, indicating

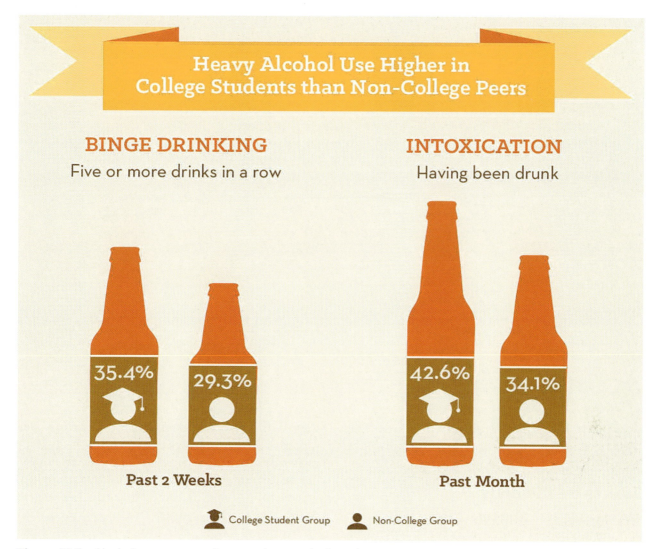

Figure 11.8 Alcohol use among college students and others their age not attending college.

Reprinted from National Institute on Drug Abuse (2016a).

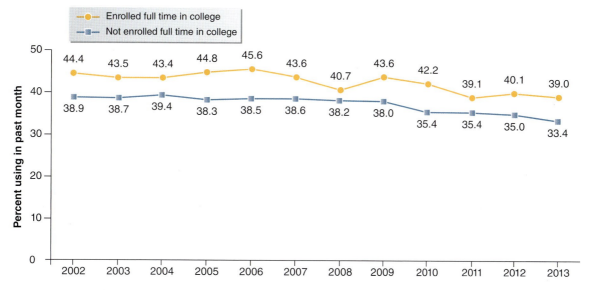

Figure 11.9 Binge alcohol use among adults aged 18 to 22, by college enrollment, 2002 to 2013.

Substance Abuse and Mental Health Services Administration (2013).

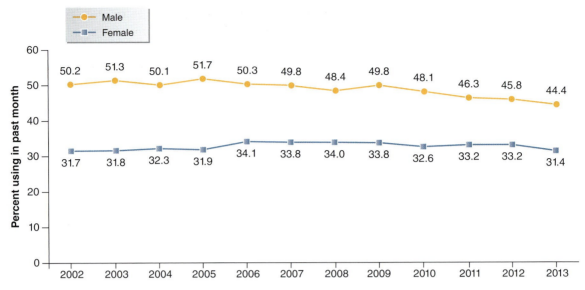

Figure 11.10   Binge alcohol use among adults aged 18 to 25, by sex, 2002 to 2013.

Substance Abuse and Mental Health Services Administration (2013).

that men drink at higher rates than women. The good news is that the rates of binge drinking have declined over time for all populations.

Effects on the Body

Alcohol can have detrimental effects on the body, and the intensities of these effects are dependent on the frequency, duration, and consumption (figure 11.11). Drinking in moderation over decades, and even binge drinking, has been associated with short-term effects on the body that include arrhythmia of the heart, hypertension, cardiomyopathy, damage to the lining of the stomach, gastritis, ulcers in the stomach, and dehydration (National Institute on Alcohol Abuse and Alcoholism n.d.). Diseases can develop due

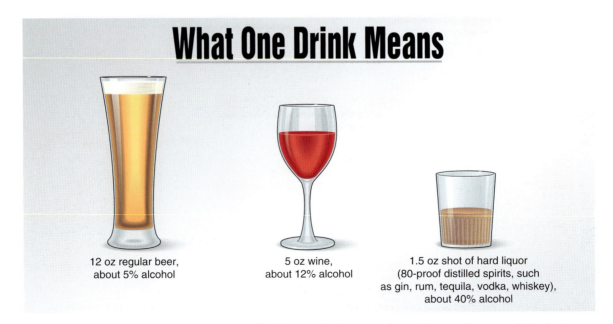

Figure 11.11   The amount of alcohol considered to be one drink varies depending on the type of alcohol.

Alcohol can damage your liver, brain, stomach, and heart and lead to high blood pressure, stroke, and heart attack.

to heavy drinking. Many of these diseases are irreversible but can be prevented by not drinking excessively. Some of the more serious diseases that result from long-term and chronic alcohol use include cirrhosis of the liver, alcoholic hepatitis, alcoholic cardiomyopathy, strokes, hypertension, severe dehydration, and pancreatitis (National Institute on Alcohol Abuse and Alcoholism n.d.).

Blood Alcohol Concentration

The effects of alcohol on the body are directly related to the amount, or level, of alcohol in the blood, typically referred to as **blood alcohol concentration (BAC)**, the higher the level of alcohol detected in the blood, the more significant and serious the impairment. It is measured from .01 to .40 (death). Specific factors that affect amount of alcohol in the blood include the type of alcohol,

the amount drunk, the time period over which the alcohol was consumed, sex, the weight of the individual, and the amount of food in the stomach. An individual who weighs more and has eaten before consuming alcohol will have a lower blood alcohol level. If a man and a woman consume the same number of drinks per hour and weigh exactly the same amount, the woman will have a higher blood alcohol level because women have a lower percentage of body water than men, which causes women to absorb more alcohol. Figure 11.12 illustrates the physical effects of blood alcohol concentration on driving. Lab 11.2 in the web study guide will help you understand the implications of drinking and its physical effects on the body, especially the blood alcohol concentration and the ability to make decisions.

Combating Binge Drinking With Drinking Responsibly

Binge drinking is when someone consumes five or more alcoholic drinks on an occasion. In order for college students to reduce their chances of

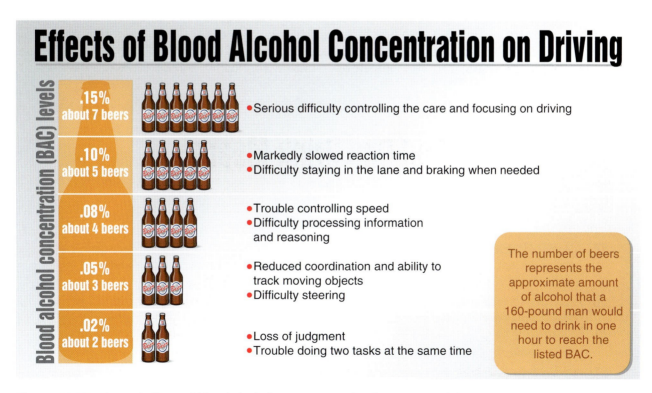

Effects of Blood Alcohol Concentration on Driving

Blood alcohol concentration (BAC) levels

.15% about 7 beers
- Serious difficulty controlling the care and focusing on driving

.10% about 5 beers
- Markedly slowed reaction time
- Difficulty staying in the lane and braking when needed

.08% about 4 beers
- Trouble controlling speed
- Difficulty processing information and reasoning

.05% about 3 beers
- Reduced coordination and ability to track moving objects
- Difficulty steering

.02% about 2 beers
- Loss of judgment
- Trouble doing two tasks at the same time

The number of beers represents the approximate amount of alcohol that a 160-pound man would need to drink in one hour to reach the listed BAC.

Figure 11.12   Physical effects of blood alcohol concentration levels on impaired driving.

Adapted from Centers for Disease Control and Prevention, *Drinking and Driving* (2011). https://www.cdc.gov/vitalsigns/drinkinganddriving/.

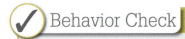

What Is Alcoholism?

Alcoholism, or alcohol dependence, includes four symptoms. Do you have any of these? Think about each of these and your behaviors related to the use of alcohol. If you answered yes to more than one of these symptoms, seek the help of a counselor on your campus or in your community (National Institute on Alcohol Abuse and Alcoholism 2012):

- **Craving**—having a strong need, or urge, to drink.
- **Loss of control**—not being able to stop drinking once you've started to drink.
- **Physical dependence**—experiencing withdrawal symptoms such as an upset stomach, shakiness, and anxiety after drinking.
- **Tolerance**—experiencing the need to drink more alcohol to get that buzzed or drunk feeling.

becoming alcoholic, they should avoid underage drinking because people who begin drinking at a younger age are more at risk for becoming an alcoholic. Second, college students who are of a legal age to drink should drink in moderation and continue this behavior well into adulthood.

Practicing drinking in moderation reduces the chances of becoming an alcoholic and reduces the risks of other social issues and diseases, such as drinking and driving, violence, personal trauma, liver disease, brain damage, and cancer (National Institute on Drug Abuse 2012a).

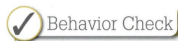

What's the Truth About Alcohol?

Which of the following statements about alcohol are myths (National Institute on Alcohol Abuse and Alcoholism n.d.)?

1. People can drink alcohol and still be in control.
2. Drinking alcohol isn't really dangerous.
3. People can sober up very quickly after drinking too much alcohol.
4. Beer has the least amount of alcohol per serving when compared to liquor or wine.
5. A few beers will not impair someone enough that he or she shouldn't drive.

The facts are as follows:

1. Alcohol reduces the chances of college students being in control because it impairs judgment and could lead to engaging in behaviors that could have serious consequences, like a car accident, risky sexual activities, or vandalism.
2. Alcohol use is dangerous. Among college students, it leads to injuries and deaths, sexual assault, and poor academic performance.
3. Sobering up takes about two hours. Nothing, not even coffee or a cold shower, can quickly eliminate alcohol from the body.
4. A 12-ounce (355 mL) glass of beer has the same amount of alcohol as a shot of 80-proof liquor or 5 ounces (148 mL) of wine (see figure 11.11).
5. Impaired driving can begin at .05 BAC, so you should not drive after drinking any amount of alcohol.

Mixing Energy Drinks and Alcohol

Although consumption of moderate amounts of caffeine is considered safe for adults, when highly caffeinated energy drinks are combined with alcohol, the effects could be fatal. According to Somogyi (2010), the average amount of caffeine consumed by the U.S. population has remained constant at about 300 milligrams per person per day, equivalent to two or three cups of regular coffee. The major sources of caffeine are beverages such as coffee, soft drinks, and tea. Teenagers and young adults consume one-third the amount of caffeine as adults. However, research has shown that many college students mix energy drinks and alcohol. In fact, 34 percent of 18- to 24-year-olds mix the two (Centers for Disease Control and Prevention 2017b). Energy drinks are beverages that increase mental alertness and physical performance and contain significantly more caffeine than a regular soft drink. These drinks can contain between 80 and 260 milligrams per 12 (355 mL) to 16 (474 mL) fluid ounce serving. Energy shots are another type of high caffeine beverage sold in smaller quantities, usually 50 milliliter bottles. They contain the same amount of caffeine as a cup of coffee.

When alcohol and energy drinks are combined, the caffeine can mask the depressant effects of the alcohol. Additionally, the caffeine does not affect the metabolism of alcohol by the liver, which increases blood alcohol concentration. Those who report mixing alcohol and energy drinks have a higher prevalence of binge drinking, sexually assaulting someone or being the victim of a sexual assault, and driving with someone who has been drinking.

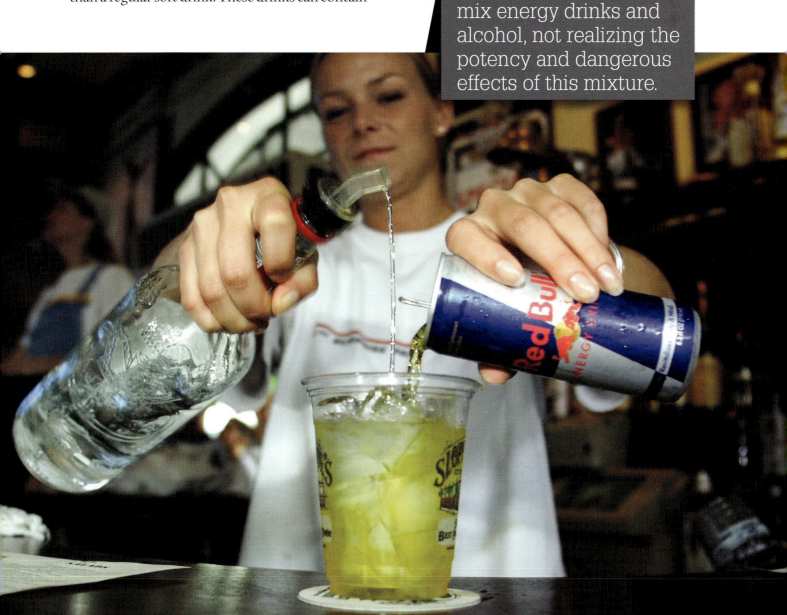

College students often mix energy drinks and alcohol, not realizing the potency and dangerous effects of this mixture.

Tobacco

Despite the efforts to reduce tobacco use in the United States, the use of these products continues to remain steady. In 2014, 25.5 percent of Americans aged 12 and older used tobacco products, including cigarettes, chewing tobacco, snuff, cigars, and pipe tobacco products (Substance Abuse and Mental Health Services Administration 2015). Of those who indicated tobacco use, 20.8 percent were current cigarette smokers. Young adults, aged 18 to 25 years old, had the highest rates of tobacco use, and their most common form of tobacco use was cigarettes. Between 2002 and 2013, the rates of cigarette use among this age group declined by 8 percent; however, smokeless tobacco use increased slightly from 4.8 percent in 2002 to 5.8 percent in 2013 (Substance Abuse and Mental Health Services Administration 2014). Full-time college students reported less cigarette use than their peers who were not enrolled full time. The rate of having used cigarettes in the past 30 days among full-time college students declined between 2002 and 2013 from 32.6 percent to 21.0 percent, respectively (figure 11.13).

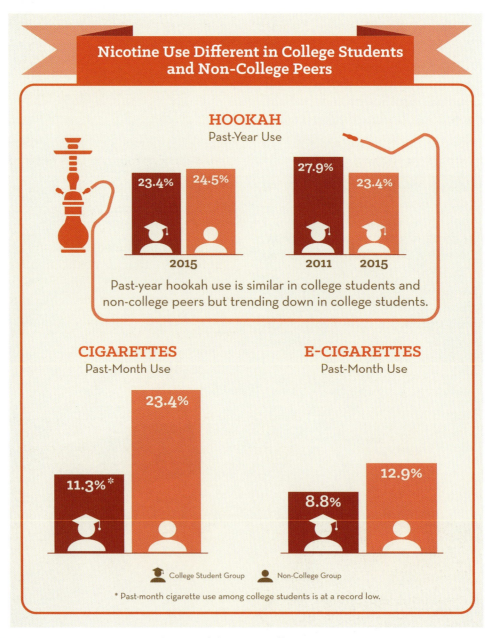

Figure 11.13   Nicotine use in college students and their non-college peers, 2015.

Reprinted from National Institute on Drug Abuse (2016a).

What Are Hookahs?

Hookahs are water pipes that are used to smoke flavored tobacco and are typically shared, passing the same mouthpiece from person to person. Using a hookah carries the same negative health risks as smoking a cigarette (Centers for Disease Control and Prevention 2016). Hookah users may absorb more toxic substances than cigarette smokers.

- **Alternate names:** Narghile, argileh, shisha, hubble-bubble, and goza.
- **Incidence:** 22 to 40 percent of college students have used hookahs (U.S. Department of Health and Human Services 2012).
- **Health effects:** Lung, bladder, and oral cancers; clogged arteries and heart disease; infections due to sharing the same mouthpiece; having babies with low birth weight; and decreased fertility.
- Hookah smoking transmits many of the same harmful chemicals as cigarettes do, including nicotine and tar. In a one-hour hookah-smoking session, users may inhale 100 to 200 times the amount of smoke as from one cigarette (U.S. Department of Health and Human Services 2012).

Chemicals in Cigarettes

Cigarettes contain over 7,000 chemicals that are harmful and poisonous and cause cancer (American Lung Association n.d.c). Cigarette smoking causes more deaths per year than HIV, illegal drugs, alcohol, motor vehicle injuries, and firearm-related incidences combined (see figure 11.14; Centers for Disease Control and Prevention 2017c). **Nicotine** is the chemical in tobacco products that causes addiction. It is found in cigars, smokeless tobacco, pipe tobacco, and e-cigarettes. Its original intended use was as an insecticide (American Lung Association n.d.b). When smoked in a cigarette or absorbed through the mucous membranes when chewing tobacco, the effects of nicotine are experienced quickly. It causes the central nervous system to increase the heart rate and blood pressure and gives the user feelings of euphoria. These elevated feelings do not last long; therefore, the user seeks more nicotine to maintain this level of stimulation. In high doses, nicotine can be poisonous. Children have died ingesting the liquid in e-cigarettes that contains nicotine.

The risks of smoking negatively affect almost every part of the body, both physically and emotionally (figure 11.15).

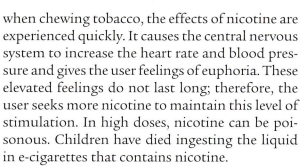

Different types of tobacco products include chew tobacco, cigarettes, electronic cigarettes, and hookahs.

Death Rates From Common Causes

Cigarette smoking causes more than

480,000

deaths each year in the U.S.

HIV-related deaths:

6,721
in 2014

Illegal drug use deaths:

45,000
in 2014

Alcohol-induced deaths:

30,722
in 2014

Firearm-related deaths:

33,736
in 2014

Motor vehicle deaths:

35.389
in 2014

Figure 11.14 Death rate from smoking compared to common death rates.

Data from https://www.cdc.gov/nchs/fastats/aids-hiv.htm; https://www.drugabuse.gov/related-topics/trends-statistics/overdose-death-rates; https://www.cdc.gov/nchs/fastats/alcohol.htm; https://www.cdc.gov/nchs/fastats/accidental-injury.htm; https://www.cdc.gov/nchs/fastats/injury.htm

Risks from Smoking

Smoking can damage every part of your body

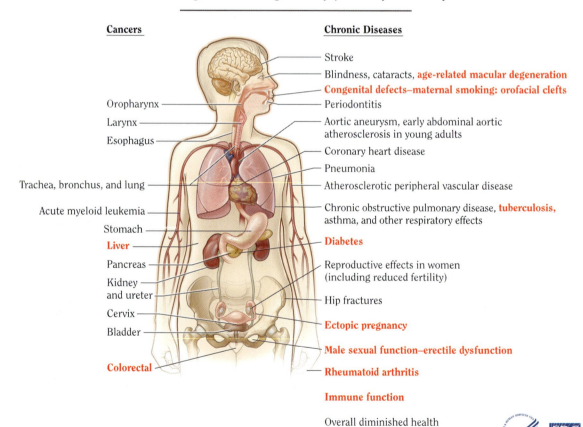

Cancers

Oropharynx

Larynx

Esophagus

Trachea, bronchus, and lung

Acute myeloid leukemia

Stomach

Liver

Pancreas

Kidney and ureter

Cervix

Bladder

Colorectal

Chronic Diseases

Stroke

Blindness, cataracts, age-related macular degeneration

Congenital defects–maternal smoking: orofacial clefts

Periodontitis

Aortic aneurysm, early abdominal aortic atherosclerosis in young adults

Coronary heart disease

Pneumonia

Atherosclerotic peripheral vascular disease

Chronic obstructive pulmonary disease, tuberculosis, asthma, and other respiratory effects

Diabetes

Reproductive effects in women (including reduced fertility)

Hip fractures

Ectopic pregnancy

Male sexual function–erectile dysfunction

Rheumatoid arthritis

Immune function

Overall diminished health

Figure 11.15 Effects of smoking on the body.

Each condition presented in bold text and followed by an asterisk (*) is a new disease causally linked to smoking in the 2014 Surgeon General's Report, *The Health Consequences of Smoking—50 Years of Progress.*

Quitting smoking and tobacco use can be very difficult because the addiction to nicotine is significant. The withdrawal symptoms, even within 24 hours of the last use of tobacco, include irritability, mood swings, aggression, and hostility. Despite the tremendous withdrawal symptoms, the body begins to heal itself within the first 24 hours after the last cigarette (see figure 11.16).

E-Cigarettes

E-cigarettes, or electronic cigarettes, are an alternative method to getting nicotine in the body. People use these devices to inhale an aerosol that contains nicotine instead of smoking a cigarette. Figure 11.17 shows the internal components of an e-cigarette and how it works to manipulate the nicotine to become an aerosol that can be inhaled into the body. Vaping is the term used to describe the act of inhaling and exhaling the water vapor produced by the electronic cigarette. E-cigarettes

are battery operated and have a heating system that heats the e-liquid from a refillable cartridge and releases the nicotine-filled aerosol (American Lung Association 2016).

Although the nicotine is not introduced into the body by a cigarette, the U.S. Surgeon General released a report indicating that e-cigarettes can still be harmful because the cartridges have additional chemicals, including carbonyl compounds and volatile organic compounds that can lead to negative health effects (U.S. Department of Health and Human Services 2016). Some of the ingredients are used in antifreeze, formaldehyde, and flavorings (American Lung Association 2016). Accidental poisoning and acute toxicity have occurred when the liquid is ingested, and some of these incidences have resulted in death. There has been an increase in the number of phone calls to poison control centers from parents concerned about their child ingesting the liquids from the e-cigarettes.

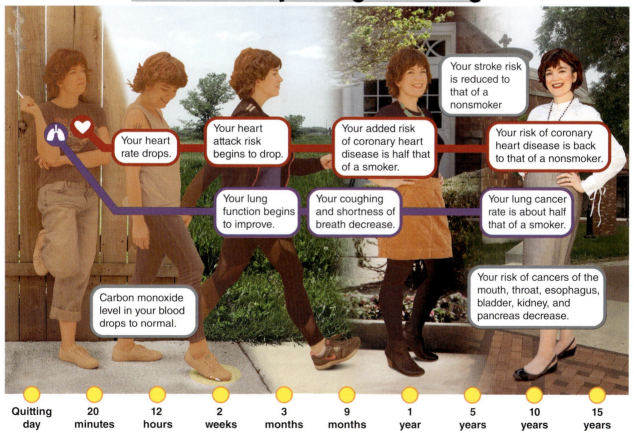

Figure 11.16   The benefits of quitting smoking are overwhelmingly positive and begin soon after quitting (Centers for Disease Control and Prevention 2017a).

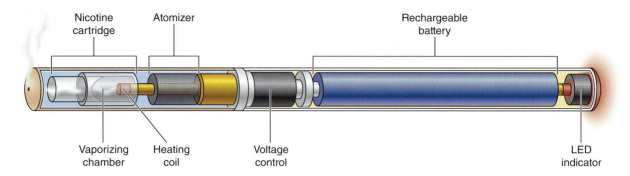

Figure 11.17   The internal parts of an e-cigarette.

Quitting Tobacco Use

Quitting smoking can be very difficult. Nicotine can be as addictive as heroin, cocaine, and alcohol (American Lung Association n.d.b). Despite the strong addiction, there are various methods for quitting tobacco. Nicotine replacement therapies include gum, patches, inhalers, nasal spray, and tablets. All these products provide low levels of nicotine that help the smoker gradually reduce the level of nicotine in the system. They help reduce the withdrawal symptoms until the smoker becomes more accustomed to a smoke-free lifestyle. Behavior modification programs provide access to support groups, counseling, and follow-up support to help participants sustain being a nonsmoker. QuitLine is a toll-free call resource for tobacco users who want to quit smoking. This resource is staffed by trained health care professionals and tobacco counselors who respond to questions about staying smoke free. In addition, counselors assist smokers in developing a personalized plan. This is a valuable resource for smokers trying to quit, but it does not replace the medical advice of the smoker's physician or health care provider. The National Cancer Institute (NCI) operates 800-QUIT-NOW, a toll-free number that will connect you directly to your state's tobacco quit line.

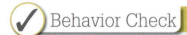 Behavior Check

The Path to Quitting Smoking

Quitting smoking is the best thing you can do for your overall health, since the body begins to heal itself after that last cigarette. Quitting can be difficult and take more than one attempt, so do not give up. Make sure you have a plan you can stick to (American Lung Association n.d.a). Ask for support from former smokers or friends and family who will be able to help you quit.

1. List the reasons you want to quit (e.g., don't want to get cancer, to save money, don't want to smell like cigarettes).
2. List the benefits of quitting smoking (e.g., breathe easier, normal heart rate and blood pressure, reduce chance of getting cancer).
3. List campus and community resources that can help you quit smoking (e.g., American Cancer Society, American Lung Association—Freedom From Smoking [http://freedomfromsmoking.org], Quit Line, College Tobacco Free Campus).
4. List specific support resources that people can provide for you (e.g., physician-NRT).
5. List the potential withdrawal symptoms, challenges, and how to prepare (e.g., combat weight gain, choose healthy snacks; if feeling anxious, go for a walk).
6. List social media outlets for support (e.g., #quitbettertogether).

Summary

Alcohol, tobacco, and marijuana are the most commonly abused drugs among young adults. The more often people use these substances, the more likely they are to develop a dependency on and tolerance to the drugs, leading to long-term use. Chronic use of these substances can lead to serious negative health effects on the body, which may include cancer, respiratory illnesses and diseases, mental health issues, violent behaviors, and poor judgment that leads to risky behaviors. Additionally, drug dependency can cause loss of jobs, failing in school, the inability to meet daily responsibilities like paying bills on time and keeping up with personal hygiene, and problems in relationships with friends, family, and partners.

You can reduce your chances of becoming dependent on drugs or alcohol by choosing not to succumb to peer pressure or to spend time around people who use drugs and in places where drugs and alcohol are easily accessible. Develop a plan in advance for how to handle situations where these substances are available and to learn how to cope with stressful situations by choosing healthier alternatives. Many community and campus resources are available for assisting students with the decision to be substance free and helping students who are dependent on substances get the help they need for recovery. Staying away from drugs, tobacco, and alcohol is a key component of living a wellness lifestyle. It's important to be present in life—to not escape it, but rather face challenges head on. This is how you learn and grow as a college student.

WEB STUDY GUIDE

Remember to complete all of the web study guide activities to further facilitate your learning, including the following lab activities:

Lab 11.1   Plan Now to Avoid Using Drugs

Lab 11.2   Blood Alcohol Concentration: Being Responsible When Drinking Alcohol

REVIEW QUESTIONS

1. What are ways to prevent becoming addicted to drugs or developing a behavioral addiction?
2. What are the criteria that are used to diagnose someone with a drug dependency?
3. What are some of the more common behavioral addictions among young adults?
4. What are the short- and long-term health effects of the following substances: marijuana, heroin, cocaine, club drugs, alcohol, and tobacco?
5. What are the physical effects of combining alcohol and energy drinks?
6. What are effective treatment options for individuals with a substance or behavioral addiction?

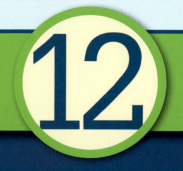

12

Sexuality and Health

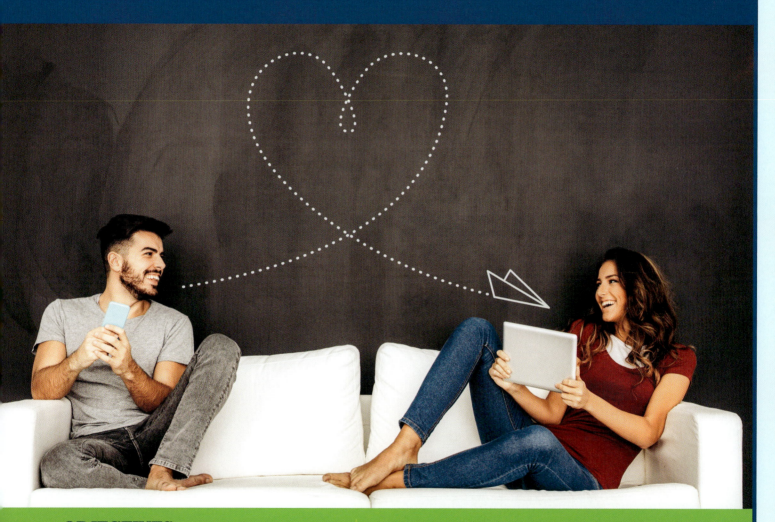

OBJECTIVES

❯ List the internal and external parts of the female and male reproductive systems.

❯ Explain how the most commonly used birth control methods prevent pregnancy. List their advantages and disadvantages.

❯ Explain the symptoms, diagnosis, treatment, prevention, and transmission of the most common bacterial and viral STIs.

❯ Define consent as it relates to sexual assault.

❯ Identify resources on college campuses that assist students in preventing and addressing sexual assault.

KEY TERMS

abstinence

areola

barrier birth control methods

birth control methods

bulbourethral glands (Cowper's glands)

circumcision

clitoris

contraception

ectopic pregnancy

ejaculation

ejaculatory duct

embryo

endometrium

epididymis

erection

Fallopian tubes

fertilization

fetus

gonads

hormonal birth control methods

hymen

labia majora

labia minora

mammary glands (breasts)

mons pubis

oocytes

ovaries

ovulation

pelvic inflammatory disease

penis

perfect use

prostate gland

scrotum

semen

seminal vesicles

seminiferous tubules

sperm

spermicide

sterilization

testes (testicles)

typical use

urethra

uterus

vagina

vas deferens

withdrawal

zygote

The chapter begins with a brief overview of the reproductive system. Next, it presents the birth control methods most commonly used by college students. This chapter discusses viral, bacterial, and other common sexually transmitted infections (STIs) in addition to prevention strategies and treatment options. It closes with information about sexual assault and resources on college campuses dedicated to educating young adults about prevention initiatives and strategies.

Sexuality as a Dimension of Health

Your sexual health is just as important as every other dimension of your health. Your sexuality is a critical and central component of who you are. This dimension of your health develops as a toddler and evolves, changes, and emerges over your lifetime. Although your sexuality is evident throughout your life, there are pivotal sexual health milestones related to developmental, emotional, and physical changes. At times, these milestones require having uncomfortable conversations. Some of these milestones are puberty, first sexual experiences with self and others, having children, and changes during aging. A personal goal for young adults should be to seek out reliable and medically accurate sources for sexual health information and become more comfortable and confident regarding these issues. This goal does not happen overnight, since it takes time to

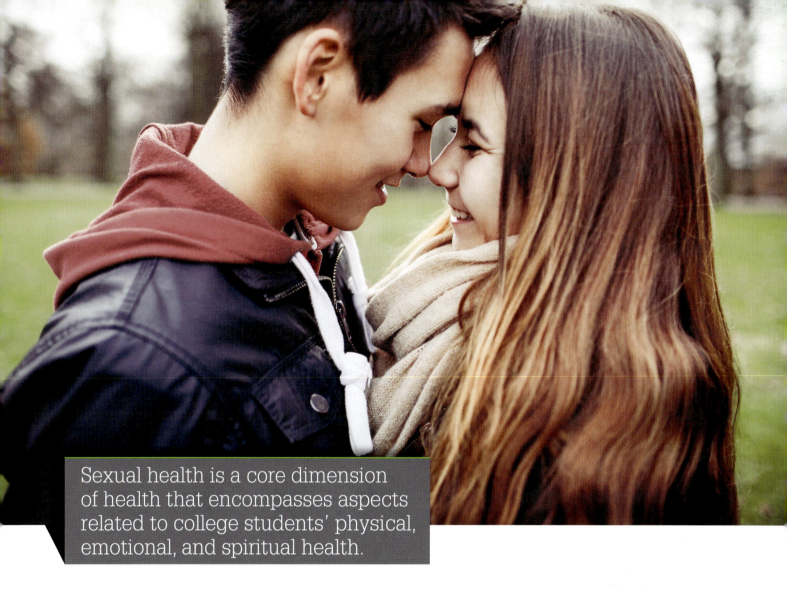

Sexual health is a core dimension of health that encompasses aspects related to college students' physical, emotional, and spiritual health.

learn about all of the sexual health issues, understand the context of these issues, and decide how to apply them to your life.

Over time, and with the addition of life experiences, you will develop specific beliefs, attitudes, feelings, morals, and behaviors that define your sexuality and how you want to express yourself. As you develop relationships with others, whether they are intimate or platonic, think about what you find physically and emotionally attractive in a partner, how to communicate effectively regarding your likes and dislikes, what it means to be sexually intimate, and how to develop empathy and understanding toward others who are not exactly like you.

This chapter focuses on the more pressing and contemporary issues that are central in a college student's life—what those issues are, how they affect college students, and what you can do to become more confident and comfortable with expressing your own sexuality and understanding others' expression of their sexuality.

Reproductive System

The primary purpose of the female and male reproductive systems is to provide the mature sexual organs, cells, and hormones needed to contribute to the next generation. In utero, the reproductive organs of fetuses of both sexes develop from the same embryonic tissues; therefore, it is difficult to identify, using ultrasound, whether the fetus has male or female genitalia until approximately the 20th week of gestation. Genetic testing can be used earlier in a pregnancy to determine the sex of the baby; however, ultrasound is the most common and inexpensive method. The homologous structures in boys and girls are the penis and clitoris and the scrotum and labia majora. Figure 12.1 shows the differences

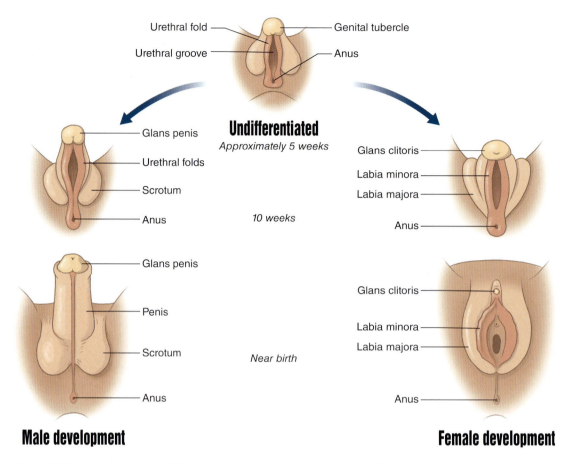

Figure 12.1   Differences in male and female reproductive organs during embryonic development.

between male and female reproductive organs during embryonic development. Note the similar tissue development between the fetuses and how there are more similarities than differences in the early stages of development.

Additional similarities that both the female and male reproductive systems share are structures called **gonads**, which are the ovaries in women and the testes in men. These organs manufacture the sex hormones that produce the eggs (**oocytes**) in the ovaries and **sperm** in the testes. Young men have the ability to produce sperm beginning at puberty, whereas women are born with a defined number of ova that are released during her reproductive years. Ovulation ends when a woman enters menopause. Puberty typically begins between ages 8 and 11 for girls and 9 and 12 for boys.

During sexual intercourse between a man and a woman, **fertilization** of the egg by the sperm normally occurs in the **Fallopian tubes**. The Fallopian tube has millions of microscopic cilia that pull the egg toward the uterus after it has been released from the ovary. The muscular wall of the Fallopian tube contracts, assists the egg in moving expeditiously to meet the sperm. If this sequence of events fails, implantation of the zygote may happen outside the uterus; this is called an **ectopic pregnancy**. A common site for an ectopic pregnancy is in the Fallopian tube; this is called a tubal pregnancy. The uterus is the intended site for implantation of the zygote and provides nourishment for the zygote as it develops into an **embryo** and then a **fetus**. The uterus sheds its inner lining every month if pregnancy does not occur.

> Women, unlike men, have an open road from the opening of the vagina to the peritoneal cavity, which increases their risks of getting pelvic inflammatory disease (PID). Bacterial infections, such as untreated sexually transmitted infections (STIs), in the Fallopian tubes can cause PID, leading to ectopic pregnancies and infertility.

Female Reproductive System

The female reproductive system is composed of internal and external organs that work together to produce the necessary hormones for typical sexual development and reproduction. Figure 12.2 shows organs of the internal and external female reproductive system. Notice that the external organs are known as the vulva, not the vagina; the vagina is an internal structure.

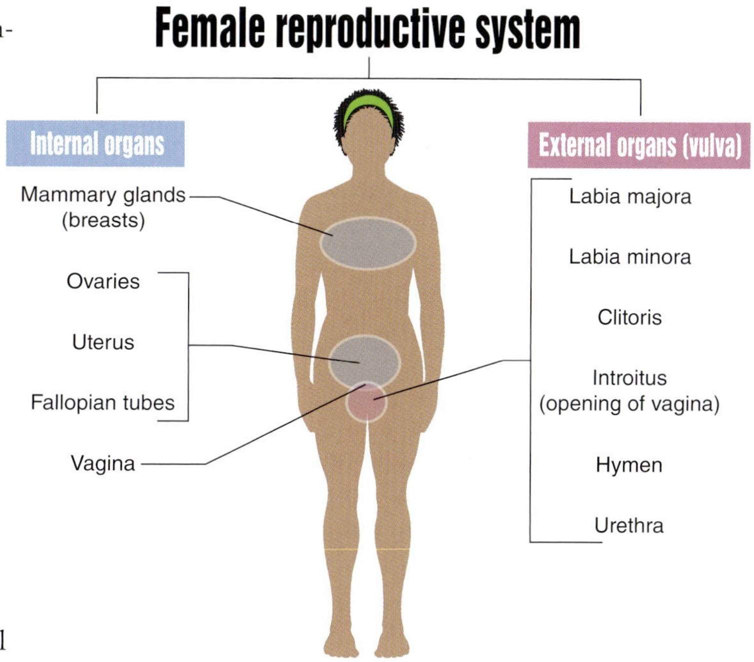

Female Internal Organs

The primary functions of the female reproductive system are to produce the oocytes (eggs or ova) and hormones necessary to support the primary and secondary reproductive sex organs that lead to a successful pregnancy. The primary sex organs are the **ovaries**, which is where the ova are produced and stored until **ovulation**, or the release of an ovum roughly once a month. The sex organs that support the transportation of the ovum out of the ovary to either unite with sperm (to create a zygote) or be expelled from the body during menstruation (if unfertilized) are the Fallopian tubes, uterus, and vagina. The ovaries are oval-shaped organs about the size of a walnut that are positioned in the upper portion of the pelvic cavity on both sides of the uterus. They are kept in place by strong, muscular ligaments. The Fallopian tubes are approximately 8 to 14 centimeters long. The end that hovers over the ovary has fingerlike projections called fimbriae. The fimbriae aid the ovum by leading it into the Fallopian tube and down to the uterus (see figure 12.3).

Female reproductive system

Internal organs
Mammary glands (breasts)
Ovaries
Uterus
Fallopian tubes
Vagina

External organs (vulva)
Labia majora
Labia minora
Clitoris
Introitus (opening of vagina)
Hymen
Urethra

Figure 12.2   The internal and external organs of the female reproductive system.

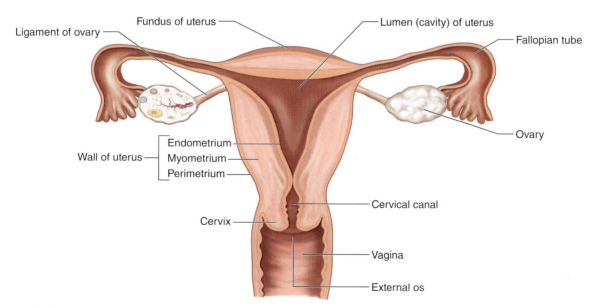

Figure 12.3   Internal female reproductive anatomy.

The **uterus** is a thick-walled muscular organ that is about the size of a fist and is shaped like an inverted pear. At the base of the uterus is the cervix. The functions of the uterus are menstruation, pregnancy, and labor. The uterus is where a fertilized egg, or **zygote**, typically implants. If a woman does not become pregnant after ovulation, then the uterine lining, called the **endometrium**, is shed as the menstrual blood approximately every 28 to 32 days. The uterus is typically in alignment with the lower body region; however, some women have a uterus that is angled forward or backward. A uterus angled toward the bladder is *anteverted* and one tilted toward the back, near the rectum, is *retroverted*. For most women, these variations in uterine placement do not cause significant problems during sexual intercourse or pregnancy.

> In endometriosis, the segments of the uterine lining end up in the peritoneal cavity and cause pain. Women who experience extreme pain and discomfort during their menstrual cycle need to consult with their physician or gynecologist.

The **vagina** is a canal-like muscular organ that receives sperm during intercourse and serves as a passageway for menstrual blood leaving the body and for a baby during delivery. For this reason, it is also called the birth canal. The vagina is about 9 centimeters (3.6 in.) long and extends from the vaginal opening to the cervix, where the uterus attaches at approximately a 90-degree angle. The vaginal opening may be partially, or completely, obstructed by a thin membrane called the **hymen**. The hymen may look different from woman to woman. Some are more intact and others have small openings. The hymen can be ruptured during first sexual intercourse, and some women will notice a small amount of blood. It can also be torn due to activities not related to sexual intercourse such as participating in recreational activities or sports. A torn or partially intact hymen does not mean a woman is no longer a virgin. Some women have a hymen that is thick, obstructing menstrual blood; in this case, the hymen may need to be removed by a physician.

Female External Genitalia (Vulva)

The external genitalia consist of the mons pubis, labia majora ("outer lips"), labia minora ("inner lips"), and clitoris. The **mons pubis** is the soft area covering the pubis bone that is made up of fatty tissue. Some women experience sexual pleasure when this region is touched. The vaginal vestibule is the region between the labia minora where the vagina, the urethra, and Bartholin's glands open. At the top of the vestibule is the clitoris. The **clitoris** is a small erectile organ and is the most sensitive area related to sexual pleasure for many women. The **labia majora** and **labia minora** are elongated folds of skin that look different in

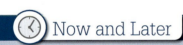

Now and Later

Preventing Pelvic Inflammatory Disease

Now

Did you know that women can get infections that cause PID that are not related to sexual activity or acquiring STIs? Recreational water sports, like water skiing or sliding down a water slide at an amusement park, can also cause PID. When going against water at a high speed, women should wear a wet suit or very tight bathing suit bottoms to prevent contaminated water from being propelled by pressure into their reproductive organs.

Later

Women need to plan on protecting their reproductive organs, beginning as a young girl, to prevent the long-term or fatal consequences of PID.

Take Home

Protect your reproductive organs, both during sexual activity and recreational activities, in order to keep them free from PID.

Female Circumcision

Female genital mutilation, or female circumcision, is a nonmedical procedure where the clitoris is partially or completely removed or the labia are sewed shut. A small opening remains for menstrual blood to leave the body. Long-term health complications of this practice include severe bleeding, problems urinating, infections, cysts, complications during childbirth, and increased risk of newborns dying. These procedures are mostly done to young girls who live in certain countries in Africa, the Middle East, and Asia. While this practice still continues today, many have fought to end female circumcision because it violates the rights of young children and women, causes lifelong health problems, is inhumane, and can be fatal to the women and their babies (World Health Organization 2017).

each woman (figure 12.4). They are composed of sensitive tissues that protect the internal organs and provide lubrication during sexual intercourse.

The **mammary glands** (**breasts**) produce and store milk to provide nourishment for babies. Milk is produced when the glands are stimulated by hormones after a woman has given birth. Each mammary gland has approximately 15 to 20 lobes that lead to the nipple. The nipple contains erectile tissue and is surrounded by the pigmented **areola**. During pregnancy, the areola becomes darker and enlarges. Breast milk is produced in the alveoli in the lobes of a lactating woman, collected into tiny ducts, and then released from the nipple (figure 12.5).

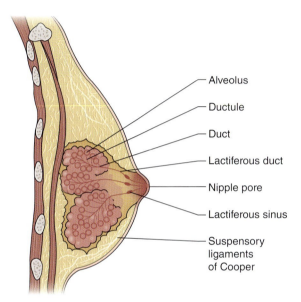

Figure 12.5 The breast is made up of mammary glands that, when stimulated by hormones, produce milk to feed a newborn baby.

Male Reproductive System

The primary role of the male reproductive system (figure 12.6) is to produce male sex hormones and to produce, store, and transport sperm and semen to aid in fertilization of the female egg. The ability for men to produce sperm begins in puberty.

Male Internal Organs

The two oval-shaped testicles are housed in the external structure called the scrotum. The testicles are where testosterone and sperm are produced. The **seminiferous tubules** are coiled tubes inside the **testes** (**testicles**), which produce sperm cells. The **epididymis** is another coiled tube (about 20 feet long when uncoiled!) that rests on the back of the testes and stores the sperm until maturation.

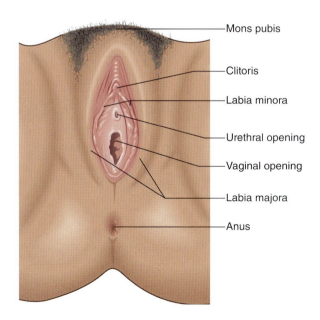

Figure 12.4 Although all women have the same external anatomy, it may look different among women.

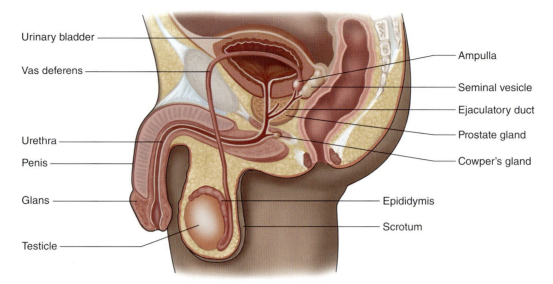

Figure 12.6   Male reproductive anatomy.

Once the sperm are mature, the epididymis aids in transporting them out of the scrotum. During sexual arousal and eventually ejaculation, sperm are forced into the **vas deferens**, a muscular tube connecting the epididymis to the urethra that is located just behind the bladder. The **urethra** is responsible for transporting urine out of the body; however, it also provides the means for the sperm and semen to leave the body during an ejaculation.

Semen is composed of sperm and secretions from the internal glands and provides the nutrients necessary for sperm motility and energy. One of the physiological responses during sexual intercourse is that urine flow to the urethra is blocked by a small valve, the **ejaculatory duct**, so that the semen can be expelled from the body. The **seminal vesicles** are small pouches attached to the vas deferens. They produce a liquid high in fructose that gives sperm the energy necessary to be motile. The **prostate gland** is shaped like a walnut and located in close proximity to the rectum and bladder. It also provides fluids that nourish the sperm. The final internal reproductive organs are the pea-sized **bulbourethral glands** (**Cowper's glands**), which excrete a fluid to help lubricate and neutralize the urethra just prior to ejaculation. An **ejaculation** is the propulsion of semen from the male reproductive system that is initiated by sexual response.

Male External Genitalia

The external organs of the male reproductive anatomy are the penis and the scrotum. The **penis** excretes urine out of the body. When erect, it is the organ necessary for sexual intercourse. The shaft of the penis has a cylindrical shape and contains three cavities made of spongelike tissue. These tissues fill with blood to achieve an **erection**. The glans is the head of the penis and is shaped somewhat like a helmet. The foreskin is a layer of skin that, when the penis is not erect, covers the glans.

The **scrotum** is an external part of the male reproductive system that holds the testicles and hangs behind the penis. The scrotum provides a nurturing environment for the testicles for optimal sperm production and maturation. It keeps the testes at a slightly cooler temperature than the rest of the body for normal sperm development.

Sperm production begins during puberty and continues throughout a man's life. A single sperm cell can take up to 74 days to mature (Encyclopaedia Britannica n.d.). Each day, a man produces around 300 million sperm cells.

Contraception and Birth Control Methods

What is the difference between contraception and birth control? Although many people use these words interchangeably, there are subtle differences between the two. Both terms are related to family planning and preventing unwanted pregnancies. **Contraception** is typically used to identify methods or devices to prevent conception, or the meeting of sperm and egg. Methods that prevent this union are gels such as spermicides, barrier methods such as condoms, hormonal methods like the birth control pill, and intrauterine devices (IUDs). Birth control pills are considered contraception because they prevent ovulation and thicken the cervical mucus to hinder sperm movement. **Birth control methods** is a broader term that typically include methods that prevent both the fertilization of an egg by the sperm (contraception) *and* the implantation of a fertilized egg into the uterine wall. Birth control methods help people plan when they want to have children and include practices (e.g., abstinence or natural

family planning) and surgeries (e.g., vasectomy or tubal ligation). Many believe these terms are interchangeable and result in the same outcomes, which are to prevent pregnancy and have more control when planning families.

According to data from the National Survey of Family Growth (Martinez and Abma 2015), two-thirds of teenagers have had sex by the time they are 19 years old. In this study, 79 percent of women and 84 percent of men said they used some type of birth control the first time they had sex. Figure 12.7 shows that young women in this age group reported condoms as the most commonly used form of birth control, followed by **withdrawal** (stopping intercourse before ejaculation), and then the birth control pill. As teenagers got older, specifically by ages 18 and 19, they were much more likely to use birth control with the first sexual encounter (figure 12.8). Among women using a contraceptive method during their reproductive years, the pill and female sterilization are the most common forms of birth control (Daniels, Daugherty, and Jones 2014).

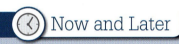
Now and Later

Male Circumcision

Now

Male babies are born with foreskin around the glans of the penis. Removal of the foreskin is called **circumcision**. The foreskin may be removed by a physician soon after birth or performed as a religious rite. Circumcision is a controversial topic for some parents since there is no medical evidence strong enough to mandate that the procedure be performed or not. The American Academy of Pediatrics recommends supporting the wishes of new parents; however, they cite some potential benefits for circumcision, such as a reduced risk of urinary tract infections, penile cancer, and transmission of some STIs and HIV for the circumcised man, as well as the possible reduced risk of cervical cancer for any female sexual partners (Healthy Children 2012). Complications of this procedure, when performed by trained health care professionals, are rare. If circumcision is to be performed, it is recommended that it be done soon after a boy is born. Parents need to consider their own medical, religious, ethical, and cultural beliefs along with the best interests of the child when making a decision.

Later

Although you may not be planning to have a child in the near future, it's important to think about whether or not you would want your son to be circumcised. What are your thoughts about circumcision? Would you have your male baby circumcised? Why or why not?

Take Home

Research the facts on male circumcision now so that you and your partner are prepared to make decisions about this issue later.

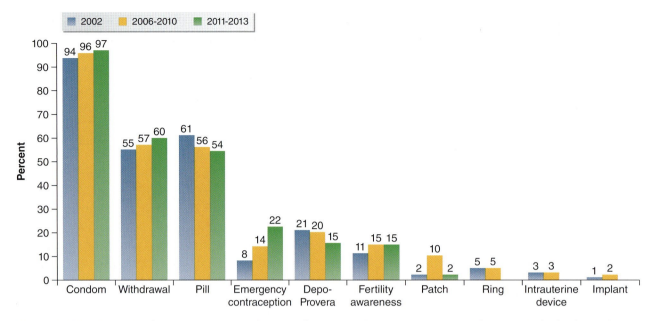

Figure 12.7 Methods of contraception used among females in the United States aged 15 to 19 who had ever had sexual intercourse. Condoms are the most common type of birth control, followed by withdrawal and the birth control pill.

Reprinted from Martinez and Abma (2015).

Almost half of all unintended pregnancies are due to inconsistent and incorrect use of birth control methods (Centers for Disease Control and Prevention 2015). Learning how to use birth control methods can help you reduce the chances of pregnancy now and increase your chances of conception if you are ready to have a baby later. The majority of college students are not planning on having children while in school; therefore, it is important to plan now if you would like to become a parent. Consider when in your life you want to begin having children and which birth control methods will help you and your partner meet this goal. If you choose not to have children, which birth control methods would be the best options for you and your partner to consider for the long term?

Being aware of birth control methods and knowing how to use them consistently and correctly with every sexual encounter is being responsible to yourself and your partner. Consider these questions when choosing a birth control method:

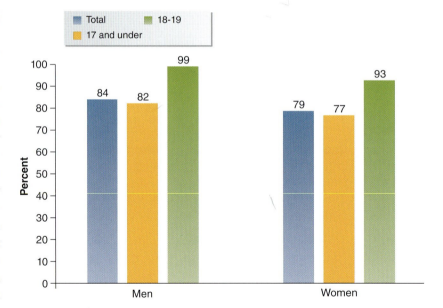

Figure 12.8. Use of contraception at first sex among men and women in the United States aged 15 to 19, by age at first sex.

Reprinted from Martinez and Abma (2015).

1. What are your and your partner's values regarding conception? What are your related opinions about the types of birth control methods?

2. Do you both know the advantages and disadvantages of each method, including side effects?

3. What are the costs of different methods? Which ones are covered by insurance plans or government plans or are available at lower costs from community health clinics? Is cost a prohibiting factor when considering birth control?

4. Which methods will require the commitment of both partners? Which methods require that only one partner be responsible?

5. Which methods can help prevent transmission of STIs?

6. Which methods require seeing a health care provider before use?

7. How long are you and your partner going to use this method?

8. When do you plan on having children?

9. Do you need a method that also protects against STIs?

10. Which methods do you and your partner consider to be convenient?

11. Which methods do you and your partner consider to be too difficult or not worth using? What are the reasons?

The implant (Nexplanon), intrauterine device (IUD), and **sterilization** (tubal ligation and vasectomy) provide the lowest failure rates because they are long-term methods that do not require attention to **perfect use**. That is, the user does not have to remember to take medication or correctly and consistently use a device or gel during every sexual encounter. Couples rarely have perfect use of birth control methods that are not considered permanent or long term. Figure 12.9 shows the percentage rates of unintended pregnancy during the first year of birth control related to **typical use** (not perfect use). You can see that it is important to learn how to use these methods correctly in order to prevent pregnancy.

Contraceptive Use by the Numbers

Check out these statistics on contraceptive use, compiled by the Guttmacher Institute (2016).

- 85%: the chance of getting pregnant with no contraceptive use
- 2 children: the average desired family size in the United States
- 3 decades: the total time a woman must use contraceptives in order to have 2 children during her childbearing years
- 62%: percentage of women of reproductive age currently using birth control
- 67%: percentage of women using contraception who choose a nonpermanent method (patch, pill, implant, shot, or ring)
- 1 in 9: sexually active women who have used emergency contraception

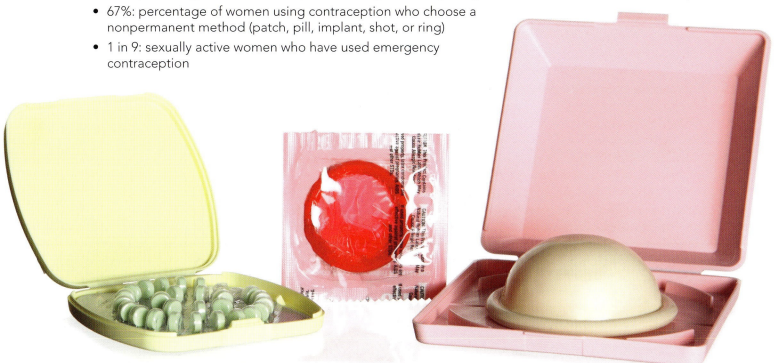

Failure Rates of Contraceptives During First Year of Use

Most effective	Method	Unintended pregnancy with typical use (%)
Less than 1 per 100	Implant	.05%
	IUD	.2%-.8%
	Male sterilization (vasectomy)	.15%
	Female sterilization (tubal ligation)	.5%
6-12 per 100	Shot (Depo-Provera)	6%
	Birth control pill	9%
	Patch	9%
	Vaginal contraceptive ring	9%
	Diaphragm	12%
18+ per 100	Male condom	18%
	Female condom	21%
	Withdrawal	22%
	Fertility-awareness-based methods	24%
	Spermicide	28%
	No method	85%

Most effective ↑ ... Least effective

Figure 12.9   If you use contraceptives, carefully evaluate which one to use, taking into account their failure rates. The percentages indicate the number of every 100 women who experienced an unintended pregnancy during the first year of typical use.

Data from Centers for Disease Control and Prevention (2015).

ABSTINENCE

Abstinence means choosing not to have sex and waiting to be sexually active until the time is right for you. For many, this means not engaging in sexual contact, sexual stimulation, kissing, oral sex, vaginal sex, or anal sex. Some people wait to engage in any or all of these activities until marriage. No one can tell you when to become sexually active or which sexual activities you should engage in. Research shows that young people who wait or postpone sexual activity between the start of a relationship and the first sexual encounter with that partner are more likely to use birth control (Manlove, Ryan, and Franzetta 2003).

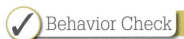 Behavior Check

Abstinence

Why do people choose abstinence? What are the pros and cons? Can you still be a sexual person if you are not sexually active? What would be the challenges to stick to a decision to be abstinent?

Abstinence provides 100 percent protection from pregnancy and STI. Abstinence means that no genital-to-genital contact occurs and there is no contact with body fluids, including vaginal secretions, semen, or blood. By not rushing into a relationship that includes sexual activities, partners can get to know each other better and build trust.

BARRIER BIRTH CONTROL METHODS

Barrier birth control methods provide a physical barrier that prevents the sperm and egg from meeting. Latex condoms (see figure 12.10), when used consistently and correctly with every sexual encounter, can provide an effective barrier and reduce the risk of acquiring many STIs that are transmitted by genital fluids, as well as HIV, the virus that causes AIDS (Centers for Disease Control and Prevention 2013b).

MALE CONDOM

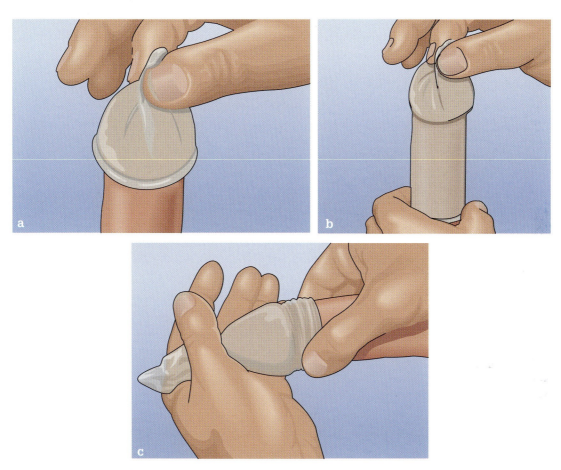

Figure 12.10a-c   Male condoms can be effective toward preventing pregnancy and STIs if they are used consistently and correctly with every sexual encounter.

Use: Read package instructions before using a condom. Check the expiration date and get a new one if the date has passed. Use latex condoms to prevent pregnancy and transmission of STIs and HIV. Place the condom over an erect penis before intercourse and pinch the tip of the condom to prevent an air bubble from forming. It is important to leave a space at the tip of the condom to collect the semen. After ejaculation, remove the condom and dispose of it in the trash, making sure the semen remains in the condom (see figure 12.10).

Advantages: Many different types are available; method available for men; partner can participate; no prescription needed.

Disadvantages: Cannot reuse condoms; need to use correctly and consistently every time; may cause irritation or allergic reactions; some men experience lack of sensation; must make sure condom is on correctly so it doesn't slip off during intercourse; can use only water-based lubricants; cannot use condoms made of animal skin (or natural condoms) because they do not prevent STIs or HIV.

FEMALE CONDOM

Use: Condom is inserted into the vagina; the smaller circle covers the cervix and the larger circle covers the vulva (see figure 12.11).

Advantages: Made of nitrile, not latex; can be inserted up to eight hours before sexual intercourse.

Disadvantages: A new condom must be used with every sexual encounter; may cause irritation or allergic reaction; user must be comfortable inserting the end of the condom in the vagina, which takes practice; cannot be used with the male condom at the same time.

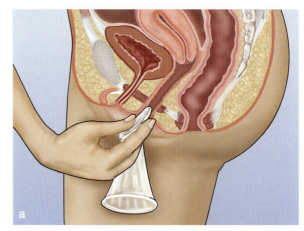

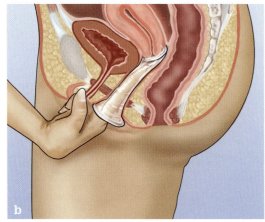

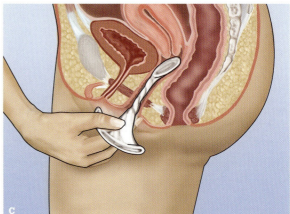

Figure 12.11a-c   A female condom can be inserted up to eight hours before intercourse.

DIAPHRAGM

Use: Fits over the cervix; must be inserted into the vagina and placed over the cervix before intercourse (see figure 12.12). A spermicide must be applied to the inside of the diaphragm before it is inserted into the vagina. A diaphragm must remain over the cervix for 6 hours after the last sexual encounter and removed within 24 hours.

Advantages: Can be reused; inserted before sexual intercourse; can be used with male condom.

Disadvantages: Must be inserted before intercourse and remain in place during intercourse; must be used with every sexual encounter; may cause irritation or allergic reaction; user must be comfortable inserting the diaphragm into the vagina, which takes practice; does not prevent HIV or STIs.

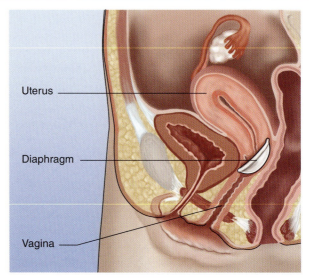

Figure 12.12   A diaphragm is a barrier method of birth control that prevents the sperm from fertilizing the egg.

CERVICAL CAP (FEM CAP)

Use: The cervical cap is smaller than the diaphragm; however, just like the diaphragm, it is used with spermicide and held in place over the cervix with suction. Must be inserted before sexual intercourse; covers the cervix and is held in place with suction; used with a spermicide.

Advantages: Can be reused; inserted before sex; can be used with male condom.

Disadvantages: Must be inserted before intercourse and remain in place during intercourse; must be used with every sexual encounter; may cause irritation or allergic reaction; user must be comfortable inserting cervical cap in the vagina, which takes practice; does not prevent HIV or STIs.

> If you are using the diaphragm or cervical cap and planning on having sex more than once in 24 hours, be sure to check the placement of these barrier methods and use more spermicide with each sexual encounter.

HORMONAL METHODS

Hormonal birth control methods contain estrogen and progestin. The hormones prevent pregnancy through various mechanisms such as preventing the egg from leaving the ovaries (i.e., preventing ovulation); thickening the cervical mucus, which prevents sperm from entering the uterus; or causing the lining of the uterus to thin, which prevents implantation of the fertilized egg. The majority of hormonal methods must be prescribed by a health care provider. One exception is the emergency contraceptive pill, which is available over the counter.

> None of the hormonal birth control methods prevent sexually transmitted infections (Centers for Disease Control and Prevention 2017h; US Department of Health and Human Services 2016b).

BIRTH CONTROL PILL

Use: A pill that usually contains progestin and estrogen taken at the same time every day to prevent fertilization and inhibit ovulation. Some pills have only one hormone. Most packs have 21 days of pills with hormones and 7 days without hormones. The seven nonhormone pills are taken when a woman's period begins. Continuous birth control pills with low estrogen may stop bleeding during the menstrual cycle; absence of a period will not cause long-term health problems. Women need to consult with their health care providers to determine which type of birth control pill is best for their overall health and quality of life.

Advantages: Does not interrupt intercourse; user can stop taking the pill at any time; may help with acne or lead to shorter and lighter periods.

Disadvantages: Requires a prescription; user must take a pill every day; missing a pill decreases the effectiveness of the method and requires using another birth control method (e.g., condom) for at least seven days; blood clotting may be an increased risk if user smokes cigarettes; may cause nausea, mood changes or depression, headaches, spotting in between periods, and breast tenderness; does not prevent HIV or STIs.

> Although the birth control pill has been used by millions of women since the 1960s and is considered very safe, be sure to contact your health care provider if you take the birth control pill and experience any of these symptoms, or ACHES: abdominal pain, chest pain, headaches, eye problems, or severe leg pain.

IMPLANT (NEXPLANON)

Use: Progestin only; small flexible tubes are surgically placed under the skin on the underside of the upper arm; suppresses ovulation and thickens cervical mucus.

Advantages: Lasts for three years; small—size of a matchstick; fertility returns within days of removal.

Disadvantages: User must have new implants inserted every three years; side effects include irregular bleeding and spotting between periods, mood changes, weight gain, headaches, acne, depression, breast tenderness, painful periods, and nausea; does not prevent HIV or STIs.

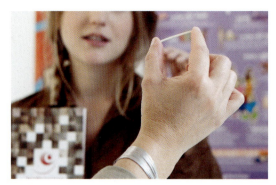

With the implant Nexplanon, the tiny rod is placed just under the skin and the body absorbs the progestin to prevent ovulation.

PATCH

Use: A small patch (1-1/2 in.; 4 cm) containing estrogen and progestin is applied to a woman's abdomen, shoulder, side of upper arm, or buttocks; prevents ovulation; thickens cervical mucus.

Advantages: Simple to use; adheres to body; user does not have to change daily.

Disadvantages: Requires a prescription; must be placed on body before intercourse and remain in place during intercourse; user must change patch weekly on the same day for three weeks, then on fourth week wear no patch to begin the menstrual cycle; patch may be less effective for obese women; side effect of skin irritation; patch may become detached from skin; contains higher levels of estrogen than the birth control pill; may be less effective for women who weigh over 198 pounds (90 kg); does not prevent HIV or STIs.

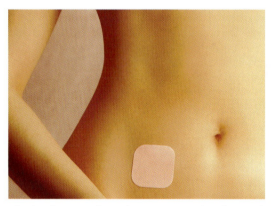

The birth control patch is worn on the skin and delivers hormones that prevent ovulation.

VAGINAL RING

Use: A flexible ring is inserted into the vagina. This method releases low doses of estrogen and progestin and stops ovulation. Unlike other hormonal birth control methods, this method requires the woman to insert the ring into the vagina. If user experiences some discomfort, then the ring is not in place. Most male partners have indicated that they cannot feel the ring during intercourse.

Advantages: Remains in place for three weeks and is removed during the woman's period; user does not have to change daily.

Disadvantages: Must be inserted before intercourse and remain in place during intercourse; user must be comfortable inserting and removing the ring; user must replace ring every month; possibility of irritation; does not prevent HIV or STIs.

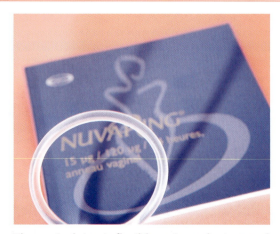

The vaginal ring is flexible so it can be inserted into the vagina and placed around the cervix.

SHOT (DEPO-PROVERA)

Use: A progestin-only shot given to women in the upper arm or buttocks every three months.

Advantages: No estrogen; begins providing protection against pregnancy within 24 hours of the first injection; no menstrual bleeding after one year of use.

Disadvantages: Injection every three months; must see a health care provider to get the injection; possible weight gain, hair loss, and mood changes; bone density decreases after long-term use; does not prevent HIV or STIs.

IUD (INTRAUTERINE DEVICE)

Use: A tiny, T-shaped device is inserted (and removed) into the uterus by a health care provider; different types are available with and without hormones (copper T); works by thickening cervical mucus and inhibiting fertilization (see figure 12.13).

Advantages: Lighter periods; less cramping during periods; some can be in place for 3 to 12 years; convenient—user does not have to do anything once it is inserted; easily removed.

Disadvantages: Some IUDs may increase bleeding and cramps during period; may cause irregular menstrual cycle, pelvic discomfort, acne, headaches, nausea, and breast tenderness; does not prevent HIV or STIs.

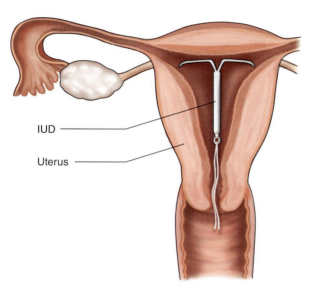

IUD

Uterus

Figure 12.13   The IUD is placed in the uterus by a health care provider to prevent pregnancy. Three different types are available that can stay in the uterus for 3, 5, or 10 years.

EMERGENCY CONTRACEPTION (MORNING-AFTER PILL)

Use: Taken after unprotected intercourse to prevent pregnancy; should be taken within three days for optimal effectiveness; delays or prevents ovulation to prevent fertilization; inhibits the Fallopian tubes from drawing the egg toward the uterus.

Advantages: An option for women who have been sexually assaulted; helpful for when a birth control method was not used, the method failed to work as intended, or the method was used incorrectly; can be up to 95 percent effective in preventing pregnancy if taken within the first 24 hours after unprotected sex.

Disadvantages: Loses effectiveness if taken more than three days after unprotected intercourse; ineffective for women who weigh more than 165 pounds (75 kg); will not work if the woman is already pregnant; cannot be taken before intercourse as a birth control method; may cause nausea and vomiting; does not prevent HIV or STIs.

In 2013, emergency contraception became available over the counter for anyone at any age. It must be displayed on store shelves for easy access.

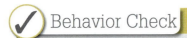

Behavior Check

Reasons for Not Using Birth Control

With all of the reliable and affordable birth control methods available to both men and women for preventing pregnancy, why do you think sexually active college students choose not to use them? Which of the following reasons are ones you have heard from your friends?

- Lack of information and knowledge about methods and how to use them.
- Too embarrassed to talk to their sexual partner or their health care provider.
- Don't want others to know they are sexually active.
- Afraid of the side effects like potential weight gain or mood swings.
- Methods are too expensive.
- Methods may reduce sexual desire, excitement, or pleasure.
- Methods are too complicated and bothersome.
- Sexually active friends use drugs or alcohol, which prevents them from using birth control methods.
- Religious or cultural reasons.
- Not sure where to get them.

Now that you know about the methods of birth control, if you are sexually active or when you become sexually active, which of these excuses have been resolved for you?

OTHER METHODS

Other types of birth control do not require the use of a barrier method or hormones. These options are available for couples who want to use a method that is in alignment with their religious and personal values. They do not require getting a prescription or using a medication or products that may cause irritations or allergies. None of these methods protect against sexually transmitted infections.

FERTILITY AWARENESS, OR NATURAL FAMILY PLANNING

Use: Users recognize ovulation and fertile days during the menstrual cycle and abstain from intercourse during those days, charting changes in cervical mucus and basal body temperature during ovulation (slightly elevated during this time). To use this method correctly, it's best to get training from a health care professional.

Advantages: Involves both partners; avoids the side effects of other methods; helps to plan a pregnancy; women and their partners learn to understand a woman's menstrual cycle.

Disadvantages: Cannot have spontaneous sex and must plan according to the menstrual cycle and ovulation; need to keep track of ovulation; will have to use alternate birth control methods if choosing to have sex during ovulation days; hard to track ovulation with an irregular menstrual cycle; does not prevent HIV or STIs.

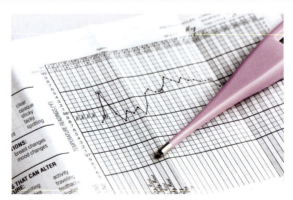

Fertility awareness requires the careful calculation and charting of ovulation during a woman's menstrual cycle. Couples who do not want children abstain from sexual intercourse during these days.

WITHDRAWAL

Use: Male withdraws penis from the woman's vagina before ejaculation; may prevent fertilization.

Advantage: No prescription or devices needed; may be better than no method.

Disadvantages: Requires cooperation of both partners; may disrupt sexual pleasure; pre-ejaculatory fluid from previous ejaculations during this sexual encounter may contain sperm; does not prevent HIV or STIs.

SPERMICIDES

Use: Spermicide contains a chemical that kills sperm. It comes in the form of foam, jelly, cream, or film that is placed inside the vagina before sex. Some types must be put in place 30 minutes ahead of time but no more than 1 hour before intercourse. Spermicides are most often used along with other birth control methods such as the male condom, diaphragm, or cervical cap.

Advantages: Easy to use, inexpensive, available at most drug stores.

Disadvantages: May cause irritations; could increase risk of getting HIV or STIs.

STERILIZATION: VASECTOMY

Use: Permanent surgical procedure that severs the vas deferens; prevents sperm from leaving the testicles (see figure 12.14).

Advantages: Permanent procedure; highly effective; does not alter sexual pleasure or desire.

Disadvantages: Surgical procedure; user experiences soreness at incision site, some swelling in the testicles; user must submit semen samples to health care provider to make sure semen no longer contains sperm; not intended to be a reversible procedure (U.S. Department of Health and Human Services 2016c); does not prevent HIV or STIs.

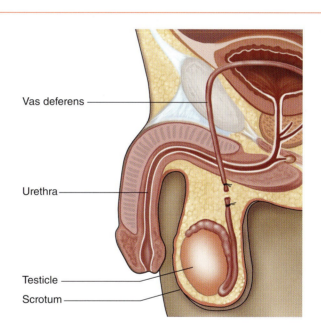

Figure 12.14 A vasectomy is a permanent surgical procedure where the vas deferens are cut and sealed to prevent the sperm from leaving the testicles.

STERILIZATION: TUBAL LIGATION

Use: Permanent surgical procedure that severs the Fallopian tubes and prevents eggs from entering the uterus (see figure 12.15).

Advantages: Permanent procedure; highly effective; does not alter sexual pleasure or desire.

Disadvantages: Surgical procedure; user experiences soreness at incision site; not intended to be a reversible procedure (U.S. Department of Health and Human Services 2016a); does not prevent HIV or STIs.

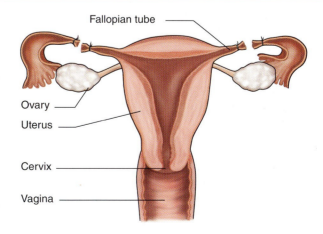

Figure 12.15 A tubal ligation is a permanent surgical procedure for women who do not want to have children.

Sexually Transmitted Infections

Talking to sexual partners about your sexual history can be uncomfortable, but it is necessary to make sure you are taking care of yourself and practicing responsible behaviors. Understanding more about your body, recognizing when something just isn't right, and knowing how to communicate about your sexual health can help you make responsible decisions. Sexually transmitted infections (STIs) can cause a lifetime of health problems; therefore, you should have conversations about preventing these infections with all sexual partners. Knowing your STI status, as well as that of your partner, is sexually responsible and important for remaining infection free throughout your life.

Sexually transmitted infections are common diseases caused by viruses, bacteria, and parasites that are transmitted through vaginal intercourse, anal intercourse, and oral sex. Most, if caught early, can be treated with antibiotics. However, viral STIs are with you for life. Some can lead to further complications, such as cancers, infertility, and problems during pregnancy and childbirth. Unfortunately, some infections do not lead to obvious symptoms, leaving the host unaware of his or her status and thus infecting sexual partners with the infection; symptoms do not have to be present for an infection to be transmitted to another person. Women are more susceptible to acquiring STIs than men are.

> Most STIs, if detected early, can be treated. Some, though, can lead to cancer, infertility, complications during pregnancy and childbirth, and death. Viral STIs are with you for life.

Approximately 19.7 million new cases of STIs are reported annually in the United States (Satterwhite et al. 2013). Of these reported cases, they are diagnosed more often among teen and young adults between the ages of 15 and 25 (figure 12.16). The most commonly diagnosed bacterial STIs are chlamydia, gonorrhea, and syphilis, and the most common viral STIs are genital herpes simplex virus (HSV), HIV/AIDS, and human papilloma virus (HPV). In 2015, the Centers for Disease Control and Prevention (2016b) released the following data indicating that reported STIs are at an unprecedented high in the United States:

- Americans aged 15 to 24 years old accounted for nearly two-thirds of chlamydia diagnoses and half of gonorrhea diagnoses.

- Men who have sex with men (MSM) accounted for the majority of new gonorrhea and primary and secondary syphilis cases (82 percent of male cases with known sex of partner). Antibiotic-resistant gonorrhea may be higher among MSM.

- Women's rates of syphilis diagnosis increased by more than 27 percent from 2014 to 2015 and accounted for less than 10 percent of new primary and secondary syphilis infections.

- More than 1.2 million people in the United States are living with HIV, and one in eight of them doesn't know it.

- From 2005 to 2014, the annual number of new HIV diagnoses declined 19 percent.

- Gay and bisexual men, particularly young African American gay and bisexual men, are most affected by STIs and HIV/AIDS (Centers for Disease Control and Prevention n.d.).

STI Treatment for Partners

Did you know that if you are diagnosed with an STI, in some states, you can get medication to give to your sexual partner? Ask your health care provider about expedited partner therapy when diagnosed with gonorrhea, chlamydia, or trichomoniasis. After you have taken the prescribed medication and no longer have symptoms, you and your partner need to see a health care provider to make sure the infection is gone (Guttmacher Institute 2018).

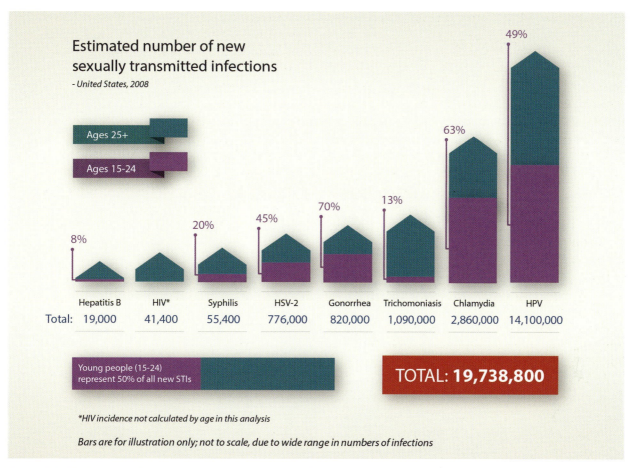

Figure 12.16   Estimated number of new STI infections, United States, 2008.
Centers for Disease Control and Prevention (2013a).

MOST COMMON VIRAL STIS

Viral STIs enter the body through skin or body fluids. A virus can survive only by attaching to living cells in the body. STIs that are classified as viral are those that can be treated but not cured. For example, herpes is a viral STI that can be successfully treated with medications prescribed by a physician to alleviate the symptoms, which may include reducing the frequency of the outbreaks (e.g., sores or blisters) in addition to reducing their severity and duration. Hepatitis and human papilloma virus are the only viral STIs that can be prevented with a vaccine.

HIV/AIDS

Facts: The human immunodeficiency virus (HIV) causes acquired immunodeficiency syndrome (AIDS). The virus is transmitted in the following body fluids: breast milk, vaginal secretions, semen, and blood. HIV attacks the body's immune system and affects its ability to fight infections. The body becomes susceptible to serious opportunistic infections that are typically rare in people without HIV. Examples of these unique infections are a skin cancer called Kaposi's sarcoma and pneumocystis pneumonia.

Prevalence: According to Hall and colleagues (2015), by the end of 2013, approximately 1.2 million people aged 13 and older were living with HIV in the United States, and 13 percent were not aware of their HIV status. Figure 12.17 shows the highest concentration of HIV diagnosis by age is in the 20- to 29-year-old age group.

Transmission: The primary modes of transmission are sharing injection-drug needles and having anal intercourse, vaginal intercourse, or oral sex with an HIV-infected person where these body fluids come in contact with a mucosal lining or damaged tissues. These delicate membranes are in the rectum, vagina, penis, and mouth. Detectable amounts of the virus show up on blood or oral secretion tests between one week and three months after exposure. The virus can be transmitted to another person by someone who is HIV positive but does not show any specific symptoms of infection.

Symptoms: When a person has been diagnosed with HIV or is known to be HIV positive, he or she may be symptom free for many years. As the infection progresses, symptoms may include fevers, weight loss, swollen lymph nodes, or oral yeast infections. A person is diagnosed with AIDS based on the progression of the disease and its toll on the immune system, causing opportunistic infections, increased levels of HIV in the body, and lower levels of infection-fighting antibodies.

Treatment: No treatment or vaccine exists to prevent HIV; however, medications can help HIV-positive individuals live a long and productive life. HIV/AIDS was first discovered in the early 1980s. At that time, when someone was diagnosed with HIV, the infection progressed very rapidly to AIDS, and many died within a few years after diagnosis. Today, with our better understanding of how the virus affects the immune system and access to medications, HIV is no longer the death sentence it once was.

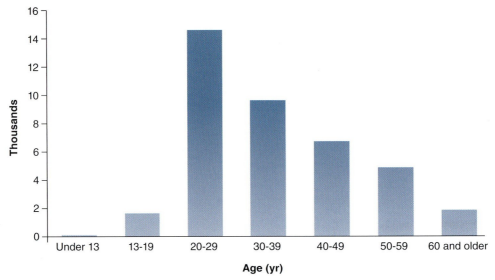

Figure 12.17   Diagnoses of HIV infection by age, United States.

Data from Centers for Disease Control and Prevention (2017e).

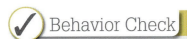 Behavior Check

HIV Testing and Prevention

The Centers for Disease Control and Prevention's Get Tested program is focused on motivating people to learn their HIV status. Knowing your status enables you to get the medical care you need to treat these infections or prevent their progress, inform your sexual partners so they can be treated, and remain infection free. On the CDC website, you can locate a testing site in your community and learn the specific types of testing you need by answering a few questions related to your sex, age, and sexual behaviors and history. Behaviors that can put you at risk for HIV are having more than one sexual partner, engaging in sexual activities without knowing your partner's sexual health history, not using condoms, having been diagnosed with other STIs, and sharing needles or syringes. The CDC recommends that everyone between the ages of 13 and 64 get tested for HIV as part of a routine health examination. For more information about getting tested, visit the CDC's website at https://gettested.cdc.gov.

PrEP (pre-exposure prophylaxis) is a relatively new prevention method for people who are not HIV positive but engage in behaviors that may put them at risk of acquiring HIV. This medication works to prevent the virus from becoming a permanent infection in the body and can reduce the risk of HIV infection by up to 92 percent, combined with using condoms, not sharing injectable drugs, and visiting a health care provider every three months (Centers for Disease Control and Prevention 2017j).

HUMAN PAPILLOMA VIRUS (HPV)

Facts: HPV is so common that most sexually active people will be diagnosed with the virus at some point (Centers for Disease Control and Prevention n.d.).

Prevalence: HPV is not a reportable STI to health departments or the CDC; therefore, it is estimated that 79 million Americans currently have HPV. Approximately 14 million new infections are diagnosed annually (Centers for Disease Control and Prevention 2017d).

Symptoms: Warts appear internally or externally in the genital area between six weeks and eight months after exposure, although some people never develop the warts.

Diagnosis: Visual examination or biopsy of the warts. For women: a Pap smear of the cervix; colposcopy (microscopic examination) of cervix.

Treatment: The warts can go away on their own without treatment, but the virus never goes away. A health care provider can remove the warts through cryotherapy (freezing) with liquid nitrogen, burning them off with a topical solution like trichloroacetic acid, cauterization with electrical heat, or a laser treatment. A prescription topical cream can also be applied to the warts if they are external.

Complications: Women are at an increased risk of cervical cancer when exposed to certain HPV strains. Women with the virus will have to deliver a baby by cesarean section if warts are present during delivery. Men can develop anal and penile cancers; men and women can develop throat cancers.

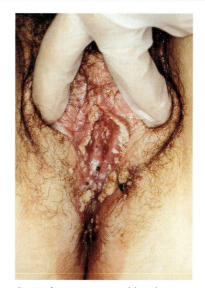

Genital warts, caused by the HPV, are typically flesh colored. They can be found in the genital (internal and external), anal, mouth, and throat regions.

Vaccine: The HPV vaccine for boys and girls, Gardasil 6, protects against six types of the virus that are linked to cancers. The vaccine is now only two doses, with the second dose given 6 to 12 months after the first dose. The CDC recommends that boys and girls be vaccinated between ages 11 and 12; however, people vaccinated as young adults can still benefit from the vaccine's protective factors if they have never been exposed to HPV or the specific types that can cause cancer (Centers for Disease Control and Prevention 2017d).

HERPES SIMPLEX VIRUS (HSV)

Facts: Two different types exist—herpes simplex virus type 1 (HSV1; oral) and herpes simplex virus type 2 (HSV2; genital). HSV1 can be transferred from the mouth to the genitals and HSV2 can be transferred from the genitals to the mouth through oral sex or if an infected person touches the infected genitals and then touches the mouth (or vice versa). Most fever blisters or cold sores on the mouth are HSV1 and tend to flare up during very stressful times. This virus can be transmitted when symptoms are not present.

Prevalence: Since HSV is not a reportable STI by law to health departments or the CDC, it is estimated that one out of six people between the ages of 14 and 49 have genital herpes (Centers for Disease Control and Prevention 2017c).

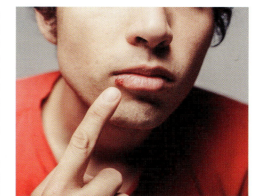

HSV type 1, a cold sore on the lip, tends to reoccur in the same place during each outbreak.

Symptoms: For both men and women, small sores or lesions (outbreaks) appear around the mouth or genitals, depending on the type of contact, 2 to 12 days after exposure. Sores can last up to two weeks. When the sores are gone, the virus remains dormant until the next outbreak.

Diagnosis: Examination of the sores and lesions and viral culture of the lesions, which involves taking a sample of the lesion tissue (Centers for Disease Control and Prevention 2017c).

Treatment: Herpes cannot be cured because it is a virus; however, medications can reduce the intensity and frequency of the outbreaks and may reduce the chances of the virus being spread to a sexual partner (Centers for Disease Control and Prevention n.d.).

Complications: Pregnant women who have an active outbreak may not be able to deliver vaginally.

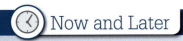 Now and Later

HPV Vaccine

The HPV vaccine is the best method for preventing many types of cancers, including cervical, penile, anal, and throat cancers. About 6 out of 10 girls and 5 out of 10 boys have been vaccinated against specific strains of HPV covered by the vaccine (see figure 12.18).

Now

The HPV vaccine was approved by the FDA in June 2006. When it was first introduced as a safe and effective method for preventing women from getting cervical cancer caused by certain strains of the virus, many parents were concerned that the primary message their young daughters would receive is that this vaccine would be that it is safe for them to become sexually active at an earlier age. Some of the controversial aspects of the vaccine included the mandate that all girls must get the vaccine. Parents thought the age at which to give the vaccine, 11 to 12 years old, was premature because girls are typically not sexually active at this age. Parents who are against the vaccine often express their concerns about their child's sexual development and are not ready to deal with such uncomfortable issues with their preteens.

Later

The vaccine is safe and effective for young women through age 26 and young men through age 21 (Centers for Disease Control and Prevention 2017g); however, the vaccines should be given at age 11 or 12, which consists of two shots given 6 to 12 months apart (CDC 2017l). You may be a parent in the future, so what are your thoughts about the HPV vaccine? How will you plan to protect your children from HPV in the future?

- Should the HPV vaccine be a mandatory vaccine for all boys and girls? Why or why not?
- Why should preteens get the HPV vaccine if they are not yet sexually active?

Take Home

Learn more about the HPV vaccine so that you can be protected from acquiring the virus.

ZIKA

Facts: Zika was first discovered in 1947, but very few cases were reported until recently. It is transmitted when an infected *Aedes* species mosquito bites a human (figure 12.19). Once Zika infects a human, it can be passed from a pregnant woman to her fetus, through sexual activity, and perhaps through blood transfusions. Zika infections are primarily concentrated in certain areas of the world, specifically in tropical Africa, Southeast Asia, and the Pacific Islands (Centers for Disease Control and Prevention 2017i). Zika transmission has been reported in the United States, specifically in south Florida and Texas (Centers for Disease Control and Prevention 2017a).

Research studies are being conducted in the United States and other countries to determine how long Zika can remain in semen and vaginal fluids, how long Zika can be passed to sexual partners, and whether there is a difference in the risk for birth defects if the pregnant woman acquires Zika during sex rather than directly from a mosquito bite (Centers for Disease Control and Prevention 2017k).

Prevalence: Zika is a notifiable infection and is reported to health departments and the CDC. As of March 22, 2017, there were 5,158 cases in the United States. The majority (94 percent) were travelers returning from countries with high rates of infection. Four percent acquired Zika from a local mosquito in Florida

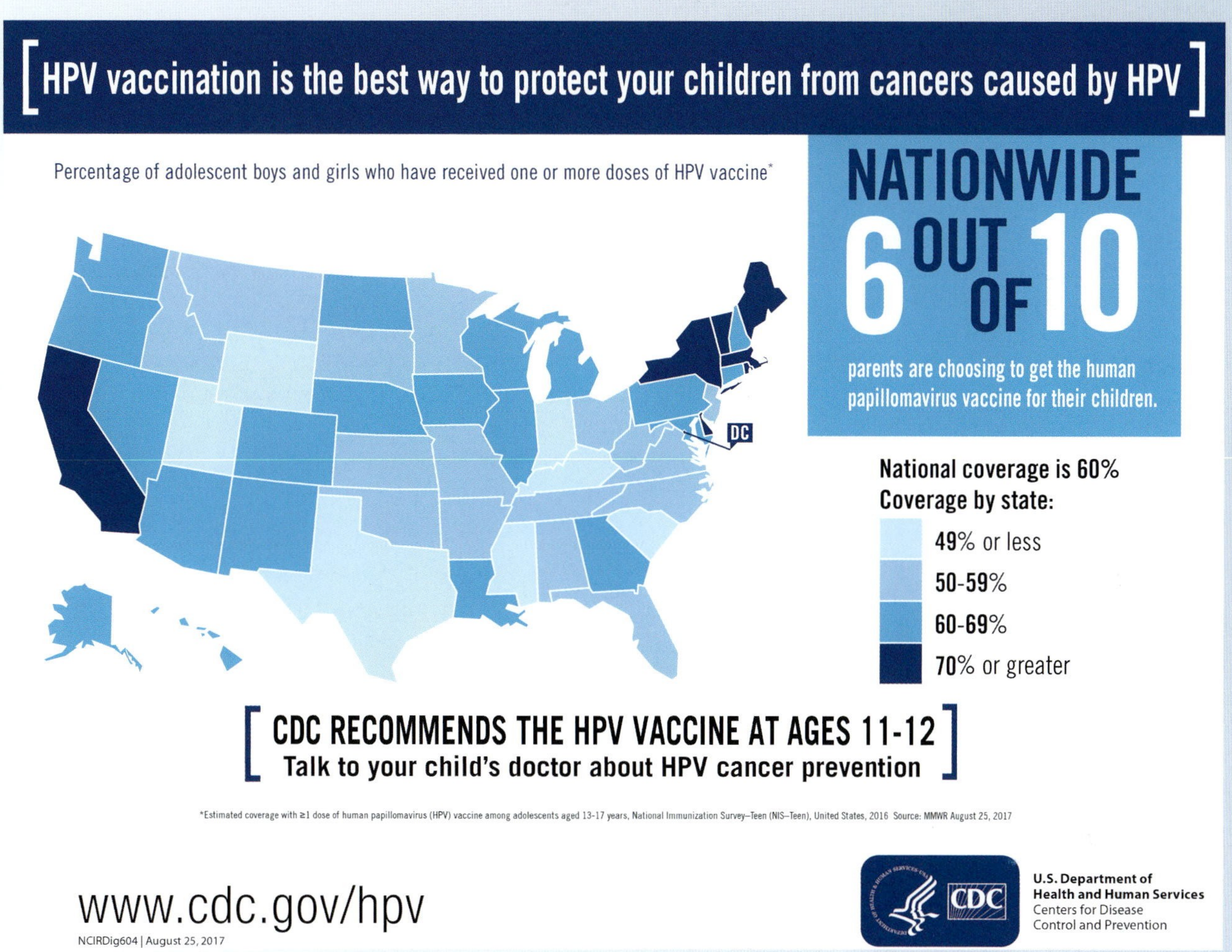

Figure 12.18 HPV vaccination rates for girls and boys, United States, 2016.

Reprinted from Centers for Disease Control and Prevention (2017d).

and Texas, and the remaining 2 percent acquired it through sexual contact, from mother to baby, and in unknown ways.

Symptoms: Most people infected with Zika have no symptoms. When experienced, symptoms are mild and last for several days to weeks. The most commonly reported symptoms are fever, rash, joint pain, red eyes, muscle pain, and headaches. Zika is not considered fatal (figure 12.19).

Diagnosis: Zika is diagnosed through a comprehensive health and travel history, especially to countries with high rates such as tropical Africa, Southeast Asia, and the Pacific Islands. A blood or urine test will confirm the infection.

Treatment: Currently, no vaccine or medication is available to treat or cure Zika.

Complications: In pregnant women who are infected with Zika, the virus causes a birth defect called microcephaly (the baby's head and brain are smaller than they should be at birth), eye and hearing defects, and compromised growth.

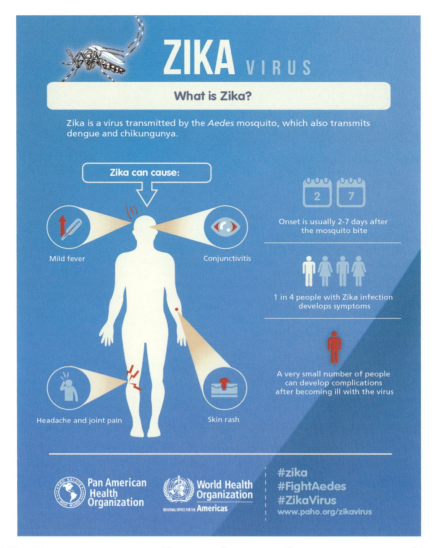

Figure 12.19   Zika is a virus transmitted by a specific species of mosquito. It causes mild symptoms that include fever, eye infections, joint pain, and skin rashes. For most people, this infection is not fatal, but it can cause serious birth defects in children born to infected mothers.

Reprinted by permission from the Pan American Health Organization, "What is Zika?" http://new.paho.org/hq/images/stories/AD/HSD/IR/Viral_Diseases/Zika-Virus/8x11introENG.png.

MOST COMMON BACTERIAL STIS

Bacterial STIs come from cells that cause infection and enter the body through the skin or body fluids (e.g., semen or vaginal fluids). If the bacterial infection is detected early, it can be successfully treated and often cured with antibiotics; however, if the infection is not treated, it could lead to long-term negative health consequences like sterility or death. Medications that treat the infection do not prevent recurrence if exposed to the bacteria in the future. Therefore, if you are sexually active, it is important to protect yourself from acquiring an STI by using condoms or other barrier methods that prevent the exchange of body fluids. See a health care provider if you are concerned about any abnormal symptoms such as discharge from the genitals or if a sexual partner has been diagnosed with a bacterial STI so that you can be diagnosed and treated in the early stages of the infection.

CHLAMYDIA

Facts: Most commonly reported STI in the United States (Centers for Disease Control and Prevention n.d.).

Prevalence: Reported cases are the highest among people aged 15 to 24 years old. In 2015, this age group accounted for 39 percent of chlamydia cases (see figure 12.20).

Symptoms: Appear 7 to 30 days after exposure; many people do not experience symptoms.

- *Men:* discharge from penis, pain in testicles, swollen testicles, painful urination
- *Women:* odorous discharge from vagina, midcycle bleeding

Diagnosis: Everyone who is sexually active should be tested. Sexually active women age 25 and younger need to be tested annually. Testing methods involve urine analysis or testing of discharge for the bacteria.

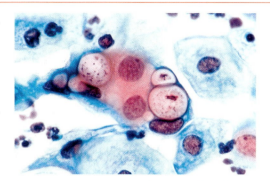

A Pap smear showing chlamydia. Not all people infected with chlamydia will have symptoms, but those who do may have an odorous or purulent discharge from the cervix (vagina) or penis.

Treatment: Can be easily cured with antibiotics if diagnosed in early stages.

Complications: If not detected and treated in the early stages of the infection, women can develop PID, which can lead to infertility. Men can develop infertility.

GONORRHEA

Facts: Known as "the clap" or "the drip," gonorrhea is the second most commonly reported STI in the United States (Centers for Disease Control and Prevention n.d.). It can infect not only the genital but also the rectum and throat.

Prevalence: High rates in teens and college-age individuals, who accounted for 32 percent of the reported cases in 2015 (see figure 12.20).

Symptoms: Appear two to seven days after exposure.

- *Men:* white or yellowish discharge from penis, pain when urinating, fever
- *Women:* white or yellowish vaginal discharge, midcycle bleeding, pain when urinating, fever, severe abdominal pain

Diagnosis: Urine analysis.

Treatment: Can be easily cured with antibiotics if diagnosed in early stages.

Complications:

- *Men:* infertility, inflammation of the urinary tract and organs (prostate gland, seminal vesicles, bladder, and epididymis)
- *Women:* PID and infertility; infection can be transmitted to a baby during childbirth

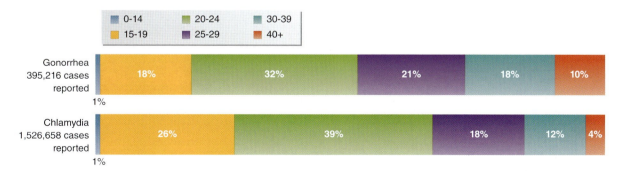

Figure 12.20 Chlamydia and gonorrhea infections, United States, 2015. Americans aged 15 to 24 account for half of the estimated 20 million new cases of STIs in the United States each year. Data show that both the numbers and rates of reported cases of chlamydia and gonorrhea are concentrated among 15- to 24-year-olds.

Reprinted from Centers for Disease Control and Prevention (2016b).

PELVIC INFLAMMATORY DISEASE (PID)

Pelvic inflammatory disease is a serious, and sometimes fatal, complication that affects women due to undiagnosed and untreated chlamydia or gonorrhea. These bacteria make their way to a woman's reproductive organs. Many women do not experience obvious signs of infection. The Fallopian tubes are the most vulnerable organs to these bacteria, which cause inflammation, severe abdominal pain, fever, and possible scarring of the tubes (see figure 12.21). Scarring of the Fallopian tubes leads to infertility because it blocks the sperm from meeting the egg or can cause the fertilized egg to get caught in the tubes, causing an ectopic pregnancy. Women who are diagnosed with PID may have to undergo a hysterectomy due to the irreversible damage to the reproductive organs.

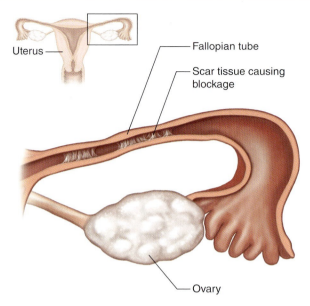

Figure 12.21   Scarring of the Fallopian tubes due to PID. PID is a leading cause of female infertility. It is typically caused by bacterial STIs that lead to scarring of the Fallopian tubes, preventing the sperm from fertilizing the egg.

SYPHILIS

Facts: Epidemics of syphilis have surfaced in the United States a number of times in the past few decades, primarily among men who have sex with men (Centers for Disease Control and Prevention n.d.). This infection is transmitted by direct contact with the chancre lesion.

Prevalence: The occurrence of syphilis has increased at a high rate. It is concentrated among men (90 percent); of those diagnosed, 82 percent of cases are among men who have sex with men. Figure 12.22 shows the steady increase of syphilis rates among gay and bisexual men since 2007 (Centers for Disease Control and Prevention 2016b).

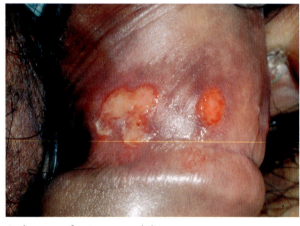

A chancre of primary syphilis.

Symptoms: For both men and women, symptoms develop over time and in stages. Symptoms of primary syphilis include a painless chancre, or ulcer, at the site of the infection; examples are on the glans (head of the penis) and labia minora. In the secondary stages of syphilis, a distinctive rash may appear on the palms of the hands and soles of the feet.

- *Primary stage:* A painless lesion, called a chancre, appears at the site of sexual contact 10 to 90 days after exposure and goes away in approximately 3 weeks.
- *Secondary stage:* The bacteria spreads in the body and causes a painless rash on the body, swollen glands, fever, sore throat, weight loss, and low energy. Symptoms can last two to six weeks.
- *Tertiary stage:* The infection will continue to spread throughout the body and cause permanent organ damage.

Diagnosis: Blood test or culture from chancre sore.

Treatment: Can be cured with penicillin in the primary and secondary stages if the infection does not spread to other parts of the body, causing irreversible organ damage.

Complications: It can take years for the bacteria to reach the tertiary stage, leading to paralysis, strokes, blindness, and heart damage. A pregnant woman with syphilis can transmit the bacterium to her fetus (Centers for Disease Control and Prevention n.d.).

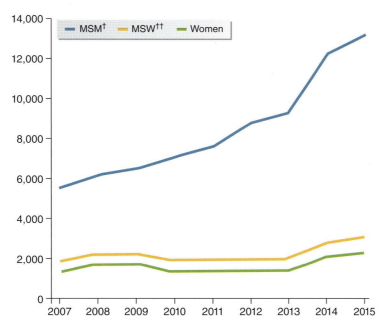

Figure 12.22   Syphilis rates among gay and bisexual men, United States, 2007 to 2015. Trend data show that rates of syphilis are increasing at an alarming rate (19 percent in 2015). Men account for a large majority (90 percent) of all primary and secondary syphilis cases, and men who have sex with men (MSM) account for 82 percent of male cases where the sex of the sex partner is known.

+Men who have sex with men.

++Men who have sex with women.

Note: Based on available data from states reporting sex of sex partners.

Reprinted from Centers for Disease Control and Prevention (2016a).

Reducing the Risks

Sexual activity can positively influence emotional and spiritual development and intimate relationships with others, but it brings the risk of sexually transmitted infections and other negative outcomes, such as a broken heart. Therefore, you need to make decisions now about how you plan to reduce your risks for STIs. Risk reduction methods include abstinence, mutual monogamy (reducing multiple sexual partners), using condoms, communicating and having honest conversations with partners, and reducing or eliminating the use of alcohol and drugs.

Routine Testing

Getting tested is the only way you can know your STI status, so begin getting tested for HIV and STIs as part of your routine medical examinations with your health care provider. Knowing your status can help you and your partners be safe and reduce the infection rates among young people.

Who should be tested? Recommendations from the Centers for Disease Control and Prevention (n.d.) are as follows:

- All adolescents and adults aged 13 to 64 should be tested at least once for HIV.

STI symptoms include pain with urination, urethra or vaginal discharge that may have an odor, sores in the genital or mouth area, or pain in the pelvic region. Be sure to see a health care provider if you or a partner experience any of these symptoms.

- Annual chlamydia screening should be done for all sexually active women younger than 25 years, as well as for older women who have new or multiple sex partners or a sex partner who has a sexually transmitted infection.

- Annual gonorrhea screening should be done for all sexually active women younger than 25 years, as well as for older women who have new or multiple sex partners or a sex partner who has a sexually transmitted infection.

- To protect the health of mothers and their infants, all pregnant women should be screened for syphilis, HIV, chlamydia, and hepatitis B. At-risk pregnant women should be screened for gonorrhea starting early in pregnancy, with repeat testing done as needed.

- All sexually active gay and bisexual men and any other men who have sex with men (MSM) should be screened at least once a year for syphilis, chlamydia, and gonorrhea. MSM who have multiple or anonymous partners should be screened more frequently for STIs (i.e., at three- to six-month intervals). Sexually active gay and bisexual men may benefit from frequent HIV testing (e.g., every three to six months).

- Anyone who has unsafe sex or shares injection drug equipment should get tested for HIV at least once a year.

- After treatment for an STI, go back to your health care provider for another test once you have completed any medications and your symptoms are gone to make sure that you are no longer infected.

How to Talk With Partners About STI History

Communicating with current or potential sexual partners about sexual history can be

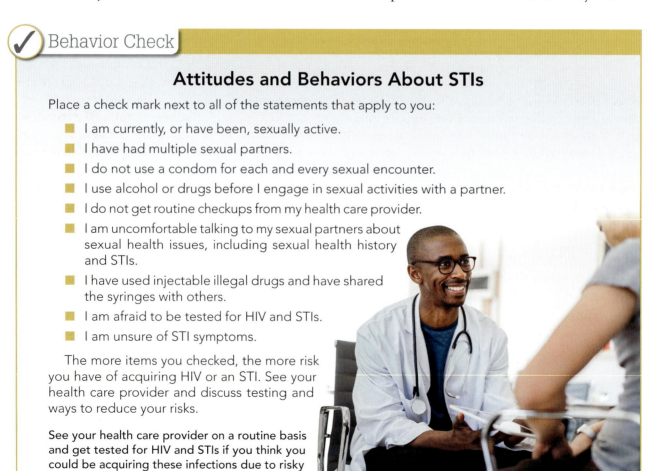

✓ Behavior Check

Attitudes and Behaviors About STIs

Place a check mark next to all of the statements that apply to you:

- I am currently, or have been, sexually active.
- I have had multiple sexual partners.
- I do not use a condom for each and every sexual encounter.
- I use alcohol or drugs before I engage in sexual activities with a partner.
- I do not get routine checkups from my health care provider.
- I am uncomfortable talking to my sexual partners about sexual health issues, including sexual health history and STIs.
- I have used injectable illegal drugs and have shared the syringes with others.
- I am afraid to be tested for HIV and STIs.
- I am unsure of STI symptoms.

The more items you checked, the more risk you have of acquiring HIV or an STI. See your health care provider and discuss testing and ways to reduce your risks.

See your health care provider on a routine basis and get tested for HIV and STIs if you think you could be acquiring these infections due to risky sexual and drug abuse behaviors.

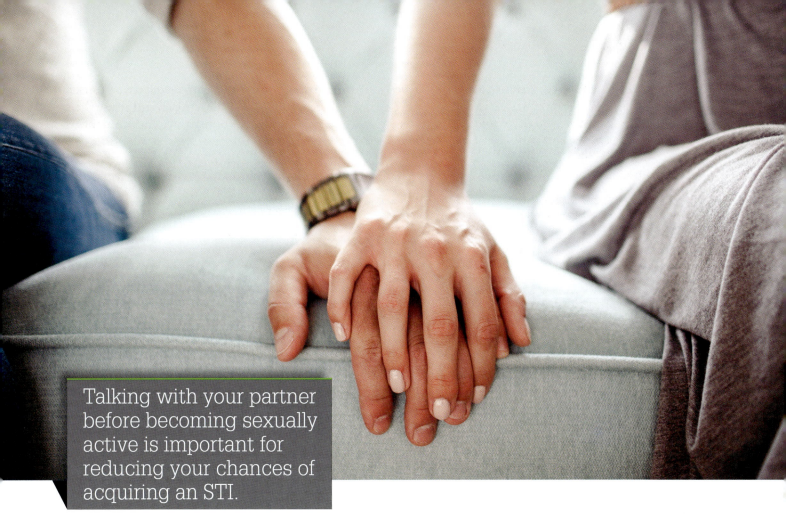

Talking with your partner before becoming sexually active is important for reducing your chances of acquiring an STI.

uncomfortable and difficult. What are ways you can begin a conversation with a partner about behaviors that put him or her at risk for HIV and STIs? In addition to discussing higher-risk sexual behaviors, consider asking partners about their number of sexual partners, diagnoses of HIV and STIs, successful treatment, follow-up with a health care provider, and STI prevention methods.

When and how will you tell a future partner if you have been diagnosed with HIV or an STI? Think about the differences between viral and bacterial STIs and how that would affect the conversation.

It is a felony for someone with HIV to knowingly transmit the infection to a sexual partner without prior notification. Some infections do not have outward signs or symptoms and are spread unknowingly. What would you do if your sexual partner gave you HIV or another STI? How would you respond?

Prevention of STIs

In short, follow these steps in order to prevent acquiring or spreading an STI (figure 12.23).

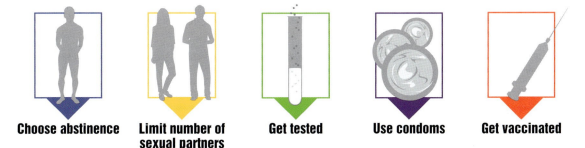

Choose abstinence   Limit number of sexual partners   Get tested   Use condoms   Get vaccinated

Figure 12.23   Following these steps will help you prevent an STI.

- Choose to be sexually abstinent.
- If you are sexually active, limit the number of sexual partners.
- Know your and your partners' STI status.
- Get routine medical exams that include STI screenings.
- Use condoms consistently and correctly with every sexual encounter.
- Get vaccinated against HPV.

Sexual Assault

(Much of the material in this section is reprinted from the Office on Women's Health in the Department of Health and Human Services at www.womenshealth.gov.)

Sexual assault is any type of sexual contact or behavior that happens without consent. Sexual assault includes rape and attempted rape, child molestation, and sexual harassment or threats. Sexual assault can happen to anyone of any age, race or ethnicity, religion, ability, appearance, sexual orientation, or gender identity. However, women have higher rates of sexual assault than men (see figure 12.24). In the United States, nearly one in five women has been raped, and almost half of women have experienced another type of sexual assault. If you have been sexually assaulted, it is not your fault (Office on Women's Health 2017; Office of Women's Health 2015).

How to Recognize and Prevent Sexual Assault: It's Everyone's Responsibility

All college students have a responsibility to recognize and prevent sexual assault on their campuses. This can begin by attending educational programs or joining organizations on your campus that focus on understanding your personal responsibility toward preventing sexual assault. So, what exactly is sexual assault? Sexual assault means that there was sexual contact or behavior that occurred without the explicit consent from the person who was sexually assaulted. It includes attempted rape; fondling or unwanted sexual touching; forcing the

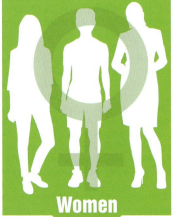
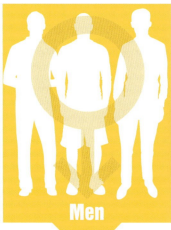
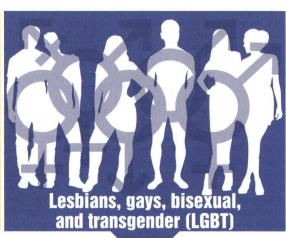

Women
- >23 million women have been raped
- Most were under the age of 25
- 1 in 5 African American women
- 1 in 8 Hispanic women

Men
- 2 million men have been raped
- 6% have experienced sexual coercion
- 11% have experienced unwanted sexual contact

Lesbians, gays, bisexual, and transgender (LGBT)
- Bisexual women have higher rates of sexual assault
- Nearly half of all bisexual women have been raped
- Lesbians and bisexual women have higher rates
- More than half of transgender people have been sexually assaulted

Figure 12.24   Who is sexually assaulted?
Data from Office on Women's Health (2015).

victim to perform sexual acts, such as oral sex or penetrating the perpetrator's body; and penetration of the victim's body, which is defined as rape (Rape, Abuse and Incest National Network n.d.).

Rape is defined by the FBI as "The penetration, no matter how slight, of the vagina or anus with any body part or object, or oral penetration by a sex organ of another person, without the consent of the victim" (US Department of Justice 2017). Force does not have to be physical; it can also be emotional, manipulating or intimidating the victim into nonconsensual sexual activity. Explicit, affirmative consent must be obtained before engaging in sexual activity. Silence is not consent. Finally, consent cannot be given when someone is mentally or physically helpless, is under the influence of drugs or alcohol, or is unconscious (Holcomb 2016).

One example of an organization that helps men understand their role in the prevention of sexual assault is Male Athletes Against Violence. This is an initiative on many college campuses focused on educating and involving men in understanding how to recognize and prevent sexual assaults. These men take a pledge to be a positive role model, educate others, have the courage to correct the violent behaviors of others, support all victims of sexual assault, and implement strategies to reduce and end sexual violence. In 2014, eight leading national fraternities also joined together to address sexual misconduct, hazing, and binge drinking by forming the Fraternal Health and Safety Initiative (FHSI; Market Wired 2014). The goal of this initiative is educate fraternity members to make positive and healthy decisions, understand the risks and consequences of their actions, and recognize and intervene during potential harmful situations. It is important for men to participate in educational programs and initiatives on campus that emphasize their roles and responsibilities related to the prevention of sexual assault. Sexual assault is a campus-wide issue that can be solved only when everyone works together toward solutions.

Another campus initiative that may exist on your campus for all students is the It's On Us campaign (www.itsonus.org). The goals of this college-based campaign

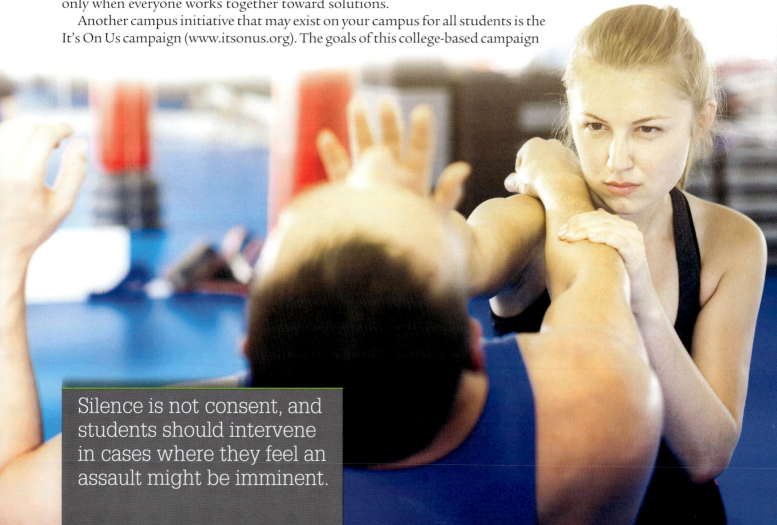

Silence is not consent, and students should intervene in cases where they feel an assault might be imminent.

are to recognize that nonconsensual sex is sexual assault, identify situations in which sexual assault may occur, intervene in situations where consent has not or cannot be given, and create an environment in which sexual assault is unacceptable and survivors are supported. See lab 12.1 in the web study guide for ways you can become an advocate for sexual assault prevention by working with your campus administrators and peers.

Consent

Consent is a clear yes to sexual activity. Just because someone has not said no does not mean she or he has given consent. Consent means the following:

- You know and understand what is going on (you are not unconscious or blacked out or intellectually disabled).
- You know what you want to do.
- You are able to say what you want to do.

- You are sober (not under the influence of alcohol or drugs).

Sometimes you cannot give legal consent to sexual activity or contact. For example, you cannot consent in any of the following conditions:

- You are threatened, forced, or manipulated into agreeing.
- You are physically unable to (drunk, high, drugged, passed out, or asleep).
- You are mentally unable to (due to illness or disability).
- You are younger than 16 (in most states) or 18 (in other states).

Getting Help

If you are in danger or need medical care, call 9-1-1. If you can, get away from the person who assaulted you and go to a safe place as fast as you can. After a sexual assault, you may feel fear,

---

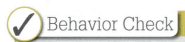

Reduce Your Risk of Sexual Assault

Take an active role in reducing sexual assault by incorporating safety strategies. You cannot always prevent sexual assault. However, you can take the following steps to help stay safe in general:

- **Go to parties or gatherings with friends.** Arrive together, check in with each other, and leave together.
- **Look out for your friends and ask them to look out for you.** If a friend is acting out of character or seems too drunk to stay safe in general, get her or him to a safe place.
- **Have a code word you can text to your family and friends** that means, "Come get me, I need help" or "Call me with a fake emergency."
- **Download a safety app on your phone.** Some apps share your location with your friends or the police if you need help. You can also set up an app to send you texts throughout the night to make sure you're safe. If you don't respond, the app will notify police.
- **Avoid drinks in punch bowls or other containers that can be easily spiked** (when alcohol is added to a drink without permission). If you think that you or one of your friends has been drugged, call the police. Tell them what happened so that you can be tested for the right drugs.
- **Know your limits when using alcohol or drugs.** Don't let anyone pressure you into drinking or doing more than you want to.
- **Trust your instincts.** If you find yourself alone with someone you don't know or trust, leave. If you feel uncomfortable in any situation for any reason, leave.
- **Be aware of your surroundings.** Especially if you are walking alone, avoid talking on your phone or listening to music with headphones. Stay in busy, well-lit areas (Office on Women's Health 2015).

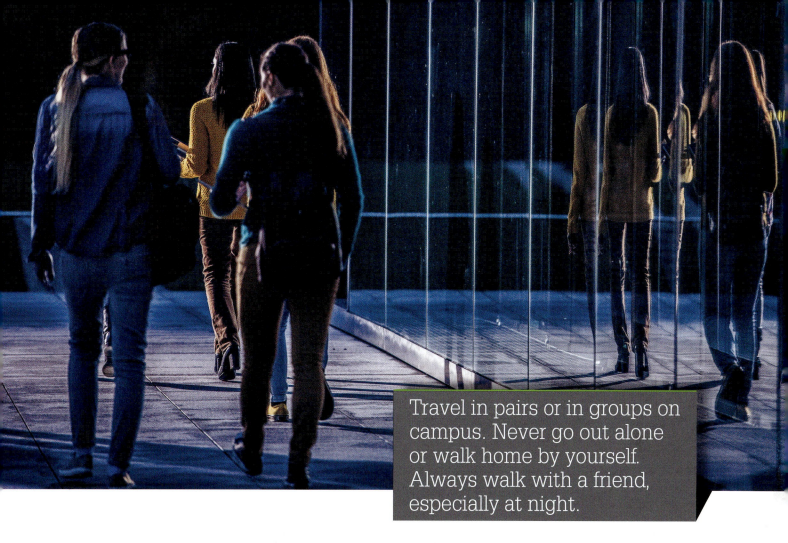

Travel in pairs or in groups on campus. Never go out alone or walk home by yourself. Always walk with a friend, especially at night.

shame, guilt, or shock. These feelings are normal. You might be afraid to talk about the assault, but it is important to get help. You can call these organizations at any time, day or night:

- National Sexual Assault Hotline, 800-656-HOPE (4673)
- National Domestic Violence Hotline, 800-799-SAFE (7233) or 800-787-3224 (TTY)

Summary

This chapter focuses on how college students can develop and sustain a sexually healthy lifestyle. Sexuality is a part of your life that begins when you are an infant and continues throughout your entire life. In order to be sexually healthy, you must understand your own reproductive anatomy and physiology, as well as those of others. Knowing more about how your body works allows you to become aware of how your body matures, changes, and develops over your lifetime. This information can prepare you for preventing or planning to have a child. A variety of methods are available for both sexually active men and women to reduce the chances of an unintended pregnancy and plan for the future. When used consistently and correctly, these methods are very reliable.

Being sexually healthy also means learning more about the risks associated with sexually transmitted infections. Keep in mind that some STIs cannot be cured and could be fatal. Knowing your partner's sexual health history and practicing safe sex (e.g., using a condom) can reduce your chances of acquiring a sexually transmitted infection. Lab 12.2 in the web study guide poses a number of questions related to how you can plan in advance to develop and sustain a healthy sexuality. Take time to think about these questions before you become sexually active. If you are currently sexually active, think about how many ways you can discuss sexual health issues with your partner, share how you plan on preventing acquiring STIs, and consider how you can plan for children in the future.

Finally, preventing sexual assault must be a collective effort among all college students. Make a commitment to learn how to prevent sexual assault, educate others, and stand up against these violent behaviors that have lifelong negative consequences. Prioritizing your sexual health can help you develop positive and respectful relationships, reduce your chances of negative physical and emotional health outcomes, plan pregnancies, and enjoy sex.

WEB STUDY GUIDE

Remember to complete all of the web study guide activities to further facilitate your learning, including the following lab activities:

Lab 12.1   Advocating for Sexual Assault Prevention

Lab 12.2   Your Personal Plan for a Healthy Sexuality

REVIEW QUESTIONS

1. How does conception happen?
2. What are examples of barrier birth control methods?
3. What are examples of hormonal birth control methods?
4. Which birth control methods have the highest rate of preventing pregnancy with typical use?
5. Which birth control methods also protect against STIs?
6. What are the symptoms of chlamydia, gonorrhea, and syphilis?
7. What are the symptoms of HPV and HSV?
8. Which STIs can be cured?
9. Which STIs can be treated but not cured?
10. What is PID?
11. What are ways to prevent sexual assault?
12. What is consent?

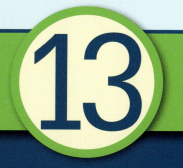

Reducing the Risks for Metabolic Syndrome

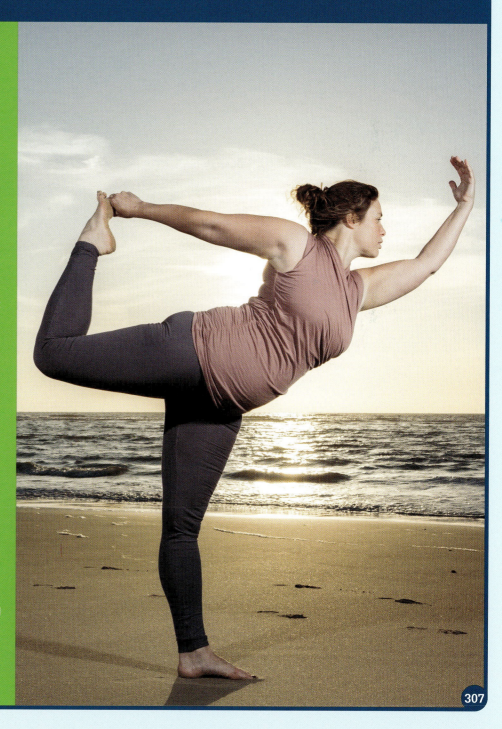

OBJECTIVES

- ❱ Define metabolic syndrome and understand the risk factors for it.

- ❱ Appreciate that metabolic syndrome increases the risk for other chronic diseases, including type 2 diabetes and cardiovascular disease.

- ❱ Understand that healthy dietary and physical activity habits can reduce the risk for type 2 diabetes.

- ❱ Know the main cardiovascular diseases, the risk factors for them, and strategies for protecting yourself from these diseases.

- ❱ Recognize that preventing metabolic syndrome early in life can influence your risk of cardiovascular disease as you age.

KEY TERMS

angina

arrhythmias

arteriosclerosis

atherosclerosis

cardiovascular disease (CVD)

cholesterol

chronic diseases

chronic systemic inflammation

coronary artery (heart) disease (CAD or CHD)

C-reactive protein (CRP)

diabetes

endothelium

gestational diabetes

heart failure

hemorrhagic stroke

high-density lipoprotein cholesterol (HDL-C)

hypercholesterolemia

hyperglycemia

hyperlipidemia

hypertension

ischemic stroke

low-density lipoprotein cholesterol (LDL-C)

metabolic syndrome (MetS)

myocardial infarction (heart attack)

pathophysiology

peripheral arterial disease (PAD)

polycystic ovary syndrome

prediabetes

stroke

triglycerides

type 1 diabetes

type 2 diabetes (T2D)

Do you know someone who has diabetes or has suffered a heart attack? Although these health conditions typically occur in middle-aged or older adults, the disease process begins earlier in life than you may realize. Your genetics, weight status, and current health behaviors, especially your diet and physical activity habits, can greatly influence your health later in life. This chapter introduces you to metabolic syndrome and how it increases a person's risk for both diabetes and cardiovascular disease. An overview of diabetes and cardiovascular disease follows with a focus on risk factors. Finally, the chapter concludes with a reinforcement that regular physical movement is essential for reducing your risk of these chronic conditions.

Are You at Risk for Metabolic Syndrome?

Many young adults are at risk for developing **metabolic syndrome (MetS)** due to the epidemic of overweight and obesity in our society. If you have been or are one day diagnosed with MetS, think of it as a wake-up call to reassess your health status and behaviors. However, be confident that you can get back on track.

Definition and Diagnosis

Metabolic syndrome can be thought of as a clustering of biological factors that raise your risk for other chronic conditions, especially diabetes and cardiovascular disease. Recall that the term *metabolic* refers to your biochemical processes and energy production systems. A syndrome is a set of signs and symptoms related to each other or occurring simultaneously. A risk factor is a trait, condition, or habit that increases your risk of developing a disease.

Although what causes metabolic syndrome and its components is complex, it is well established that central obesity is a key factor (International Diabetes Federation 2006). To be diagnosed with MetS, a person has to have central obesity (defined by a high waist circumference based on ethnicity-specific values) plus two of the four other factors, including unhealthy blood lipids, high blood pressure, and high blood glucose, listed as follows.

High Waist Circumference:

- **Men:** ≥94 centimeters (37 in.) for Caucasians; ≥90 centimeters (35.4 in.) for most Asians

- **Women:** ≥80 centimeters (31.4 in.)

Plus Two of These Four Factors:

- *Elevated triglycerides:* ≥150 mg/dL or taking medication for this condition
- *Low HDL cholesterol:* <40 mg/dL for women and <50 mg/dL for men or people on medication for this condition
- *Elevated blood pressure:* Systolic ≥ 130 mmHg or diastolic ≥ 85 mmHg or people diagnosed with hypertension or taking medication to control it
- *Elevated fasting blood glucose:* ≥100 mg/dL or people diagnosed with type 2 diabetes or taking medication to control it

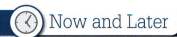 Now and Later

MetS Can Lead to the Big Metabolic Three

Now

Do you think that heart attacks, diabetes, and cancer happen only to older adults? Do you ever rationalize putting off exercise with the thought that you'll have more time to take care of your health later? In fact, the risk for these primary causes of death begin fairly early in life and is often linked to MetS. Due to the obesity epidemic and our sedentary lifestyles, approximately 10 percent of young adults and over one-third of the adult population have MetS (Moore, Chaudhary, and Akinyemiju 2017). Do you know anyone your age who has been diagnosed with MetS? You or some of your friends may have it and not even know it.

Later

As part of the aging process (e.g., hormone changes), body composition changes (e.g., abdominal fat increases) and physical activity goes down. Therefore, the rates for MetS increase even more with age. For example, approximately 50 percent of middle-aged adults have MetS, and the rates climb to nearly 65 percent for adults over age 70 (Moore, Chaudhary, and Akinyemiju 2017). MetS rates are predicted to reach 25 percent of the Earth's population in the near future (International Diabetes Federation 2006). When people are lean and highly physically active, their chance of having MetS is reduced drastically to nearly zero. MetS is another example of how our genetics unfavorably interact with our environment.

Take Home

Take steps now to know your risk factors for MetS. If you are at risk, make lifestyle changes to reduce your risk and prevent risk factors for other chronic conditions, especially the Big Metabolic Three. Invest in your health as if you were investing in a retirement account.

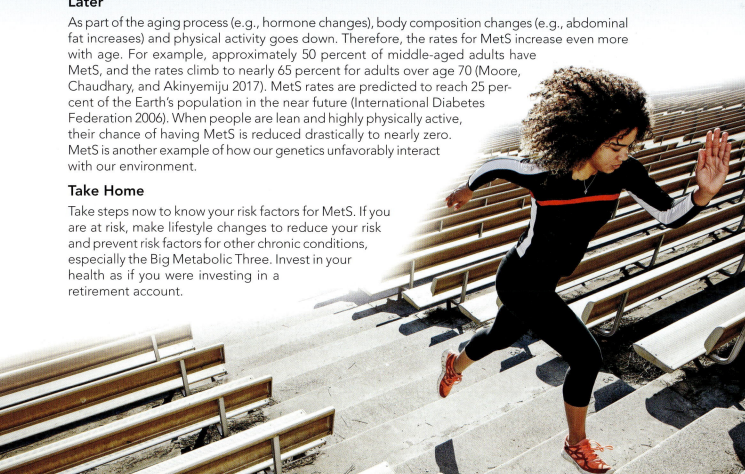

Why Do We Care About MetS?

Being diagnosed with MetS is not the critical issue. We care about MetS because if you have a number of metabolic risk factors, your chances of developing one of the Big Metabolic Three increases substantially. A person who has MetS has at least a fivefold greater risk of developing **type 2 diabetes (T2D)**. T2D is one of the worldwide major causes of premature illness and death, primarily because it increases the risk of **cardiovascular disease (CVD)**, which is responsible for at least 80 percent of all deaths. Thus, MetS and T2D are currently driving the CVD epidemic (International Diabetes Federation 2006). Finally, much emerging research also supports a link between MetS and several cancers (Stocks et al. 2015). If you want to avoid the Big Metabolic Three, you need to avoid MetS. This means that, first and foremost, you need to learn personal strategies for managing your waistline.

Your Traits, Conditions, and Habits = Risk of MetS

The risk for MetS is a complex mix of genetic factors, certain conditions, and your habits. For example, if your family tree has many people with MetS, your risk increases. However, if you eat a relatively clean and balanced diet, engage in regular physical activity and exercise, and manage your weight, you will go a long way toward preventing MetS. These key health choices also help you lower **chronic systemic inflammation**.

Chronic Inflammation: A Flame for Chronic Diseases

Chronic diseases such as T2D are considered to be so because they are lifelong or recurrent, unlike communicable diseases such as the flu or genetic diseases. Rather, chronic diseases are caused by the interaction between our genes, our environment, and our health behaviors. Nearly everyone who gets diagnosed with a chronic disease develops a subclinical (i.e., undetectable) disease first. There may not be any signs and symptoms, but the **pathophysiology** associated with the disease is present, often many years prior to diagnosis. A low-level chronic systemic inflammation is often related to this subclinical disease state.

Cellular Inflammation Basics

If you have ever scraped your knee, sprained your ankle, or had strep throat, you have probably become aware of acute inflammation. White blood cells travel to the scene to destroy bacteria and the immune process repairs your tissues. This healing process is termed the *inflammatory response* and is one of the body's most basic survival mechanisms. Typically, this response stays local and then resolves after the injury or infection heals, which you recognize when the pain and swelling go away. However, sometimes the system does not shut off and inflammatory-promoting compounds spread throughout the body, damaging cells and tissues. In this case, our defense mechanisms have turned against us. This low-level systemic inflammation can simmer for years, contributing to a range of chronic conditions, including T2D, CVD, and some cancers (Libby, Ridker, and Hansson 2009). Understanding the role that inflammation plays in your risk for chronic disease is important. Even more critical is the need to recognize how your health behavior choices influence your levels of inflammation (see figure 13.1).

Detection of Chronic Inflammation

To detect this silent inflammation, physicians might measure levels of **C-reactive protein (CRP)** or other markers in the blood. If the levels are elevated, they will conduct additional testing to determine what is triggering the inflammation and then pursue treatment. Inflammation is a key cause or factor in almost all chronic degenerative and lifestyle diseases, especially vascular diseases such as atherosclerosis (Roitman and LaFontaine 2012). Obesity, especially abdominal obesity, diet quality, physical activity or exercise, physical fitness, and smoking are key factors associated with this stealthy condition. See figure 13.1 and ask yourself if you might be igniting your inflammatory flame.

Evaluating Your Risk for Diabetes Mellitus

Diabetes is a chronic disease that occurs when the pancreas cannot make the hormone insulin or when the insulin the body produces does not work very well (American Diabetes Association n.d.).

Inflammation Fuels Chronic Disease

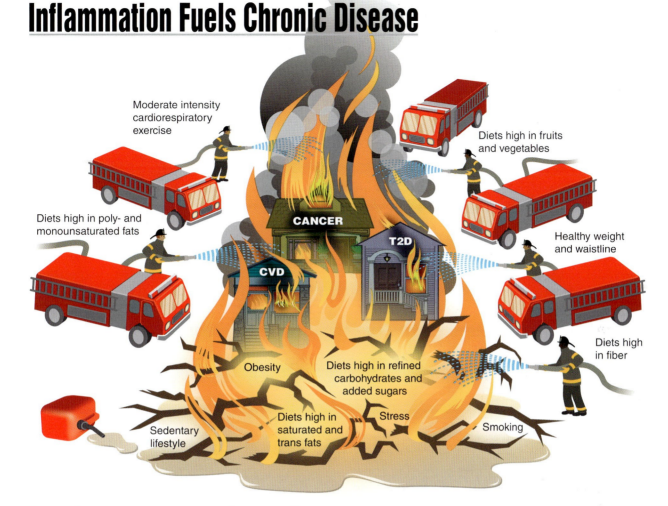

Figure 13.1 Are you igniting your inflammatory flame or putting it out?

All carbohydrate foods are broken down and released as glucose into the blood. Insulin helps glucose get into the cells and produce energy (those energy bucks). When insulin is not available or it cannot be used effectively, glucose cannot enter cells; thus, glucose begins to build up in the blood. This condition is called **hyperglycemia** (high blood sugar). If these high-glucose conditions continue for long periods of time, tissues and organs get damaged. The following is a list of primary conditions that often occur with long-term diabetes if it is not well controlled with diet, exercise, and medication:

> Keeping your blood sugar under control not only helps prevent diabetes but also reduces the risk for many other chronic health conditions.

- **Cardiovascular disease**. High blood glucose is linked to artery vessel damage, which accelerates risk for cardiovascular disease.
- **Eye complications**. Many eye conditions that increase in prevalence with age (such as glaucoma) are also increased in people with diabetes.
- **Kidney disease**. Kidneys are large filters with millions of tiny blood vessels. Because small blood vessels are more likely to be damaged with high blood glucose, kidney failure is common in people with diabetes.
- **Neuropathy**. Nerves become damaged, resulting in loss of feeling and often pain.

- *Skin changes*. People with diabetes often have more bacterial and fungal infections and itching skin.

If possible, it is best to avoid diabetes. But if you have diabetes, good blood sugar control is essential for preventing numerous other chronic conditions, many of which can be fatal, such as CVD.

Types and Definitions

Two main types of diabetes exist. First, **type 1 diabetes**, which affects only ~5 percent of the people with diabetes, is caused by the body's inability to produce insulin. Your health behaviors are mainly linked to the most common type of diabetes, type 2 diabetes (T2D), which is primarily due to insulin resistance. A less common and very specific type of diabetes is **gestational diabetes**, which develops in pregnant women due to many factors, including pregnancy-related hormones and insulin resistance. Insulin resistance means that the body's tissues, especially the muscles, become less receptive to the action of insulin. In response, the pancreas has to make more insulin in order to maintain blood glucose in the normal range. Over time, the pancreas becomes exhausted and is unable to manage blood sugar levels, so blood sugar begins to rise (Centers for Disease Control and Prevention 2017a).

Note that there is also a **prediabetes** category related to T2D, which is when a person has a level of elevated glucose that is above normal but not yet

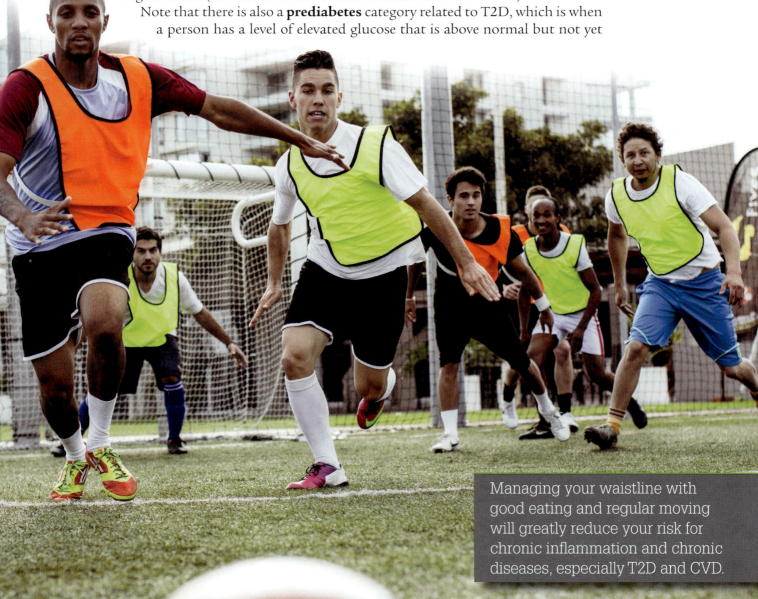

Managing your waistline with good eating and regular moving will greatly reduce your risk for chronic inflammation and chronic diseases, especially T2D and CVD.

to the level defined for having diabetes. This is important because before people develop T2D, they almost always have prediabetes. In fact, more than one-third of the population has prediabetes, and most of those people have no idea they have it. Similar to MetS, prediabetes also increases your risk for T2D and CVD (Centers for Disease Control and Prevention 2017b).

Diagnosis

All types of diabetes are diagnosed with blood tests using several well-established clinical techniques (American Diabetes Association 2014). When reviewing table 13.1, notice how the normal, prediabetes, and diabetes categories are ranked in order of increasing A1C, or blood glucose levels.

Symptoms and Risk Factors for Prediabetes

Similar to MetS, prediabetes should be a wake-up call, a louder one, to make some changes in your lifestyle so you can prevent the progression to T2D. If you have several of the following risk factors, you are advised to consult your physician (Centers for Disease Control and Prevention 2017b). Remember, often there are no symptoms of prediabetes or T2D until the disease becomes advanced.

- *Age*. Being 45 years or older.
- *Family history*. Having a parent or sibling with T2D.
- *Race or ethnicity*. African Americans, Hispanic and Latino Americans, American Indians, Pacific Islanders, and some Asian Americans are at higher risk.
- *Overweight*. Having a high BMI (and also a high waist circumference).
- *Physical activity*. Being physically active fewer than three times per week.
- *Gestational diabetes*. Being diagnosed with gestational diabetes or having a baby who weighs more than 9 pounds (4 kg) at birth.
- *Polycystic ovary syndrome*. A hormonal disorder characterized by higher than normal levels of androgens that causes enlarged ovaries and leads to infertility and insulin resistance.

Treatment Options

Treatment options for prediabetes and T2D center around lifestyle changes and medication.

- *Weight loss*. If a person has prediabetes and is overweight, losing a small amount of weight can greatly improve the chance of

Table 13.1   Common Clinical Tests for Diabetes

Test	Brief description	Normal	Prediabetes	Diabetes
A1C	A marker that measures your average blood glucose for the past 2 to 3 months. *Does not require you to fast or drink anything.	<5.7%	5.7-6.5%	≥6.5%
Fasting plasma glucose (FPG)	Tests your fasting glucose. *Requires you not to drink or eat for at least 8 hours (typically completed in the morning before breakfast).	<100 mg/dL	100-126 mg/dL	≥126 mg/dL
Oral glucose challenge test (OGTT)	A test that checks how your body handles a glucose load. *Requires you to fast and then drink a sweet drink (a glucose beverage) and then have your blood tested again in 2 hours.	<140 mg/dL	140-200 mg/dL	≥200 mg/dL

the progression to T2D. This small amount can be as little as 5 percent of body weight. For a 200-pound (91 kg) person, that means losing 10 to 14 pounds (4.5 to 6.4 kg; Centers for Disease Control and Prevention 2017b).

- *Regular physical activity*. Engaging in activities that cause muscular contraction on most days of the week and meeting the physical activity guidelines can greatly reduce the risk of prediabetes in general and the progression to T2D specifically. Muscle contraction increases the action of insulin that helps move blood glucose into cells, thereby lowering blood glucose.

- *Diet quality*. In addition to reducing caloric intake to cause weight loss, improving diet quality can help manage blood glucose. Be sure to limit added sugars and refined carbohydrates.

- *Medications*. If a person does not adhere to lifestyle changes or if the condition has progressed too far, oral medications or injectable insulin may be needed to control his or her blood sugar.

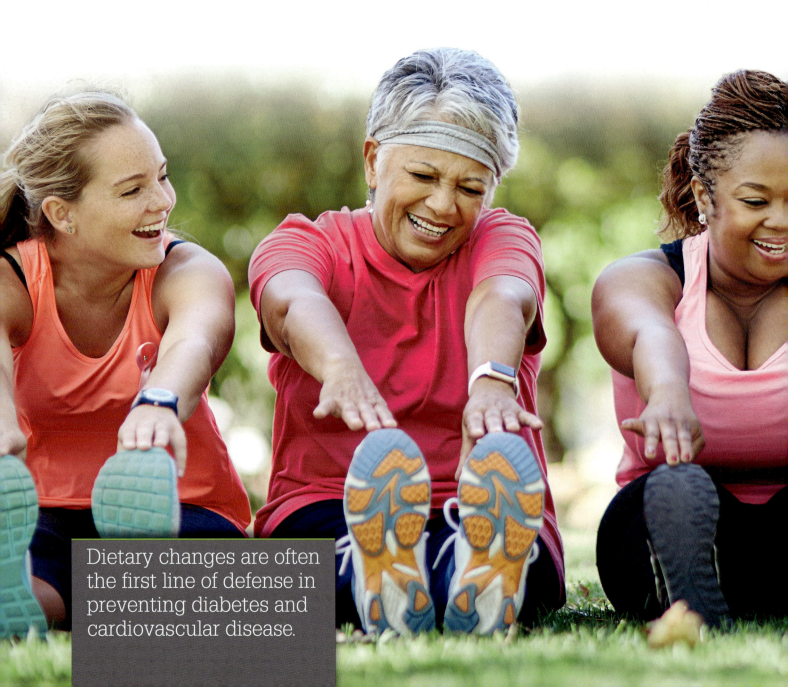

Dietary changes are often the first line of defense in preventing diabetes and cardiovascular disease.

Prevent and Manage T2D With Quality Resources

You have likely heard that an ounce of prevention is worth a pound of cure. This is absolutely true for your blood glucose management and the prevention of MetS, prediabetes, and T2D (figure 13.2). Unfortunately, if you are genetically predisposed to be at high risk for hyperglycemia, you will need to be extra vigilant about your diet, physical activity, and waistline. The majority of adults diagnosed with T2D will have to manage this disease for the rest of their lives. If you are at high risk for diabetes, keeping your blood glucose in the healthy range is critical for preventing comorbidities later in life. An excellent resource for more information is the American Diabetes Association (www.diabetes.org).

Cardiovascular Disease: Our Number One Killer

Cardiovascular disease (CVD)—which includes **coronary artery (heart) disease (CAD or CHD)**, and **stroke**—has been the largest cause of death worldwide for the past several decades (World Health Organization 2017). Over half of young adults have at least one risk factor for CAD and almost 25 percent have plaque buildup in their arteries, which indicate that this age group has risk factors

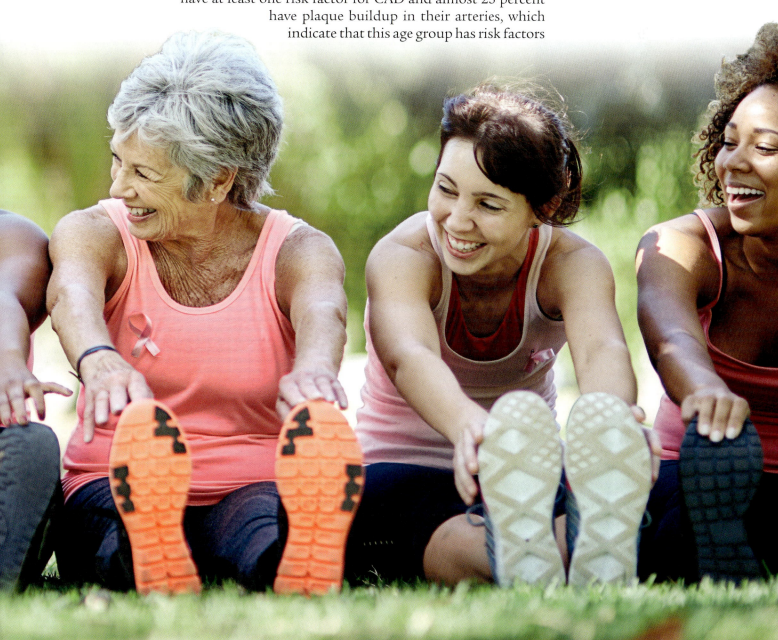

Will You Get Type 2 Diabetes?

Exercise and physical activity

Physical Activity: Being physically active less than 3 times per week.

Weight and waist line

Age: Being 45 years or older.

Overweight: Having a high BMI (and also a high waist circumference).

Gestational diabetes: Being diagnosed with gestational diabetes or having a baby greater than 9 pounds.

Genetics

Family history: Having a parent or sibling with T2D.

Polycystic Ovary Syndrome: A hormonal disorder characterized by higher than normal levels of androgens, which causes enlarged ovaries and leads to infertility and insulin resistance.

Race/ethnicity: African Americans, Hispanic/Latino Americans, American Indians, Pacific Islanders, and some Asian Americans are at higher risk.

?

Figure 13.2   Progression from metabolic health to MetS to prediabetes to T2D involves a complex mix of your genetics, exercise and physical activity habits, and how well you manage your waistline.

that may lead to CVD, especially CHD (Arts, Fernandez, and Lofgren 2014). Therefore, in order to reduce your chances of developing CVD later in life, you should examine your lifestyle factors now, along with your genetics and family history. Evaluating your personal risk for CVD, including talking to your parents and family members about your family history, is a critical first step toward prevention.

Major Forms of Cardiovascular Disease: Definitions and Diagnosis

CVD is defined as a variety of conditions that can prevent the heart from circulating blood and oxygen throughout the body. Without blood flow, and hence oxygen delivery, tissues and cells die. Although most situations occur in the heart itself, which is why many people refer to CVD as heart disease, blood-flow problems can occur all over the body. Major sites of concern are the neck,

brain, and large arteries in the arms, abdomen, and legs. Although blood flow can be reduced by **arrhythmias** (abnormal rhythms of the heart) or heart valve problems, the majority of CVD is caused by **atherosclerosis**, which is when plaque builds up on the walls of arteries, reducing blood flow (figure 13.3). The plaque causes the arteries to become narrower, preventing optimal blood flow to all tissues downstream. Most heart attacks and strokes are caused by a plaque rupture and a blood clot that gets caught in the narrowed artery, which prevents blood from flowing.

Another factor that alters the work of the heart and cardiovascular system is **arteriosclerosis**, more commonly known as hardening of the arteries. Arteriosclerosis is a condition where the walls of the arteries are thickened and hardened, which reduces blood flow to organs and tissues. Arteriosclerosis is related to atherosclerosis and typically occurs due to the aging process.

Progression of Plaque Buildup

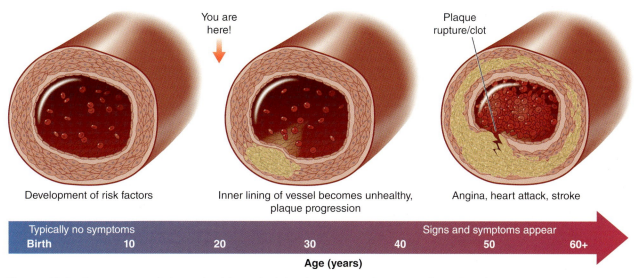

Figure 13.3 Progression of plaque buildup, which leads to angina, heart attack, and stroke.

Atherosclerotic Heart Disease: The Heart Attack

When the atherosclerosis process progresses in the arteries of the heart and the artery becomes very narrow, a ruptured plaque or a blood clot often completely blocks a heart artery and stops blood flow. This is called a **myocardial infarction (heart attack)**. A heart attack occurs when the heart tissue supplied by the blocked artery begins to die. Because various arteries deliver oxygen-rich blood to different parts of the heart, where the clot occurs has major implications for recovery and survival. Sometimes people will refer to a mild or massive heart attack to describe the extent of the damage based on the size of the vessel and the chamber of the heart it supplies. Know the common signs of a heart attack and act quickly.

CHD can be completely silent, with no symptoms, or it might present with **angina** (chest pain), especially under conditions of higher oxygen demand for the heart when heart rate and blood pressure increase, such as during exercise or emotional distress (e.g., anger or anxiety). Sometimes CHD is suspected when routine activities start to cause breathlessness and chest heaviness. A physician might have a person complete a graded exercise stress test by walking on a treadmill, which increases demand on the heart through increasing the speed and grade. During this physical challenge, the patient is monitored for arrhythmias, heart rate, blood pressure, and any other signs and symptoms like chest pain. Medical imaging techniques are often used to determine if there are blood-flow issues due to blocked arteries or value abnormalities.

Stroke

Stroke is the second leading cause of death in the world (World Health Organization 2017). Similar to CHD, 80 percent of strokes are preventable and high blood pressure is the number one cause of a stroke (American Stroke Association n.d.). High blood pressure is a modifiable risk factor: You can lower it. Strokes can be caused by a blood vessel bursting (**hemorrhagic stroke**), but the great majority of strokes are caused by a clot (**ischemic stroke**). This latter type of stroke is very similar to a heart attack, but the clot occurs in the brain and not the heart. Thus, instead of heart cells dying, the brain cells die if they are deprived of blood and oxygen for long enough. If blood flow is restored quickly, the good news is that some of the brain cells may only be injured and over time can self-repair in response to therapy and time, which allows speech, memory, and body movement and functioning to improve. Unfortunately, stroke is the leading cause of disability in middle-aged and older adults. High blood pressure can lead to either cause.

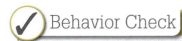 Behavior Check

Automatic External Defibrillator (AED)

Defibrillators can save lives by restoring a normal heart rhythm, especially after a heart attack. They are found in schools, airports, fitness centers, and public buildings. Do you see any AEDs on campus? The American Red Cross and the American Heart Association offer courses on how to use AEDs. We recommend becoming trained so you can save a life.

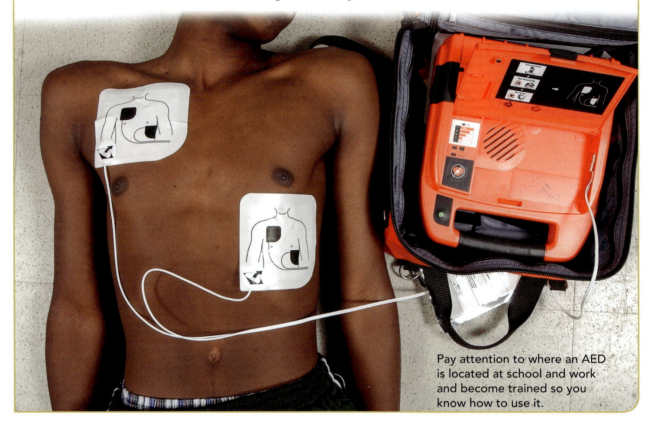

Pay attention to where an AED is located at school and work and become trained so you know how to use it.

Detecting Strokes

Strokes can be very evident or hard to detect (see figure 13.4). The Stroke Association uses an acronym of FAST:

- **Face drooping.** Does one side of the face droop or is it numb? Ask the person to smile and check to see if the face is uneven or lopsided.

- **Arm weakness.** Is one arm weak or numb? Ask the person to raise both arms and check to see if one arm drifts downward.

- **Speech difficulty.** Is speech slurred? Is the person unable to speak or hard to understand? Ask the person to repeat a simple sentence like "The sky is blue." See if he or she is able to correctly repeat the words.

- **Time.** If the preceding symptoms are present, even if they appear to be going away, call 911 to get help. Time is of the essence, since the sooner the treatment can be started, the less permanent damage will occur for the brain cells. Also note the time you think the symptoms started so you can inform the emergency responders.

Warning Signs of Heart Attack and Stroke

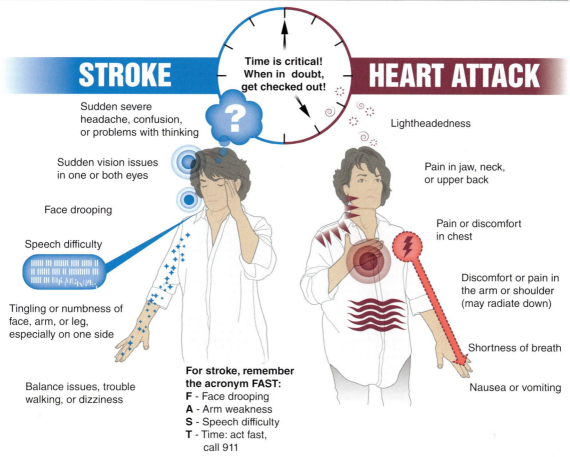

Figure 13.4   Know the warning signs of a heart attack and stroke. If you suspect someone is experiencing any of these symptoms, call 911 immediately. Minutes may save lives!

Additional clues might be remembered as STROKE:

- **Speech.** Trouble speaking or understanding speech.
- **Tingling.** Sudden numbness or weakness of face, arm, or leg, especially on one side.
- **Remember.** Sudden confusion and problems with thinking.
- **Off balance.** Trouble walking, dizziness, or loss of balance or coordination.
- **Killer headache.** Sudden severe headache with no known cause.
- **Eyes.** Sudden trouble seeing in one or both eyes.

Peripheral Artery Disease (PAD)

Peripheral arterial disease (PAD), sometimes referred to as peripheral vascular disease, is a lesser-known form of CVD. It is often caused by a process of atherosclerosis similar to that connected with CHD and stroke. PAD is the narrowing of the peripheral arteries, which reduces blood flow and oxygen delivery and occurs mainly in major vessels of the legs where symptoms are noticed. When we walk, our leg muscles have greater need for oxygen and hence blood flow. Classic symptoms of PAD include cramping, pain, or tiredness in the legs when walking that subside when resting. Over and above the reduction in physical function and pain that occurs with this condition, the presence of PAD also increases the risk for CHD and stroke (American Heart Association 2016).

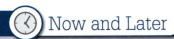 Now and Later

Heart-Healthy Behaviors

Now

The atherosclerosis process begins very early in life. By making good behavior choices now, you can prevent plaque buildup that might cause a heart attack or stroke later in your life. Understanding your risk factors related to your genetics is also important. Having candid conversations with parents and grandparents about their health can help you understand your personal risk of CVD. Finally, getting regular medical checkups is key. Most checkups provide a screening for CVD by assessing weight, blood pressure, and your blood lipid profile.

Later

Once you have graduated, try to keep a regular schedule for medical checkups. Adherence to a heart-healthy lifestyle can often become challenging as your life gets more complicated with employment, families, hobbies, and friends. Remember that healthy habits will make you feel great in the short term and can also increase your chances of having a long and disability-free life.

Take Home

Atherosclerosis, the major cause of CVD, begins early in life and, beyond genetics, is greatly influenced by your health behaviors. CVD can largely be prevented. If detected early, it can be treated to avoid a severe cardiovascular event such as a heart attack or stroke. Taking care of your arteries now can save your life later.

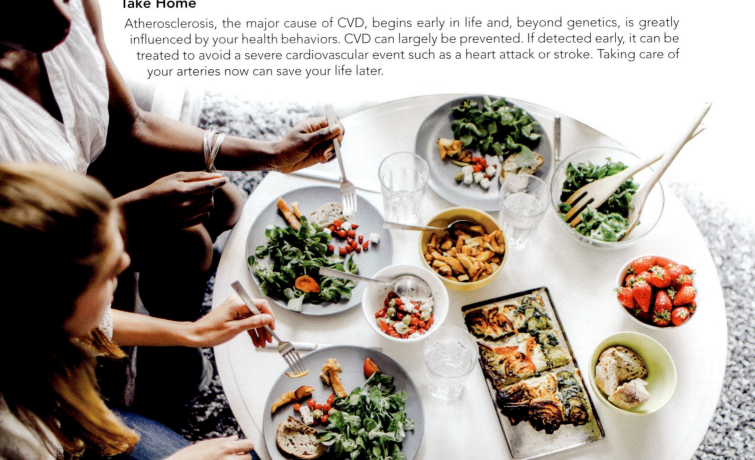

Heart Failure

Heart failure does not mean that the heart stops beating. Heart failure typically occurs when the heart muscle has been permanently damaged from several conditions, including atherosclerosis, a heart attack, chronic uncontrolled high blood pressure, birth defects, and other less common factors. This results in a less-than-optimal pumping action and can greatly limit the amount of physical activity or exercise a person can perform, including basic activities around the house. When the heart rate and contraction force is compromised to a certain degree, fluids can start to back up in the lungs or in the lower legs, which can make breathing or walking very difficult. In addition to a heart-healthy lifestyle, this condition requires medications to help the heart pump effectively and control the fluid. Unfortunately, people with heart failure have a high level of disability and mortality.

Address Risk Factors to Prevent Future Disease

Several factors can increase your risk for CVD in general and CHD and heart attack specifically. These can be categorized into major risk factors that you cannot change, behaviors that you can change, and conditions *that are related to your behaviors* that you can manage. Check out tables 13.2 and 13.3 to get an overview of these factors. Essentially, the more risk factors you have and the greater the level of each risk factor, the higher chance of a future heart attack. You will explore your personal risk factors for cardiometabolic diseases in lab 13.1 in the web study guide. Because the presence of a

> Preventing CVD begins with knowing your personal CVD risk factors, especially the ones that are under your control. Know your numbers!

Table 13.2 Nonmodifiable Risk Factors for Coronary Heart Disease and Heart Attack

Factors you cannot change	
Age	Risk increases with age, with the majority of heart attacks occurring after the age of 65.
Sex	Men have a greater risk of CVD and CHD compared to women, and they have heart attacks at an earlier age than women do.
Family history	Risk increases if you have a parent or sibling who developed CVD or CHD.
Race or ethnicity	African-Americans and non-Hispanic blacks are at a greater risk than whites/non-Hispanic whites. Rates among Hispanics, American Indians, native Hawaiians, and some Asian Americans are higher than among whites in part due to obesity rates.

Data from American Heart Association (2018); Centers for Disease control and Prevention (2015).

Table 13.3 Modifiable Risk Factors for Coronary Heart Disease and Heart Attack

Factors you can manage over time (with behavior and medications)	Factors you can manage today (with lifestyle choices)
Overweight and obesity (see chapter 9)	Diet quality and alcohol (see chapter 8)
MetS, prediabetes, and type 2 diabetes (see previous text in this chapter)	Smoking (see chapters 11 and 14)
High blood pressure (see following section)	Stress (see chapter 10)
High cholesterol (see following section)	Exercise, physical activity, and fitness (see chapter 4)

Data from American Heart Association (2018); Centers for Disease Control and Prevention (2015).

strong family history (a risk factor in itself) will mean you need to work harder to prevent these chronic diseases as you age, lab 13.2 in the web study guide will involve exploring your genetic family tree for risk factors and known diseases, including diabetes and CVD.

Chronic Conditions to Be Managed

Several of the risk factors that you can manage on a daily basis with your lifestyle choices are discussed in other chapters (cardiorespiratory fitness, nutrition, weight management, stress, and smoking) or previously in this chapter (MetS, T2D). These factors often co-exist with the other risk factors of high blood pressure and an unhealthy blood lipid profile. When people cannot manage high blood pressure or their blood lipid profile with lifestyle changes, these conditions are often treated with medications.

High Blood Pressure

Blood pressure (BP) is the pressure exerted against the arteries during heart contraction (systolic blood pressure; the upper number) and relaxation (diastolic blood pressure; the lower number). **Hypertension** is the medical term to describe chronically elevated resting blood pressure. Chronic high blood pressure increases the heart's workload with each beat and causes the heart muscle to adapt in an unhealthy way, contributing to many forms of heart disease, including risk for a heart attack. Hypertension can also increase risk for stroke. Hypertension can be completely silent, even if it is quite high. Thus, it is important to monitor your resting blood pressure on at least an annual basis. Getting your blood pressure monitored is a quick, simple, pain-less procedure that is included in routine visits to the doctor as a vital sign. Blood pressure machines are also conveniently located in grocery stores with clinics, at pharmacies, and often at worksites. Remember that your target is to keep your

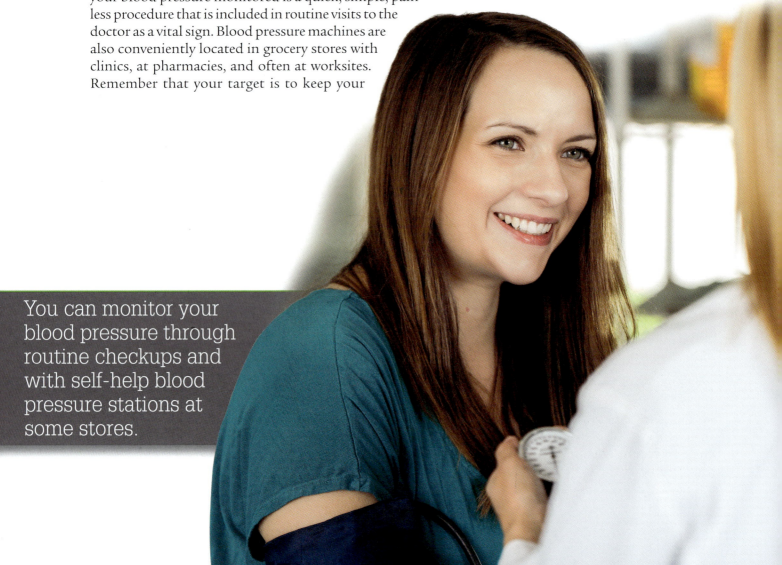

You can monitor your blood pressure through routine checkups and with self-help blood pressure stations at some stores.

resting blood pressure below 120/80 mmHg (American Heart Association 2017 and American Stroke Association):

- *Normal:* systolic BP < 120 mmHg *and* diastolic BP < 80 mmHg
- *Elevated:* systolic BP 120 to 129 mmHg *and* diastolic BP < 80 mmHg
- *Stage 1 hypertension:* systolic BP 130 to 139 mmHg *or* diastolic BP 80 to 89 mmHg
- *Stage 2 hypertension:* systolic BP ≥ 140 mmHg *or* diastolic BP ≥ 90 mmHg

Hypertension can be caused by genetics, certain medications, or lifestyle behaviors. For most college students, the latter is generally the cause. You can help prevent hypertension by making healthy lifestyle choices in the following areas:

- *Weight management*. Maintaining a healthy weight and keeping your waistline in check is important for managing blood pressure.
- *Diet quality*. Over and above managing your diet to help manage your weight, high-quality dietary fuel reduces your risk for hypertension. This involves consuming a variety of fruits and vegetables, choosing low-fat dairy products, and reducing the amount of sodium in your diet. DASH (Dietary Approaches to Stop Hypertension) is a popular and well-researched diet that reinforces many of the healthy dietary strategies discussed in chapter 8 (see www.dashdiet.org).
- *Regular physical activity and exercise*. Beyond weight management, regular activity, especially cardiorespiratory exercise that is moderate to vigorous in intensity, is effective for reducing the risk for hypertension.
- *Stress*. Chronic stress can increase risk for hypertension. Managing your stress, including getting high-quality sleep, is important for managing your blood pressure.

If you are diagnosed with hypertension, in addition to the lifestyle factors just described, your doctor will prescribe one or more of a number of medications to keep your blood pressure in the normal range.

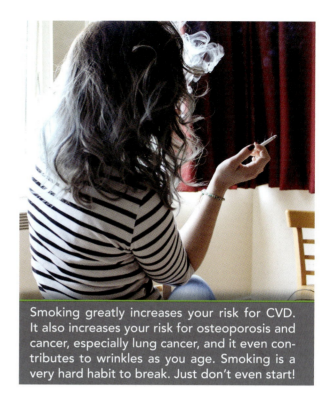

Smoking greatly increases your risk for CVD. It also increases your risk for osteoporosis and cancer, especially lung cancer, and it even contributes to wrinkles as you age. Smoking is a very hard habit to break. Just don't even start!

High Cholesterol

Blood **cholesterol**, a waxy, fatlike substance, is an important factor for the process of atherosclerosis. Your body needs some cholesterol to function; however, too much cholesterol in your blood, termed **hypercholesterolemia**, can accelerate the atherosclerosis process. **Hyperlipidemia** is the medical term for when your blood has too many lipids (fats), including cholesterol and triglycerides. A simple way to think about blood lipids is that too many of them in the blood provide material for plaques to develop (i.e., they can clog your arteries).

A simple blood test, called a lipid profile, provides measurements that help assess your risk for CVD. A conventional lipid profile includes total cholesterol, **high-density lipoprotein cholesterol (HDL-C)**, or "good cholesterol," **low-density lipoprotein cholesterol (LDL-C)**, or "bad cholesterol," and triglycerides.

High cholesterol is affected by more than weight management. You can also maintain healthy blood lipids by improving the quality of your diet, being physically active, and not smoking.

- HDL-C is a good cholesterol. It carries the LDL away from the arteries; therefore, higher levels are protective against CVD.

- LDL-C is the primary type of cholesterol that contributes to the buildup of plaque in the arteries that can cause a heart attack or stroke.

- Finally, **triglycerides**, although needed for energy production, increase the risk of a heart attack or stroke if levels are too high.

Blood cholesterol levels have traditionally been evaluated using specific ranges of values. However, recent scientific advances now use the various blood values in context with other risk factors (e.g., age, sex) to predict a 10-year risk for atherosclerotic CVD. The guidelines provide specific recommendations for primary prevention (i.e., person has not been diagnosed with CVD) and secondary prevention (i.e., a person already has been diagnosed with CVD) and for treatment in people 20 to 79 years old (Stone et al. 2014). For young adults who are not yet 20 years old, specific blood lipid values are still evaluated (see table 13.4). Importantly, the clinical significance of your personal blood lipid values, including the treatment plan, should be evaluated by a physician familiar with your health history, including your family history.

Hyperlipidemia can be genetic or caused by lifestyle behaviors. Similar to hypertension, lifestyle choices are the primary way you can change an unhealthy lipid profile, even if someday you are put on medications:

- **Weight management**. Being overweight or obese tends to raise LDL-C and lower HDL-C. Managing your weight and waistline is critical for preventing hyperlipidemia.

- **Diet quality**. From a dietary standpoint, the best strategy for lowering your cholesterol is to reduce the intake of your saturated and trans fats. Another key is to have a diet high in fiber, which can lower cholesterol, sometimes up to 10 percent. Of course, other recommendations include following a healthy diet by eating fruits, vegetables, whole grains, poultry, fish, and nuts and limiting foods and beverages with added sugars. A diet high in refined carbohydrates and added sugars can elevate triglycerides. High levels of alcohol in the diet can also increase triglycerides. Fuel quality greatly affects your blood lipids.

- **Regular physical activity and exercise**. A sedentary lifestyle is linked with lower HDL-C, which means there is less good cholesterol to combat the bad cholesterol. Regular physical activity also helps reduce triglycerides in the blood.

- **Smoking**. Smoking also lowers HDL-C, the good cholesterol. This is another great reason to never light up.

If you are diagnosed with hyperlipidemia and you are unable to improve your blood values with lifestyle changes, you might be prescribed one or more medications, such as statin drugs, which are very effective for the treatment of dyslipidemia (Stone et al. 2014).

Exercise and Physical Activity as Key Prevention Behaviors

It should be clear that exercise and physical activity are critical for preventing MetS, T2D, and CVD, especially CHD. It is nearly impossible to have cardiovascular health without doing a relatively

Table 13.4   Blood Cholesterol Levels for Young Adults < 20 Years Old

	Acceptable	Borderline risk	High
Total cholesterol	<170	170-199	≥200
LDL	<110	110-129	≥130
HDL	>45	40-45	<40
Triglycerides	<90	90-129	≥130

Data from U.S. Department of Health and Human Services (2012).

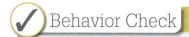
✓ Behavior Check

Know Your Numbers

Many young adults think if their weight is reasonably managed, they must have good blood pressure and blood lipid numbers and are therefore protected from chronic diseases like CHD. To some degree this is true; however, some people can reasonably manage their weight without eating very well (i.e., they manage their calories but their fuel quality is low). A diet high in saturated fats, refined carbohydrates and simple sugars, sodium, and alcohol can negatively affect the blood lipid profile even when a person is not overweight or obese. If a person also has chronically high stress and does not engage in regular cardiorespiratory exercise, the lipid profile and blood pressures might not be in the   healthy range. If you have a strong family history of hyperlipidemia or hypertension,   get tested and know your numbers.

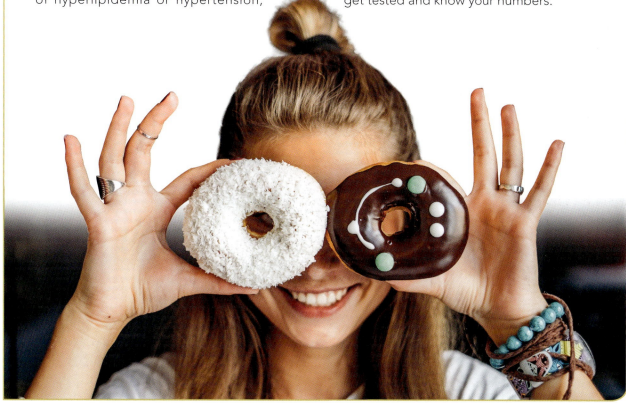

high amount of intentional exercise. People who have cardiorespiratory fitness greatly reduce their risk for obesity, hypertension, hyperlipidemia, and T2D. The majority of the beneficial effects of exercise and physical activity for preventing CHD can be explained *indirectly* through their positive influence on these traditional risk factors.

Cardiorespiratory exercise and fitness also *directly* reduce risk of CVD through their effects on the walls of the arteries and the chambers of the heart. The very inner lining of the arteries, called the **endothelium**, controls physiological functions such as blood flow, which is linked to wear and tear on the lining of the vessel and risk for hypertension, and vessel permeability, which is important to the atherosclerotic process and plaque buildup. Exercise training produces many positive changes on the endothelium, making the vessels more flexible in response to physical demand and also facilitating repair processes. The chambers of the heart are also favorably affected by regular exercise, especially the left ventricle, which is responsible for pumping oxygenated blood to the body (Roitman and LaFontaine 2012).

Thus, as a lifestyle choice to prevent a future heart attack, exercise and physical activity provide powerful indirect *and* direct benefits for your arteries.

Figure 13.5 summarizes the keys to reducing your risk of having a heart attack.

Prevention of CVD Starts Early in Life

Although it should be clearly evident by now, the prevention of CVD and its risk factors, including MetS, prediabetes, and T2D, are key to cardiovascular health. Maintaining good cardiovascular health comes down to these top strategies:

1. Do not smoke (not even a little bit!).
2. Eat clean and balanced (most of the time!).
3. Have a high level of physical activity (especially cardiorespiratory exercise of a moderate to vigorous intensity!).
4. Manage your waistline (which should happen if you follow 2 and 3 on this list!).

Unless you happen to have genetics that are working against you, if you invest in these strategies, you can greatly increase your chance of preventing CVD. It will also be very unlikely that you will develop high blood pressure, hyperlipidemia, or MetS (or prediabetes or T2D).

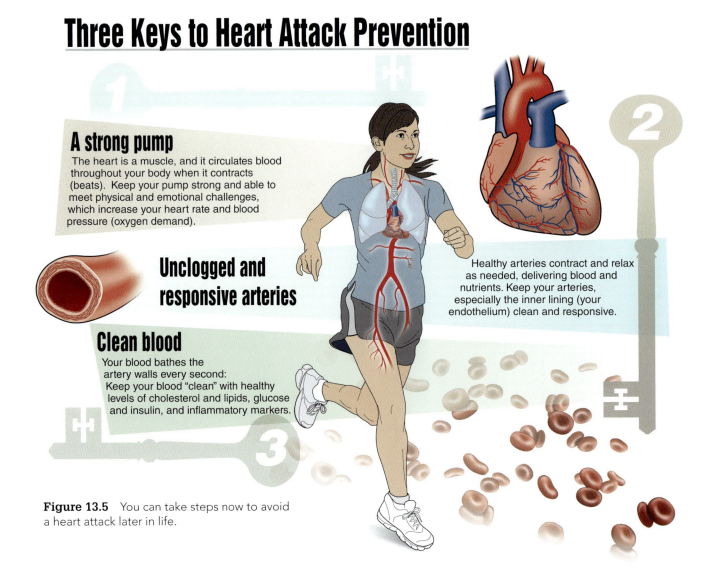

Three Keys to Heart Attack Prevention

A strong pump
The heart is a muscle, and it circulates blood throughout your body when it contracts (beats). Keep your pump strong and able to meet physical and emotional challenges, which increase your heart rate and blood pressure (oxygen demand).

Unclogged and responsive arteries

Healthy arteries contract and relax as needed, delivering blood and nutrients. Keep your arteries, especially the inner lining (your endothelium) clean and responsive.

Clean blood
Your blood bathes the artery walls every second: Keep your blood "clean" with healthy levels of cholesterol and lipids, glucose and insulin, and inflammatory markers.

Figure 13.5 You can take steps now to avoid a heart attack later in life.

Summary

The cornerstone of prevention strategies for T2D and CVD is your lifestyle choices, including avoiding smoking and second-hand smoke, limiting alcohol consumption, and, most importantly, eating a balanced and healthy diet, engaging in regular moderate- to vigorous-intensity cardiorespiratory exercise, and managing your weight and waistline. T2D and CVD disease processes often start at a very young age with MetS. As the decades progress, MetS becomes prediabetes, which becomes T2D, which leads to CVD in the following decade. Prevention starts today. Know the risk factors for these diseases, know your personal family history, and chart your risk numbers for life. Investing in heart-healthy behaviors will help you feel good today and prevent chronic diseases in the decades to come.

www WEB STUDY GUIDE

Remember to complete all of the web study guide activities to further facilitate your learning, including the following lab activities:

Lab 13.1   Your Personal Risk Profile for Cardiometabolic Diseases

Lab 13.2   Your Cardiometabolic Family Tree

REVIEW QUESTIONS

1. How does MetS influence the risk for T2D and CVD?

2. List the risk factors for T2D and CVD. Which factors are the same and which are different?

3. What are the primary risk factors for T2D and CVD that you can change through your lifestyle choices?

4. Which type of exercise is most effective for enhancing your cardiovascular health? Describe the specifics of the exercise in terms of FITT.

5. Which specific components of a healthy diet help reduce the risk of CVD?

6. When does the atherosclerotic process for CHD typically begin? Explain how early health choices can prevent subclinical disease with respect to this process.

7. How does habitual cardiorespiratory exercise directly and indirectly reduce the risk for CHD?

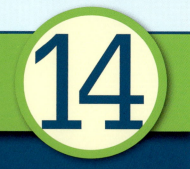

Reducing the Risks for Cancer

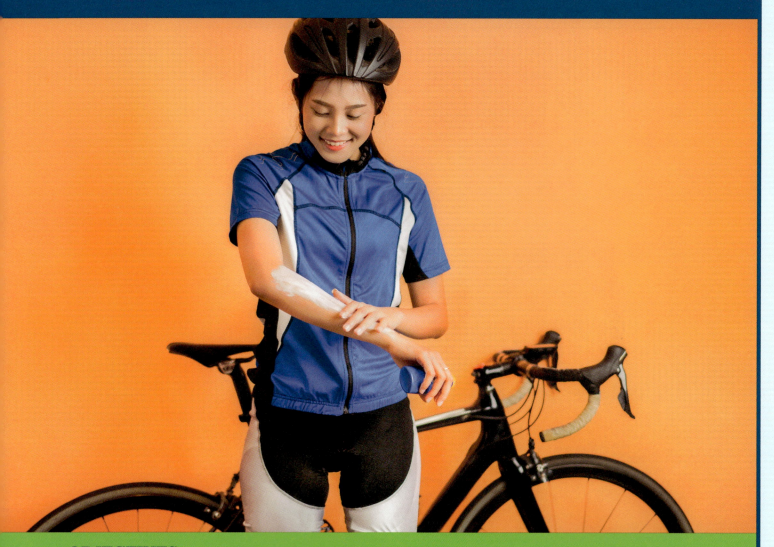

OBJECTIVES

❭ Define how cancer develops in the body.

❭ Identify the most commonly diagnosed cancers in the United States.

❭ Identify the cancers that cause the highest mortality rates in the United States.

❭ Explain how cancer develops related to genetics, lifestyle, and personal behaviors.

❭ Explain the different types of cancer treatments.

❭ Develop a plan to prevent cancer.

KEY TERMS

benign

biopsy

cancer

carcinogen

carcinogenesis

carcinoma in situ

chemotherapy

endoscopy

fecal occult blood test

malignant

melanoma

metastasis

mutation

polyp

prognosis

radiation therapy

surgery

TNM system

Cancer affects one in three people and is the second leading cause of death in the United States. This chapter provides a basic explanation of what cancer is; how it develops related to genetics, lifestyle, and behaviors; how it is detected; and how it is treated. The chapter includes information about commonly diagnosed cancers and what you can do to prevent cancer.

Cancer has been a medical mystery for centuries. Tumors were described in pictures and written records in many ancient civilizations in Asia, South America, and Egypt. In 400 BC, Hippocrates observed abnormal growths from breast tumors in his patients that looked like limbs of a crab. In 1700, an Italian physician named Bernardino Ramazzini noticed an increased incidence of breast cancer among Catholic nuns. He speculated that this may be related to their oath of celibacy and childlessness and thus questioned whether there was a direct cause-and-effect relationship between lifestyle and cancer. Another interesting connection between cancer and lifestyle emerged in 1775 with the observations of British physician Percivall Pott. He had many young patients in their 20s who worked as chimney sweepers. In this job, workers were lowered into chimneys to

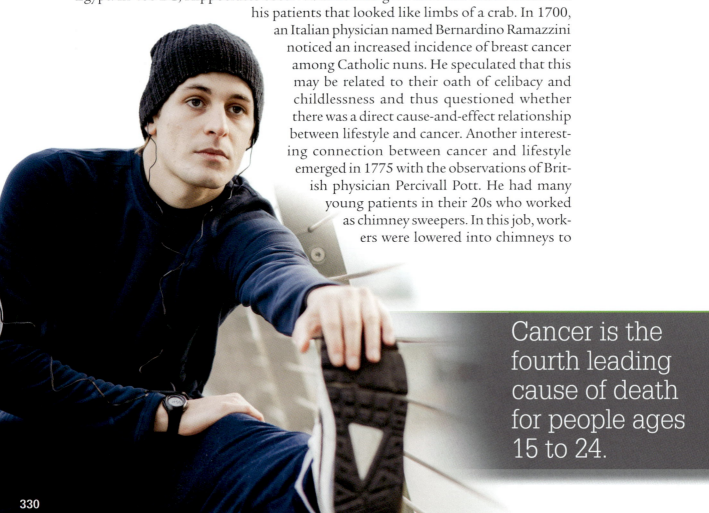

Cancer is the fourth leading cause of death for people ages 15 to 24.

scrub the soot off the interior walls. These young men were being diagnosed with cancers of the scrotum at a very high rate. Dr. Pott concluded that the chimney soot, or tar, was the causative agent and recommended that the men wash their hands and body and change their clothes after cleaning chimneys to reduce their exposure to the tar. These simple recommendations reduced the rates of cancer. In more recent history, in 1971, President Richard Nixon signed the National Cancer Act with the goal of eradicating cancer as a leading cause of death.

The Nature of Cancer

Cancer is a significant leading cause of death and disability. Over 87 percent of all cancers are diagnosed at age 50 and older (American Cancer Society 2017a), and our country's older population is increasing as the many baby boomers who were born between 1942 and 1964 are aging. Despite the current numbers, the overall number of cancer cases and deaths have followed a steady decline. Some of this is due to changes in lifestyle behaviors such as a decreased tobacco use. Advanced medical technology that detect cancer in the earlier stages and improved treatment options specific to the type of cancer that lead to a longer survival rate have also helped many people live cancer free.

Figure 14.1 shows the leading causes of death in 2014 in the United States according to the Centers for Disease Control and Prevention (2015). Cancer is the second leading cause of death overall and the fourth leading cause of death for young people ages 15 to 24. It accounts for 22.5 percent of all deaths. The relative survival rate for cancer is calculated based on the percentage of people who are still alive five years after their cancer diagnosis and gives us an idea about what we can expect related to life expectancy. Since the early 1970s, the five-year survival rate for all cancers has increased 20 percent among white people and 24 percent among black people (68 percent and 61 percent, respectively; American Cancer Society 2017a). The cancers with the most significant survival rates over the past five decades are prostate, breast, colon, and rectum cancers, and leukemia. Certain cancers can be defined as curable if they are detected early and have not spread to other parts of the body and if the treatment options are successful.

Cancer is a malignant tumor and is not considered a single disease. It is many diseases; well over 100 different types of cancer exist. The common factors in these diseases are the characteristics of the cells. Cancer develops from an abnormal growth in healthy cells that the body is unable to stop from growing; the spread of the growth can become uncontrollable. Some of the distinct

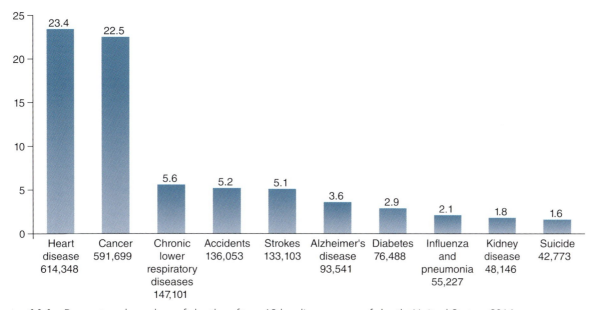

Figure 14.1   Percent and number of deaths of top 10 leading causes of death, United States, 2014.

Data from Kochanek et al. (2016).

characteristics of these abnormal cells are large nuclei, larger than normal cell size, and variations in shape and size. Eventually, these cells multiply and divide, invading the space in which the cancer began. In many cases, if the disease is not detected early, these cells spread to other parts of the body.

Tumors: Benign Versus Malignant

A **benign** tumor is still a tumor. It is described as an abnormal growth that is not cancer; the cells do not break off of the primary tumor and spread to other parts of the body (figure 14.2). These types of tumors are encapsulated, meaning that

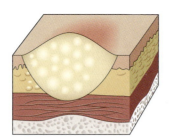

Type: Tumor
Description: A swelling or enlargement, any mass lesion; may be either malignant or benign
Examples: Lipoma, inflammatory reaction

Figure 14.2   Cross-section of a benign tumor.

they have a defined border that does not allow the cells to break free and spread. Although these types of tumors are not cancer, they can still be fatal if left untreated or not removed from the site. An untreated tumor may still grow and become larger in the site, taking up space and potentially preventing normal body functioning. For example, a tumor located in the lower abdominal cavity could fill that space as it becomes larger, which could affect the ability to urinate or have a bowel movement.

A **malignant** tumor is also a mass of abnormal cells; however, the cells look and act different than those of benign tumors (figure 14.3). Malignant tumors have the ability to grow in size and shape, and the cells can separate from the primary tumor and spread to other parts of the body. These cells invade nearby tissue and then spread by way of the circulatory (blood) or the lymphatic system. This is a multistage and multiyear process.

How Does Cancer Develop?

Chemicals, radiation, viruses, and heredity all cause changes to the cell's genes that lead to cancer. Chemicals (such as those in cigarettes), radiation, and viruses invade normal cells. This leads to abnormal cell growth, or a **mutation**, which is the alteration of the genetic makeup of a normal cell. Specific cancers have been identi-

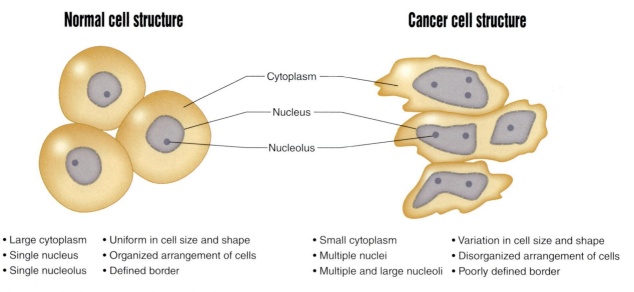

Normal cell structure

Cytoplasm
Nucleus
Nucleolus

• Large cytoplasm   • Uniform in cell size and shape
• Single nucleus   • Organized arrangement of cells
• Single nucleolus   • Defined border

Cancer cell structure

• Small cytoplasm   • Variation in cell size and shape
• Multiple nuclei   • Disorganized arrangement of cells
• Multiple and large nucleoli • Poorly defined border

Figure 14.3   Comparison of normal cells and cancer cells.
Reprinted from National Cancer Institute (1990).

fied as hereditary; genes are passed on that make people more susceptible to cancer. The development of cancer, **carcinogenesis**, is a multistep process consisting of a series of mutations over many years.

A **carcinogen** is an agent that is capable of causing permanent damage to the molecular structure of the cell's DNA. This initiating agent is either inherited or acquired though carcinogenic chemicals, radiation, or viruses. Exposure is often repeated over time. Initiating agents include the chemicals in cigarettes, UVA radiation from the sun, air pollution, or the human papilloma virus (which can cause cervical cancer).

Who Gets Cancer?

Information from the American Cancer Society (2017a, b) gives us insight on who develops cancer. In the United States in 2017, there were 1.6 million new cancer cases and almost 601,000 deaths. This is equivalent to approximately 5,000 new cases and over 1,600 deaths every day. Figure 14.4 shows the leading sites of new cancer cases

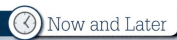 Now and Later

Should You Fear Cancer?

Now

Should you fear cancer? Let's put it in perspective. Are you more afraid of a shark attack, being in an airplane crash, contracting the West Nile Virus, or being diagnosed with cancer, heart disease, or Alzheimer's disease? Many fears are rooted in emotions rather than facts. Cancer can be caused by genetics or lifestyle behaviors such as a poor diet or using tobacco products. Knowing the causes now can help you reduce the chances of developing cancer in the future. Let's add some perspective. Table 14.1 shows the odds over a lifetime that a U.S. citizen will die by certain causes.

Table 14.1 Odds of Dying

What we fear: actual death rates	What we should fear: actual death rates
Shark attack: 1 in 3.7 million	Cancer: 1 in 4
Bear attack: 1 in 1.2 million	Heart disease: 1 in 4
Amusement park rides: 1 in 950,000	Stroke: 1 in 23
Anthrax: 1 in 730,000	Diabetes: 1 in 53
Fireworks: 1 in 340,733	Alzheimer's disease: 1 in 75
Lightning: 1 in 161,856	Intentional self-harm (suicide): 1 in 95
Commercial airplane: 1 in 40,000	Kidney disease: 1 in 97
West Nile Virus: 1 in 15,000	Vehicle accident: 1 in 114

Data from Ropeik and Gray (2002); American Cancer Society (2016a): National Safety Council (2017); The Wildlife Museum (2017).

Later

Cancer develops over time and is more likely to develop if someone is repeatedly exposed to cancer-causing chemicals or substances, like radiation from the sun or the toxic chemicals in cigarettes. What can you do to reduce your odds of dying from one of the leading causes of death in the United States in the future?

Take Home

Although cancer can take years to develop and is typically thought of as a disease of older people, you can take steps now, as a college student, to prevent your chances of being diagnosed with cancer. Begin setting your cancer prevention goals now: It's never too early to use sunscreen, limit alcohol, quit smoking, and begin age-appropriate health screenings like breast self-exams. Do all you can to learn how to prevent cancer from starting in your body and what you can do to increase your survival by catching cancer early.

in women and men. Cancer rates were the highest during the 20th century primarily due to high rates of tobacco use and its relationship to lung cancer. Since 1991, the death rate has declined 25 percent, which means that there have been more than 2.1 million fewer deaths due to cancer in the past 20 years. Older people are at a higher risk of developing cancer; 41 out of 100 men and 38 out of 100 women will be diagnosed with cancer at some point in their lifetime. Lifestyle and behaviors also affect the development of cancer among those who smoke, eat an unhealthy diet, and are not regularly physically active. See lab 14.1 in

the web study guide to determine which lifestyle behaviors contribute to specific types of cancer. Knowing which behaviors can lead to certain cancers will help you plan ways to reduce your chances of developing cancer.

Cancer: Race and Ethnicity

Cancer affects all populations and groups in the United States. However, specific groups have higher incidence rates, more cancer-related health complications, decreased survival rate and quality of life after treatment, more incidences of late-stage diagnosis, and higher mortality rates than

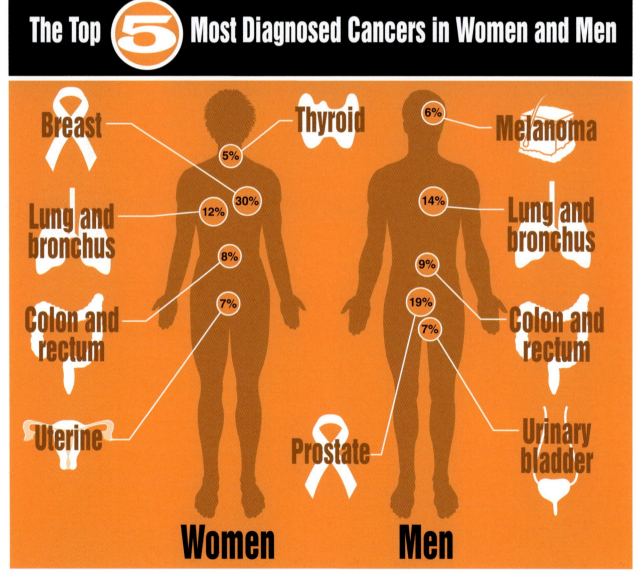

Figure 14.4   Leading types of cancer diagnosed in women and men, by percentage of new cancer cases.

Data from American Cancer Society (2017a).

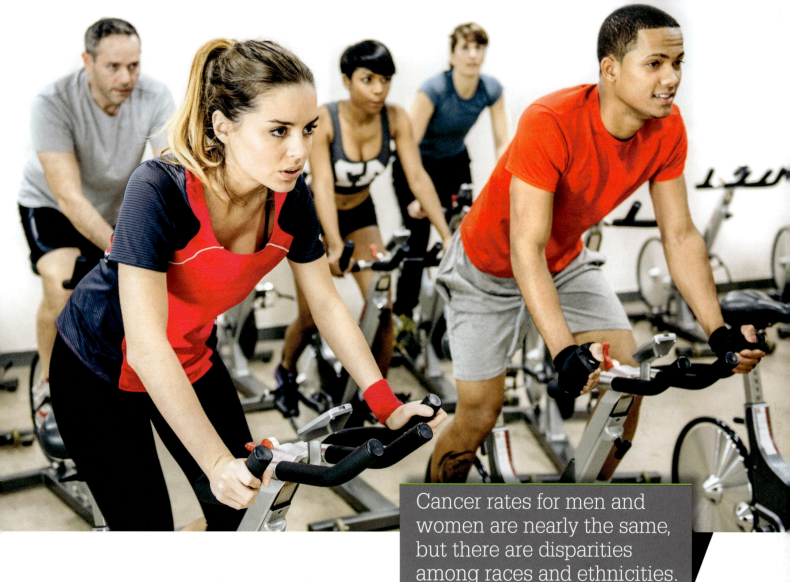

Cancer rates for men and women are nearly the same, but there are disparities among races and ethnicities.

others. Certain types of cancers are diagnosed more often among people of color than white people. While the information shown in this section focuses on race and ethnicity, disparities exist among other population groups, defined by disability, sex, sexual identity, geographic location, income level, and educational attainment (National Cancer Institute 2016a). Figures 14.5 and 14.6 show that the incidence of cancer and the death rates are highest among non-Hispanic black men.

Cancer: Disparities in the United States (National Cancer Institute 2016a)

- Black people have higher death rates than all other groups for many, although not all, cancer types.

- Black women are much more likely than white women to die of breast cancer.

- Black people are more than twice as likely as whites to die of prostate cancer and nearly twice as likely to die of stomach cancer.

- Colorectal cancer incidence is higher in black people than in whites.

- Hispanic, Latina, and black women have higher rates of cervical cancer than women of other racial and ethnic groups.

- Black women have the highest rates of death from cervical cancer.

- Hispanic and Latino people, American Indians, and Alaska natives have the highest rates of liver and intrahepatic bile duct cancer, followed by Asian Pacific Islanders.

- American Indians and Alaska natives have higher death rates from kidney cancer than people of other racial and ethnic groups.

- Both the incidence of lung cancer and death rates from the disease are higher in black men than in men of other racial and ethnic groups.

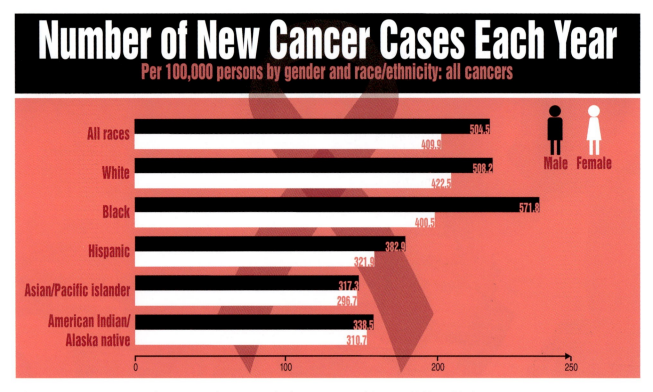

Figure 14.5 Cancer incidence rates by race and ethnicity, United States, 2009 to 2013.

Reprinted from National Cancer Institute (2016a).

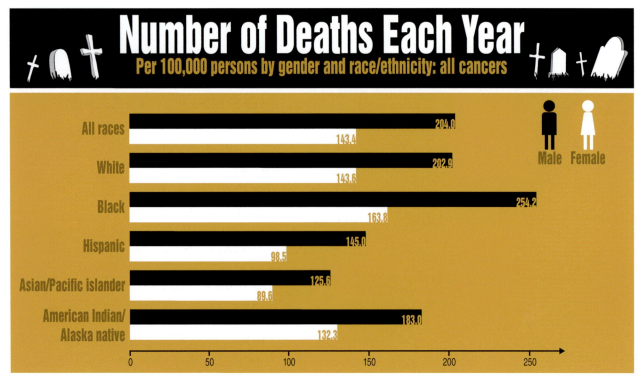

Figure 14.6 Cancer death rates by race and ethnicity, United States, 2009 to 2013.

Reprinted from National Cancer Institute (2016a).

The Risks Change Over Your Lifetime

Review table 14.2 and look at the risks of developing cancer as a young adult and then over one's lifetime. Then, look at the differences between men and women in the same age categories. Women have a higher overall lifetime risk of developing cancer than men, and their risk is higher than men for some specific cancers as well. Why do you think men have a higher risk of developing lung cancer at a younger age than women, but the overall lifetime risk is higher for women than for men? This is the same trend regarding skin cancer, except in the reverse: Women are more likely to develop skin cancer at a younger age than men, but the overall lifetime risk is higher for men than for women. What are your hypotheses related to these differences?

The incidence rates of lung cancer among women began to rise in the early 1980s due to more women smoking, but

Table 14.2 Probability (%) of Developing Invasive Cancers by Age and Sex, U.S., 2011 to 2013*

Site	Sex	Birth to 49	Birth to death
All sites^	M	1 in 30	1 in 2
	F	1 in 18	1 in 3
Breast	F	1 in 52	1 in 8
Prostate	M	1 in 354	1 in 8
Colon and rectum	M	1 in 294	1 in 22
	F	1 in 318	1 in 24
Lung	M	1 in 643	1 in 14
	F	1 in 598	1 in 17
Skin+	M	1 in 220	1 in 28
	F	1 in 155	1 in 44

*For those who are cancer-free at the beginning of each age interval.
^ All sites exclude basal cell and squamous cell skin cancers and in situ cancers except urinary bladder.

+ Statistic is for non-Hispanic whites.

Reprinted from National Cancer Institute (2016b).

these rates surpassed men. Studies have been conducted to determine why women are more susceptible to lung cancer. The results are still inconclusive, but the explanation could be related to hormonal interactions or women's metabolism of nicotine (Blot and McLaughlin 2004).

For skin cancer, women and non-Hispanic whites are more likely to be diagnosed with skin cancer, but the rates among men increase after age 65. This is most likely due to men working in occupations and participating in recreational activities where they are exposed to ultraviolet radiation over many years.

Why Do Specific Racial and Ethnic Groups Have Higher Incidence and Mortality Rates?

The most common reasons why other races and ethnic groups have higher cancer incidence and death rates than whites are due to lack of health care coverage and low socioeconomic status (National Cancer Institute 2008). Due to their limited opportunities for quality health care and the lack of financial means to afford medical care, people from these racial and ethnic groups are less likely to receive the recommended screenings and are more likely to be diagnosed with a late-stage cancer. Research related to racial and ethnic differences have discovered that biological differences may also play a role; black men have the higher rates of prostate cancer that may be due to a genetic or biological difference (National Cancer Institute 2016a). Understanding the role biological differences play among various popula-

tions can help researchers develop early screening and interventions to prevent late-stage diagnosis and improve quantity and quality of life for black men.

Approaches to Reducing the Cancer Disparities

- Provide health care to all regardless of one's ability to pay.
- Fund screening programs to be implemented in specific geographical locations where programs are scarce or do not exist.
- Implement educational programs in community-based organizations that increase knowledge and teach skills for reducing behavioral and lifestyle factors that contribute to developing cancer.
- Allocate additional funding that supports understanding the role of biological differences across all racial and ethnic groups.

Detection, Staging, and Treatment of Cancer

Learning about health screenings and the early detection of cancer will increase our chances of surviving the disease, should we ever have it. Once a cancer has been detected, determining its size and location and whether it has spread to other locations in the body will help guide the treatment plan and prognosis. All of this information helps the cancer patient and the team of health care providers determine the appropriate treatment plan that supports an optimal quality of life.

Early Detection of Cancer

The chances of survival increase when cancer is detected early. Also, the types of treatments with early detection are less invasive and do not greatly affect quality of life. Early-detection techniques do not prevent the cancer from developing, but detecting the disease in its early stages leads to a better prognosis and quality of life (figure 14.7). When early-detection techniques are implemented as part of routine medical care, you and your physician can note immediate changes. The cancer is most likely to be localized rather than distant. Cancer treatment involves removal of the tumors and use of medications or radiation to prevent the cancer cells from dividing and spreading.

The most common types of early-detection techniques for many types of cancers that are conducted by medical professionals are biopsies, X-rays, genetic testing, endoscopy, and blood tests. However, you can do certain techniques yourself on a monthly basis. Talk with your doctor about the need for additional medical screenings.

Biopsy

A **biopsy** is when a physician or surgeon removes a sample of cells or tissues from the tumor site. A screening of the cells or tissue will allow the health care provider to determine whether the tumor is malignant or benign and the type of cancer.

- *Fine-needle aspiration.* A small sample of cells is taken from the tumor with a syringe. This technique removes the least amount of cells compared to the others. Typically, no scarring or damage occurs to the surrounding area.
- *Core needle biopsy.* A small core sample of cells is removed from the tumor. There may be a small scar and the potential need for stitches.
- *Incisional.* A small wedge sample of cells is taken from the tumor. There may be a somewhat large scar and the need for stitches or other treatment to close the incision site.

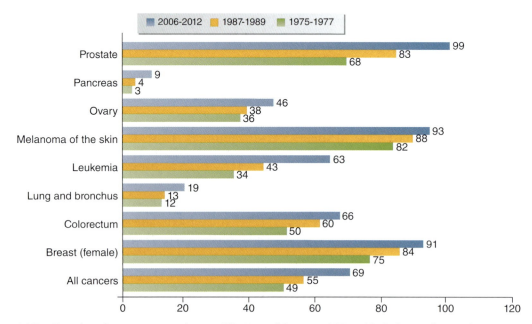

Figure 14.7   Trends in five-year survival rates (%), United States, 1975 to 2012. Survival rates for most cancers have increased due to earlier detection and advances in treatment.

Data from American Cancer Society (2017).

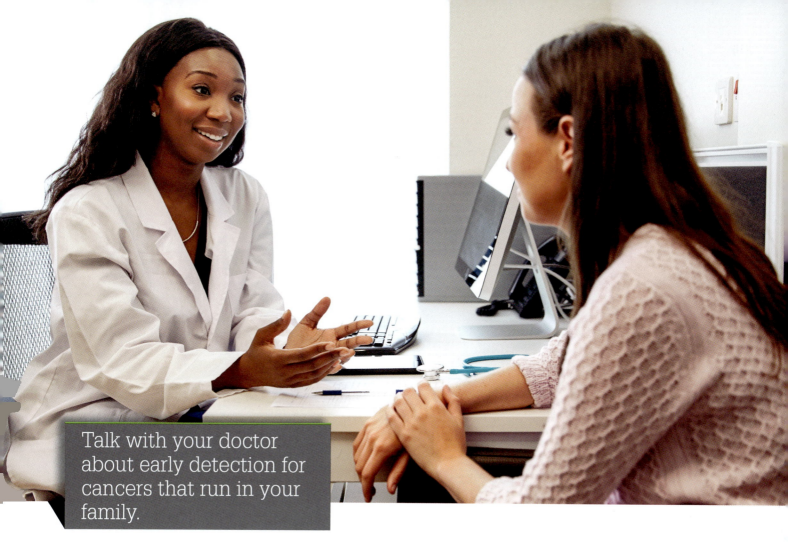

Talk with your doctor about early detection for cancers that run in your family.

- **Excisional.** The entire tumor area is extracted and no surrounding tissue remains. There will be a noticeable scar and the need for stitches or another treatment to close the incision site.
- **Ductal lavage.** Cells are extracted from milk ducts in the breast with a syringe.

X-Rays

Table 14.3 shows the various types of imaging techniques and technology that allow health care providers to determine the location and size of tumors in the body.

Genetic Testing

Hereditary cancers can be detected early through medical techniques such as chromosome analysis. Some of these tests are covered by insurance and others are not. It is important to discuss options with your health care and insurance providers. Lab 14.2 in the web study guide will help you determine if you have a predisposition to cancer based on your family history of cancer. Share the results of this activity with your health care provider so he or she can discuss which tests may be able to help you prevent and detect cancers early. According to the American Cancer Society

Table 14.3 Types of Imaging Used to Detect Cancer

Type of imaging	Description
Ultrasound	Use of a device called a transducer that transmits high-frequency soundwaves to examine the inside of the body
Mammogram	X-ray of the breast
Magnetic resonance imaging (MRI)	Magnet and radio waves to examine the inside of the body
Computed tomography (CT)	Scanning X-ray technique of cross-sectional photos of the body

(2017c), you should consider genetic testing if you have any of the following:

- Several first-degree relatives (mother, father, sister, brother) with cancer, especially the same type of cancer
- Family members who developed cancer at a young age
- Close relatives with rare cancers
- A known genetic mutation in the family

Endoscopy

Physicians can insert a thin, flexible illuminated tube, called an endoscope, into internal body cavities to check for cancer. This procedure is called **endoscopy**. Common sites where these flexible tubes can be inserted are the throat, esophagus, bladder, colon, and rectum. Endoscopies allow physicians to detect and locate possible tumors, ulcers, **polyps**, and areas of inflammation or bleeding, and remove tissue samples or the suspicious tumor during the procedure. Endoscopes are used for colon cancer screenings to detect cancers in the large intestine (figure 14.8).

Self-Detection Techniques

You can take an active part in early detection by examining your body on a monthly basis so that you are aware of what is normal and what is not. The American Cancer Society developed the acronym CAUTION to help people identify signs and symptoms of cancer (figure 14.9).

Both women and men can do monthly breast and skin self-examinations, and men can conduct a monthly testicular self-examination. See figures 14.10 and 14.11 for instructions on how to do these self-exams.

Staging of Cancer

Once someone is diagnosed with cancer, the physician or oncologist (a physician who specializes in cancer) will determine the stage, or seriousness, of the disease. They will stage the malignant tumor based on the extent to which the cancer cells have spread throughout the body. This assists the physician in determining the types of treatments and the **prognosis**, which is the physician's best estimate of the time it can take to recover from the treatments and how the cancer may affect the patient's quality of life. The stage of the cancer is based on the size of the primary tumor, the extent to which it has invaded the space where it is located, and if it has spread to lymph nodes or other locations in the body.

Staging is based on the level to which the cancer cells have invaded, or penetrated, layers of tissue.

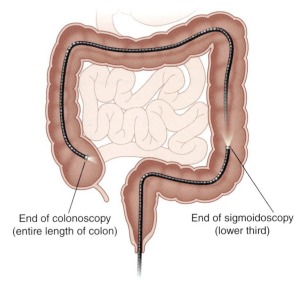

Figure 14.8 Both a colonoscopy and a sigmoidoscopy use a thin, flexible tube with a light and camera to examine the colon. A colonoscopy examines the entire length of the colon whereas the sigmoidoscopy examines only the lower third of the colon (MedlinePlus 2017).

End of colonoscopy (entire length of colon)

End of sigmoidoscopy (lower third)

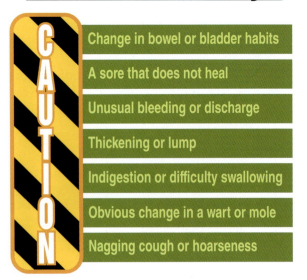

The CAUTION Acronym

C Change in bowel or bladder habits

A A sore that does not heal

U Unusual bleeding or discharge

T Thickening or lump

I Indigestion or difficulty swallowing

O Obvious change in a wart or mole

N Nagging cough or hoarseness

Figure 14.9 The acronym CAUTION can help you notice changes that you should report to your doctor.

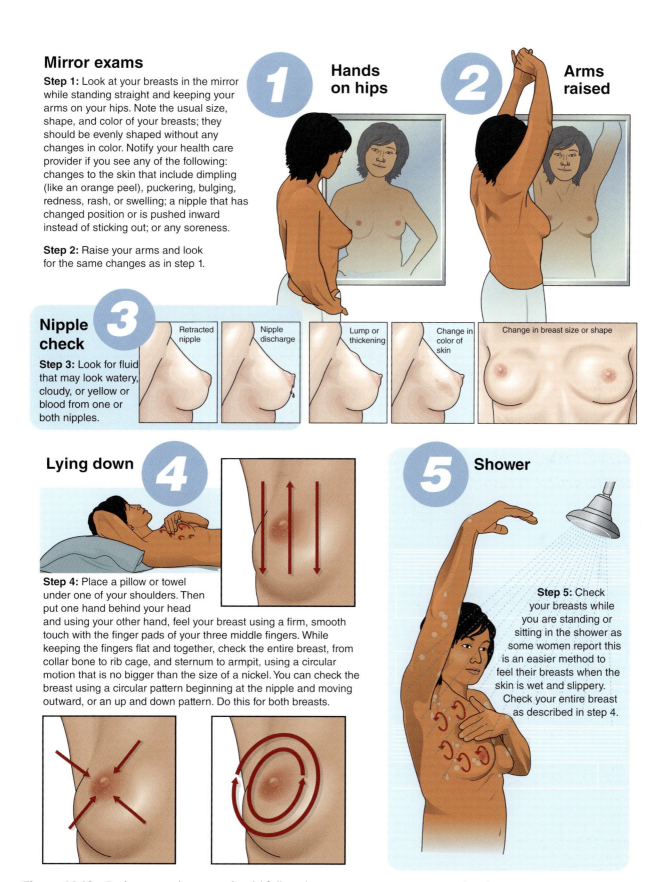

Mirror exams

Step 1: Look at your breasts in the mirror while standing straight and keeping your arms on your hips. Note the usual size, shape, and color of your breasts; they should be evenly shaped without any changes in color. Notify your health care provider if you see any of the following: changes to the skin that include dimpling (like an orange peel), puckering, bulging, redness, rash, or swelling; a nipple that has changed position or is pushed inward instead of sticking out; or any soreness.

Step 2: Raise your arms and look for the same changes as in step 1.

1 **Hands on hips**

2 **Arms raised**

Nipple check **3**

Step 3: Look for fluid that may look watery, cloudy, or yellow or blood from one or both nipples.

Retracted nipple

Nipple discharge

Lump or thickening

Change in color of skin

Change in breast size or shape

Lying down **4**

Step 4: Place a pillow or towel under one of your shoulders. Then put one hand behind your head and using your other hand, feel your breast using a firm, smooth touch with the finger pads of your three middle fingers. While keeping the fingers flat and together, check the entire breast, from collar bone to rib cage, and sternum to armpit, using a circular motion that is no bigger than the size of a nickel. You can check the breast using a circular pattern beginning at the nipple and moving outward, or an up and down pattern. Do this for both breasts.

5 Shower

Step 5: Check your breasts while you are standing or sitting in the shower as some women report this is an easier method to feel their breasts when the skin is wet and slippery. Check your entire breast as described in step 4.

Figure 14.10   Both men and women should follow these instructions to examine their breasts.

Breastcancer.org. 2017. "The Five Steps of a Breast Self-Exam." Last modified February 22, 2017. www.breastcancer.org/symptoms/testing/types/self_exam/bse_steps.

Testicular Self-Exam

Step 1: While standing, move your penis out of the way so you can see your scrotum. Examine the scrotum for any changes in skin color, swelling, soreness, or thickening. It is normal for one testicle to be slightly larger than the other and for one of the testicles to hang a bit lower than the other.

Step 2: Using both hands, specifically your thumbs and fingers, locate one of the testicles and begin to gently roll the testicle between your fingers and thumbs noticing any changes which may include hard lumps, painless lumps, smooth rounded bumps, swelling, shape, or consistency. Do this for both testicles.

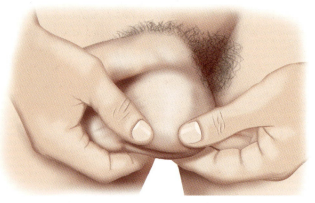

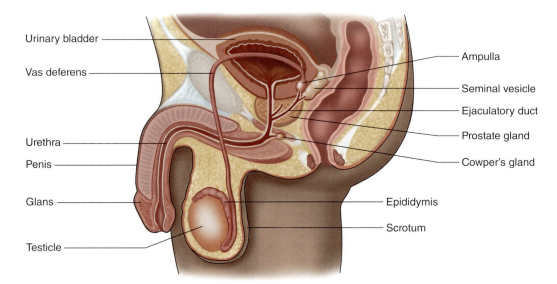

Figure 14.11   Men should follow these instructions to examine their testicles.

American Cancer Society. 2016b. "Do I Have Testicular Cancer?" Last modified May 23, 2016. www.cancer.org/cancer/testicular-cancer/do-i-have-testicular-cancer.html.

If the cells have not spread or penetrated any layers of tissues, and are confined to the original cells, then this is known as **carcinoma in situ**. If the cells have gone beyond the original layer of cells, then the cancer is defined as invasive. The physician will need to determine if the cancer is localized, regional, or distant and will use different imaging techniques to determine the extent of the invasiveness. Some primary cancers have a distinctive path where they have traditionally been known to spread to other parts of the body by invading the lymph or circulatory system (through the blood vessels). For example, metastatic lung cancer tends to spread to other lobes of the lung and the bones, liver, or brain (Simon and Brustugun 2015). Metastatic breast cancer spreads to the bones, lungs, liver, and brain (Naume 2014).

The **TNM system** is used to determine the extent or size of the primary tumor (T), whether or not the cancer cells have spread to lymph nodes (N), and if **metastasis** (M) has occurred, that is, the cells have traveled to other parts of

World War II sailors were accidentally exposed to mustard gas, which resulted in low white blood cell counts. This led to the discovery of medications that slow down or stop the division of cancer cells (Nordqvist 2015).

the body. Based on the TNM findings, the patient will be given a diagnosis and prognosis of a stage of 0, I, II, III, or IV. Stage 0 is carcinoma in situ, meaning that the cancer has not spread and is not invasive. Stage I indicates the cancer is in the very early stages, and stage IV is the most advanced. For example, if a woman is diagnosed with stage IV breast cancer, then a malignant tumor (T) of any size has been diagnosed, the cancer has most likely spread to local or distant lymph nodes (N), and the cancer has metastasized (M) to distant sites in the body (American Cancer Society 2017d).

Common Treatments of Cancer

The most common treatments for most cancers are surgery, chemotherapy, and radiation. **Surgery** involves the removal of the malignant tumor. For more advanced cancers, it may also require

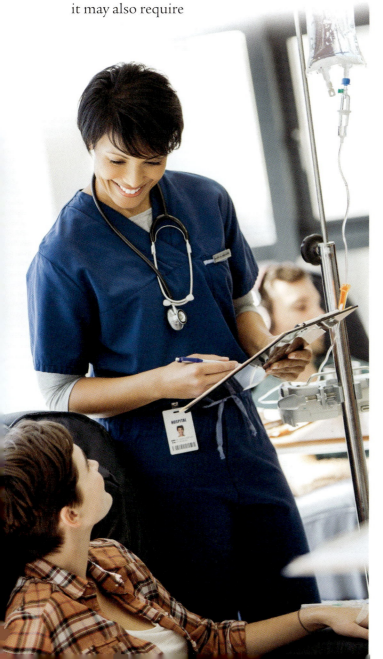

the removal of surrounding tissues and lymph nodes. The goal of **chemotherapy** is to introduce powerful medications into the body that stop the cancer cells from reproducing and the tumor from growing larger, thus preventing the cancer from spreading to other sites in the body. Chemotherapy can be administered by pill, liquid medications that are given through an IV or infusion, or injections through the skin or in muscles. In many cases, oncologists use chemotherapy medications in conjunction with other treatments such as surgery or radiation. However, in some cases, chemotherapy alone can treat cancer; no other treatments are necessary. Additionally, chemotherapy may be prescribed on a long-term basis to prevent the recurrence of cancer. **Radiation therapy** involves the use of radioactive waves, such as X-rays, gamma rays, neutrons, and protons, to kill cancer cells or shrink the size of the tumor. The radioactive beams can target specific cancer cells from a machine that delivers the beam either externally (outside of the body) or internally in the form of a small pellet that is placed in the body near the cancer cells (National Cancer Institute 2017).

Causes of Cancer

Do we have the ability to prevent cancer? More than half of all cancer deaths in the United States are preventable because they are related to lifestyle causes that can be altered to reduce the risks (American Association for Cancer Research 2014). Approximately 5 percent of all cancers are clearly hereditary; the majority of cancers, up to 95 percent, are due to genetic mutations caused by exposure to environmental toxins and lifestyle factors such as tobacco use, sun exposure, alcohol, drugs, not eating healthy foods, and lack of physical activity (American Cancer Society 2017a). Figure 14.12 shows the top causes of cancer.

Heredity

You have no control over your genetics and what you have inherited from your parents. You have inherited your parent's eye color, hair color, and body build. You can also inherit their cancer genes. Overall, inherited cancers are rare and many are diagnosed in childhood. Some inherited cancers show up in adulthood. An example of a childhood

Preventable Causes of Cancer (%)

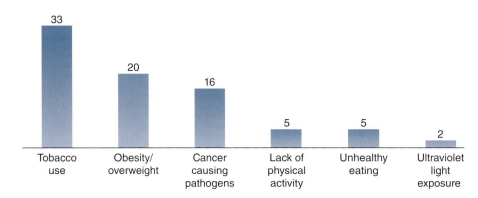

33	20	16	5	5	2
Tobacco use	Obesity/ overweight	Cancer causing pathogens	Lack of physical activity	Unhealthy eating	Ultraviolet light exposure

Figure 14.12   Most cancers are due to genetic mutations caused by lifestyle factors that could be altered to reduce the risk.

Data from Colditz and Wei (2012).

inherited cancer is retinoblastoma, an eye tumor. If detected early, it can be successfully treated. Adult inherited cancers include some types of breast and colon cancer. It is important to know your family medical history and understand your risks of developing cancer in your lifetime. The risks of developing some inherited cancers can be determined through screenings such as blood tests that can be discussed with your health care provider.

Lifestyles, Behaviors, and Cancer

Diet and tobacco use are the leading causes of cancer, and tobacco use is the leading cause of cancer deaths in the United States. An unhealthy diet, lack of physical activity, excessive sun expo-

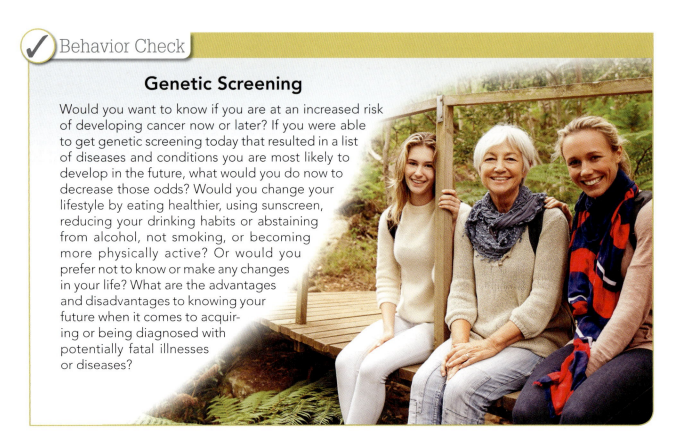

✓ Behavior Check

Genetic Screening

Would you want to know if you are at an increased risk of developing cancer now or later? If you were able to get genetic screening today that resulted in a list of diseases and conditions you are most likely to develop in the future, what would you do now to decrease those odds? Would you change your lifestyle by eating healthier, using sunscreen, reducing your drinking habits or abstaining from alcohol, not smoking, or becoming more physically active? Or would you prefer not to know or make any changes in your life? What are the advantages and disadvantages to knowing your future when it comes to acquiring or being diagnosed with potentially fatal illnesses or diseases?

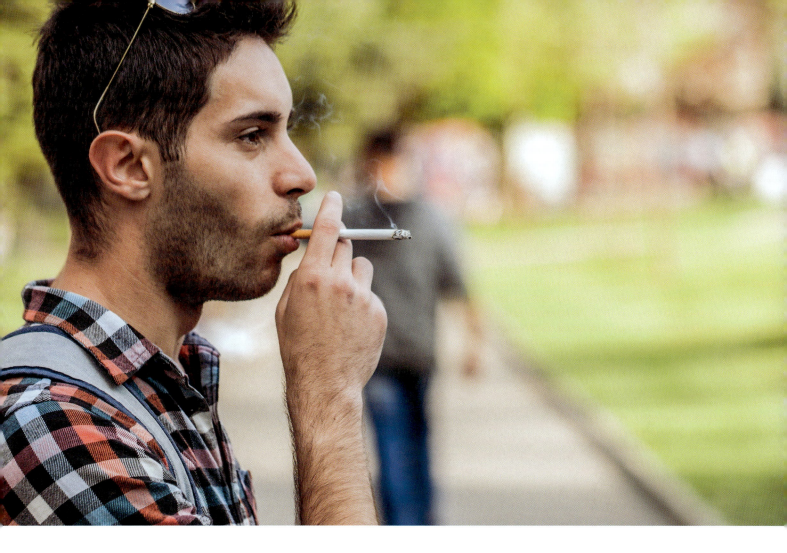

sure, and pollutions in the environment also contribute to cancer deaths. Learning more about your own lifestyle and behaviors can help you make choices to reduce your risks of developing cancer in the future.

Tobacco Use

Tobacco use has significantly declined in the United States since the early 2000s. The first Surgeon General's report related to smoking and tobacco, *Smoking and Health: Report of the Advisory Committee of the Surgeon General of the Public Health Service*, was published on January 11, 1964 (Centers for Disease Control and Prevention 2016) in response to the increase in the number of lung cancer cases and deaths among men. Fortunately, these rates have since declined. One out of every three cancer deaths in the United States is related to tobacco use (U.S. Department of Health and Human Services 2014).

Smoking is known to be linked to 13 different types of cancer (U.S. Department of Health and Human Services 2014), including lung, upper respiratory tract, esophagus, oral, tongue, bladder, pancreas, stomach, liver, and kidney. It may also contribute to cancers of the colon and rectum. The many chemicals found in cigarettes and other tobacco products are the causes of cancer. When the cancer is detected is based on how long someone has smoked and how many cigarette or tobacco products were used each day. Men and women who smoke are approximately 25 times more likely to develop lung cancer than those who do not smoke (American Cancer Society 2017a). Between 2010 and 2014, smoking caused more than 87 percent of all lung cancer deaths. Despite

It is never too late to quit smoking or quit using tobacco products! The body begins to heal within 20 minutes of that last cigarette! Talk to your health care provider, call 800-QUIT-NOW, or go to www.smokefree.gov for help.

efforts to reduce the number of current and new smokers, smoking continues to be the leading cause of preventable disease and death in the United States (U.S. Department of Health and Human Services 2014).

Diet and Physical Activity

Being overweight or obese is linked to risk for certain types of cancers. Figure 14.13 shows the sites in the body that may develop cancer due to being overweight or obese. The rates of obesity in the United States have increased dramatically since 1960, with the largest increases occurring between the years 1990 and 2006. Between 2011 and 2012, 35 percent of adults and 17 percent of youth ages 2 to 19 years were obese (Ogden et al. 2014).

The cancers most likely associated with overweight are breast, kidney, bowel, and uterine. Other parts of the body that are also at risk are the brain, thyroid, liver, stomach, gallbladder, pancreas, ovaries, and bones. The American Cancer Society recommends eating five or more servings of fruits and vegetables per day to help prevent cancer. Between 2007 and 2010, 76 percent of the total U.S. population did not meet dietary recommendations for fruit intake recommendations and 87 percent did not meet vegetable intake recommendations (National Cancer Institute 2015). Eating a variety of fruits and vegetables may prevent cancers of the mouth and pharynx, esophagus, lungs, stomach, and colon and rectum. So, eat your fruits and veggies!

In order to get a head start on preventing cancer, try to be

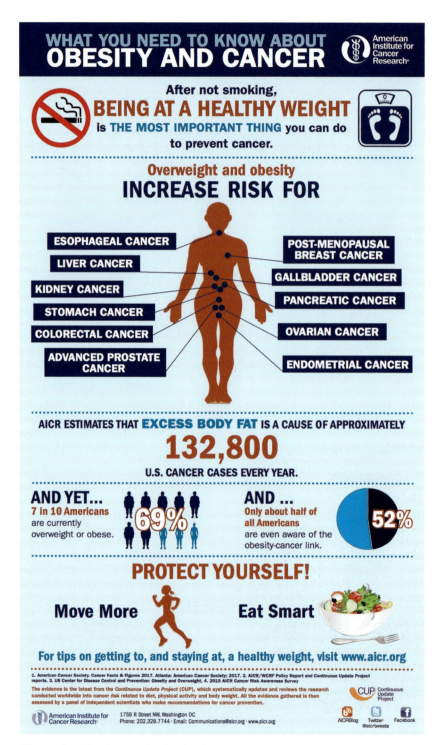

Figure 14.13   Sites in the body where cancer may develop due to being overweight or obese.

Reprinted from American Institute for Cancer Research (2017).

physically active most days for a weekly total of approximately 150 minutes. Maintaining a weight that is healthy for your body will decrease your chances of developing one of the cancers associated with being overweight or obese. According to research, college students have an average of 42 hours a week that they can devote to leisure activities. According to Yarnal and colleagues (2013), some college students spend these hours engaging in activities that improve their mood and increase coping skills, participating in physical activities, and becoming more involved in community and academic engagement programs. You can increase your physical activity on campus by walking to class, riding your bike, taking advantage of campus recreational facilities, or joining an intramural sport.

Sun Exposure

Spring break is typically a time for college students to hit the road and head to sunny beaches. The majority of skin cancers are due to spending too much time unprotected in the sun during the hours of 10 a.m. to 2 p.m., when ultraviolet radiation exposure is at the highest and sunburns are most likely to occur. Sunburn is the reddening of the skin that feels hot to the touch after too much exposure to ultraviolet light from the sun or other sources such as sunlamps or tanning beds. Sunburns increase one's chances of developing skin cancer.

Skin cancer is the most commonly diagnosed cancer in the United States. The American Cancer Society (2017a) estimates that ultraviolet exposure is linked to over a million cases of basal and squamous cell skin cancers (non-melanoma skin cancers). In 2017, 87,110 new cases of malignant **melanoma** were diagnosed. Malignant melanoma is the most dangerous type of skin cancer and the most likely to metastasize quickly if not detected early. Melanoma can develop from existing moles or as a new mole. Conducting monthly skin self-examinations using the ABCDE signs and symptoms rule (figure 14.14) can help detect skin cancer in early stages. Figure 14.14 provides examples of suspicious moles that need to be examined by a health care provider. Treatment of skin cancer involves the removal by electrocautery (burning), cryotherapy (freezing), or excision (cutting or shaving) of the suspicious lesion and perhaps an additional margin of skin and tissue around the mole.

Environment

Carcinogens in the environment that have been known to cause cancer include arsenic, asbestos,

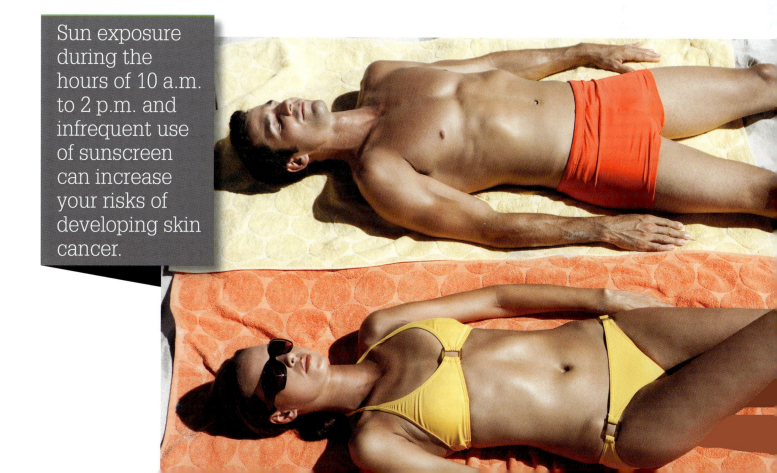

Sun exposure during the hours of 10 a.m. to 2 p.m. and infrequent use of sunscreen can increase your risks of developing skin cancer.

Signs and Symptoms of Skin Cancer

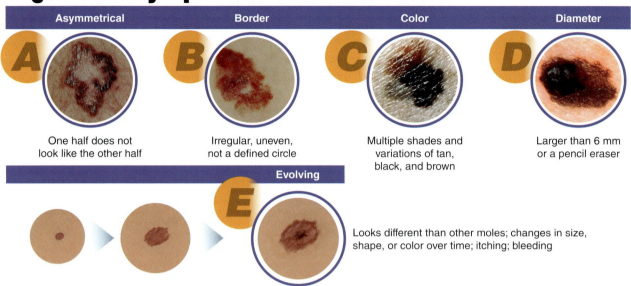

Asymmetrical	Border	Color	Diameter
One half does not look like the other half	Irregular, uneven, not a defined circle	Multiple shades and variations of tan, black, and brown	Larger than 6 mm or a pencil eraser

Evolving

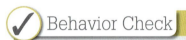

Looks different than other moles; changes in size, shape, or color over time; itching; bleeding

Figure 14.14 Use the ABCDE method of checking moles for signs and symptoms of skin cancer.

Reprinted from National Cancer Institute (1990).

✓ Behavior Check

Reduce Your Risk of Skin Cancer

College students and young adults spend a lot of time in the sun and at tanning salons because being tan is perceived as looking attractive and healthy. However, overexposure to ultraviolet radiation over many years causes not only skin cancer, but also premature aging and wrinkles, damage to the eyes, and other types of infections. You are at an increased risk of developing skin cancer if you have any of the following traits or behaviors (Centers for Disease Control and Prevention 2017):

- A lighter natural skin color
- Family history of skin cancer
- A personal history of skin cancer
- Exposure to the sun through work and play
- A history of sunburns, especially early in life
- A history of indoor tanning
- Skin that burns, freckles, reddens easily, or becomes painful in the sun
- Blue or green eyes
- Blond or red hair
- Certain types and a large number of moles

Think about your exposure to ultraviolet radiation and make a commitment to check your body every month for changes in moles or the development of new moles. Wear sunscreen and apply it often and try to stay out of the sun during the hottest times of the day, between 10 a.m. and 2 p.m.

benzene, radon, soot, tar, vinyl chloride, and ultraviolet light. The implementation of strict policies and laws preventing the use of these chemicals and substances has reduced the rates of some cancers associated with their use and long-term exposure. Until the 20th century, asbestos was used as insulation in homes, schools, and buildings. Many construction workers exposed to this substance developed lung cancer. Benzene causes an increase of leukemia, a blood cancer. Radon is a naturally occurring odorless gas that also increases the risk of lung cancer. It's found underground and can leak through the foundation in homes. Many health departments in the United States offer homeowners radon gas testing kits. Soot and tar can be found in many industrial settings. They cause lung, skin, and liver cancers. Environmental and occupational specialists work closely with businesses to make sure their employees are using protective gear, including masks, clothing, and sunscreen, to reduce their exposure to these chemicals and substances.

> Women who have a mother, sister, or daughter who has been diagnosed with breast cancer are about two times more likely to develop breast cancer when compared to women who do not have a family history (ACS 2017a).

Most Commonly Diagnosed Cancers

Tables 14.4 and 14.5 present the incidence, risk factors, warning signs, detection, treatment, and survival rates for the most commonly diagnosed cancers. You

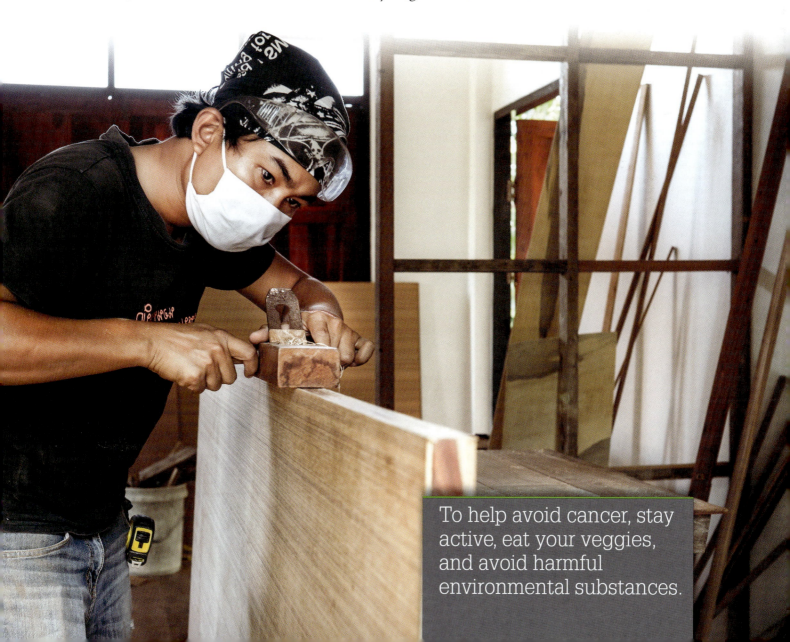

To help avoid cancer, stay active, eat your veggies, and avoid harmful environmental substances.

Table 14.4 Selected Cancers: Incidence, Risk Factors, and Warning Signs

Cancer site	Incidence trends	Risk factors	Warning signs
Lung Second most commonly diagnosed cancer and leading cause of cancer death in men and women	Rates declining annually: 2% in men and 1% in women	80% of lung cancer cases are caused by cigarette smoking and cigar and pipe use. Other causes are exposure to radon gas, second-hand smoke, organic chemicals, air pollution, and diesel exhaust; occupational hazards such as paving, roofing, painting, and chimney sweeping; and genetic predisposition	Symptoms appear in late stages: persistent cough, blood in mucus, chest pain, voice changes, shortness of breath, and recurrent pneumonia or bronchitis
Breast Most frequently diagnosed cancer in women Second leading cause of death in women	Rates stable in white women Increased .05% in black women	Overweight/obesity, postmenopausal hormone use (estrogen and progestin), physical inactivity, alcohol use, smoking, family history, genetic predisposition, high breast tissue density, type 2 diabetes, younger age at first menstrual period (before age 12) or late menopause (after age 55), use of oral contraceptives, never having had children or having a child after age 30	Lump or mass in breast; persistent changes in breast: thickening, swelling, distortion, tenderness, skin irritation, redness, scaliness, nipple abnormalities, nipple discharge
Colon/rectum Third most common cancer in men and women	Diagnosis rates have declined by 3% since 2004	Obesity, physical inactivity, smoking, high consumption of red meats, low calcium intake, alcohol use, diet low of fruits and vegetables, family history, genetic predisposition, history of ulcerative colitis or Crohn's disease	Typically does not have early symptoms; symptoms include rectal bleeding, blood in stool, change in bowel habits or stool shape, cramping in lower abdomen, decreased appetite, weight loss
Prostate Most commonly diagnosed cancer and third leading cause of cancer deaths in men	Risk is 74% higher in black men than white men	Increasing age, African heritage, family history, genetic predisposition, smoking	Early symptoms typically not present; advanced symptoms include weak or interrupted urine flow, urge to urinate more frequently, difficulty starting or stopping urine flow, blood in urine, pain or burning sensation when urinating, pain in hips, spine, or ribs
Cervix Increased cases due to infection with human papilloma virus (HPV)	Rates have declined by half since 1975	HPV, sexual intercourse beginning at an early age, multiple sexual partners, suppressed immune system, multiple childbirths, smoking, long-term oral contraceptive use	Abnormal vaginal bleeding, midcycle bleeding, menstrual bleeding that is heavier and longer than normal, bleeding or vaginal discharge after menopause, bleeding after intercourse, douching, or a pelvic exam

Data from American Cancer Society (2017a).

Table 14.5 Select Cancers: Screening Procedures, Detection, Treatment, and Survival Rate

Who should be screened	Test or procedure	Detection recommendation	Treatment options (always dependent on the stage of the cancer)	5-year survival rate
Lung Current or former smokers with a history of smoking 30+ packs per year	Low-dose helical CT	Begin at age 55 and continue through age 77 if patient is in good health; current smokers or those who have quit within the last 15 years should be screened	Surgery, radiation, chemotherapy, immunotherapy, targeted therapy	15% for men, 21% for women 55% if localized
Breast Women ages 40+	Mammography	Regular screening starting at age 45 Ages 45-54: screen annually Ages 55+: screen every 1 or 2 years	Surgical removal of tumor (lumpectomy), mastectomy (removal of breast), radiation post mastectomy, chemotherapy	90% 99% if localized
Colon/rectum Men and women ages 50+	gFOBT (Guaiac-based **fecal occult blood test**) or FIT (fecal immunochemical test) OR	Annual testing of stool; if positive, follow up with colonoscopy	Surgery is most common; chemotherapy alone or in combination with radiation	65% 90% if localized
	Stool DNA test OR	Every 3 years: if positive, follow up with colonoscopy		
	Flexible sigmoidoscopy OR	Every 5 years: if positive, follow up with colonoscopy		
	Double-contrast barium enema OR	Every 5 years: if positive, follow up with colonoscopy		
	Colonoscopy OR	Every 10 years		
	CT colonography	Every 5 years		
Prostate Age 50+ for men who are at average risk of prostate cancer and are expected to live at least 10 more years Age 45 at high risk: African Americans and men who have a first-degree relative (father, brother, or son) diagnosed with prostate cancer at an early age (younger than age 65) Age 40 higher risk: more than one first-degree relative who had prostate cancer at an early age	Prostate-specific antigen (PSA) with or without digital rectal examination (DRE)	Negative result: Future screenings depend on a PSA of less than 2.5 ng/mL retested every 2 years. Annual test if PSA level is 2.5 ng/mL or higher. Prostate cancer advances slowly. Men without symptoms with a life expectancy of less than 10 years would not benefit from PSA screening. Health status is the primary consideration related to screenings.	Depends on age; younger men and early stages: observation over time instead of treatment; surgery; external beam radiation, radioactive seed implants (brachytherapy), hormonal therapy with surgery or radiation	92% 100% if localized

> *continued*

Table 14.5 > *continued*

Who should be screened	Test or procedure	Detection recommendation	Treatment options (always dependent on the stage of the cancer)	5-year survival rate
Cervix Ages 21-29	Pap test	Every 3 years	Loop electrosurgical excision procedure (LEEP) to remove abnormal tissue, cryotherapy (destroy cells with extreme cold), laser ablation, conization (cone-shaped removal of abnormal tissue); invasive treated with surgery or radiation with chemotherapy; targeted therapy	69% for white women, 57% for black women 91% if localized
Ages 30-65	Pap test and HPV DNA test	Every 5 years		
Ages 66+	Pap test and HPV DNA test	No screenings recommended if results for at least 3 consecutive Pap tests were negative within the last 10 years or if results for more than 2 Pap and HPV tests were negative within the past 5 years		
Women who have had a total hysterectomy		No cervical cancer screenings recommended		

Data from American Cancer Society (2017a).

can discuss this information with your health care provider to decide when you should begin screenings based on your age, sex, lifestyle, and health behaviors.

Summary

So, now what? The bad news is that cancer can be fatal and not all cancers can be cured. Many research efforts are still focused on the prevention, detection, and treatment of cancers. The good news is that we know how to prevent many cancers, and there have been significant medical advancements in the early detection of cancer. More treatments exist that are specific to the type and stage of cancer, as well as new and improved medications and complementary therapies. Reducing your cancer risks means reducing your chances of getting cancer and having a great quality of life for decades to come!

WEB STUDY GUIDE

Remember to complete all of the web study guide activities to further facilitate your learning, including the following lab activities:

Lab 14.1   Preventing Cancer and Detecting It Early as a College Student

Lab 14.2   How Does Your Family Cancer History Affect Your Risk of Developing Cancer?

REVIEW QUESTIONS

1. What is the difference between benign and malignant tumors?
2. What does the acronym CAUTION mean?
3. List and describe the primary ways cancer can be treated.
4. What are the most commonly diagnosed cancers among men and among women?
5. Which cancers have the highest mortality rates?
6. What are the reasons for health disparities related to cancer prevention and treatment?
7. List environmental chemicals and substances that are linked to cancer.
8. What are the primary causes of cancer?

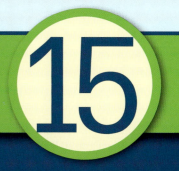

15

Fitness and Wellness: Today and Beyond

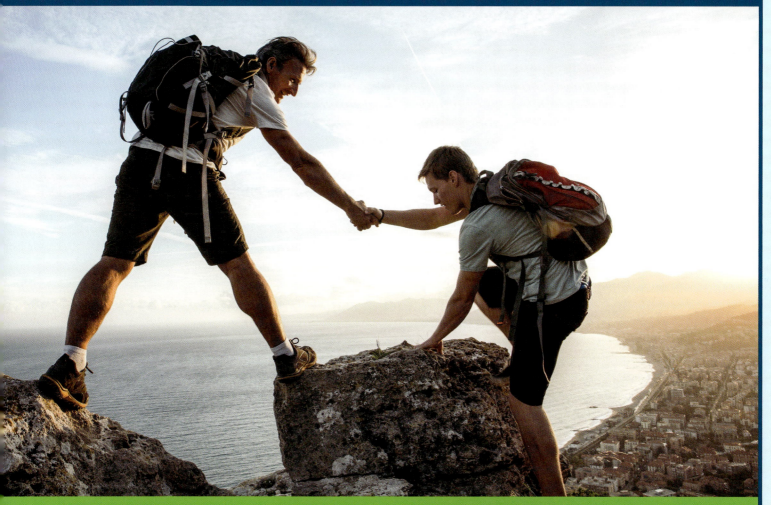

OBJECTIVES

❱ Revisit wellness concepts and SMART goals and apply them to future lifestyle choices.

❱ Understand the differences between chronological age, functional age, biological age, and psychological age.

❱ Define and discuss differences between conventional medical practices and complementary and alternative medicine (CAM).

❱ Introduce the use of activity trackers for measuring health parameters.

❱ Analyze the differences between fitness coaching and training.

❱ Map out a fitness and wellness plan for life.

KEY TERMS

activity trackers

biological age

chronological age

complementary and alternative medicine (CAM)

conventional medical practices

functional age

lifestyle coach

personal training

procrastination

psychological age

Living Well Over the Life Span

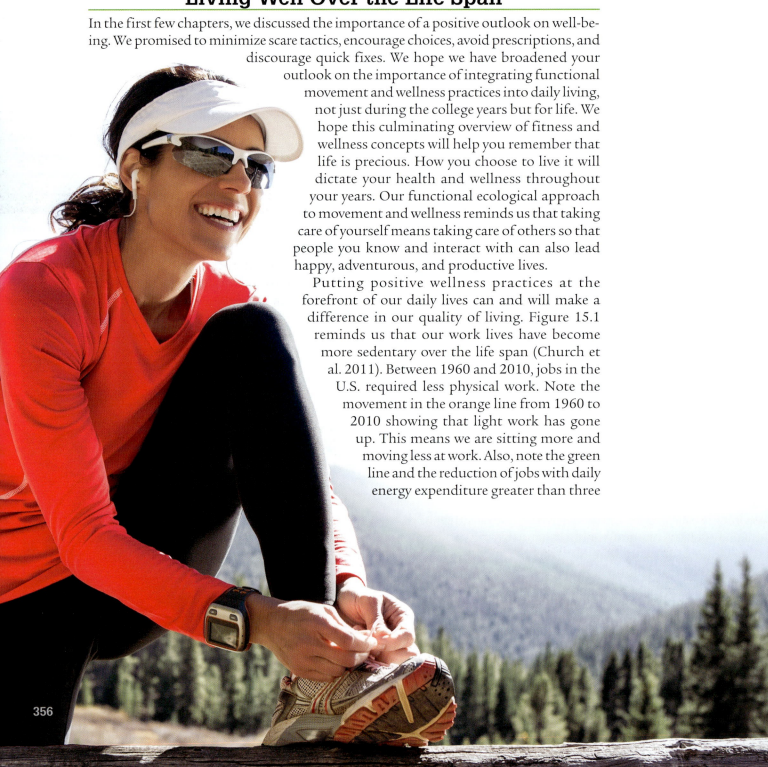

In the first few chapters, we discussed the importance of a positive outlook on well-being. We promised to minimize scare tactics, encourage choices, avoid prescriptions, and discourage quick fixes. We hope we have broadened your outlook on the importance of integrating functional movement and wellness practices into daily living, not just during the college years but for life. We hope this culminating overview of fitness and wellness concepts will help you remember that life is precious. How you choose to live it will dictate your health and wellness throughout your years. Our functional ecological approach to movement and wellness reminds us that taking care of yourself means taking care of others so that people you know and interact with can also lead happy, adventurous, and productive lives.

Putting positive wellness practices at the forefront of our daily lives can and will make a difference in our quality of living. Figure 15.1 reminds us that our work lives have become more sedentary over the life span (Church et al. 2011). Between 1960 and 2010, jobs in the U.S. required less physical work. Note the movement in the orange line from 1960 to 2010 showing that light work has gone up. This means we are sitting more and moving less at work. Also, note the green line and the reduction of jobs with daily energy expenditure greater than three

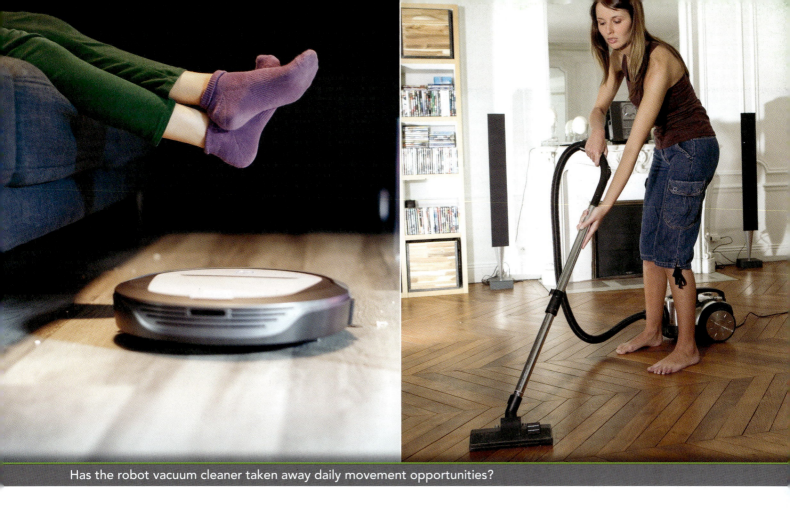

Has the robot vacuum cleaner taken away daily movement opportunities?

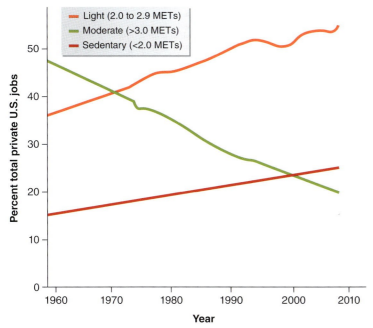

Figure 15.1 The reduction of activity levels in the workplace. Between 1960 and 2010, U.S. jobs required less physical work. Note the increase in light daily work versus the decrease in moderate daily work.

Reprinted by permission from T.S. Church et al., "Trends over 5 Decades in U.S. Occupation-Related Physical Activity and Their Associations with Obesity," *PLOS ONE* 6, no. 5 (2011): e19657. This is an open-access article distributed under the terms of the Creative Commons Attribution License.

METs from approximately 50 percent of U.S. jobs to less than 20 percent. Our jobs require less physical energy daily and involve more sitting.

In our daily lives, we also use dishwashers and robot vacuum cleaners, clap to turn our lights on and off, and have Alexa give us input instead of talking with a friend or colleague. The majority of the research introduced in this book tells us that in order to be well, we need to move more and sit less. The human movement paradigm introduced in chapter 2 reminds us of the triad of human movement: Daily movement, sitting less, and exercising are all a part of living well.

U.S. obesity rates are at an all-time high due to the decline in daily movement practices combined with poor nutritional choices. According to the Centers for Disease Control and Prevention (CDC), in the United States, obesity rates are less than 25 percent only in the states of Colorado, Hawaii, Massachusetts, and the District of Columbia (see figure 15.2).

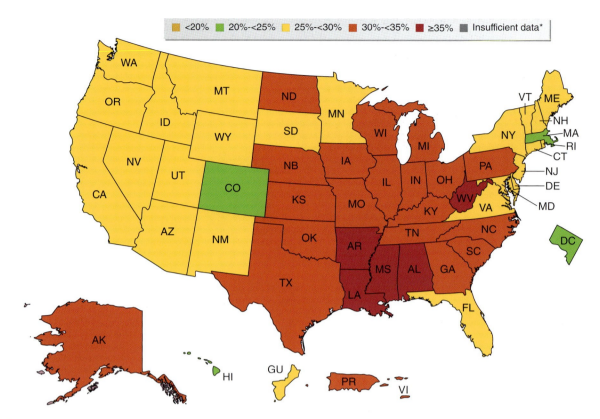

Figure 15.2 Obesity is on the rise in most U.S. states.

Reprinted from Centers for Disease Control and Prevention (2017).

Living Longer or Living Better?

In addition to moving less, we are living longer, but not necessarily better. According to the United Nations (2005), the number of elderly people will increase to 22 percent of the total U.S. population by 2050. Daley and Spinks (2000) reported that the average terminal age for men and women in 1980 was 69.8 and 77.5, respectively. They also reported that in 2040, life expectancy will be 75 years for men and 83 years for women. The choices you make now will dictate how well you live later in life. The landmark study by Paffenbarger and others (1986) that followed Harvard alumni ages 35 to 74 taught us that moving throughout the life span might add more years to your life.

> It is up to you to move more so that you can overcome the trend of sedentary living and live a longer, more independent life.

Consider figure 15.3. What will your life curve look like? The dotted green curve where you are active and healthy throughout your life span? The

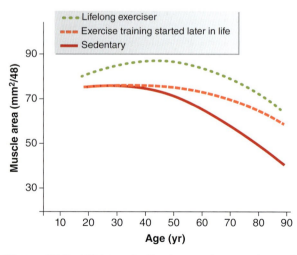

Figure 15.3 Lifelong decline in muscle area, depending on activity level. Starting and sticking with an active lifestyle will prolong physical decline later in life and can give you more years of life.

Reprinted by permission from J.F. Signorile, *Bending the Aging Curve: The Complete Exercise Guide for Older Adults* (Champaign, IL: Human Kinetics, 2011), 13.

orange dashed curve where you start moving later in life when you have a life event? The red curve where you have fewer years of life due to sedentary living? The choices you make throughout the life span matter in the grand scheme of a life well lived.

Differences Between Physiological and Chronological Age

According to Stanton (1996), there are differences between **chronological age**, **functional age**, **biological age**, and **psychological age**. Figure 15.4 provides definitions and examples of these terms. Think about what you want people to say about you as you go through various life stages. Do you want to be known as someone who has energy and zest for life or someone who has aches, pains, and physical and emotional problems?

Many of us have older relatives who constantly talk about their frequent visits to traditional medical facilities. We say to ourselves, "I'm not going to be like that when I am older." Yet if you do not take care of yourself now, that may be who you become. Based on the direction you are heading with your focus on your personal health and wellness, what do you think people will say about your chronological, biological, functional, and psychological age? Which of these categories would you say your parents or relatives fit into? Consider now the steps you want to take so that your various "ages" are not any older than your actual chronological age. What changes do you want to make in activity level, healthy eating, and stress management?

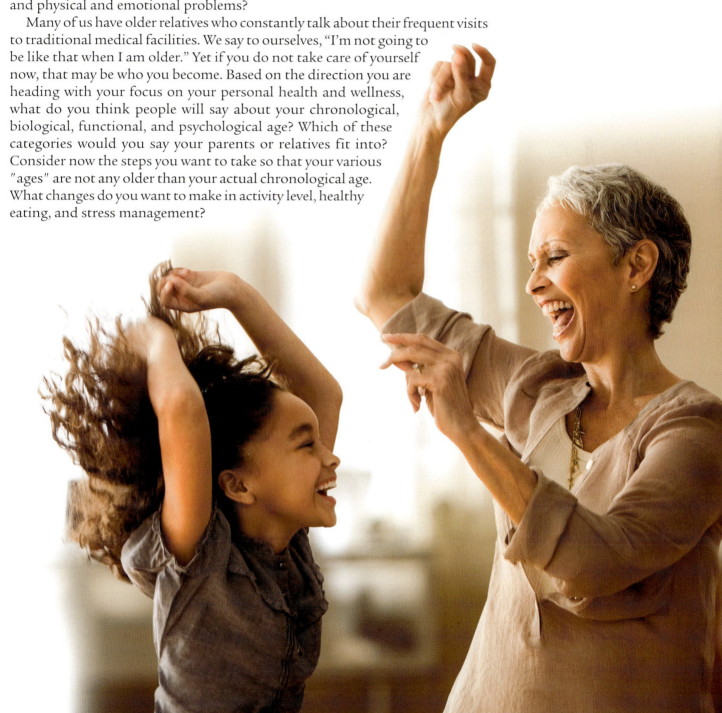

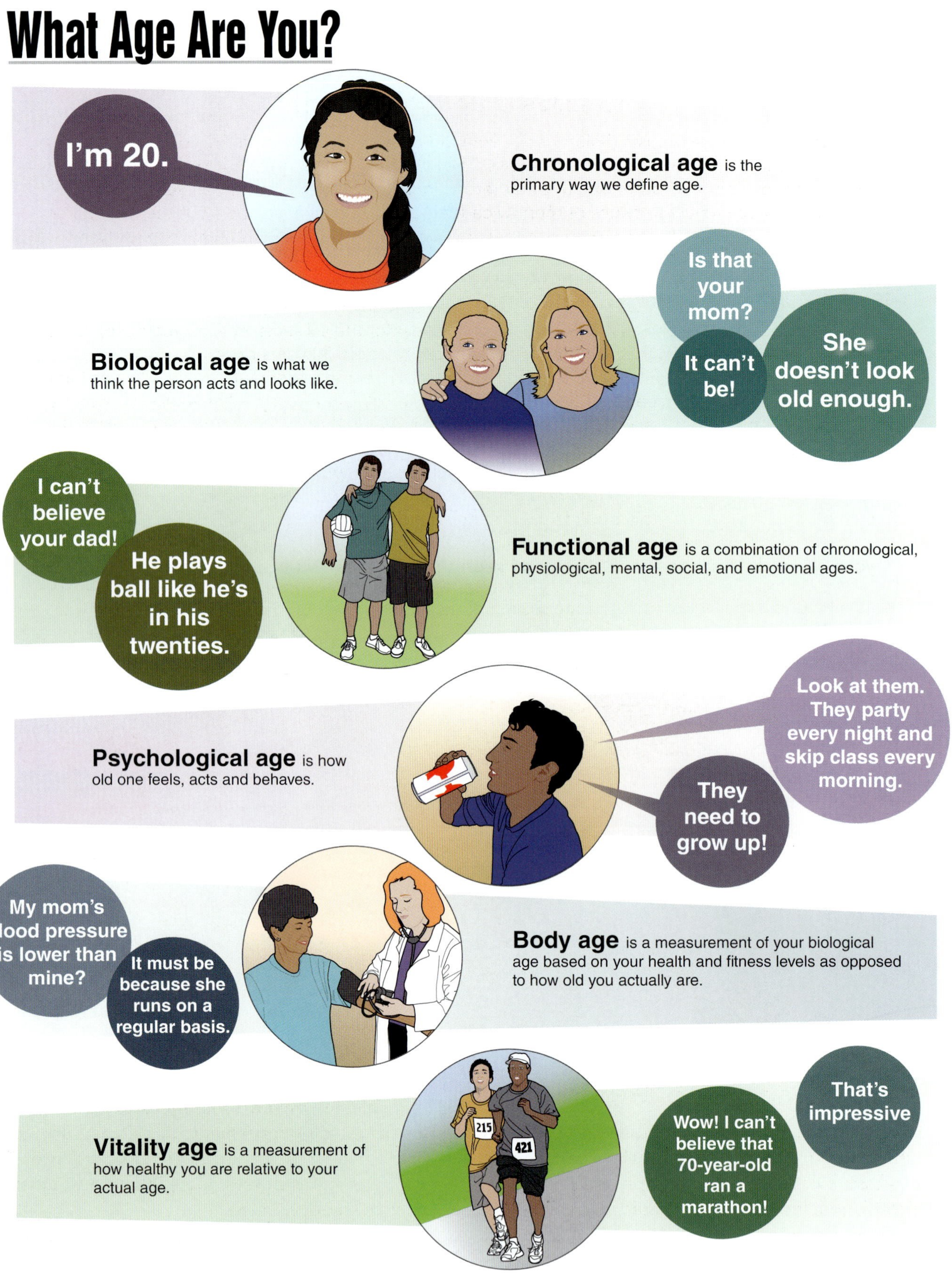

What Age Are You?

Chronological age is the primary way we define age.

I'm 20.

Biological age is what we think the person acts and looks like.

Is that your mom? It can't be! She doesn't look old enough.

Functional age is a combination of chronological, physiological, mental, social, and emotional ages.

I can't believe your dad! He plays ball like he's in his twenties.

Psychological age is how old one feels, acts and behaves.

Look at them. They party every night and skip class every morning. They need to grow up!

Body age is a measurement of your biological age based on your health and fitness levels as opposed to how old you actually are.

My mom's blood pressure is lower than mine? It must be because she runs on a regular basis.

Vitality age is a measurement of how healthy you are relative to your actual age.

Wow! I can't believe that 70-year-old ran a marathon! That's impressive

Figure 15.4 Age can be quantified in many different ways: chronological, biological, functional, and even psychological.

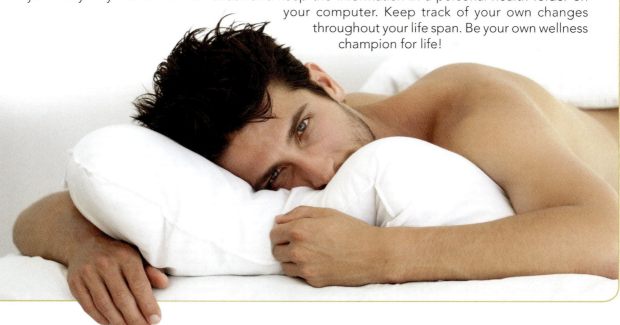

✓ Behavior Check

The Dallas Bed-Rest Study

In 1966, a group of scientists (Saltin et al. 1968) did an experiment where they paid five healthy 20-year-old men to lie in bed for three weeks. The scientists then analyzed the subjects' $\dot{V}O_2$max, body composition, and other health parameters. In just three weeks, these 20 year olds developed physiologic characteristics of men twice their age. The scientists then put the men on an eight-week exercise-training program following the bed rest. Exercise did more than reverse the bed-rest deterioration. This study was a demonstration of the dramatic effects of not moving followed by exercise training on fitness and health parameters.

Another identical study was performed on these same five men 30 years later (McGuire et al. 2001). The scientists found that three weeks of bed rest for the subjects, now 50 years old, had a more profound effect on their physical work capacity than did 30 years of aging.

Finally, McGavock and colleagues (2009) repeated this same experiment again 10 years later when the men were 60 years old: three weeks of bed rest followed by eight weeks of exercise training. The men's decline in cardiorespiratory fitness ($\dot{V}O_2$max) was comparable with what they experienced after three weeks of strict bed rest when they were 20.

These studies have influenced health care practices. Patients are now up and walking rather quickly post-surgery. The study also reminds us of the importance of exercising over the life span. Chapters 1 through 7 of this book focus on and test your physical capacity. Now that you have acquired this personal information on your physical abilities at a young age, consider retesting yourself yearly. Perform a well-check and keep the information in a personal health folder on your computer. Keep track of your own changes throughout your life span. Be your own wellness champion for life!

Approaches to Medicine

Conventional Western medicine is a system in which medical doctors and other health care professionals (such as nurses, pharmacists, physician's assistants, and therapists) treat symptoms and diseases. For example, if you need a knee replacement, the painful knee is thought to be fixed once it has been replaced and you have completed therapy after surgery. This type of medicine is also called allopathic medicine, biomedicine, **conventional medical practices**, or just plain mainstream medicine. Medical doctors, doctors of osteopathy, and allied health professionals, such as nurses and physical therapists, practice standard care.

Complementary and alternative medicine (CAM) can be used as an approach that honors your body as a system and works with it to heal you. Examples of alternative practices include homeopathy, nontraditional medicine, chiropractic treatment, yoga and tai chi practices, and acupuncture. According to the National Center for Complementary and Integrative Health (2017), almost 38 percent of adults and 12 percent of children have used some form of CAM. Figure 15.5 lists the 10 most common complementary healthy approaches for adults.

The type of complementary and alternative medicine that has seen the greatest increase is yoga (Clark et al. 2015). The use of yoga, tai chi, and qigong has increased linearly, with yoga accounting for approximately 80 percent of the prevalence. Yoga has also seen the highest improvement in percentage of adult participation since 1999.

Finally, as shown in figure 15.5, individual dietary supplements remained the most popular complementary health approach used. The use of some supplements such as glucosamine chondroitin, ginseng, and ginkgo have decreased. However, since 2002 the use of fish oil and omega-3 have nearly quadrupled (Barnes, Powell-Griner, McFann, and Nahin, 2004), and since 2007 the use of melatonin and probiotics and prebiotics have also increased (Barnes,

Bloom, and Nahin, 2008; Clarke, Black, Stussman, Barnes, and Nahin, 2015). Nearly 8 percent of Americans supplement with fish oil or omega-3, and nearly 2 percent use probiotics or prebiotics. Chapters 8 and 9 provide many details on nutrition practices. Many people use alternative nutritional approaches to stay healthy over their lifetime that are based on both traditional medical recommendations and a CAM practioner's advice.

CAM approaches have not gone through the same research rigor as double-blind clinical research trials of conventional medical practices. However, traditional approaches involving lab research may not fully apply to CAM because benefits of CAM involve not only physical health, but also mental and psychological health. It is difficult to conduct rigorous studies that evaluate both physical and social or psychological issues. Plus, CAM approaches tend to be more individual in their outcomes. Many people who feel better after CAM treatments cannot explain why. You may want to consider options for wellness that are less invasive. However, given the lack of research on the benefits, this is a choice best left up to the consumer at this point.

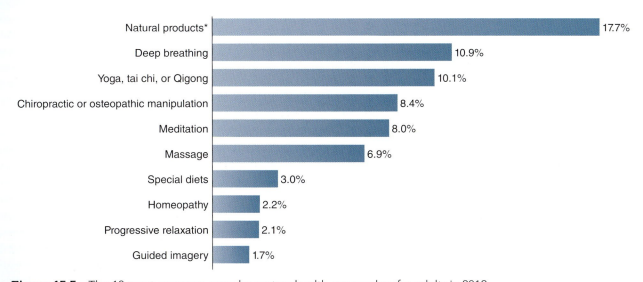

Figure 15.5   The 10 most common complementary health approaches for adults in 2012.
*Dietary supplements other than vitamins and minerals.
Reprinted from National Center for Complementary and Integrative Health (2016).

Finding Resources to Enhance Your Fitness and Wellness

One traditional way to improve your fitness and wellness is to hire a personal trainer to help you learn how to exercise. Fitness facilities across the nation offer **personal training**. Recall that the human movement paradigm discussed in chapter 2 includes physical activity, exercise, and minimal sedentary living (see figure 15.6). Personal trainers might speak with you about sedentary living

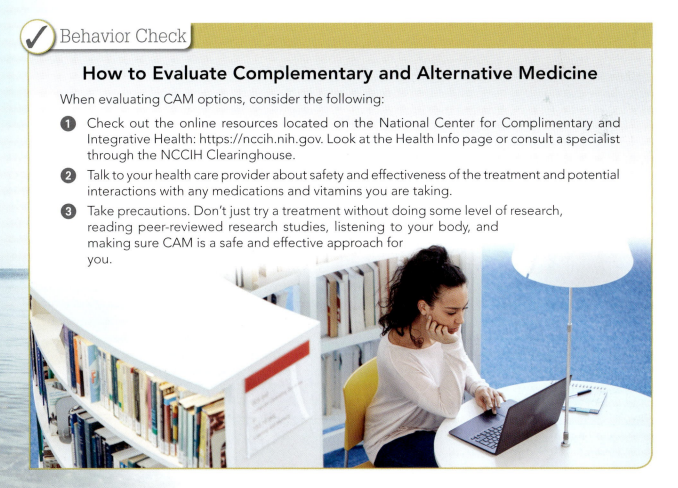

✓ Behavior Check

How to Evaluate Complementary and Alternative Medicine

When evaluating CAM options, consider the following:

1 Check out the online resources located on the National Center for Complimentary and Integrative Health: https://nccih.nih.gov. Look at the Health Info page or consult a specialist through the NCCIH Clearinghouse.

2 Talk to your health care provider about safety and effectiveness of the treatment and potential interactions with any medications and vitamins you are taking.

3 Take precautions. Don't just try a treatment without doing some level of research, reading peer-reviewed research studies, listening to your body, and making sure CAM is a safe and effective approach for you.

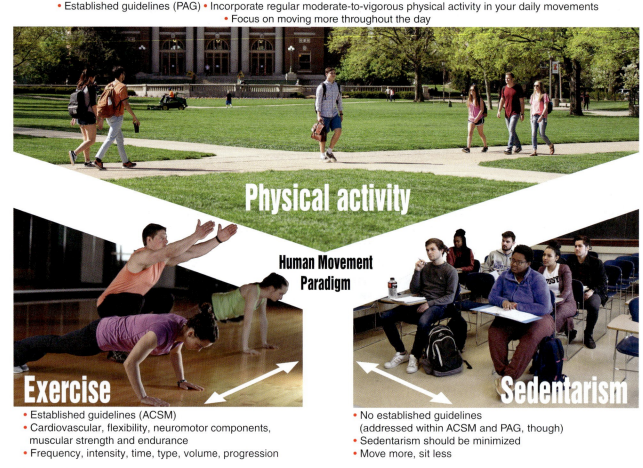

Figure 15.6 The human movement paradigm, incorporating physical activity, exercise, and minimal sedentary living.

and physical activity, but remember that they are employed by exercise facilities, so they often focus on exercise routines using the facility's equipment. Consider purchasing an activity tracker to monitor your sedentary living and daily physical movement habits.

Activity Trackers

The ACSM named wearable technology within the top five trends for 2018 (Thompson 2017). Sales of **activity trackers** have tripled (Endeavour Partners 2014), and by 2019, the smart wearable market could generate $53 billion in sales. The wearable technology revolution is changing from day to day, making it challenging to find evidence-based research. Research is generally not keeping up with the technology changes. A review by Duncan and colleagues (2017) revealed that activity trackers hold promise for increasing physical activity, but much more research is needed to analyze the long-range effect of these

devices on movement behavior and outcomes. Wrist-worn devices have become the most predominant choice of consumers. Activity trackers can be multidimensional, focusing on many of the behavioral aspects that affect a person's health and well-being beyond movement, including sleep and nutrition tracking.

Michelle Segar's 2015 book, *No Sweat*, describes numerous accounts of clients who did not know that moving throughout the day counted toward health and fitness. Many of her clients thought the only way to get fit was to join a fitness facility. Activity trackers can offer you objective accountability as well as a social outlet. They may be a game changer for a population-based explosion of movement.

Activity Trackers as an Alternative to Fitness Centers?

The majority of Americans have not joined a fitness center or facility. According to Tharrett and

Peterson (2017), less than 22 percent of the U.S. population has joined and regularly attended a fitness facility in the last 25 years. The obvious barriers to using a formal fitness program or facility are cost, discomfort using equipment, or difficulty attending classes at a specific time or day. A recognized benefit to using activity trackers is the reduction of many of these barriers. Inactive people might find using an activity tracker less intimidating than joining a fitness facility. Technology experts believe that wearable activity trackers will be important for facilitating physical movement among people who do not use traditional physical activity and fitness services (Herz 2014).

Activity Trackers in Combination With Coaching

Personal activity trackers combined with professional coaching may have the potential to change behavior (Sforzo et al. 2015), although a solid evidence-based research study is lacking at this time. Theoretically, personal activity trackers promote awareness, hold users accountable for movement goals, and record movement in an easy and convenient manner. Research suggests that fitness professionals lack the knowledge about tracker usage to facilitate movement change with their clients (Green 2015); therefore, you should look for a professional who not only knows how activity trackers work but also understands the human movement paradigm and coaching concepts. Research found that coaches had more success working with clients who had activity trackers after both parties had acquired personal experience using the devices (Kiessling and Kennedy-Armbruster 2016). Activity trackers can assist you in behavior change by helping you set more realistic movement goals that are specific to how you move within the demands of your own life. They can also prompt you to move more and sit less. For example, Mandic and others (2009) found that people on the low end of the fitness spectrum who used activity trackers to increase habitual movement gained confidence to exercise more.

Personal Trainers

If you are already physically active and want to enhance your exercise options, working with a personal trainer may be effective for you. Working with a personal trainer can be especially helpful if you join a fitness facility and want to learn how to use equipment to train.

Personal Training Credentialing Process

Before you hire a personal trainer, be sure that he or she has a professional fitness certification approved by the National Commission for Certifying Agencies (NCCA). Many national certifications include both written and practical examinations for which a fitness professional must demonstrate basic skills in exercise leadership and knowledge of its related components (e.g., anatomy and physiology, intensity

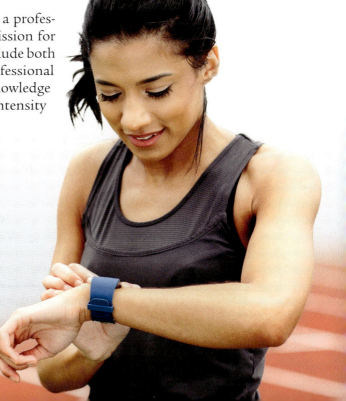

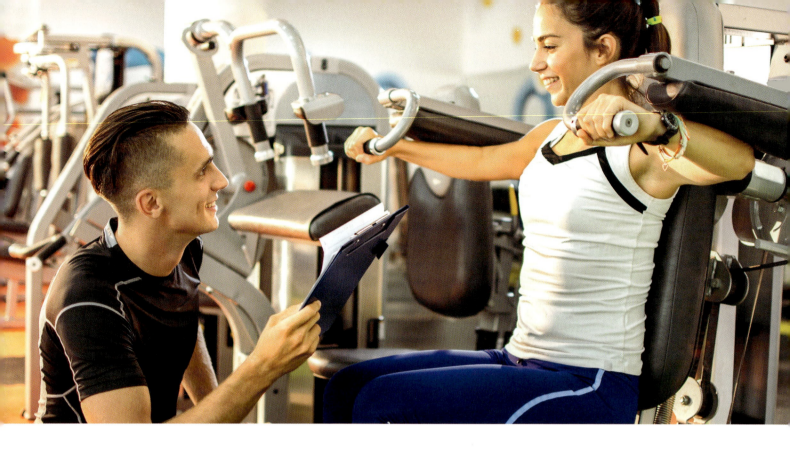

monitoring, injury prevention). NCCA-accredited certification tests are developed by exercise and fitness professionals based on specific knowledge, skills, and attributes necessary to enhance healthy movement practices and prevent injury. Local or in-house certifications or training programs may not be rigorous enough to meet clinical practice standards. All NCCA-accredited fitness certifications also involve cardiopulmonary resuscitation (CPR) and automated external defibrillator (AED) training.

CREP is a nonprofit corporation composed of organizations that offer NCCA-accredited exercise certifications. Coalition members collectively seek to advance the fitness profession. The mission of CREP is to secure recognition of registered exercise professionals for their distinct roles in medical, health, fitness, and sports performance fields. Use both the NCCA accreditation and CREP websites when looking for fitness professionals. If you already have a personal trainer, look them up on this registry and see if they are certified by an accredited organization.

> One of the best ways to know if an exercise professional has an NCCA-accredited certification is to check the United States Registry of Exercise Professionals at www.usreps.org.

Personal Training and Lifestyle Coaching

Once you have determined that your hired personal trainer is qualified and trained, the next step is to do an interview to see if he or she is more of a personal trainer, a **lifestyle coach**, or both. If you prefer instruction and motivation, check out a facility that offers small group training. It helps to be trained in a small group so you can venture out on your own eventually. New HIIT programs and facilities that offer group instruction and motivation (like Orangetheory Fitness) are popping up. Personal trainers will help you learn how to use equipment correctly and can also help design a training program for you, but once you know what to do, motivation and commitment become the key drivers of success. You can stay motivated and committed by having a friend work out with you or working with a coach who checks in on your goals and holds you accountable to them.

When you look into a personal trainer's background, be sure to look for coaching training. Certified coaches are trained differently than certified personal fitness trainers. Coaches are trained in behavioral theory that is grounded in holding you accountable to your own goals. Personal trainers can teach you how to do movements in a strength and conditioning area and also adapt a fitness program to your needs. Certified coaches, on the other hand, work more on the behavioral aspects of changing your perspective on movement and exercise and setting realistic goals. Make sure you know the ultimate goal of the personal trainer you select and also check to see if he or she has been trained in coaching techniques. This will help you find out if you are getting the instruction you need to continue on the pathway toward consistent movement and exercise adherence.

Specific Wellness Concepts and SMART Goals Revisited

Let's take a moment to revisit the SMART fitness and wellness goals you established earlier in chapters 2 and 3. Look at your goal or goals. Did you accomplish them? Most of us start our fitness and wellness journeys with physical goals because they seem to be the easiest to start with. Now that you have learned more about broader wellness concepts such as healthy body composition, stress, addiction, sexuality, and metabolic syndrome, you can reflect on how these concepts fit into your overall fitness and wellness plan. This reflection will help you complete lab 15.1.

Wellness is more than looking good and being fit; it is about pondering your dreams and looking at your values while setting specific SMART goals to help you on your journey.

- Imagine that for body composition, you set a weight range of 10 to 15 pounds (4.5 to 6.8 kg) that you want to try to stick with over your lifetime. Hold yourself accountable to that range by weighing yourself monthly.

- For stress, consider getting an activity tracker that tracks sleep so you can see if you are sleeping well.

- What kind of overall life changes are you going to make to reduce metabolic syndrome in your lifetime?

- Are you determined to improve your daily food choices to make the healthy choice the easy choice? What specific behaviors will you work on first?

These ideas are larger picture items to ponder as you finalize your thoughts on *Fitness and Wellness: A Way of Life*. Lab 15.1 relates to revisiting your SMART goals from chapters 2 and 3, keeping them in a place where you can continually revisit them. Let's take a minute to think about procrastination before we finish with a review of your SMART goals.

Procrastination

Now that we have reviewed some of the larger wellness concepts related to living well throughout the life span, let's focus on a specific trait that can sabotage you from "just doing it." That trait is **procrastination**. You

> Personal training is about transferring knowledge and skills related to fitness instruction and goal setting, while lifestyle coaching is about behavioral skill development and being coached to set your own personal goals.

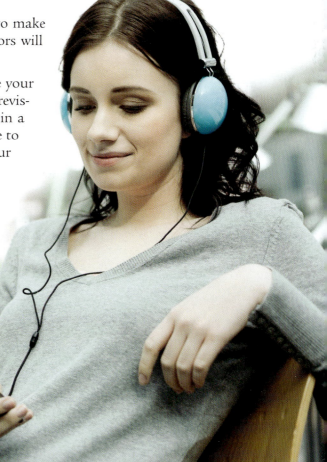

> Every day spent procrastinating is another day spent worrying about that thing. Do it *now* and move on with your life.

may be thinking, "It's all fine and good that we've learned about wellness concepts, but I think I'll start working on my wellness tomorrow." Lack of motivation is a key factor in procrastination.

It is generally quite easy to work on wellness concepts when you are with a group or enrolled in a class; goal setting on your own can be a bigger challenge. Think about one or two specific things related to your own personal wellness that you procrastinate on. If you are not a procrastinator, think of a time in the past when this was a problem for you. Do you know why you procrastinate? For many people, it a puzzle. You tell yourself that you really want to work on a wellness lifestyle, but for some mysterious reason, you just cannot seem to get around to it. We all have our own reasons why we tend to forget about our fitness and wellness goals. There are many online procrastination tests that you can take if this is something you feel you need to consider. Perform a Google search of procrastination short tests, and see how you fair on this issue, if you feel it might affect your overall goal setting in lab 15.1.

Healthy People 2030 and Beyond

As health care continues to evolve as a result of the political system, it is hard to predict what will happen to the larger picture of health insurance in the United States. Young adults under the age of 26 years old are able to stay on their parent's health care plan for now. Therefore, this section does not discuss how to make sure you have medical insurance but rather encourages you to ask questions and know where your health insurance is coming from.

Planning for Healthy People 2030, the fifth edition of the initiative, is underway. It will continue to produce new challenges and build on lessons learned from the past. The initiative began in 1979 when the Surgeon General issued a report on reducing preventable death and injury. This report included objectives for national health promotion and disease-prevention goals for the United States. The report continues to be updated. Visit www.healthypeople.gov for the most recent progress update.

It is important to think globally but work locally. What each person contributes is what make us better as a whole. How will you continue to contribute to your health and well-being?

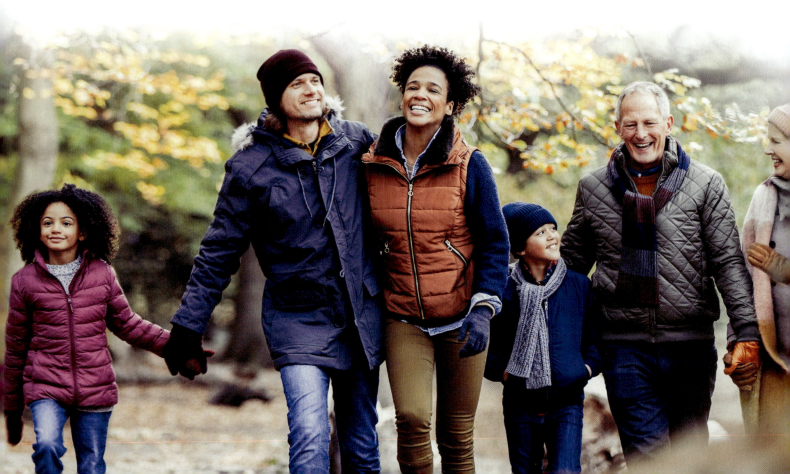

Fitness and Wellness: A Way of Life

The goal of this book is to provide you with information and experiences to help you set your own goals and priorities related to fitness and wellness daily practices. If you have implemented any of the information from this book, you are on your way to attaining a higher quality of life. Just as the section on Functional Movement Training after chapter 6 gives you choices for fitness movements, you, too, have a choice whether to make your health and wellness a lifelong priority.

Take a moment to reflect back on the initial goal you set based on your fitness pre- and post-testing goals. How did you do? Did you meet your goals or not? What worked and what did not work? How will you continue your goals in the future? What did you implement that really worked? Your next steps might be integrating this fitness goal into a wellness goal, thus considering content from the wellness portion in the later chapters of the book. Do you want to reduce stress, improve your nutrition practices, sleep better, or improve your relationships with others?

The following are ideas for wellness goals:

- Reduce stress by organizing a walking study session with friends.
- Consider activities where you might meet a life partner, such as through a volunteer activity where you are helping others rather than drinking in a bar.
- Make healthy eating choices 80 percent of the time so you feel and think better.
- Walk to your classes so your body will be physically tired at the end of the day, allowing you to sleep better.

What do you need to do to stay healthy and well? How might you overcome life's challenges in the future to keep your health a priority? In lab 15.1, you will map your integrated fitness and wellness plan. We hope as you chart your life career path, you will also integrate your fitness and wellness plan. Finding a career is one aspect of college life. Fitting your personal fitness and wellness goals into your life plan helps you bridge the gap between these two important life happenings. Keep in mind that doing fitness and wellness best practices is a process. We are all a work in progress. If you continue to put your best foot forward and work to improve the quality of your life (which ultimately may improve your longevity), you will reap the benefits of a life well lived. We wish you well as you continue to make forward-thinking choices toward your own fitness and wellness way of life.

WEB STUDY GUIDE

Remember to complete all of the web study guide activities to further facilitate your learning, including **Lab 15.1: Mapping Your Fitness and Wellness Plan for Life**.

REVIEW QUESTIONS

1. Between 1960 and 2010 (Church et al., 2011) found some interesting findings about our daily movement habits. What did their research discover?

2. Lists three things that have been invented to save time and energy and replace something we used to do physically ourselves (no specific right answer here; please list examples).

3. What happened to the men tested in the Dallas Bedrest study when they were 20 years old, 50 years old, and 60 years old?

4. What's the difference between chronological age and biological age?

5. What's the difference between functional age and psychological age?

6. "I think I'll start on that goal tomorrow" is an example of what personal trait?

7. How is a personal trainer different from a lifestyle coach?

GLOSSARY

abstinence—The choice not to engage in any type of sexual activity, which may include oral sex, anal intercourse, or vaginal intercourse.

ACSM exercise guidelines—The American College of Sports Medicine (ACSM) provides evidence-based recommendations categorized into cardiorespiratory exercise, resistance exercise, flexibility exercise, and neuromotor exercise to help the general public approach intentional exercise practices.

action stage of change—A process of change within the TTM theory of behavior change. In this stage, the behavior change is attained and you are actively engaged in the behavior change.

activity trackers—A device or application for monitoring and tracking fitness-related data such as distance walked or run, nutritional information, and in some cases heartbeat and quality of sleep.

addiction—When someone becomes dependent on a drug, alcohol, or a behavior (e.g., exercising) and cannot stop despite the negative effects.

adenosine triphosphate (ATP)—The energy source for cellular processes.

adenosine triphosphate–phosphocreatine (ATP-PC) system—The energy system that supplies immediate but limited energy to muscle cells through the breakdown of cellular stores of ATP and creatine phosphate (CP).

adiposity—An expression of how much stored energy, or fat, the body contains, similar to the term *body fat*.

adrenal glands—Endocrine glands are located near the kidneys that produce several hormones important for the stress response, including adrenaline and cortisol.

adrenocorticotropic hormone (ACTH)—In the stress cascade, ACTH stimulates the release of cortisol from the cortex of the adrenal gland.

air displacement plethysmography—A technique for measuring body density that uses air displacement rather than water.

allostatic balance (allostasis)—The process of achieving stability (or balance), or homeostasis, through physiological or behavioral change.

allostatic load—The wear and tear on the body that results from chronic stress; the physiological consequences of chronic exposure to changing or elevated neuroendocrine response.

anabolic-androgenic steroids (AAS)—Synthetic variations of the male hormone testosterone that both build muscle and provide male sexual characteristics.

angina—A condition caused by a reduced blood supply to the heart muscle; typically characterized as severe pain or pressure in the chest that often spreads to the shoulders, arms, and neck.

anorexia—An eating disorder characterized by low weight, fear of gaining weight, and a strong desire to be thin that results in food restriction.

antioxidants—Substance found in food that can block the formation and action of free radicals and repair damage that they cause.

areola—Darker skin around the nipple of the breast.

arrhythmias—A condition in which the heartbeats with an irregular or abnormal rhythm.

arteriosclerosis—A condition whereby the walls of the arteries are thickened and hardened; typically occurs with advanced age.

atherosclerosis—A disease of the arteries that can occur anywhere in the body; characterized by the deposition of plaques of fatty material on the inner walls of the vessels that, when advanced, reduces blood flow.

autonomic nervous system (ANS)—The main branch of the nervous system that is responsible for control of bodily functions not under direct conscious control, such as breathing, heart beating, and digestion.

barrier birth control methods—Pregnancy prevention methods that provide a barrier that inhibits sperm from fertilizing the egg (e.g., male or female condom).

behavioral addiction—Certain behaviors, like gambling or compulsive shopping, that become chronic and out of control; can cause the same euphoric feelings as abusing drugs or other substances.

benign—A tumor that is not cancerous.

binge drinking—Drinking alcohol with the intention of getting drunk by consuming large quantities over a short period of time.

binge-eating disorder—An eating disorder characterized by frequent and recurrent episodes of eating much faster than normal, until uncomfortably full, when not hungry, and sometimes with subjective loss of control.

bioelectrical impedance analysis (BIA)—A technique that measures body composition by sending a small electrical current through the body and measuring the resistance to the current, which relates to water content of the body.

biological age—A measure of how well or poorly your body is functioning relative to your actual calendar age.

biopsy—The surgical removal of a benign or malignant tumor.

birth control methods—Methods that prevent a fertilized egg from implanting into the uterine wall.

blood alcohol concentration (BAC)—The level of alcohol that can be detected in the blood after drinking.

body composition—The makeup of the body; often expressed in percentages of fat, muscle, and bone.

body dysmorphic disorder—A mental disorder characterized by the obsessive idea that some aspect of one's own appearance is severely flawed and requires exceptional measures to hide or fix it. The appearance flaw is either imagined or severely exaggerated.

body image—How you see yourself in the mirror or when you picture yourself in your mind; encompasses your beliefs about your appearance, how you evaluate yourself, and how you sense and control your body.

body mass index (BMI)—A weight-to-height ratio calculated by dividing weight in kilograms by height in meters squared; used to assess weight status.

bone density T-score—The number of standard deviations that your bone density is above or below what is normal for a healthy young adult of your sex (i.e., someone with peak bone mass); a proxy for bone strength.

bulbourethral glands (Cowper's glands)—Small glands in men that contribute to the fluid in semen.

bulimia nervosa—An eating disorder characterized by binge eating followed by purging, either by vomiting or laxatives.

cancer—A mass of cells that have characteristics of uncontrolled growth and large nuclei, vary in shape and size, and develop into a malignant tumor.

carbohydrates—An essential nutrient typically found in sugar, starch, or dietary fiber; provides 4 kilocalories per gram.

carcinogen—An agent that is capable of causing permanent damage to the molecular structure of the cell's DNA, causing cancer.

carcinogenesis—The process in which healthy cells become cancerous cells.

carcinoma in situ—Cancerous cells that have not penetrated any layers of tissues and are confined to the area of the originating cells.

cardiorespiratory endurance—The ability of the circulatory and respiratory systems to supply oxygen during sustained physical activity.

cardiorespiratory fitness—The ability to perform large muscle movements during exercise or physical activity for a sustained period of time.

cardiovascular disease (CVD)—Most often refers to conditions that involve narrowed or blocked blood vessels that lead to a reduction in blood flow.

central nervous system (CNS) depressants—A drug that lowers or depresses normal functioning in the body along the central nervous system of the brain and spinal cord.

chemotherapy—Powerful medications that are introduced into the body in the form of pills or liquids administered through an IV, infusion, or injection; designed to stop the cancer cells from reproducing, which prevents the tumor from growing larger and spreading to other sites in the body.

cholesterol—A waxy, fatlike substance that is found in cells of the body and acts as precursor of steroid compounds; an important part of cell membranes.

chronic diseases—A disease that lasts greater than three months, cannot be prevented with vaccines or cured by medication, and does not go away on its own.

chronic systemic inflammation—A condition due to the release of pro-inflammatory cytokines from immune system cells and the chronic elevation of the innate immune system that can contribute to the development or progression of chronic diseases, including heart disease.

chronological age—The number of years a person has been alive.

circumcision—Surgical removal of the extra skin (foreskin) around the glans (head) of the penis.

clitoris—Small organ made of erectile tissue located at the top of the vulva that develops from the same embryonic tissue as the penis. Its only function is sensitivity to sexual stimulation.

club drugs—Psychoactive drugs that cause hallucinogenic effects and lowered inhibitions; examples include MDMA and Rohypnol.

cocaine—A psychoactive drug that is very addictive and derived from coca leaves.

complementary and alternative medicine (CAM)—Medical products and practices that are not part of standard medical care.

complete protein—A protein that contains all of the essential amino acids.

complex carbohydrates—Made of sugar molecules connected together in long, complex chains.

connective tissue—The parts of the body (such as ligaments, tendons, and cartilage) that support and hold together the other parts of the body (such as muscles, organs, and bones).

contemplation stage of change—A process of change within the TTM theory of behavior change. In this stage, you are intending to start the healthy behavior in the next six months.

contraception—Devices and techniques used to prevent pregnancy, specifically preventing the sperm and egg from uniting.

conventional medical practices—The current form of medical treatment, focused on treating illnesses, that is widely used and practiced by health care professionals.

coronary artery (heart) disease (CAD or CHD)—Commonly called heart disease, CAD is the blockage of arteries that supply the heart muscle due to atherosclerosis.

corticotropin-releasing hormone (CRH)—In response to stress, CRH is released from the hypothalamus; it binds to corticotropic-releasing hormone receptors and stimulates the release of adrenocorticotropic hormone from the pituitary gland.

cortisol—In the glucocorticoid class of hormones; primarily released from the adrenal glands during the stress response and often called the stress hormone.

C-reactive protein (CRP)—A common marker of chronic systemic inflammation; located in the blood.

decisional balance—A method of weighing the pros and cons of making an individual change to see if you are ready to invest the time and effort to do it.

dependence—When someone who uses addictive substances cannot stop using them, is unable to complete daily tasks, and has mental health problems as a result of substance use.

depression—A common but serious mood disorder with symptoms presenting for at least two weeks that affects how a person feels, thinks, or handles daily activities such as sleeping, eating, or working.

diabetes—A chronic disease that occurs when the pancreas cannot make insulin or when the insulin the body produces does not work very well, resulting in high blood sugar.

diastole—Relaxation or filling phase of the heart.

dietary fats—Also commonly called dietary lipids, this nutrient class typically comes from tropical oils and animal and plant sources in our contemporary diets; provides 9 kilocalories per gram.

dose–response association—Concept related to physical activity and exercise whereby a greater volume or intensity of training causes greater health and fitness benefits.

drug abuse—When an individual takes a drug not as prescribed or intended consistently and over a long period of time.

drug misuse—When a drug is taken for reasons other than as intended.

dual-energy X-ray absorptiometry (DEXA)—A technique that measures body composition (fat, lean soft tissue [muscle], and bone mass) and density using a small dose of radiation to produce an image of the body.

dynamic stretching—A type of movement routine in which momentum and active muscular effort are used to stretch a muscle and the end position is not held (e.g., walking lunges).

ectopic fat—Fat depots in the body that are not primary and are located in an abnormal place, such as in the liver or around the heart.

ectopic pregnancy—When a fertilized egg settles in the Fallopian tube or the peritoneal cavity instead of the uterus.

ejaculation—The ejection of semen from a man's body through the penis.

ejaculatory duct—Small vessels that transport the sperm out of a man's body through the prostate and the urethra.

embryo—The beginning stage of cells that represent an undeveloped fetus that has implanted into the uterine wall.

endocrine system—The glands in the body that secrete hormones directly into the circulatory system to be carried to target organs.

endometrium—The lining of the uterus where an embryo implants for nourishment and grows; a blood lining that is released during a woman's period if no embryo is present.

endoscopy—A physician inserts a thin, lighted, flexible tube, called an endoscope, into internal body cavities to check for cancer.

endothelium—A thin layer of cells that lines the interior surface of the blood vessels and lymphatic vessels, forming an interface between circulating blood and the rest of the vessel wall.

energy balance—The relationship between calories taken in through foods and drinks and energy expended, typically expressed as calories per day.

energy density—The number of calories per gram of food.

epididymis—System of small ducts that is the site of sperm maturation in the testes.

epinephrine—Sometimes called adrenalin; a hormone secreted by the medulla of the adrenal glands that is responsible for increased heart rate and blood pressure and other responses that prepare the body for fight or flight.

erection—When the cavernous tissue in the penis becomes dilated with blood and the penis becomes hard.

ergogenic—In the context of exercise or sport, a technique or substance that enhances performance.

essential fat—Minimally required fat for health, especially reproductive function in women.

exercise—Bodily exertion for the sake of developing and maintaining physical fitness. Specific guidelines have been established by the ACSM.

exercise addiction—A state characterized by a compulsive engagement in any form of physical exercise, despite having negative consequences that could include physical injuries or problems in one's professional life or personal relationships.

Fallopian tubes—Pair of tubes along which eggs travel from the ovaries to the uterus.

fast-twitch fiber—White muscle fibers that have a faster contraction speed but fatigue more easily.

fecal occult blood test—A test physicians recommend to check for blood in stool (fecal matter).

female athlete triad—A syndrome of three interrelated conditions, including energy deficiency with or without disordered eating, menstrual disturbances, and bone loss or osteoporosis.

fertilization—The process of the combining of the sperm and egg.

fetus—Term used to describe a baby in utero during the gestational period spanning from two months after conception to birth.

fight-or-flight response—Also termed the acute stress response, this is a physiological reaction coordinated by the neurological and endocrine systems that occurs in response to an actual or perceived harmful event or threat to survival.

flexibility—The range of motion in a joint or group of joints or the ability to move joints effectively through a complete range of motion.

free radical—A chemically unstable molecule produced from natural metabolic processes of various fats and proteins that, once formed, can react with other fats, proteins, and DNA, damaging cell membranes and mutating genes; have been implicated in aging, cancer, and other degenerative diseases.

functional age—An idea that rests on the premise that a measure other than chronological age could better reflect one's position in the aging process.

functional fitness—Sometimes referred to as neuromotor training; involves balance, agility, coordination, and proprioceptive training in combination.

functional movement—The choices you make on a regular basis related to incorporating movement into daily living activities.

functional fitness training—Training your core and assisting muscles to work together by simulating common movements you might do at home, at work, or in sports; helps with stability and prepares the body for daily tasks.

generalized anxiety disorder—A disorder when a person feels extremely worried or nervous about events in life when there is little reason to worry; causes uncontrollable anxiety and reduces focus on daily tasks.

gestational diabetes—A specific type of diabetes that occurs during pregnancy and is a result of pregnancy hormones and other lifestyle behaviors that contribute to insulin resistance.

glucose—A simple sugar within the bloodstream that is broken down to produce ATP.

glycemic index—A relative ranking of carbohydrate in foods based on how slowly or quickly the foods cause increases in blood glucose levels. A value of 100 represents the standard, an equivalent of pure glucose.

glycogen—The form of glucose stored in the liver and skeletal muscles for rapid delivery to muscles; it is broken down to produce ATP.

gonads—Sex organs in men (testes) and women (ovaries).

health span—The length of time that a person is not only alive but also healthy.

heart failure—Sometimes referred to as chronic or congestive, this condition is due to an impairment in the pumping ability of the heart due to structural or functional abnormalities. This impairment compromises blood circulation to the rest of the body and causes abnormal fluid levels within various tissues, including in the lower legs and lungs.

heart rate reserve (HRR) method—HRR is the difference between maximal heart rate and resting heart rate; often used to determine exercise intensity.

hemorrhagic stroke—Occurs when a blood vessel in the brain breaks or ruptures, causing damage to brain cells; most commonly occurs due to high blood pressure and a weakness in the artery wall.

heroin—A highly addictive white powder derived from morphine that has a sedative effect on the body but causes a euphoric feeling.

HHS Physical Activity Guidelines—This organization recommends performing 150 minutes of cumulative movement per week in any sequence of bouts, focusing on moving more throughout the day.

high-density lipoprotein cholesterol (HDL-C)—A subtype of cholesterol in the blood known to act as a scavenger to remove LDL-C.

high-intensity interval training (HIIT)—Form of cardiorespiratory training that alternates high-intensity activities of a shorter duration with longer lower-intensity activities in a repetitive sequence.

hormonal birth control methods—Pregnancy prevention methods that require the use of hormones (e.g., birth control pill or patch).

human movement paradigm—A diagram depicting the interrelationship of exercise, physical activity, and sedentarism.

hydrodensitometry (underwater weighing)—A technique for measuring body density (the mass per unit of a living human being) that is a direct application of Archimedes' principle that an object displaces its own volume of water.

hydrogenated oils—Created by a chemical process whereby hydrogen is added to liquid oils to create a solid form; partially hydrogenated oils contain trans fats.

hymen—A thin membrane that surrounds the opening to the vagina.

hypercholesterolemia—An excess of cholesterol in the bloodstream.

hyperglycemia—High blood sugar.

hyperlipidemia—An abnormally high concentration of fats or lipids in the blood.

hypertension—Abnormally high blood pressure.

hypothalamus—A region of the forebrain that coordinates the autonomic nervous system and the activity of the pituitary gland, controlling body temperature, thirst, hunger, and other homeostatic systems; also involved in the control of sleep and emotional activity.

hypothalamus-pituitary-adrenal axis (HPA axis)—A major neuroendocrine system that controls reactions to stress, and many other body processes, using a complex set of direct influences and negative feedback control mechanisms among the hypothalamus, the pituitary glands, and adrenal cortex

illegal drugs—Drugs that are regulated and considered illegal by government; examples include cocaine, LSD, and heroin.

illicit drugs—Drugs that are used for nonmedical reasons; making, selling, or using them is prohibited by law (examples include cocaine, heroin, and opioids).

incomplete protein—Plant food lacking in one or more amino acids that can be eaten with another incomplete protein to make a complete protein; the two foods are then considered complementary proteins.

intermuscular adipose tissue—An ectopic fat depot located beneath the fascia of the muscle; generally considered to be located between muscle groups and within the muscle itself.

ischemic stroke—This stroke type, where a clot occurs in a blood vessel in the brain, is the most common and is similar to a heart attack.

isometric—A type of muscle contraction where the muscle lengthens or the joint angle does not change.

isotonic concentric—A type of muscle contraction where the muscle shortens and the joint angle decreases.

isotonic eccentric—A type of muscle contraction that is the opposite movement of isotonic concentric contractions: The muscle lengthens and the joint angle increases.

kilocalorie (calorie)—A unit of food energy of 1,000 calories. The term calorie is a simplified or abbreviated term that represents a kilocalorie, or 1,000 calories; 1 kilocalorie is the amount of heat needed to raise the temperature of 1 liter of water 1 degree Celsius.

labia majora—The outer skin folds of the vulva that are composed of fatty tissue and covered with pubic hair.

labia minora—The inner skin folds of the vulva; are not covered with pubic hair.

licensed dietitian (LD)—In addition to the RDN credentialing, many states have regulatory laws for dietitians and nutrition practitioners.

life expectancy—The average life span of an individual.

life span—The length of time a person lives.

lifestyle coach—A profession, different from counseling, that addresses specific personal conditions and encourages personal discovery in order to make the individual's life what he or she wants it to be.

low back pain—A common disorder involving the muscles, nerves, and bones of the back. Pain can vary from a dull constant ache to a sudden sharp feeling.

low-density lipoprotein cholesterol (LDL-C)—A subtype of cholesterol in the blood known to accelerate the atherosclerotic process.

macronutrients—Chemical compounds found in food, primarily carbohydrate, protein, and fat; provide humans with the majority of their energy.

magnetic resonance imaging (MRI)—A noninvasive medical test that that uses a magnetic field and pulses of radio-wave energy to map structures inside the body, including the location and amount of adipose, muscle, and bone tissues.

maintenance stage of change—A process of change within the TTM theory of behavior change. In this stage, you continue your healthy behavior for at least two years.

malignant—A tumor that is diagnosed as cancer based on an abnormal mass of cells that have the ability to grow in size and shape and separate from the primary tumor and spread to other parts of the body. These cells invade nearby tissue and then spread by way of the circulatory (blood) and lymphatic systems.

mammary glands (breasts)—Located on the chest, when stimulated by pregnancy hormones, these organs secrete milk to provide nourishment for a baby.

mantra—A word or phrase that is repeated, often during meditation, that enables the mind and body to get to a calm state.

marijuana—A drug made from dried leaves of the hemp, or cannabis plant that is illegal in most U.S. states; typically smoked to get a euphoric feeling.

maximal oxygen consumption ($\dot{V}O_2max$)—The maximal amount of oxygen the body can take in and use during maximal physical effort; provides the best objective measure of cardiorespiratory fitness.

medical model—A health model used by trained medical experts that focuses on prescribing drugs and procedures when illness is the cause of a lifestyle change.

melanoma—A type of dangerous skin cancer; the most commonly diagnosed cancer in the United States.

metabolic equivalence (METs)—The ratio of rate of energy expenditure during an activity compared to the rate of energy expended at rest. A measure of exercise intensity based on the assumption that a single MET is equal to the amount of oxygen a person consumes (i.e., energy expended) per unit of body weight while at rest.

metabolic syndrome (MetS)—A clustering of biological factors that raises your risk for other chronic conditions, especially diabetes and cardiovascular disease.

metabolism—The breakdown of food and its transformation into energy.

metastasis—When cancer cells have left the original site and traveled to other parts of the body through the circulatory or lymphatic system.

micronutrients—Chemical elements or substances required in very small amounts for healthy growth, development, and physiological function.

mindfulness meditation—A meditation technique that focuses on reducing psychological stress through being mindful of the present moment rather than thinking about the past or future.

minerals—An inorganic compound required by living organisms that must be obtained through the diet.

mons pubis—Soft area covering the pubis bone that is composed of fatty tissue; some women experience sexual pleasure when this region is touched.

muscle capacity—The maximum amount that a muscle or muscle group can physically perform.

muscle dysmorphia—Sometimes called body dysmorphic disorder, a subtype of body dysmorphic disorder where a person obsesses about being small and undeveloped or frail.

muscle fiber—An individual muscle cell.

muscular endurance—The ability of the muscle to hold or repeat a contraction without fatigue.

muscular power—The rate at which muscle force can be executed; alternatively, muscle force production (strength) expressed relative to time.

muscular strength—The amount of force that can be produced with a single maximum effort.

mutation—Abnormal cell growth that leads to the alteration of the genetic makeup of a normal cell.

myocardial infarction (heart attack)—A life-threatening condition that occurs when blood flow to the heart is abruptly stopped, most often due to a clot that has blocked a narrowed artery.

neuromotor exercise—Involves motor skills such as balance, agility, coordination, gait, and proprioceptive training.

nicotine—A substance derived from a tobacco plant that causes smokers to become addicted to cigarettes.

nonoxidative (anaerobic) energy system—The energy system that supplies rapid but also limited energy to muscle cells through the breakdown of glucose and glycogen; does not need oxygen to function; also produces lactic acid.

norepinephrine—Sometimes called noradrenaline; a neurotransmitter that is released primarily from the sympathetic nerve fibers and secondarily from the adrenal glands during the fight-or-flight response, increasing arousal, reaction time, heart rate, and blood glucose levels.

obesity—Being above a weight that is considered normal or desirable for a given height, typically defined as a body mass index of greater than 30 kilograms per square meter for adults. Also indicates having too much stored fat mass.

obesogenic environment—A term used to describe how our genetics have not evolved with our socially and physically built environment, which predisposes a large portion of the population to store too much energy or become obese.

oocytes—Immature egg in the ovary.

opioids—A highly addictive drug that is derived from opium and prescribed to treat and manage pain.

osteoporosis—A bone disease whereby bone mass and density loss results in an increased risk of fracture from everyday activities and nontraumatic injuries such as falling.

ovaries—A reproductive organ in women that produces the egg (oocytes) and hormones.

overweight—Being above a weight that is considered normal or desirable for a given height, typically defined as a body mass index of greater than 25 kilograms per square meter for adults.

ovulation—When a mature egg (ovum) is expelled from the ovaries.

oxidative (aerobic) system—The energy system that supplies energy more slowly but for a longer duration to working muscles through the breakdown of glucose or glycogen and fats; this system requires oxygen.

panic disorder—An anxiety disorder characterized by unexpected and repeated episodes of intense fear accompanied by physical symptoms that may include chest pain, heart palpitations, shortness of breath, dizziness, or abdominal distress.

parasympathetic nervous system—The division of the ANS that slows the heart rate, increases intestinal and glandular activity, and relaxes sphincter muscles; responsible for the rest and digestion functions of the body.

PAR-Q+—A self-administered form that contains screening questions focused on symptoms of heart disease and bone or joint problems; this questionnaire accesses your readiness to perform physical activity.

pathophysiology—Disordered physiological processes associated with disease or injury.

pelvic inflammatory disease—Infection of a woman's reproductive organs due to untreated chlamydia or gonorrhea; can lead to sterility.

penis—The erectile organ in men; urine and semen are expelled from the body through the penis.

percent body fat—The relative amount of fat contained in the body; calculated as fat mass divided by body mass and often abbreviated as %Fat.

perfect use—When a contraception method is used correctly during every sexual encounter.

peripheral arterial disease (PAD)—Sometimes referred to as peripheral vascular disease, this occurs with narrowing or occlusion of arteries outside the heart or brain due to atherosclerotic plaques; typically most evident in the legs.

personal training—Training provided by an individual certified in general fitness who provides an exercise prescription through one-on-one exercise instruction.

personality—Individual differences in patterns of thinking, feeling, and behaving.

physical activity—Any bodily movement produced by skeletal muscles that requires energy expenditure.

phytochemicals—Substances that are found in plant foods that may help prevent chronic diseases; include antioxidants.

pituitary gland—Sometimes called the master gland as it controls other hormone glands, including the adrenals, thyroid, and ovaries and testes, this endocrine gland is located at the base of the brain.

polycystic ovary syndrome—A hormonal disorder characterized by higher-than-normal levels of androgens that causes enlarged ovaries and leads to infertility and insulin resistance.

polyp—Areas of inflammation or bleeding in certain body cavities that could become cancerous tumors.

posture—The position in which someone holds his or her body when standing or sitting.

precontemplation stage of change—A process of change within the TTM theory of behavior change. In the precontemplation stage of change, you are not even thinking about changing a given behavior.

prediabetes—A condition when blood glucose levels are not normal but not quite high enough to be diagnosed as diabetes.

preparation stage of change—A process of change within the TTM theory of behavior change. In the preparation stage, you begin the process of the change and make changes to prepare for the change.

Prochaska's transtheoretical model (TTM)—An integrative theory of behavior change that assesses your readiness to act on a new, healthier behavior and provides strategies to guide your change process.

procrastination—The act of delaying or postponing something.

prognosis—A physician's best estimate of the time it can take to recover from the treatments and how having cancer may affect the patient's quality of life.

proprioceptors—A sensory receptor located in subcutaneous tissues capable of detecting movement and position of the body through a stimulus produced within the body.

prostate gland—A male organ that provides the majority of the fluid in semen.

protein—An essential nutrient composed of amino acids that are literally the building blocks of our body, forming muscles, bones, and cell membranes; provides energy to the body when needed at 4 kilocalories per gram.

psychoactive drugs—Drugs that alter consciousness, moods, and thoughts; examples include alcohol, cocaine, tobacco, and cannabis.

psychological age—A measure of how you perceive your body is functioning relative to your actual chronological age.

radiation therapy—The use of radioactive waves (such as X-rays, gamma rays, neutrons, or protons) to kill cancer cells or shrink the size of the tumor by targeting specific cancer cells; treatment comes either from a machine that delivers the beam externally, or outside of the body, or in the form of a small pellet that is placed in the body, near the cancer cells.

rating of perceived exertion (RPE)—A scale that allows a numerical estimation of the feelings of exertion during physical activity or exercise.

refined carbohydrates—Grain products that have been processed by a food manufacturer so that the whole grain is no longer intact and is missing the bran and germ.

registered dietitian nutritionist (RDN)—Food and nutrition experts who have met the rigorous criteria to earn the RDN credential, including a bachelor's degree, a supervised practice program, a national examination, and continuing professional educational requirements.

resting metabolic rate (RMR)—The minimal amount of energy needed to support basic physiological processes when the body is completely at rest.

RICE principle—A way to think about first aid for musculoskeletal injuries. The acronym RICE stands for rest, ice, compression, elevation.

sarcopenia—Loss of mass, quality, and strength of skeletal muscle; associated with the normal aging process.

satiety—The feeling of fullness that is related to the suppression of hunger for a period of time after a meal.

saturated fatty acids—A type of fat in which the fatty acid chains have all or predominantly single bonds; are typically solid at room temperature.

scrotum—Sac that holds the testes; located behind the penis.

sedentarism—Habits and routines associated with relatively low levels of activity and movement, which could lead to health-related problems.

self-confidence—Belief in your ability to succeed at what you put your mind to. It is a combination of self-esteem and general self-efficacy.

self-efficacy theory—Belief in your ability to succeed in specific situations or accomplish a task. Your sense of self-efficacy can play a large role in how you approach goals, tasks, and challenges.

self-efficacy—Belief in your ability to perform specific behaviors in order to produce the outcomes you desire.

semen—A whitish fluid that contains sperm; primarily produced by the prostate gland and seminal vesicles.

seminal vesicles—Vesicles that provide the sugar and protein fluid that contribute to the components of semen.

seminiferous tubules—Coiled tubules where sperm are produced.

simple carbohydrates—Sugars made of just one or two sugar molecules.

skinfold thickness—A measurement taken with a caliper that corresponds to the amount of subcutaneous fat a person has at a given region of the body.

slow-twitch fiber—Red muscle fibers that are fatigue resistant but have a slower contraction speed.

SMART goals—A process used for accountability in goal setting; SMART stands for specific, measurable, attainable, realistic, and time bound.

social anxiety disorder—Sometimes referred to as social phobia, this disorder is characterized by a persistent, intense, and chronic fear of being watched and judged by others and feeling embarrassed or humiliated to the degree that it interferes with work, school, and other activities and may negatively affect the person's ability to form relationships.

social ecological model—Focuses on both population-level and individual-level determinants of health and interventions. Your health is determined by influences at many levels, including public policy, community, institutional, interpersonal, and intrapersonal factors.

specificity of training—Training principle that developing a particular fitness component requires performing exercises or activities specifically designed for that component in terms of muscle groups, muscle actions, and energy systems.

sperm—A cell in men that contributes to reproduction.

spermicide—A substance (e.g., foams, creams, gels) that contains chemicals that can kill sperm to prevent pregnancy.

static stretching—A stretch that is held in a challenging but comfortable position for a period of time, usually somewhere between 10 to 30 seconds.

sterilization—A surgical procedure that is intended to be permanent that prevents the sperm from leaving the testicles (vasectomy) or the egg from leaving the ovaries (tubal ligation).

stimulants—Drugs that cause an increase to physiological responses in the body, which may include a rapid heart rate and increases in blood pressure, breathing, alertness and attention, and energy.

stress—A condition or feeling experienced when we perceive that demands in a physical, mental, or emotional domain exceed our personal or social resources to meet them.

stressor—An event or situation that potentially triggers the stress response.

stretch reflex—Sometimes called the myotatic stretch reflex; a muscle contraction in response to stretching within the muscle that provides automatic regulation of skeletal muscle length.

stroke—A condition where atherosclerosis or a clot blocks the blood vessels in the brain to the point that blood flow is restricted enough to cause brain cells to die.

subcutaneous fat—A primary fat depot located just under the skin.

substance abuse—When someone takes a drug not as prescribed or intended over a long period of time.

surgery—The removal of the malignant tumor; for more advanced cancers, it may require the removal of surrounding tissues and lymph nodes.

sympathetic nervous system—The division of the ANS that speeds up the heart rate, depresses secretion, and reduces tone and contractility of smooth muscle; responsible for the fight-or-flight response.

systole—Contraction or ejection phase of the heart.

talk test—Another valid method for assessing exercise intensity that involves monitoring the difficulty of talking while exercising.

testes (testicles)—Reproductive organs in men that produce and hold sperm.

theory of planned behavior (TPB)—Theory that links one's beliefs and behavior. The theory states that attitude toward behavior, subjective norms, and perceived behavioral control in combination shape your behavioral intentions and behaviors.

thermic effect of activity (TEA)—Energy expended above RMR due to skeletal muscle contraction, including while sitting, standing, fidgeting, and doing intentional exercise.

thermic effect of meals (TEM)—Energy expended associated with digestion, absorption, transport, metabolism, and storage of digested food.

time management—The ability to successfully prioritize and schedule one's time in an efficient manner to maintain productivity toward goals.

TNM system—A diagnostic system used to determine the extent or size of the primary tumor (T), whether or not the cancer cells have spread to lymph nodes (N), and if the cells have traveled to other parts of the body—that is, metastasized (M).

trans fatty acids—An unsaturated fatty acid that occurs as a result of the hydrogenation process, with a trans arrangement of the carbon atoms adjacent to its double bonds; often found in margarines and manufactured cooking oils.

Transcendental Meditation—A meditation technique that involves repetition of a word or phrase while sitting with the eyes closed to quiet the mind.

triglycerides—Formed from glycerol and three fatty acid groups; high concentrations in the blood elevates risk for CVD.

type 1 diabetes—A metabolic disorder that is characterized by high blood sugar due to lack of insulin; occurs most commonly as a result of beta-cell destruction in the pancreas.

type 2 diabetes (T2D)—A metabolic disorder characterized by high blood sugar, insulin resistance, and a relative lack of insulin.

typical use—Average, real-life use of birth control methods; accounts for human error (as opposed to correct, exact use with every sexual encounter, as occurs during clinical trials, for example).

unsaturated fatty acids—A type of fat in which there is at least one double bond; typically liquid at room temperature.

urethra—Tubular structure through which urine exits the body.

uterus—Muscular organ in the lower abdominal cavity of women where an embryo develops into a fetus.

vagina—A cylindrical space that begins at the opening of the vulva and ends at the opening of the cervix; the space for the penis during intercourse.

vas deferens—Tubular structure in men that transports semen out of the body.

visceral fat—A primary fat depot located deep within the abdominal cavity beneath the muscle wall.

vitamins—An organic compound that is an essential nutrient and is required in limited amounts; must be obtained through the diet.

wellness model—A health model that focuses on living well and encourages personal lifestyle choices and the use of self-management skills for preventing disease.

whole grains—A grain that is intact and contains the endosperm, germ, and bran.

withdrawal—A birth control method that requires a man to remove his penis from his partner's vagina before ejaculation.

zygote—The organism that develops after the blending of an egg and sperm.

REFERENCES

Chapter 1

Arloski, M. 2014. *Wellness Coaching for Lasting Lifestyle Change.* (2nd ed.). Duluth, MN: Whole Person Associates.

Archer, S. 2007. "Fitness and Wellness Intertwine: A Major industry Arises." *IDEA Fitness Journal* July-August: 36-47.

Åstrand, P. 1992. "Why Exercise?" *Medicine & Science in Sports & Exercise* 24(2): 153-62.

Baer, D. 2014. "Harvard Psychologist Says These 8 Principles Will Bring You the Most Happiness for Your Money." *Business Insider.* www.businessinsider.com/harvard-dan-gilbert-money-happiness-principles-2014-10.

Biswas, A., P. Oh, G. Faulkner, R. Bajaj, M. Silver, M. Mitchell, and D. Alter. 2015. "Sedentary Time and Its Association With Risk for Disease Incidence, and Hospitalization in Adults: A Systematic Review and Meta-Analysis." *Annals of Internal Medicine* 162(2): 123-32. doi:10.7326/M14-1651.

Blair, S., H. Kohl III, and N. Gordon. 1992. "Physical Activity and Health: A Lifestyle Approach." *Medicine, Exercise, Nutrition, and Health* 1: 1, 54-56.

Boseley, S. 2016. "Global Life Expectancy Increases to 71.4 Years." *The Guardian.* www.theguardian.com/world/2016/may/19/global-life-expectancy-increases-by-five-years-to-71-who.

Buettner, D. 2015. *The Blue Zones Solution: Eating and Living like the World's Healthiest People.* Washington, DC: National Geographic Society.

Chetty, R., M. Stepner, S. Abraham, S. Lin, B. Scuderi, N. Turner, A. Bergeron, and D. Cutler. 2016. "The Association Between Income and Life Expectancy in the United States, 2001-2014." *Journal of the American Medical Association* 315(16): 1750-66.

Gilbert, D. 2007. *Stumbling on Happiness.* New York: Random House.

Hauser, A. 2016. "Do You Live in the Saddest State?" *Inside Business.* https://weather.com/health/news/gallup-healthways-well-being-report.

Healy, G., N. Eakin, A. Owen, M. Lamontage, E. Moodie, B. Winkler, G. Fjeldsoe, L. Wiesner, D. Willenberg, and A. Dunstan. 2016. "A Cluster Randomized Controlled Trial to Reduce Office Workers Sitting Time Effect on Activity Outcomes." *Medicine & Science in Sports & Exercise* 48: 9, 1787-1797.

Gallup-Healthways. 2017. *State of American Well-Being: 2016 State Well-Being Rankings.* http://info.healthways.com/hubfs/Gallup-Healthways%20State%20of%20American%20Well-Being_2016%20State%20Rankings%20vFINAL.pdf.

Jay, M. 2012. *The Defining Decade: Why your Twenties Matter and How to Make the Most of Them Now.* New York: Hachette Book Group.

Katzmarzyk, T. 2014. "Standing and Mortality in a Prospective Cohort of Canadian Adults." *Medicine & Science in Sports & Exercise* 46(5): 940-46.

Khalid, A. 2016. "Here Are the Happiest—and Most Miserable—States in America." *The Daily Dot.* www.dailydot.com/irl/what-are-the-happiest-and-unhappiest-states-in-america.

Levine, J. 2014. *Get Up: Why Your Desk Chair Is Killing You and What You Can Do About It.* New York: Palgrave McMillian.

McCoy, K. 2009. "Burning Calories with Everyday Activities." *Everyday Health.* www.everydayhealth.com/weight/everyday-activities-that-burn-calories.aspx.

Ming Wei, M.D., J.B. Kampert, C.E. Barlow, M.Z. Nichaman, L.W. Gibbons, R.S. Paffenbarger, Jr., and S.N. Blair. 1999. "Relationship Between Low Cardiorespiratory Fitness and Mortality in Normal Weight, Overweight and Obese Men." *Journal of the American Medical Association* 1999:282(16): 1547-53. doi:10.1001/jama.282.16.1547.

Perkins, D. 2009. *Making Learning Whole: How Seven Principles of Teaching Can Make Learning Whole.* San Francisco: Jossey-Bass.

Pina, P. 2016. "2016 Food Trends From Google Search Data: The Rise of Functional Foods." *Think With Google.* www.thinkwithgoogle.com/articles/2016-food-trends-google.html.

Rogers, R.G., B.G. Everett, A. Zajacova, and R.A. Hummer. 2010. "Educational Degrees and Adult Mortality Risk in the United States." *Biodemography and Social Biology* 56(1): 80-99.

Schlossberg, M. 2016. "The Diet Industry Is Dying as a New Mentality Takes Hold in America." *Business Insider.* www.businessinsider.com/the-death-of-the-diet-industry-2016-7.

Seligman, M. E.P. 2011. *Flourish.* New York: Free Press: A Division of Simon and Schuster.

Segar, M. 2015. *No Sweat: How the Simple Science of Motivation Can Bring You a Lifetime of Fitness.* New York: AMACOM.

Springbuk. 2017. "2017 Health and Wellness Statistics." www.springbuk.com/2017-health-wellness-statistics.

Well People. 2011. "A New Vision of Wellness." www.wellpeople.com/What_Is_Wellness.aspx.

U.S. National Prevention Health Promotion and Public Health Council (2016). Accessed January 20, 2018. www.surgeongeneral.gov/priorities/prevention/about/healthy-aging-in-action-final.pdf.

Xu, J.Q., S.L. Murphy, K.D. Kochanek, and E. Arias. 2016. *Mortality in the United States, 2015. NCHS Data Brief, no. 267.* Hyattsville, MD: National Center for Health Statistics.

Chapter 2

American College of Sports Medicine. 1978. "American College of Sports Medicine Position Statement: The Recommended Quantity and Quality of Exercise for Developing and Maintaining Fitness in Healthy Adults." *Medicine & Science in Sports & Exercise* 10: vii-x.

American College of Sports Medicine. 1990. "American College of Sports Medicine Position Stand: The Recommended Quantity and Quality of Exercise for Developing and Maintaining Cardiorespiratory and Muscular Fitness in Healthy Adults." *Medicine & Science in Sports & Exercise* 43(7): 1334-59.

American College of Sports Medicine. 1998. "American College of Sports Medicine Position Stand: The Recommended Quantity and Quality of Exercise for Developing and Maintaining Cardiorespiratory and Muscular Fitness, and Flexibility in Healthy Adults." *Medicine & Science in Sports & Exercise* 30(6): 975-91.

American College of Sports Medicine. 2006. *ACSM's Guidelines for Exercise Testing and Prescription* (7th ed.). Baltimore: Lippincott Williams & Wilkins.

American College of Sports Medicine. 2018. *ACSM's Guidelines for Exercise Testing and Prescription* (10th ed.). Philadelphia: Wolters Kluwer.

Brown, E. 2013. "AMA to Offices: Don't Make Workers Sit All Day!" *Los Angeles Times*, June 18, 2013. www.latimes.com/science/sciencenow/la-sci-sn-ama-policy-sitting-20130619-story.html.

Carroll A. 2016. "Closest Thing to a Wonder Drug? Try Exercise." *The New York Times*, June 20, 2016. www.nytimes.com/2016/06/21/upshot/why-you-should-exercise-no-not-to-lose-weight.html?_r=0.

Centers for Disease Control and Prevention. 2016. "Exercise or Physical Activity." *National Center for Health Statistics.* www.cdc.gov/nchs/fastats/exercise.htm.

Hamilton, M., G. Healy, D. Dunstan, T. Zderic, and N. Owen. 2008. "Too Little Exercise and Too Much Sitting: Inactivity Physiology and the Need for New Recommendations on Sedentary Behavior." *Current Cardiovascular Risk Reports* 2(4): 292-8. doi: 10.1007/s12170-008-0054-8.

Healy G.N., S.P. Lawler, A. Thorp, M. Neuhaus, E.L. Robson, N. Owen, and D.W. Dunstan. 2012. "Reducing Prolonged Sitting in the Workplace. (An Evidence Review: Full Report)."

Isaacson, W. 2011, *Steve Jobs*. New York: Simon & Schuster.

Melbourne, Australia: Victorian Health Promotion Foundation. Available at www.vichealth.vic.gov.au/search/creating-healthy-workplaces-publications.

Katzmarzyk, P., T. Church, C. Craig, and C. Bouchard. 2009. "Sitting Time and Mortality From all Causes, Cardiovascular Disease, and Cancer." *Medicine & Science in Sports & Exercise* 41(5): 998-1005.

Kohl, H., C. Craig, E. Lambert, S. Inoue, J. Alkandari, G. Leetongin, S. Kahlmeier, and L. Landro. 2012. "The Pandemic of Physical Inactivity: Global Action for Public Health." *The Lancet* 380(9838): 294-305.

Levine, J. 2014. *Get Up: Why Your Desk Chair Is Killing You and What You Can Do About It.* New York: Palgrave McMillian.

Matthews, C., K. Chen, P. Freedson, M. Buchowski, B. Beech, R. Pate, and R. Troiano. 2008. "Amount of Time Spent in Sedentary Behaviors in the United States." *American Journal of Epidemiology* 167(7): 875-81.

Matthews, C., S. Moore, J. Sampson, A. Blair, Q. Ziao, S. Keadle, A. Hollenbeck, and Y. Park. 2015. "Mortality Benefits for Replacing Sitting Time With Different Physical Activities." *Medicine & Science in Sport and Exercise* 47(9): 1833-40.

National Physical Activity Plan. n.d. "About the Plan: Vision and Background." Accessed December 2, 2017. www.physicalactivityplan.org/theplan/about.html.

National Physical Activity Plan. n.d. Columbia, SC. Accessed January 22, 2018. www.physicalactivityplan.org/theplan/about/knowledge.html.

Office of Disease Prevention and Health Promotion (2018). Part A. Executive Summary. Accessed March 4, 2018. https://health.gov/paguidelines/second-edition/report/pdf/02_A_Executive_Summary.pdf.

Pate, R., M. Pratt, and S. Blair. 1995. "Physical Activity and Public Health: A Recommendation From the Centers for Disease Control and Prevention and the American College of Sports Medicine." *Journal of the American Medical Association* 273(5): 402-7.

Pronk, N., A. Katz, M. Lowry, and J. Payfer. 2012. "Reducing Occupational Sitting Time and Priming Working Health: The Take-A-Stand Project, 2011." *Preventing Chronic Disease* 9(11): 323.

Ognibene, G., W. Torres, R. von Eyben, and K. Horst. 2016. "Impact of a Sit-Stand Workstation on Chronic Low Back Pain: Results of a Randomized Trial." *Journal of Occupational & Environmental Medicine* 58(3): 287-93.

Shah, S., M. O'Byrne, M. Wilson, T. Wilson. 2011. "Elevator or Stairs?" *Canadian Medical Association Journal* 183(18): E1353-E1355. doi: 10.1503/cmaj.110961.

Smart Growth America. June 2016. "Foot Traffic Ahead: 2016." https://smartgrowthamerica.org/resources/foot-traffic-ahead-2016/.

Trost, S., N. Owen, A. Bauman, J. Sallis, and W. Brown. 2002. "Correlates of Adults' Participation in Physical Activity: Review and Update." *Medicine & Science in Sports & Exercise* 34(12): 1996-2001.

U.S. Burden of Disease Collaborators. 2013. "The State of Health in the United States." *Journal of the American Medical Association* 310(6): 585-6. doi:10.1001/jama.2013.13809.

United States Department of Health and Human Services. 1996. *Physical Activity and Health: A Report of the Surgeon General.* Atlanta: Author.

U.S. Department of Health and Human Services. 2008. *2008 Physical Activity Guidelines for Americans.* Washington (DC): U.S. Department of Health and Human Services; ODPHP Publication No. U0036. Accessed January 20, 2018. Available at www.health.gov/paguidelines.

Xu, J.Q., S.L. Murphy, K.D. Kochanek, and E. Arias. 2016. *Mortality in the United States, 2015. NCHS Data Brief, no 267.* Hyattsville, MD: National Center for Health Statistics.

Young, D., M-F. Hivert, S. Alhassan, S.M. Camhi, J.F. Ferguson, P.T. Katmarzyk, C.E. Lewis, et al. 2016. "Sedentary Behavior and Cardiovascular Morbidity and Mortality: A Science Advisory from the American Heart Association." *Circulation* 134(13): e262-79. doi: 10/1161/CIR.0000000000000440.

Chapter 3

Ajzen, I., and B. Driver. 1992. "Application of the Theory of Planned Behavior to Leisure Choice." *Journal of Leisure Research* 24: 207-24.

Bandura A. 1977. "Self-Efficacy: Toward a Unifying Theory of Behavioral Change." *Psychological Review* 84: 191-215.

Bauman, A., R. Reis, J. Sallis, J. Wells, R. Loos, and B. Martin. 2012. "Correlates of Physical Activity: Why Are Some People Physically Active and Others Not?" *The Lancet* 380(9838): 258-71.

Berry, T., and B. Howe. 2004. "Effects of Health-Based and Appearance-Based Exercise Advertising on Exercise Attitudes, Social Physique Anxiety and Self-Presentation in an Exercise Setting." *Social Behavior and Personality International Journal* 32(1): 1-12.

Deci, E.L., and R.M. Ryan. 1985. *Intrinsic Motivation and Self-Determination in Human Behavior.* New York: Plenum.

Downs, D.S., and H.A. Hausenblas. 2005. "The Theories of Reasoned Action and Planned Behavior Applied to Exercise: A Meta-Analytic Update." *Journal of Physical Activity and Health* 2: 76-97.

Duhigg, C. 2014. *The Power of Habit: Why We Do What We Do in Life and Business.* New York: Random House.

Fishman, E. 2016. "Bikeshare: A review of recent literature." *Transport Reviews*, 36(1): 92-113.

Kilpatrick, M., E. Hebert, and D. Jacobsen. 2002. "Physical Activity Motivations: A Practitioner's Guide to Self-Determination Theory." *Journal of Physical Education, Recreation, and Dance* 73: 36-41.

Levine, J. 2014. *Get Up: Why Your Chair Is Killing You and What You Can Do About It.* New York: Palgrave McMillan.

McAuley, E. 1994. "Enhancing Psychological Health Through Physical Activity." In *Toward Active Living: Proceedings of the International Conference on Physical Activity, Fitness and Health,* edited by H. Quinney, L. Gauvin, and A. Wall, 83-90. Champaign, IL: Human Kinetics.

National Physical Activity Plan. n.d. "About the Plan: Vision and Background." Accessed December 2, 2017. www.physicalactivityplan.org/theplan/about.html.

Nigg, C. 2014. *ACSM's Behavioral Aspects of Physical Activity and Exercise.* Philadelphia, PA: Wolters Kluwer/Lippincott Williams and Wilkins.

Prochaska, J.O., and C.C. DiClemente. 1984. *The Transtheoretical Approach: Towards a Systematic Eclectic Framework.* Homewood, IL: Dow Jones Irwin.

Sallis, J., M. Floyd, D. Rodriguez, and B. Saelens. 2012. "Role of Built Environments in Physical Activity, Obesity, and Cardiovascular Disease." *Circulation* 125: 729-37.

Sallis, J., N. Owen, and E. Fisher. 2015. *Health Behavior: Theory, Research and Practice* (5th ed.). San Francisco: Jossey-Bass.

Segar, M. 2015. *No Sweat: How the Simple Science of Motivation Can Bring You a Lifetime of Fitness.* New York: AMACOM.

Tudor-Locke, C., C. Leonardi, W.D. Johnson, P.T. Katzmarzyk, and T.S. Church. 2011. "Accelerometer Steps/Day Translation of Moderate-to-Vigorous Activity." *Preventive Medicine* 53: 31-3. doi:10.1016/j.ypmed.2011.01.014.

Valliant, G. 2002. *Aging Well: Surprising Guideposts to a Happier Life From the Landmark Harvard Study of Adult Development.* New York: Hachette Book Group.

Van Cappellen, P., E.L. Rice, L.I. Catalino, and B.L. Fredrickson. 2017. "Positive Affective Processes Underlie Positive Health Behaviour Change." *Psychology & Health* May 12: 1-21. doi: 10.1080/08870446.2017.1320798.

Warburton, D., V. Jamnik, S. Bredin, and N. Gledhill. 2011. "The Physical Activity Readiness Questionnaire for Everyone (PAR-Q+) et Electronic Physical Activity Readiness Medical Examination (ePARmed-X+)." *The Health & Fitness Journal of Canada* 4(2): 3-23.

Zenko, Z., P. Ekkekakis, and G. Kavetsos. 2016. "Changing Minds: Bounded Rationality and Heuristic Processes in Exercise-Related Judgments and Choices." *Sport, Exercise, and Performance Psychology* 5(4): 337-51.

Chapter 4

American College of Sports Medicine. 2018. *ACSM's Guidelines for Exercise Testing and Prescription* (10th ed.). Philadelphia: Wolters Kluwer Health.

Donnelly, J.E., C.H. Hillman, D. Castelli, J.L. Etnier, S. Lee, P. Tomporowski, K. Lambourne, and A.N. Szabo-Reed. 2016. "Physical Activity, Fitness, Cognitive Function, and Academic Achievement in Children: A Systematic Review." *Medicine & Science in Sports & Exercise* 48(6): 1197-1222.

Garber, C.E., B. Blissmer, M.R. Deschenes, B.A. Franklin, M.J. Lamonte, I.M. Lee, D.C.

Martin, S.A., B.D. Pence, and J.A. Woods. 2009. "Exercise and Respiratory Tract Viral Infections." *Exercise and Sport Sciences Reviews* 37(4): 157-64.

Milanovic, Z., G. Sporis, and M. Weston. 2015. "Effectiveness of High-Intensity Interval Training (HIT) and Continuous Endurance Training for $\dot{V}O_2$max Improvements: A Systematic Review and Meta-Analysis of Controlled Trials." *Sports Medicine* 45(10): 1469-81.

Nichol, K.L., S.D. Heilly, and E. Ehlinger. 2005. "Colds and Influenza-Like Illnesses in University Students: Impact on Health, Academic and Work Performance, and Health Care Use. *Clinical Infectious Diseases* 40(9): 1263-70.

Nieman, and D.P. Swain. 2011. "American College of Sports Medicine Position Stand. Quantity and Quality of Exercise for Developing and Maintaining Cardiorespiratory, Musculoskeletal, and Neuromotor Fitness in Apparently Healthy Adults: Guidance for Prescribing Exercise." *Medicine & Science in Sports & Exercise* 43(7): 1334-59.

Ratey, J. 2008. *SPARK: The Revolutionary New Science of Exercise and the Brain.* New York: Little Brown.

Tudor-Locke, C., C. Leonardi, W.D. Johnson, P.T. Katzmarzyk, and T.S. Church. 2011. "Accelerometer Steps/Day Translation of Moderate-to-Vigorous Activity." *Preventive Medicine* 53:31-33. doi:10.1016/j.ypmed.2011.01.014.

U.S. Department of Health and Human Services. 2008. *2008 Physical Activity Guidelines for Americans.* Washington, DC: Author. https://health.gov/paguidelines/pdf/paguide.pdf.

Chapter 5

Aagaard, P., C. Suetta, P. Caserotti, S.P. Magnusson, and M. Kjær. 2010. "Role of the Nervous System in Sarcopenia and Muscle Atrophy With Aging: Strength Training as a Countermeasure." *Scandinavian Journal of Medicine & Science in Sports* 20: 49-64. doi:10.1111/j.1600-0838.2009.01084.x.

American College of Sports Medicine. 2018. *ACSM's Guidelines for Exercise Testing and Prescription* (10th ed.). Philadelphia: Wolters Kluwer.

American Council on Exercise. 2011. *Essentials of Exercise Science for Fitness Professionals.* San Diego: Author.

American Council on Exercise. 2014. *Personal Trainer Manual* (5th ed.). San Diego: Author.

Cook, G. 2010. *Movement: Functional Movement Systems.* Santa Cruz, FL: On Target Publications.

Garber, C.E., B. Blissmer, M.R. Deschenes, B.A. Franklin, M.J. Lamonte, I.M. Lee, D.C. Nieman, and D.P. Swain. 2011. "American College of Sports Medicine Position Stand. The Quantity and Quality of Exercise for Developing and Maintaining Cardiorespiratory, Musculoskeletal, and Neuromotor Fitness in Apparently Healthy Adults: Guidance for Prescribing Exercise." *Medicine & Science in Sports & Exercise* 43(7): 1334-59.

Kennedy-Armbruster, C.A., and M.M. Yoke. 2014. *Methods of Group Exercise Instruction* (4th ed.). Champaign, IL: Human Kinetics.

Kurtz, S., K. Ong, E. Lau, F. Mowat, and M. Halpern. 2007. "Projections of Primary and Revision Hip and Knee Arthroplasty in the United States from 2005-2030." *Journal of Bone & Joint Surgery* 89(4): 780-5. doi: 10.2106/JBJS.F.00222.

Schoenfeld, B.J., Z.K. Pope, F.M. Benik, G.M. Hester, J. Sellers, J.L. Nooner, J.A. Schnaiter, et al. 2016. "Longer Interset Rest Periods Enhance Muscle Strength and Hypertrophy in Resistance-Trained Men." *Journal of Strength and Conditioning Research* 30(7): 1805-12.

Varma, V., D. Dey, A. Leroux, J. Di, J. Urbanek, L. Ziao, and V. Zipunnikov. 2017. "Re-Evaluating the Effect of Age on Physical Activity Over the Lifespan." *Preventive Medicine* 101(August): 102-8. https://doi.org/10.1016/j.ypmed.2017.05.030.

Westcott, W. 1996. *Building Strength and Stamina: New Nautilus Training for Total Fitness.* Champaign, IL: Human Kinetics.

Chapter 6

American College of Sports Medicine. 2018. *ACSM's Guidelines for Exercise Testing and Prescription* (10th ed.). Philadelphia: Wolters-Kluwer.

Anderson, G.B. 1998. "Epidemiology of Low Back Pain." *Acta Orthopaedica Scandinavia* 281(Suppl): 28-31.

Centers for Disease Control and Prevention. 2001. "Prevalence of Disabilities and Associated Health Conditions Among Adults—United States, 1999." *Journal of the American Medical Association* 285(12): 1571-2.

Clarke, T.C., R.L. Nahin, P.M. Barnes, and B.J. Stussman. 2016. *Use of Complementary Health Approaches for Musculoskeletal Pain Disorders Among Adults: United States, 2012. National Health Statistics Reports; no 98.* Hyattsville, MD: National Center for Health Statistics.

https://www.cdc.gov/nchs/data/hus/2014/046.pdf.

Cooper, R., R. Hardy, and K. Patel. 2014. "Physical Capacity in Mid-Life and Survival Over 13 years of Follow-Up: British Birth Cohort Study." *British Medical Journal* 2014(348): g2219. https://doi.org/10.1136/bmj.g2219.

Deyo, R.A., D. Cherkin, D. Conrad, and E. Volinn. 1991. "Cost, Controversy, Crisis: Low Back Pain and the Health of the Public." *Annual Review of Public Health* 1991(12): 141-56.

Friedman, H.S., and L.R. Martin. 2012. *The Longevity Project: Surprising Discoveries for Health and Long Life From the Landmark Eight-Decade Study.* New York: Penguin.

Katz, J.N. 2006. "Lumbar Disc Disorders and Low-Back Pain: Socioeconomic Factors and Consequences." *The Journal of Bone and Joint Surgery, American volume* 88(Suppl 2): 21-4.

National Institutes of Neurological Disorders and Strokes. 2014. *Low Back Pain Fact Sheet.* www.ninds.nih.gov/Disorders/Patient-Caregiver-Education/Fact-Sheets/Low-Back-Pain-Fact-Sheet.

Rapoport, J., P. Jacobs, N.R. Bell, and S. Klarenbach. 2004. "Refining the Measurement of the Economic Burden of Chronic Diseases in Canada." *Chronic Diseases in Canada* 25(1): 13-21.

Ricci, J.A., W.F. Stewart, E. Chee, C. Leotta, K. Foley, and M.C. Hochberg. 2006. "Back Pain Exacerbations and Lost Productive Time Costs in United States Workers." *Spine* 31(26): 3052-60.

Rubin, D.I. 2007. "Epidemiology and Risk Factors for Spine Pain." *Neurologic Clinics* 25(2): 353-71. https://doi.org/10.1016/j.ncl.2007.01.004.

Chapter 7

American College of Sports Medicine. 2018. *ACSM's Guidelines for Exercise Testing and Prescription.* Philadelphia: Wolters Kluwer Health.

Addison, O., R.L. Marcus, P.C. Lastayo, and A.S. Ryan. 2014. "Intermuscular Fat: A Review of the Consequences and Causes." *International Journal of Endocrinology* 2014: 309570.

Bouchard, C., and L. Perusse. 1988. "Heredity and Body Fat." *Annual Review of Nutrition* 8: 259-77.

Gallagher, D., S.B. Heymsfield, M. Heo, S.A. Jebb, P.R. Murgatroyd, and Y. Sakamoto. 2000. "Healthy Percentage Body Fat Ranges: An Approach for Developing Guidelines Based on Body Mass Index." *The American Journal of Clinical Nutrition* 72(3): 694-701.

Heymsfield, S.B., C.B. Ebbeling, J. Zheng, A. Pietrobelli, B.J. Strauss, A.M. Silva, and D.S. Ludwig. 2015. "Multi-Component Molecular-Level Body Composition Reference Methods:

Evolving Concepts and Future Directions." *Obesity Reviews* 16(4): 282-94.

Heymsfield, S.B., T.G. Lohman, Z. Wang, and S.B. Going. 2005. *Human Body Composition*. Champaign IL: Human Kinetics.

Joy, E., M.J. De Souza, A. Nattiv, M. Misra, N.I. Williams, R.J. Mallinson, J.C. Gibbs, et al. 2014. "2014 Female Athlete Triad Coalition Consensus Statement on Treatment and Return to Play of the Female Athlete Triad." *Current Sports Medicine Reports* 13(4): 219-32.

Kohrt, W. 2010. "Physical Activity and Risk of Obesity in Older Adults." In *Physical Activity and Obesity*, edited by C. Bouchard and P.T. Katzmarzyk, 117-120. Champaign IL: Human Kinetics.

Lee, S.Y., and D. Gallagher. 2008. "Assessment Methods in Human Body Composition." *Current Opinion in Clinical Nutrition & Metabolic Care* 11(5): 566-72.

Looker, A.C., L.J. Melton, III, T. Harris, L. Borrud, J. Shepherd, and J. McGowan. 2009. "Age, Gender, and Race/Ethnic Differences in Total Body and Subregional Bone Density." *Osteoporosis International* 20(7): 1141-9.

Pietrobelli, A., S.B. Heymsfield, Z.M. Wang, and D. Gallagher. 2001. "Multi-Component Body Composition Models: Recent Advances and Future Directions." *European Journal of Clinical Nutrition* 55(2): 69-75.

Pollock, M.L., and A.S. Jackson. 1984. "Research Progress in Validation of Clinical Methods of Assessing Body Composition." *Medicine & Science in Sports & Exercise* 16(6): 606-15.

Shapses, S.A., and D. Sukumar. 2012. "Bone Metabolism in Obesity and Weight Loss." *Annual Review of Nutrition* 32: 287-309.

Slaughter, M.H., and T.G. Lohman. 1976. "Relationship of Body Composition to Somatotype." *American Journal of Physical Anthropology* 44(2): 237-44.

Weaver, C.M., C.M. Gordon, K.F. Janz, H.J. Kalkwarf, J.M. Lappe, R. Lewis, M. O'Karma, T.C. Wallace, and B.S. Zemel. 2016. "The National Osteoporosis Foundation's Position Statement on Peak Bone Mass Development and Lifestyle Factors: A Systematic Review and Implementation Recommendations." *Osteoporosis International* 27: 1281-1386.

Xiao, J., S.A. Purcell, C.M. Prado, and M.C. Gonzalez. 2017. "Fat Mass to Fat-Free Mass Ratio Reference Values From NHANES III Using Bioelectrical Impedance Analysis." *Clinical Nutrition* pii: S0261-5614(17)31353-5.

Chapter 8

American College of Sports Medicine. 2011. *Selecting and Effectively Using Hydration for Fitness*. Indianapolis: Author. www.acsm.org/docs/brochures/selecting-and-effectively-using-hydration-for-fitness.pdf.

Institute of Medicine. 2004. *Dietary Reference Intakes: Water, Potassium, Sodium, Chloride and Sulfate*. Washington, DC: The National Academies Press. www.nationalacademies.org/hmd/Reports/2004/Dietary-Reference-Intakes-Water-Potassium-Sodium-Chloride-and-Sulfate.aspx.

Institute of Medicine. 2005. *Dietary Reference Intakes for Energy, Carbohydrate, Fiber, Fat, Fatty Acids, Cholesterol, Protein,* *and Amino Acids*. Washington, DC: The National Academies Press. https://doi.org/10.17226/10490.

Institute of Medicine. 2006. *Dietary Reference Intakes: The Essential Guide to Nutrient Requirements*. Washington, DC: The National Academies Press. https://doi.org/10.17226/11537.

Kamper, A.L., and S. Strandgaard. 2017. "Long-Term Effects of High-Protein Diets on Renal Function." *Annual Review of Nutrition* 37: 347-69.

Melina, V., W. Craig, and S. Levin. 2016. "Position of the Academy of Nutrition and Dietetics: Vegetarian Diets." *Journal of the Academy of Nutrition and Dietetics* 116(12): 1970-80.

Palmer, S. 2014. *RD Resources for Consumers: Protein in Vegetarian and Vegan Diets*. Chicago: Academy of Nutrition and Dietetics. https://vegetariannutrition.net/docs/Protein-Vegetarian-Nutrition.pdf.

Phillips, S.M., S. Chevalier, and H.J. Leidy. 2016. "Protein 'Requirements' Beyond the RDA: Implications for Optimizing Health." *Applied Physiology, Nutrition, and Metabolism* 41(5): 565-72.

U.S. Department of Agriculture. n.d.a. "Interactive DRI for Healthcare Professionals." Accessed December 18, 2017. www.nal.usda.gov/fnic/interactiveDRI.

U.S. Department of Agriculture. n.d.b. "Vitamins and Minerals." Accessed December 17, 2017. www.nal.usda.gov/fnic/vitamins-and-minerals.

U.S. Department of Health and Human Services and U.S. Department of Agriculture. 2015. *2015-2020 Dietary Guidelines for Americans* (8th ed.). Washington, DC: Author. http://health.gov/dietaryguidelines/2015.

U.S. Food and Drug Administration. n.d. *FDA Vitamins and Minerals Chart*. Silver Spring, MD: Author. www.accessdata.fda.gov/scripts/InteractiveNutritionFactsLabel/factsheets/Vitamin_and_Mineral_Chart.pdf.

U.S. Food and Drug Administration. 2014. "Nutrition Labeling and Education Act (NLEA) Requirements—Attachment 1." Last modified November 25, 2014. www.fda.gov/ICECI/Inspections/InspectionGuides/ucm114045.htm.

U.S. Food and Drug Administration. 2017a. "Changes to the Nutrition Facts Label." Last modified November 11, 2017. www.fda.gov/Food/GuidanceRegulation/GuidanceDocumentsRegulatoryInformation/LabelingNutrition/ucm385663.htm.

U.S. Food and Drug Administration. 2017b. "Information for Consumers on Using Dietary Supplements." Last modified November 29, 2017. www.fda.gov/Food/DietarySupplements/UsingDietarySupplements/default.htm.

U.S. Food and Drug Administration. 2018. "Final Determination Regarding Partially Hydrogenated Oils (Removing Trans Fat)." Last modified January 4, 2018. www.fda.gov/Food/IngredientsPackagingLabeling/FoodAdditivesIngredients/ucm449162.htm.

Whole Grains Council. n.d. "Whole Grains 101." Accessed December 16, 2017. https://wholegrainscouncil.org/wholegrains-101.

Wolfram, T. 2017. "Food Allergies and Intolerances." *Academy of Nutrition and Dietetics*. www.eatright.org/resource/

health/allergies-and-intolerances/food-allergies/food-allergies-and-intolerances.

Chapter 9

American College of Sports Medicine. 2018. *ACSM's Guidelines for Exercise Testing and Prescription*. Philadelphia: Wolters Kluwer Health.

Bouchard, C., and P.T. Katzmarzyk. 2010. *Physical Activity and Obesity*. Champaign IL: Human Kinetics.

Bray, M.S., R.J.F. Loos, J.M. McCaffery, C. Ling, P.W. Franks, G.M. Weinstock, M.P. Snyder, J.L. Vassy, and T. Agurs-Collins. 2016. "NIH Working Group Report—Using Genomic Information to Guide Weight Management: From Universal to Precision Treatment." *Obesity (Silver Spring)* 24(1): 14-22.

Centers for Disease Control and Prevention. 2017. "Adult Obesity Causes And Consequences." Accessed November 28, 2017. https://www.cdc.gov/obesity/adult/causes.html.

Hill, J.O., and H.R. Wyatt. 2013. *State of Slim: Fix Your Metabolism and Drop 20 Pounds in 8 Weeks on the Colorado Diet*. New York: Rodale.

Jensen, M.D., D.H. Ryan, C.M. Apovian, J.D. Ard, A.G. Comuzzie, K.A. Donato, F.B. Hu, et al. 2014. "2013 AHA/ACC/TOS Guideline for the Management of Overweight and Obesity in Adults: A Report of the American College of Cardiology/American Heart Association Task Force on Practice Guidelines and The Obesity Society." *Journal of the American College of Cardiology* 63(25 Pt B): 2985-3023.

Malhotra, R., T. Ostbye, C.M. Riley, and E.A. Finkelstein. 2013. "Young Adult Weight Trajectories Through Midlife By Body Mass Category." *Obesity (Silver Spring)* 21(9): 1923-34.

Reinehr, T. 2017. "Long-Term Effects of Adolescent Obesity: Time to Act." *Nature Reviews Endocrinology* 2017 Nov 24. doi: 10.1038/nrendo.2017.147. [Epub ahead of print].

Tremblay, A., and F. Bellisle. 2015. "Nutrients, Satiety, and Control of Energy Intake." *Applied Physiology, Nutrition, and Metabolism* 40(10): 971-9.

Chapter 10

American College Health Association. 2017. *National College Health Assessment spring 2017 Reference Group Data Report*. www.acha-ncha.org/docs/NCHA-II_SPRING_2017_REFERENCE_GROUP_DATA_REPORT.pdf.

American Psychological Association. n.d.a. "Listening to the Warning Signs of Stress." Accessed January 22, 2018. www.apa.org/helpcenter/stress-signs.aspx.

American Psychological Association. n.d.b. "Six Myths About Stress." Accessed January 22, 2018. www.apa.org/helpcenter/stress-myths.aspx.

American Psychological Association. n.d.c. "Stress: The Different Kinds of Stress." Accessed January 22, 2018. www.apa.org/helpcenter/stress-kinds.aspx.

American Psychological Association. 2014. "Stress in America: Are Teen Adopting Adults' Stress Habits?" Accessed August 10, 2017. www.apa.org/news/press/releases/stress/2013/stress-report.pdf.

American Sleep Association. n.d. "What is Sleep?" Accessed January 22, 2018. www.sleepassociation.org/patients-general-public/what-is-sleep.

Bureau of Labor Statistics. 2016. "American Time Use Survey." Accessed December 20, 2016. www.bls.gov/tus/charts/students.htm.

Centers for Disease Control and Prevention. 2016a. "Tips for Better Sleep." Last modified July 15, 2016. www.cdc.gov/sleep/about_sleep/sleep_hygiene.html.

Centers for Disease Control and Prevention. 2017a. "Coping with Stress." Accessed December 4, 2017. www.cdc.gov/features/copingwithstress/index.html.

Centers for Disease Control and Prevention. 2017b. "How Much Sleep Do I Need?" Last modified March 2, 2017. www.cdc.gov/sleep/about_sleep/how_much_sleep.html.

Centers for Disease Control and Prevention. 2017c. "Sleep and Sleep Disorders." Last modified March 9, 2017. www.cdc.gov/Sleep/index.html.

Goyal, M., S. Singh, E.M. Sibinga, N.F. Gould, A. Rowland-Seymour, R. Sharma, Z. Berger, et al. 2014. "Meditation Programs for Psychological Stress and Well-Being: A Systematic Review and Meta-Analysis." *JAMA Internal Medicine* 174(3): 357-68.

Lazarus R.S., and S. Folkman. 1984. *Stress, Appraisal and Coping*. New York: Springer.

National Institutes of Mental Health. 2016a. "Anxiety Disorders." Last modified March 2016. www.nimh.nih.gov/health/topics/anxiety-disorders/index.shtml.

National Institutes of Mental Health. 2016. "Depression." Last modified October 2016. www.nimh.nih.gov/health/topics/depression/index.shtml.

National Institutes of Health. 2017. "Stress." Last modified September 2017. https://nccih.nih.gov/health/stress.

Office of Disease Prevention and Health. 2008. *Physical Activity Guidelines for Americans*. Washington, DC: U.S. Department of Health and Human Services. https://health.gov/paguidelines.

Puetz, T.W., P.J. O'Connor, and R.K. Dishman. 2006. "Effects of Chronic Exercise on Feelings of Energy and Fatigue: A Quantitative Synthesis." *Psychological Bulletin* 132(6): 866-76.

Sapolsky, R.M. 2004. *Why Zebras Don't Get Ulcers*. New York: St. Martin's Press.

University of South Florida. n.d. "10 Steps to Successful Time Management." Accessed July 24, 2017. http://hsc.usf.edu/NR/rdonlyres/B054F50D-8B3E-4B90-9352-FEC5144E-6C04/26088/10StepstoSuccessfulTimeManagement.pdf.

Watson, N.F., M.S. Badr, G. Belenky, D.L. Bliwise, O.M. Buxton, D. Buysse, D.F. Dinges, et al. 2015. "Recommended Amount of Sleep for a Healthy Adult: A Joint Consensus Statement of the American Academy of Sleep Medicine and Sleep Research Society." *Sleep* 38(6): 843-4.

Chapter 11

Addiction Hope. 2016. "Sexual Addiction Causes, Statistics, Addiction Signs, Symptoms & Side Effects." Accessed March 4, 2017. www.addictionhope.com/sexual-addiction.

American Lung Association. 2016. "E-Cigarettes and Lung Health." Last modified December 8, 2016. www.lung.org/stop-smoking/smoking-facts/e-cigarettes-and-lung-health.html.

American Lung Association. n.d.a. "I Want to Quit Smoking." Accessed January 28, 2017. www.lung.org/stop-smoking/i-want-to-quit.

American Lung Association. n.d.b. "Nicotine." Accessed January 28, 2017. www.lung.org/stop-smoking/smoking-facts/nicotine.html.

American Lung Association. n.d.c. "What's in a Cigarette?" Accessed January 28, 2017. www.lung.org/stop-smoking/smoking-facts/whats-in-a-cigarette.html.

American Psychiatric Association. 2000. *Diagnostic and Statistical Manual of Mental Disorders* (4th ed.). Washington, DC: Author.

BBC News. 2014. "Many Young People Addicted to Net, Survey Suggests." October 15, 2014. www.bbc.com/news/technology-29627896.

Bragg, J. 2009. "Digging Out From $80,000 in Debt." *CNN: Money and Main Street*, September 22, 2009. www.cnn.com/2009/LIVING/worklife/09/21/mainstreet.digging.out.of.debt/index.html?_s=PM:LIVING.

Caba, J. 2013. "Heavy Drinking Will Lead to Divorce, Unless Both Partners Are Equally Alcoholic." www.medicaldaily.com/heavy-drinking-will-lead-divorce-unless-both-partners-are-equally-alcoholic-263648.

Center for Behavioral Health Statistics and Quality. 2016. *Key Substance Use and Mental Health Indicators in the United States: Results From the 2015 National Survey on Drug Use and Health*. HHS Publication No. SMA 16-4984, NSDUH Series H-51. www.samhsa.gov/data/sites/default/files/NSDUH-FFR1-2015/NSDUH-FFR1-2015/NSDUH-FFR1-2015.pdf.

Centers for Disease Control and Prevention. 1988. *Program Evaluation Handbook: Drug Abuse Education*. Office of Disease Prevention and Promotion, U.S. Department of Health and Human Services. Los Angeles, CA: The Associates.

Centers for Disease Control and Prevention. 2016. "Hookas." Last modified December 1. www.cdc.gov/tobacco/data_statistics/fact_sheets/tobacco_industry/hookahs.

Centers for Disease Control and Prevention. 2017a. "Benefits of Quitting." Last modified June 30, 2017. www.cdc.gov/tobacco/quit_smoking/how_to_quit/benefits/index.htm.

Centers for Disease Control and Prevention. 2017b. "Caffeine and Alcohol." Last modified June 9, 2017. www.cdc.gov/alcohol/fact-sheets/caffeine-and-alcohol.htm.

Centers for Disease Control and Prevention. 2017c. "Health Effects of Cigarette Smoking." Last modified May 15, 2017. www.cdc.gov/tobacco/data_statistics/fact_sheets/health_effects/effects_cig_smoking.

Centers for Disease Control and Prevention. 2017d. "Syringe Services Programs." Last modified September 28, 2017. www.cdc.gov/hiv/risk/ssps.html.

Cranford, J.A. 2014. "DSM-IV Alcohol Dependence and Marital Dissolution: Evidence From the National Epidemiologic Survey on Alcohol and Related Conditions." *Journal of Studies on Alcohol and Drugs* 75(3): 520-9. http://dx.doi.org/10.15288/jsad.2014.75.520.

Eating Disorder Hope. n.d. "Eating Disorder Statistics & Research." Accessed March 4, 2017. www.eatingdisorderhope.com/information/statistics-studies.

Feliz, J. 2014. "New Survey: Misuse and Abuse of Prescription Stimulants Becoming Normalized Behavior Among College Students, Young Adults."

www.drugfree.org/newsroom/adhd-survey-2014.

Foundation for a Drug-Free World. n.d. "The Truth about Crystal Meth and Methamphetamine." Accessed January 2, 2017. www.drugfreeworld.org/drugfacts/crystalmeth.html.

Grant, J., M. Potenza, A. Weinstein, and D. Gorelick. 2010. "Introduction to Behavioral Addictions." *American Journal of Drug and Alcohol Abuse* 35(5): 233-41. doi:10.3109/00952990.2010.491884.

Johnston, L.D., M. O'Malley, J.G. Bachman, J.E. Schulenberg, and R.A. Miech. 2016. *Monitoring the Future National Survey Results on Drug Use, 1975-2014: Volume 2, College students and adults ages 19-55*. Ann Arbor, MI: Institute for Social Research, The University of Michigan.

www.monitoringthefuture.org/pubs/monographs/mtf-vol2_2015.pdf.

Kilpatrick, S. 2016. "How to Help Prevent Students from Abusing Drug and Alcohol." www.campusanswers.com/prevent-student-drug-alcohol-abuse.

Koran, L.M., R.J. Faber, E. Aboujaoude, M.D. Large, and R.T. Serpe. 2006. "Estimated Prevalence of Compulsive Buying Behavior in the United States." *American Journal of Psychiatry* 163(10): 1806-12.

National Council on Alcoholism and Drug Dependence. 2015. "Drugs and Alcohol in the Workplace." www.ncadd.org/about-addiction/addiction-update/drugs-and-alcohol-in-the-workplace.

National Council on Problem Gambling. n.d. "What Is Problem Gambling?" Accessed March 4, 2017. www.ncpgambling.org/help-treatment/faq.

National Institute on Alcohol Abuse and Alcoholism. n.d. "Alcohol Myths." *College Drinking: Changing the Culture*. Accessed June 22, 2017. www.collegedrinkingprevention.gov/specialfeatures/alcoholmyths.aspx.

National Institute on Alcohol Abuse and Alcoholism. n.d. "Alcohol and You: An Interactive Body." Accessed December 31, 2016. https://www.collegedrinkingprevention.gov/SpecialFeatures/interactiveBody.aspx.

National Institute on Alcohol Abuse and Alcoholism. 2012. "A Family History of Alcoholism: Are You at Risk?" https://pubs.niaaa.nih.gov/publications/familyhistory/famhist.htm.

National Institute on Drug Abuse. 2012a. "Commonly Abused Drugs." www.drugabuse.gov/sites/default/files/cadchart_2.pdf.

National Institute on Drug Abuse. 2012b. "Research Report Series: Inhalants." https://d14rmgtrwzf5a.cloudfront.net/sites/default/files/inhalantsrrs.pdf.

National Institute on Drug Abuse. 2014. "Stimulant ADHD Medications: Methylphenidate and Amphetamines." Last modified January, 2014. www.drugabuse.gov/publications/drugfacts/stimulant-adhd-medications-methylphenidate-amphetamines.

National Institute on Drug Abuse. 2016a. "Drug and Alcohol Use in College-Age Adults in 2015." Last modified November, 2016. www.drugabuse.gov/related-topics/trends-statistics/infographics/drug-alcohol-use-in-college-age-adults-in-2015.

National Institute on Drug Abuse. 2016b. "Understanding Drug Use and Addiction." Last modified August 2016. www.drugabuse.gov/publications/drugfacts/understanding-drug-use-addiction.

National Institute on Drug Abuse. 2016c. "What is Cocaine?" www.drugabuse.gov/publications/research-reports/cocaine.

National Institute on Drug Abuse. 2017a. "College-Age and Young Adults." Last modified July, 2017. www.drugabuse.gov/related-topics/college-age-young-adults.

National Institute on Drug Abuse. 2017b. "Commonly Abused Drug Charts." Last modified July, 2017. www.drugabuse.gov/drugs-abuse/commonly-abused-drugs-charts.

National Institute on Drug Abuse. 2017c. "Cough and Cold Medicine Abuse." Last modified December, 2017. www.drugabuse.gov/publications/drugfacts/cough-cold-medicine-abuse.

National Institute on Drug Abuse. 2017d. "Heroin." Last modified July, 2017. www.drugabuse.gov/publications/drugfacts/heroin.

National Institute on Drug Abuse. 2017e. "Methamphetamine." Last modified February, 2017. www.drugabuse.gov/publications/drugfacts/methamphetamine.

National Institute on Drug Abuse. 2017f. "What is Marijuana?" Last modified August, 2017. www.drugabuse.gov/publications/drugfacts/marijuana.

National Institute on Drug Abuse for Teens. 2017. "Inhalants." Last modified March, 2017. https://teens.drugabuse.gov/drug-facts/inhalants.

Patrick, S.W., R.E. Schumacher, B.D. Benneyworth, E.E. Krans, J.M. McAllister, and M.M. Davis. 2012. "Neonatal Abstinence Syndrome and Associated Health Care Expenditures: United States, 2000-2009." *Journal of the American Medical Association* 307(18): 1934-40. doi:10.1001/jama.2012.3951.

Physicians Committee for Responsible Medicine. n.d. "Birth Defect Statistics." Accessed April 22, 2017. www.pcrm.org/research/resch/reschethics/birth-defect-statistics.

Ritalin Abuse Health. n.d. "What Are Street Names for Ritalin?" Accessed February 26, 2017. www.ritalinabusehelp.com/what-are-street-names-for-ritalin.

Rubin, J. n.d. "Compulsive Exercise." Accessed March 4, 2017. www.nationaleatingdisorders.org/compulsive-exercise.

Somogyi, L. 2010. "Caffeine Intake by the US Population." www.fda.gov/downloads/AboutFDA/CentersOffices/OfficeofFoods/CFSAN/CFSANFOIAElectronicReadingRoom/UCM333191.pdf.

Stop Medicine Abuse. n.d. "Slang Terms." Accessed February 26, 2017. http://stopmedicineabuse.org/what-does-abuse-look-like/slang-terms.

Substance Abuse and Mental Health Services Administration. 2013. *Results From the 2012 National Survey on Drug Use and Health: Summary of National Findings.* NSDUH Series H-46, HHS Publication No. (SMA) 13-4795. Rockville, MD: Author.

Substance Abuse and Mental Health Services Administration. 2014. *Results From the 2013 National Survey on Drug Use and Health: Summary of National Findings.* NSDUH Series H-48, HHS Publication No. (SMA) 14-4863. Rockville, MD: Author. www.samhsa.gov/data/sites/default/files/NSDUHresultsPDFWHTML2013/Web/NSDUHresults2013.htm.

Substance Abuse and Mental Health Services Administration. 2015. *Behavioral Health Trends in the United States: Results From the 2014 National Survey on Drug Use and Health.* HHS Publication No. (SMA) 15-4927, NSDUH Series H-50. www.samhsa.gov/data.

Substance Abuse and Mental Health Services Administration. 2016. "Racial and Ethnic Minority Populations." Last modified February 18, 2016. www.samhsa.gov/specific-populations/racial-ethnic-minority.

U.S. Department of Health and Human Services. 2012. *Preventing Tobacco Use Among Youth and Young Adults: A Report of the Surgeon General.* Atlanta: Author. www.surgeongeneral.gov/library/reports/preventing-youth-tobacco-use/full-report.pdf.

U.S. Department of Health and Human Services. 2016. *E-Cigarette Use Among Youth and Young Adults: A Report of the Surgeon General.* Atlanta: Author. https://e-cigarettes.surgeongeneral.gov/documents/2016_SGR_Exec_Summ_508.pdf.

U.S. Drug Enforcement Administration. n.d. "Total of All Meth Clandestine Laboratory Incidents Including Labs, Dumpsites, Chem/Glass/Equipment." Accessed April 30, 2017. \www.dea.gov/resource-center/meth-lab-maps.shtml.

Volkow, N.D. 2013. "Letter From the Director: Methamphetamine." *National Institute on Drug Abuse.* www.drugabuse.gov/publications/research-reports/methamphetamine.

Chapter 12

Centers for Disease Control and Prevention. n.d. "Frequently Asked Questions." Get Tested. National HIV, STD, and Hepatitis Testing. https://gettested.cdc.gov/faq-page.

Centers for Disease Control and Prevention. 2013a. "CDC Fact Sheet: Incidence, Prevalence, and Cost of Sexually Transmitted Infections in the United States." www.cdc.gov/std/stats/sti-estimates-fact-sheet-feb-2013.pdf.

Centers for Disease Control and Prevention. 2013b. "Condom Fact Sheet in Brief." Last modified March 25, 2013. www.cdc.gov/condomeffectiveness/brief.html.

Centers for Disease Control and Prevention. 2015. "Unintended Pregnancy Prevention." Last modified January 22, 2015. www.cdc.gov/reproductivehealth/unintendedpregnancy.

Centers for Disease Control and Prevention. 2016a. "2015 STD Surveillance Report." Last modified October 19, 2016. www.cdc.gov/nchhstp/newsroom/2016/2015-std-surveillance-report.html#Figures.

Centers for Disease Control and Prevention. 2016b. "Reported STDs at Unprecedented High in the US." Last modified October 19, 2016. www.cdc.gov/nchhstp/newsroom/2016/std-surveillance-report-2015-press-release.html.

Centers for Disease Control and Prevention. 2017a. "Areas With Risk of Zika" Last modified September 15, 2017. www.cdc.gov/zika/geo/index.html.

Centers for Disease Control and Prevention. 2017b. "Effectiveness of Family Planning Methods." Last modified February 9, 2017. www.cdc.gov/reproductivehealth/contraception/unintendedpregnancy/pdf/contraceptive_methods_508.pdf.

Centers for Disease Control and Prevention. 2017c. "Genital Herpes—CDC Fact sheet." Last modified September 1, 2017. www.cdc.gov/std/herpes/stdfact-herpes.htm.

Centers for Disease Control and Prevention. 2017d. "Genital HPV Infection—Fact Sheet." Last modified November 16, 2017. www.cdc.gov/std/hpv/stdfact-hpv.htm.

Centers for Disease Control and Prevention. 2017e. "HIV in the United States: At a Glance." Last modified November 29, 2017. www.cdc.gov/hiv/statistics/overview/ataglance.html.

Centers for Disease Control and Prevention. 2017f. "HPV Vaccine Coverage Maps—Infographic." Last modified August 24, 2017. www.cdc.gov/hpv/infographics/vacc-coverage.html.

Centers for Disease Control and Prevention. 2017g. "HPV Vaccine Information for Young Women." Last modified January 3, 2017. www.cdc.gov/std/hpv/STDFact-HPV-vaccine-young-women.htm.

Centers for Disease Control and Prevention. 2017h. "How Effective are Birth Control Methods?" Last modified February 9, 2017. www.cdc.gov/reproductivehealth/contraception.

Centers for Disease Control and Prevention. 2017i. "How Zika Spreads." Last modified August 28, 2017. www.cdc.gov/zika/about/overview.html.

Centers for Disease Control and Prevention. 2017j. "Pre-Exposure Prophylaxis (PrEP)." Last modified August 31, 2017. www.cdc.gov/hiv/risk/prep/index.html.

Centers for Disease Control and Prevention. 2017k. "Sexual Transmission and Prevention." Last modified August 2, 2017. www.cdc.gov/zika/prevention/sexual-transmission-prevention.html.

Centers for Disease Control and Prevention. 2017l. "HPV Vaccines: Vaccinating Your Preteen or Teen." Last modified August 24, 2017. www.cdc.gov/hpv/parents/vaccine.html.

Daniels, K., J. Daugherty, and J. Jones. 2014. *Current Contraceptive Status Among Women Aged 15-44: United States, 2011-2013. NCHS data brief, no. 173.* Hyattsville, MD: National Center for Health Statistics. www.cdc.gov/nchs/data/databriefs/db173.pdf.

Encyclopedia Britannica. n.d. "Spermatogenesis." Accessed July 8, 2017. www.britannica.com/science/spermatogenesis.

Guttmacher Institute. 2016. "Contraceptive Use in the United States." www.guttmacher.org/fact-sheet/contraceptive-use-united-states.

Guttmacher Institute. 2018. "Partner Treatment for STIs." Last modified January 1, 2018. www.guttmacher.org/state-policy/explore/partner-treatment-stis.

Hall, H.I., Q. An, T. Tang, R. Song, M. Chen, T. Green, and J. Kang. 2015. "Prevalence of Diagnosed and Undiagnosed HIV Infection—United States, 2008-2012." *MMWR* 64(24): 657-62. www.cdc.gov/mmwr/preview/mmwrhtml/mm6424a2.htm?s_cid=mm6424a2_e.

Healthy Children. 2012. "Should the Baby Be Circumcised?" Last modified August 27, 2012. www.healthychildren.org/English/ages-stages/prenatal/decisions-to-make/Pages/Should-the-Baby-be-Circumcised.aspx.

Holcomb, J.S. 2016. "10 Things You Should Know About Sexual Assault." www.crossway.org/articles/10-things-you-should-know-about-sexual-assault.

Manlove, J.S., S. Ryan, and K. Franzetta. 2003. "Patterns of Contraceptive Use Within Teenagers' First Sexual Relationships." *Perspectives on Sexual and Reproductive Health* 36(6): 246-55. doi: https://doi.org/10.1363/3524603.

Market Wired. 2014. "Eight Leading National Fraternities Form a Historic Consortium to Address Important Issues of Sexual Misconduct, Hazing and Binge Drinking Head On." https://finance.yahoo.com/news/eight-leading-national-fraternities-form-133500836.html.

Martinez, G.M., and J.C. Abma. 2015. *Sexual Activity, Contraceptive Use, and Childbearing of Teenagers Aged 15-19 in the United States. NCHS data brief, no 209.* Hyattsville, MD: National Center for Health Statistics.

Office on Women's Health. 2015. "Sexual Assault Fact Sheet." Last modified on September 18, 2015. www.womenshealth.gov/files/assets/docs/fact-sheets/sexual-assault-factsheet.pdf.

Office on Women's Health. 2017. "Sexual Assault." Last modified April 28, 2017. www.womenshealth.gov/a-z-topics/sexual-assault.

Pan American Health Organization. n.d. "What Is Zika?" Accessed March 9, 2017. http://new.paho.org/hq/images/stories/AD/HSD/IR/Viral_Diseases/Zika-Virus/8x11intro-ENG.png.

Rape, Abuse, and Incest National Network. n.d. "Sexual Assault." Accessed July 11, 2017. www.rainn.org/articles/sexual-assault.

Satterwhite, C.L., E. Torrone, E. Meites, E.F. Dunne, R. Mahajan, M.C. Ocfemia, J. Su, F. Xu, and H. Weinstock. 2013. "Sexually Transmitted Infections among US Women and Men: Prevalence and Prevalence Estimates, 2008." *Sexually Transmitted Diseases* 40(3): 187-93.

Trussell, J. 2011. "Contraceptive Failure in the United States." *Contraception* 83(5): 397-404.

US Department of Health and Human Services. 2016a. "Female Sterilization." Last modified August 16, 2016. www.hhs.gov/opa/pregnancy-prevention/sterilization/female-sterilization/index.html.

US Department of Health and Human Services. 2016b. "Hormonal Methods." Last modified August 25, 2016. www.hhs.gov/opa/pregnancy-prevention/hormonal-methods/index.html.

US Department of Health and Human Services. 2016c. "Male Sterilization." Last modified August 16, 2016. www.hhs.gov/

opa/pregnancy-prevention/sterilization/male-sterilization/index.html.

US Department of Justice. 2017. "An Updated Definition of Rape." Last modified April 7, 2017. www.justice.gov/archives/opa/blog/updated-definition-rape.

World Health Organization. 2017. "Female Genital Mutilation." Last modified March 26, 2017. www.who.int/mediacentre/factsheets/fs241/en.

Chapter 13

American Diabetes Association. n.d. "Diabetes Basics." Accessed December 30, 2017. www.diabetes.org/diabetes-basics.

American Diabetes Association. 2014. "Diagnosing Diabetes and Learning About Prediabetes." Last modified December 9, 2014. www.diabetes.org/are-you-at-risk/prediabetes/?loc=a-trisk-slabnav.

American Heart Association. 2016. "Peripheral Artery Disease." Last modified October 2016. www.heart.org/HEART-ORG/Conditions/VascularHealth/PeripheralArteryDisease/Peripheral-Artery-Disease-PAD_UCM_002082_SubHome-Page.jsp.

American Heart Association. 2018. "Understand Your Risks to Prevent a Heart Attack." www.heart.org/HEARTORG/Conditions/HeartAttack/UnderstandYourRiskstoPreventaHeartAttack/Understand-Your-Risks-to-Prevent-a-Heart-Attack_UCM_002040_Article.jsp#.WkOraN-nGUk.

American Heart Association and American Stroke Association. 2017. *Highlights From the 2017 Guideline for the Prevention, Detection, Evaluation and Management of High Blood Pressure in Adults.* http://professional.heart.org/idc/groups/ahamah-public/@wcm/@sop/@smd/documents/downloadable/ucm_497445.pdf.

American Stroke Association. n.d. "About Stroke." www.strokeassociation.org/STROKEORG/AboutStroke/About-Stroke_UCM_308529_SubHomePage.jsp. Accessed December 30, 2017.

Arts, J., M.L. Fernandez, and I.E. Lofgren. 2014. "Coronary Heart Disease Risk Factors in College Students." *Advances in Nutrition* 5(2): 177-87.

Centers for Disease Control and Prevention. 2015. "Heart Disease Risk Factors." www.cdc.gov/heartdisease/risk_factors.htm.

Centers for Disease Control and Prevention. 2017a. "Diabetes Basics." www.cdc.gov/diabetes/basics/index.html.

Centers for Disease Control and Prevention. 2017b. "Prediabetes." www.cdc.gov/diabetes/basics/prediabetes.html.

International Diabetes Federation. 2006. *The IDF Consensus Worldwide Definition of the Metabolic Syndrome.* Brussels: IDF Communications. www.idf.org/e-library/consensus-statements/60-idfconsensus-worldwide-definitionof-the-metabolic-syndrome.html.

Libby, P., P.M. Ridker, and G.K. Hansson. 2009. "Inflammation in Atherosclerosis: From Pathophysiology to Practice." *Journal of the American College of Cardiology* 54(23): 2129-38.

Moore, J.X., N. Chaudhary, and T. Akinyemiju. 2017. "Metabolic Syndrome Prevalence by Race/Ethnicity and Sex in the United States, National Health and Nutrition Examination Survey, 1988-2012." *Preventing Chronic Disease* 14: E24.

National Heart, Lung, and Blood Institute. 2012. *Expert Panel on Guidelines for Cardiovascular Health and Risk Reduction in Children and Adolescents.* NIH Publication No. 12-7486. Bethesda, MD: Author. www.nhlbi.nih.gov/files/docs/guidelines/peds_guidelines_full.pdf.

Roitman, J.L., and T. LaFontaine. 2012. *The Exercise Professional's Guide to Optimizing Health.* Baltimore: Lippincott Williams & Wilkins.

Stocks, T., T. Bjorge, H. Ulmer, J. Manjer, C. Haggstrom, G. Nagel, A. Engeland, et al. 2015. "Metabolic Risk Score and Cancer Risk: Pooled Analysis of Seven Cohorts." *International Journal of Epidemiology* 44(4): 1353-63.

Stone, N.J., J.G. Robinson, A.H. Lichtenstein, C.N. Bairey Merz, C.B. Blum, R.H. Eckel, A.C. Goldberg, et al. 2014. "2013 ACC/AHA Guideline on the Treatment of Blood Cholesterol to Reduce Atherosclerotic Cardiovascular Risk in Adults: A Report of the American College Of Cardiology/American Heart Association Task Force on Practice Guidelines." *Circulation* 129(25 Suppl 2): S1-45.

World Health Organization. 2017. "The Top 10 Causes of Death." www.who.int/mediacentre/factsheets/fs310/en.

Chapter 14

American Association for Cancer Research. 2014. "AACR Cancer Progress Report 2014." *Clinical Cancer Research* 20(Supplement 1): SI-S124.

American Cancer Society. n.d. "Nutrition and Activity Quiz." Accessed May 10, 2017. www.cancer.org/healthy/eat-healthy-get-active/nutrition-activity-quiz.html.

American Cancer Society. 2016a. "Lifetime Risk of Developing or Dying From Cancer." Last modified March 23, 2016. www.cancer.org/cancer/cancer-basics/lifetime-probability-of-developing-or-dying-from-cancer.html.

American Cancer Society. 2016b. "Do I Have Testicular Cancer?" Last modified May 23, 2016. www.cancer.org/cancer/testicular-cancer/do-i-have-testicular-cancer.html.

American Cancer Society. 2017a. *Cancer Facts & Figures 2017.* Atlanta: American Cancer Society.

American Cancer Society. 2017b. "2017 Estimates." *Cancer Statistics Center.* https://cancerstatisticscenter.cancer.org/#/.

American Cancer Society. 2017c. "Understanding Genetic Testing for Cancer." Last modified April 10, 2017. www.cancer.org/cancer/cancer-causes/genetics/understanding-genetic-testing-for-cancer.html#written_by.

American Cancer Society. 2017d. *American Joint Committee on Cancer: Breast Cancer Staging* (7th ed.). https://cancerstaging.org/references-tools/quickreferences/Documents/BreastSmall.pdf.

American Institute for Cancer Research. 2017. "What You Need to Know About Obesity and Cancer." www.aicr.org/learn-more-about-cancer/infographics/infographic-obesity-and-cancer.html.

Blot, W.J., and J.K. McLaughlin. 2004. "Are Women More Susceptible to Lung Cancer?" *Journal of the National Cancer Institute* 96(11): 812-3. doi: 10.1093/jnci/djh180.

Breastcancer.org. 2017. "The Five Steps of a Breast Self-Exam." Last modified February 22, 2017. www.breastcancer.org/symptoms/testing/types/self_exam/bse_steps.

Centers for Disease Control and Prevention. 2015. *Health, United States, 2015: With Special Feature on Racial and Ethnic Health Disparities*. Hyattsville, MD: Author.

Centers for Disease Control and Prevention. 2016. "Surgeon General's Reports on Smoking and Tobacco Use." Last modified December 8, 2016. www.cdc.gov/tobacco/data_statistics/sgr/.

Centers for Disease Control and Prevention. 2017. "What Are the Risk Factors for Skin Cancer?" Last modified April 25, 2017. www.cdc.gov/cancer/skin/basic_info/risk_factors.htm.

Colditz, G.A., and E.K. Wei. 2012. "Preventability of Cancer: The Relative Contributions of Biologic and Social and Physical Environmental Determinants of Cancer Mortality." *Annual Review of Public Health* 33: 137-56.

Kochanek, K.D., S.L. Murphy, J. Xu, and B. Tejada-Vera. 2016. "Deaths: Final Data for 2014." *National Vital Statistics Reports* 65(4). Hyattsville, MD: National Center for Health Statistics. www.cdc.gov/nchs/data/nvsr/nvsr65/nvsr65_04.pdf.

National Cancer Institute. 1990. "Normal and Cancer Cells Structure." Last modified January 1, 2001. https://visualsonline.cancer.gov/details.cfm?imageid=2512.

National Cancer Institute. 2008. "Cancer Health Disparities." Last modified March 11, 2008. www.cancer.gov/about-nci/organization/crchd/cancer-health-disparities-fact-sheet.

National Cancer Institute. 2015. "Usual Dietary Intakes: Food Intakes, U.S. Population, 2007-10." Last modified May 20, 2015. http://epi.grants.cancer.gov/diet/usualintakes/pop/2007-10.

National Cancer Institute. 2016a. "Cancer Disparities." Last modified October 21, 2016. www.cancer.gov/about-cancer/understanding/disparities.

National Cancer Institute. 2016b. "Probability of Developing or Dying of Cancer." Statistical Research and Applications Branch. www.srab.cancer.gov/devcan.

National Cancer Institute. 2017. "Radiation Therapy. NCI Dictionary of Cancer Terms." www.cancer.gov/publications/dictionaries/cancer-terms?cdrid=44971.

National Safety Council. 2017. "Injury Facts: The Source for Safety Data." www.nsc.org/learn/safety-knowledge/Pages/injury-facts.aspx.

Naume, B. 2014. "Metastatic Patterns of Breast Cancer." Last modified March 26, 2014. http://oncolex.org/Breast-cancer/Background/MetastaticPatterns.

Nordqvist, C. 2015. "Chemotherapy: Types, Uses, Side Effects." *Medical News Today*. Last modified July 8, 2015. www.medicalnewstoday.com/articles/158401.php.

Ogden, C.L., M.D. Carrol, B.K. Kit, and K.M. Flegal. 2014. "Prevalence of Childhood and Adult Obesity in the United States, 2011-2012." *Journal of the American Medical Association* 311(8): 806.

Ropeik, D., and G. Gray. 2002. *Risk: A Practical Guide for Deciding What's Really Safe and What's Really Dangerous in the World Around You*. New York: Houghton Mifflin.

Simon, G.R., and O.T. Brustugun. 2015. "Metastatic Patterns of Lung Cancer." Last modified August 7, 2015. http://oncolex.org/Lung-cancer/Background/MetastaticPatterns.

The Wildlife Museum. n.d. "What Are the Odds of a Shark Attack?" Accessed April 18, 2017. www.thewildlifemuseum.org/exhibits/sharks/odds-of-a-shark-attack.

U.S. Department of Health and Human Services. 2014. *The Health Consequences of Smoking: 50 Years of Progress. A Report of the Surgeon General*. Atlanta: Author. www.surgeongeneral.gov/library/reports/50-years-of-progress/front-matter.pdf.

Yarnal, C., X. Qian, J. Hustad, and D. Sims. 2013. "Intervention for Positive Use of Leisure Time Among College Students." *Journal of College and Character* 14(2): 171-6. doi:10.1515/jcc-2013-0022.

Chapter 15

Barnes, P.M., B. Bloom, and R. Nahin. 2008. https://nccih.nih.gov/sites/nccam.nih.gov/files/news/nhsr12.pdf. *National Health Statistics Report* 2008 December 10(12): 1-23.

Barnes, P., E. Powell-Griner, K. McFann, and R. Nahin. 2004. https://nccih.nih.gov/sites/nccam.nih.gov/files/news/camstats/2002/report.pdf. *Advance Data* 2004 May 27(343): 1-19.

Centers for Disease Control and Prevention. 2017. "Adult Obesity Prevalence Maps." Last modified August 31, 2017. www.cdc.gov/obesity/data/prevalence-maps.html.

Church, T.S., D.M. Thomas, C. Tudor-Locke, P.T. Katzmarzyk, C.P. Earnest, R.Q. Rodarte, C.K. Martin, S.N. Blair, and C. Bouchard. 2011. "Trends Over 5 Decades in U.S. Occupation-Related Physical Activity and Their Associations With Obesity." *PLoS ONE* 6(5): e19657. https://doi.org/10.1371/journal.pone.0019657.

Clarke, T.C., L.I. Black, B.J. Stussman, P.M. Barnes, and R.L. Nahin. 2015. http://www.cdc.gov/nchs/data/nhsr/nhsr079.pdf. *National Health Statistics reports; no. 79*. Hyattsville, MD: National Center for Health Statistics.

Daley, M.J., and W.L. Spinks. 2000. "Exercise Mobility and Aging." *Sports Medicine* 29(1): 1-12.

Duncan, M., B. Murawski, C.E. Short, A.L. Rebar, S. Schoeppe, S. Alley, C. Vandelanotte, and M. Kirwan. 2017. "Activity Trackers Implement Different Behavior Change Techniques for Activity, Sleep, and Sedentary Behaviors." *Interactive Journal of Medical Research* 6(2): e13. http://doi.org/10.2196/ijmr.6685.

Endeavour Partners. (2014, August 15). "Endeavour Partners' Consumer Behavior Study Points to Uncertain Future of Wearable Devices." *Marketwired*. www.marketwired.com/press-release/endeavour-partners-consumer-behavior-study-points-uncertain-future-wearable-devices-1938954.htm.

Green, D.J. 2015. *How Will Wearable Activity Devices Impact the Fitness Industry?* https://acewebcontent.azureedge.net/certifiednews/images/article/pdfs/ACE_WearableStudy.pdf.

Herz, J.C. (2014, November 6). "Wearables Are Totally Failing the People Who Need Them Most." *WIRED*. www.wired.com/2014/11/where-fitness-trackers-fail.

Kiessling, P., and C. Kennedy-Armbruster. 2016. "Move More, Sit Less, Be Well: Behavioral Aspects of Activity Trackers." *ACSM's Health and Fitness Journal* 20(6): 26-31.

Mandic, S., J. Myers, R. Oliveira, J. Abella, and V. Froelicher. 2009. "Characterizing Differences in Mortality at the Low End of the Fitness Spectrum." *Medicine and Science in Sports and Exercise* 41(8): 1573-9.

McGavock, J., J. Hastings, P. Snell, D. McGuire, E. Pacini, B. Levine, and J. Mitchell. 2009. "A Forty-Year Follow-Up of the Dallas Bed Rest and Training Study: The Effect of Age on the Cardiovascular Response to Exercise in Men." *The Journals of Gerontology: Series A* 64A(2): 293-9. https://doi.org/10.1093/gerona/gln025.

McGuire, D.K., B.D. Levine, J.W. Williamson, P.G. Snell, C.G. Blomqvist, B. Saltin, and J.H. Mitchell JH. 2001. "A 30-Year Follow-Up of the Dallas Bedrest and Training Study: II. Effect of Age on Cardiovascular Adaptation to Exercise Training." *Circulation* 104(12): 1358-66.

National Center for Complimentary Medicine and Integrative Health. "The use of complementary and alternative medicine in the US. 2017." https://nccih.nih.gov/research/statistics/2007/camsurvey_fs1.htm.

National Center for Complementary and Integrative Health. 2016. "Complementary, Alternative, or Integrative Health: What's in a Name?" https://nccih.nih.gov/health/integrative-health.

National Center for Complementary and Integrative Health. 2017a. "Trends in Natural Products." https://nccih.nih.gov/research/statistics/NHIS/2012/natural-products/trends.

National Center for Complementary and Integrative Health. 2017b. "Yoga and Wellness." https://nccih.nih.gov/research/statistics/NHIS/2012/wellness/yoga.

Paffenbarger, R., M.A. Hyde, A. Wing, and C. Hsieh. 1986. "Physical Activity, All-Cause Mortality, and Longevity of College Alumni." *New England Journal of Medicine* 314(10): 605-13. doi: 10.1056/NEJM198603063141003.

Saltin, B., G. Blomqvist, J.H. Mitchell, R.L. Johnson, Jr., K. Wildenthal, and C.B. Chapman. 1968. "Response to Exercise After Bed Rest and After Training." *Circulation* 38 (suppl 5): VII1- 78.

Segar, M. 2015. *No Sweat: How the Simple Science of Motivation Can Bring You a Lifetime of Fitness*. New York: AMACOM.

Sforzo, G., M. Moore, and M. Scholtz. 2015. "Delivering Change That Lasts: Health and Wellness Coaching Competencies for Exercise Professionals." *ACSM's Health and Fitness Journal* 19(2): 20-5.

Signorile, J.F. 2011. *Bending the Aging Curve: The Complete Exercise Guide for Older Adults*. Champaign, IL: Human Kinetics.

Stanton, W.R. 1996. *From Child to Adult: The Dunedin Multidisciplinary Health and Development Study*. Oxford: Oxford University Press.

Stussman, B.J., L.I. Black, P.M. Barnes, T.C. Clarke, and R.L. Nahin. 2015. http://www.cdc.gov/nchs/data/nhsr/nhsr085.pdf. *National Health Statistics Reports; no. 85*. Hyattsville, MD: National Center for Health Statistics.

Tharrett, S., and J. Peterson. 2017. *Fitness Management* (4th ed.). Monterey, CA: Healthy Learning.

Thompson, W.R. 2017. "Worldwide Survey of Fitness Trends for 2018." *ACSM's Health & Fitness Journal* 21(6): 10-19.

United Nations. 2005. *World Population Prospects: The 2004 Revision*. New York: Author.

Warburton, D., S. Charlesworth, H. Foulds, D. McKenzie, R. Shephard, and S. Bredin. 2013. "Qualified Exercise Professionals: Best Practices for Work With Clinical Populations." *Canadian Family Physician* 59(7): 759-61.

INDEX

Note: The italicized *f* and *t* following page numbers refer to figures and tables, respectively.

A

AAS (anabolic-androgenic steroids) 103
abdominals
  daily activity and 128
  strengthening and stretching 129
abstinence 282
academic achievement, cardiorespiratory fitness and 74
Academy of Nutrition and Dietetic 194
Achilles tendon 123
acquired immunodeficiency syndrome. *See* HIV/AIDS
ACTH (adrenocorticotropic hormone) 221
action stage of change 40, 44*f*
active transportation 52*t*, 82
activity(ies) 54, 77, 79, 80, 80*f*. *See also* physical activity(ies)
activity trackers 364-365
added sugars 172, 188, 209*t*
Adderall 246, 247, 247*f*, 256
addiction 254
  college students and 246-257, 247*f*
  signs and risk factors 245-246
  types of 240-244
adductor longus 134
adductor magnus 134
adenosine triphosphate (ATP) 68-69, 68*f*, 70
adenosine triphosphate-phosphocreatine (ATP-PC system) 69*t*, 70
ADHD (attention-deficit hyperactivity disorder) 256
adipocytes 149
adiposity 149, 157-159
adolescents
  addiction in 240
  lean mass, bone mass, and density in 150
  need for sleep 232
  preventing obesity in 202
adrenal glands 221
adrenalin. *See* epinephrine
adrenocorticotropic hormone (ACTH) 221
adults
  complementary health approaches for 363*f*
  macronutrient distribution recommended for 174*f*
  overweight and obesity of 198-199, 198*f*, 346
AED (automatic external defibrillator) 318
aerosols 252

age 107, 316*f*, 337*t*
  effects on body composition 150
  functional, biological, and physiological 359, 360*f*
  osteoporosis as risk factor for 161-162
  %fat 158, 159*t*
  resting metabolic rate and 206
  weight change and 150
Aging Well (Valliant) 49
AIDS. *See* HIV/AIDS
air displacement plethysmography 152
air quality, checking 84
alcohol 184
  abuse 241, 248
  blood alcohol concentration 261, 261*f*
  calories in 171*f*
  college students and use of 257-260, 259*f*
  effects on the body 260-261, 260*f*
  mixing energy drink and 263
  potential implications of 211-212
Alcoholics Anonymous 243
alcoholism 262
allocation of effort 224
allostasis 220
allostatic balance 220
allostatic load 224, 235
alpha linoleic acid 174
American Association for Cancer Research 343
American Cancer Society 268, 331, 333, 339, 345
American College Health Association 228
American College of Sports Medicine (ACSM)
  on cardiorespiratory fitness 71, 72
  exercise guidelines 27, 31-32, 33-34
  fluid recommendations 183
  Guidelines for Exercise Testing and Prescription 29
  on moderate-intensity activity 77, 79, 81, 97
  neuromotor exercise according to 113
  1998 position stand 29
  1RM intensity 98
  on participating in functional fitness 114
  %fat 158
  on performing aerobic activities 213
  physical activity guidelines 76
  progression of cardiorespiratory endurance program 81
  recommendations of muscular fitness volume 99-100
  on strength training 99

2018 exercise guidelines for visual summary 30, 30*f*, 33-34
2006 position stand 30
American Council on Exercise 98, 100
American Diabetes Association 311, 312
American Heart Association 318, 320
American Lung Association 265, 267, 268
American Medical Association, 2013 34, 199
American Psychiatric Association 244
American Psychological Association 219, 222, 231
American Red Cross 318
American Sleep Association 232, 234, 235
American Stroke Association 317
amino acids 177
amphetamine 247, 249, 250
anabolic-androgenic steroids (AAS) 103
anabolic steroids 249
android fat pattern 151
angina 317
anorexia 214, 242*f*
anterior deltoids 136, 137
antioxidants 181
anxiety disorder 117, 237, 238
areola 277, 277*f*
argileh. *See* hookahs
arrhythmias 316
arteriosclerosis 316, 320
Åstrand, Per-Olof 16-17
atherosclerosis 316, 317*f*
atherosclerotic heart disease 317
athletes, heavily muscled 158
ATP. *See* adenosine triphosphate (ATP)
ATP-PC system (adenosine triphosphate-phosphocreatine) 69*t*, 70
attention-deficit hyperactivity disorder (ADHD) 256
attitudes, about drug use 244
automatic external defibrillator (AED) 318
autonomic nervous system 220

B

baby boomers, intentional fitness practices and 30-31
BAC (blood alcohol concentration) 261, 262
ballistic or bouncing stretching 111
bariatric surgery 211
barrier birth control methods 283-285, 283*f*, 284*f*
beats per minute (bpm) 77
beer belly 160
behavioral addiction 240, 242-244, 242*f*
behavioral attitude 47

behavioral choices 3, 212
behavioral signs, of excessive stress 227t
behavioral theories, in social psychology 45-50
behavior change, managing 39-58
  action items in change process 44f, 45
  decisional balance 50-53
  personalizing behavior change process 53-54
  Prochaska's transtheoretical model (TTM) 40, 44-45
  reasons for change behavior 40
  self-efficacy theory 45, 46-47
  social ecological model 48-49, 48f, 49f
  stages of changes 42 43, 44, 45f
  starting with personal movement program 55-56
  theory of planned behavior 47-48
benign tumor 332, 332f
beverages 184, 203, 263
BIA (bioelectrical impedance analysis) 154, 155
biceps 142
Big Eight 190
Big Metabolic Three 73, 170, 176, 185, 309, 310
binge drinking 258, 259f, 260f, 261-262
binge-eating disorder 214, 242f, 243
bioelectrical impedance analysis (BIA) 154, 155
biofeedback 232
biopsy, cancer and 338-339
birth control 279-281, 282f, 285, 289
blood 64f, 261, 261f
blood alcohol concentration (BAC) 261, 262
blood cholesterol 323-324, 324t
blood pressure 63-64
blood stream 221
blood sugar 185, 238, 311, 312
blood vessel system 62-64, 62f
blue zones 4, 13
BMI. See body mass index (BMI)
BOD POD 152
body composition
  assessment of 151-153, 155-157
  basics of 148-151
  benefits of healthy 163-164
  components of 148, 149f
  healthy 163-164
  measuring 148
  personal measurement of weight status and 155
  portable options for assessment of 154
  program for managing 164-167
  weight status and risk of chronic disease 157-163
body density 152
body dysmorphic disorder 213, 214
body image 213, 215
body mass index (BMI) 155, 157-159, 157t, 199, 201
body size 214
body types 151

body weight, strengthening and stretching 96, 96t. See also overweight; weight; weight management
  for abdominals 129
  for back of upper arm 145
  for calf 123
  for chest and front of shoulder 137
  for front of upper arm 143
  for hams and glutes 127
  for hip abductors 133
  for hip adductors 135
  for lats and middle back 141
  for lower back 131
  for quads
  for upper back and rear shoulder 139
bone bank, deposits and withdrawals 163, 163f
bone density T-score 161
bone mass 148, 150, 165
bpm (beats per minute) 77
brain 74, 250, 251
breast cancer 335, 350t, 351t
breathing 103, 232
brevis 134
British Medical Journal 118
bulbourethral glands (Cowper's glands) 278, 278f
bulimia nervosa 214
buprenorphine 254

C
CAD (coronary artery disease) 315
caffeine 184, 235, 263
calcium 182t, 192
calcium intake 162, 186
calories 21t, 171, 171f, 178, 203. See also weight management
calves
  daily activity and 122
  strengthening and stretching 123
CAM. See complementary and alternative medicine (CAM)
cancer 73, 338-340. See also specific types
  benign vs. malignant tumors 332
  causes of 347-349
  common treatment of 343
  development of 332-333
  early detection of 338-343, 338f, 339t, 340f
  imaging used to detect 339t
  insight on development of 333-334, 334f
  most commonly diagnosed 349-352
  nature of 331-332
  race and ethnicity and 334-335, 336f
  risk cancer over lifetime 337
cannabinoids (marijuana) 249
carbohydrates 66, 171-174, 171f, 172t, 203
carcinogen 333
carcinogenesis 333
carcinoma in situ 342
cardiometabolic diseases 73, 176, 177
cardiorespiratory activity, weight-loss maintenance and 213
cardiorespiratory endurance 71-72, 80f. See also cardiorespiratory fitness
cardiorespiratory fitness

benefits of 73-75
  defined 71-72
  energy production systems 65-71
  plan to improve 75-83
  safety and getting started with 83-84
cardiorespiratory function evaluation 71-73
cardiorespiratory system 60-71, 66f
cardiovascular diseases (CVDs) 73, 310, 311, 315-326
cardiovascular fitness, Personal Movement Plan to enhance 83, 84
cardiovascular system. See cardiorespiratory system
CAUTION acronym 340, 340f, 341f, 342f
cellular inflammation 310
Center for Behavioral Health Statistics and Quality 251, 255t
Centers for Disease Control and Prevention 28, 37, 116, 198, 199, 234, 235, 244, 252, 257, 258, 263, 265, 267, 280, 283, 285, 290, 292, 293, 294, 297, 298, 299, 312, 313, 331, 345, 348
central nervous system (CNS) 253, 256, 265
certified fitness trainer, help in weight management behaviors 215-216
cervical cap (fem cap) 285f
cervix cancer 335, 350t, 351t
CHD (coronary heart disease) 315, 321t
chemotherapy 343
chest and front of shoulder
  daily activity for 136
  strengthening and stretching 137
chilling food 193
chlamydia 297, 297f, 300
chronic diseases 310
chronic sleep deprivation 235
cigarettes 263, 263f, 265-266
circumcision 277, 279
clinical depression 237
clitoris 276, 277f
club drugs (MDMA, Rohypnol, and GHB) 249, 257t
CNS. See central nervous system (CNS)
CNS depressants 249
cocaine 246, 247f, 249, 253, 253f
coconut and coconut oil 176
cognitive behavioral therapy 242, 244
cognitive evaluation, of threat 222
cold medicine with codeine (CNS depressant) 256
collars and spotters, using 103
collateral damage 224-225
college life, stressors and hassles of 225-230
college students 263f, 356
  addiction and 246-247, 247f
  alcohol use and abuse by 257-260, 259f, 260f
  drugs used by 246
  marijuana used among 250f
  mixing energy drinks and alcohol 263
  nicotine use in 263f
  rates of drinking among 258, 259f

recognizing and preventing sexual assault 302-304
College Tobacco Free Campus 268
colon/rectum cancer 350t, 351t
community-based therapies 242
complementary and alternative medicine (CAM) 361-362, 363
complete protein 178
complex carbohydrates 172
complicated dismount 225
compulsive exercising 242f, 243
compulsive shopping or buying 242f, 243
computed tomography (CT), to detect cancer 339t
computer game addictions 242f, 243
condom 282f, 284f
connective tissue, flexibility and 107
consent, to sexual activity 304
contemplation stage of change 44, 44f
contraception 279-282, 280f, 281f, 282f
conventional endurance training 82
conventional medical practices 361
cooking food 193
cool down, as strategy in injury prevention 57f
core muscle training 99
core needle biopsy 338
coronary artery disease (CAD) 315
coronary heart disease (CHD) 315, 321t
corticotropin-releasing hormone (CRH) 221
cortisol 221
C-reactive protein (CRP) 310
CRH (corticotropin-releasing hormone) 221
Crohn's disease 350t
cross-contamination, of food 193
cross-training 77, 80
CRP (C-reactive protein) 310
CT (computed tomography), to detect cancer 339t
curl-ups, body weight 120
CVDs. See cardiovascular diseases (CVDs)

D
daily functional movement 118-119
daily life 82, 95, 102, 108
daily movement 19
Dallas bed-rest study 361
DASH (Dietary Approaches to Stop Hypertension) 323
deaths 157, 183, 266f, 331, 331f, 333f, 336f. See also mortality rates
decisional balance 50-51, 51t, 58
density 150, 152
dependence 244, 251
Depo-Provera 287
depression 117, 237-238
development, of addiction to drug or behavior 246
DEXA (dual-energy X-ray absorptiometery) 153, 160
DGs (Dietary Guidelines for Americans) 186-189

diabetes mellitus 185
    definition and conditions with long-term 310-312
    diagnosis of 313, 313f
    symptoms and risk factors for prediabetes 313
    treatment options 313
    treatment options and preventing 313-315
    types and definitions 312-313
Diagnostic and Statistical Manual of Mental Disorders (American Psychiatric Association) 244
diaphragm 284f
diastole 61, 63
diet 150, 323, 324, 346, 437, 438
Dietary Approaches to Stop Hypertension (DASH) 323
dietary fats 66-67, 174-177, 209t
Dietary Guidelines for Americans (DGs) 186-189
dietary intake 209t, 231
dietary limitations, common 189-191
dietary patterns 186-187
dietary plan, balanced 192
dietary protein 178
dietary reference intakes (DRI) 185, 186
dietary supplements 179, 191-193
digestive disorders, osteoporosis and 162
disaccharides 172t
disordered eating 178
dissociative drugs (ketamine and PCP) 249, 257t
distress, eustress vs. 220, 220f
dopamine 241
dose-response association 80-81
Drex. See cold medicine with codeine (CNS depressant)
DRI (dietary reference intakes) 185, 186
driving, effects of blood alcohol concentration on 261f
Drug and Alcohol Abuse Hotline 249
drug free, information of staying 248
drug(s) 240. See also medications
    abuse 240, 248, 254
    commonly abused 257
    dissociative 257t
    hallucinogenic 267t
    illegal 250-255
    illicit 244, 245, 245f, 246
    misuse 240
    prescription 211
    psychoactive 249-257
dual-energy X-ray absorptiometer (DEXA) 153, 160
ductal lavage 339
dynamic stretching 111
dynamometers, advanced 92

E
"eating clean," expression of 170
eating disorders 214
eccentric training 103
e-cigarettes (electronic cigarettes) 263f, 267, 267f, 268f

ecstasy 246
ectomorph 151
ectopic fat 149, 159
ectopic pregnancy 274
ejaculation 278
ejaculatory duct 278, 278f
embryo 274
emergency contraception (morning-after pill) 287
emotional distress, struggle to manage weight and 200
emotional health 76
emotional responses 222
emotional signs, of excessive stress 227t
emotional stressors, roles in health and society 211
emotional wellness 9, 11
endocrine disorders, osteoporosis and 162
endocrine system 221
endometriosis 276
endometrium 276
endomorph 151
endoscopy, to detect cancer 340
endothelium 325-326
endurance training 98
energy
    balance 198, 199, 203-207
    carbohydrates as energy source 171-174
    density 203, 205, 209t
    expending 209-210
    expenditure 71, 204, 205
    needs, supply and demand 60-65
    positive 236
    potential interactive implications of 211
    production systems 65-71
    studies for enhancing 235
    systems 68-70, 69t, 71
energy drinks, mixing with alcohol 263
energy in 199, 203, 211, 212
energy intake, reducing 208, 209t
energy needs 171
energy out 199, 203, 206, 211, 212
environment 206, 229, 246, 347, 349
environmental wellness 13
epididymis 277, 278f
epinephrine 221
erection 278
erector spinae 130-131
ergogenic 103
escalator, stairs vs. 28
essential fat 149
ethnic group, osteoporosis and 162
eustress vs. distress 220, 220f
excision of tumors 339
exercise 27. See also functional movement training; physical activity(ies); strength training
    addiction 214
    cardiorespiratory systems 65, 66f, 210
    common modes of 207t
    compulsive 242f
    maximal strenuous 63, 64f, 66f
    movement mode matters 164-165

exercise *(continued)*
  multijoint or compound 99
  neuromotor 106, 113-114, 119
  osteoporosis and 162
  prescription 28, 29, 30-31
  resting metabolic rate and 206
  single-joint 99
  as stress management strategy 230-231
  weight change and 150
exercise equipment use, as activity 80
eye complications, diabetes and 311

F
fallopian tubes 274, 275, 298
family tree 201, 202
fast-food 176, 194
fast-twitch fibers 88, 89
fat depots 151, 159
fat mass 148, 150, 165
fats
  calories and energy in 171*f*
  dietary 174
  distribution, genetics and 151
  facts 149
  saturated fatty acids 174, 175*t*, 176, 188
  trans fats 174, 175*t*, 176
fat-soluble vitamins 181
fatty acids, types of 175*t*
FDA. *See* Food and Drug Administration (FDA)
female athlete triad 166-167
female circumcision 277
female condom 282*f*, 284*f*
fertility awareness (natural family planning) 288, 288*f*
fertilization 274
fetus 274
FHSI (Fraternal Health and Safety Initiative) 303
fiber 172*t*, 173-174, 209*t*
field tests, conducting 73, 84
fight-or-flight response 220, 221*f*
financial consideration, protein and 178
financial pressures, college life stressors and 230
financial wellness 14, 21
fine-needle aspiration 338
fitness 18-19, 363, 369. *See also* cardiorespiratory fitness; cardiovascular fitness; muscular fitness; wellness
  analyzing choices 101-102
  functional, neuromotor exercise and 113-114
  for health 116
  SMART goals for movement and 36-37
FITT (frequency, intensity, time, and type) 205
  in cardiorespiratory fitness 76-83
  exercise energy expenditure and 206
  flexibility 109-111, 109*f*
  in muscular fitness program 96-98, 97*f*
  neuromotor exercise 114
  for organizing exercise prescription 29
  weight-loss maintenance and 213
FITT-VPP guidelines 101-102

FITT-VP principle 83
flexibility 86, 91
  assessment 119
  benefits of 112
  definition and interaction of strength and 106-107
  physiological teamwork for 114-116
  training 29-30, 110
folate 182*t*
food allergies 189-190, 191
Food and Drug Administration (FDA) 103, 176, 189, 190*f*, 191, 192-193, 194, 211, 294
food and eating addictions 242*f*
Food and Nutrition Board 194
food intolerance 189-190, 191
food labels, reading 189-191
food processing costs 203
foods 65-67, 203, 243. *See also* food safety
food safety 193, 194*f*
Fraternal Health and Safety Initiative (FHSI) 303
free radicals 181
free weight, for strengthening and stretching
  abdominals 129
  back of upper arm 145
  calf 123
  chest and front of shoulder 137
  front of upper arm 00
  hams and glutes 127
  hip abductors 133
  hip adductors 135
  lats and middle back 141
  lower back 131
  positives and negatives of 96, 96*t*
  quads 125
  upper back and shoulder 139
frequency 76, 97, 110
fructose 172*t*
fruits 180
fuel quality, performance and 185
functional fitness 113-114, 115, 200
functional movement 16-17, 22, 26-27, 28, 117
functional movement training 17, 28, 102
  abdominals 128-129
  back of upper arm 144-145
  calves 122-123
  chest and front of shoulder 136-137
  front of upper arm 142
  hams and glutes 126-127
  hip adductors 132-133, 134-135
  holding stretches 121
  introducing neuromotor movements 120
  lats and middle back 140-141
  lower back 130-131
  number of repetitions and sets 120-121
  quads 124-125
  reasons for 120
  upper back and shoulders 138-139
  warm up before stretching and strengthening 120
function claim, structure of 189

G
galactose 172*t*
gambling 242*f*, 243
gases 252
gastrocnemius 123
generalized anxiety disorder 237
genetics 316*f*
  body type and 151
  cancer and 343-344, 344*f*
  developing an addiction and 245
  modern society and energy imbalance 201
genetic testing, cancer and 339-340
gestational diabetes 312, 316*f*
GHB 249, 257*t*
glucose 171-172, 172*t*
gluten-free diet 191
gluteus medius 133
gluteus minimus 133
glycemic index 203, 205
glycogen 70
glycolytic system 70
GMOs 194
goals 36-37, 50-55, 58, 65, 75-76, 77*f*, 95
Golgi tendon organ 112, 113*f*
gonads 274
gonorrhea 297, 297*f*, 300
Google food trends 20
goza. *See* hookahs
gracilis 134
guided imagery 232
Guttmacher Institute 281, 290
gynoid fat pattern 151

H
habitual movement 236
hallucinogens (LSD, mescaline, and psilocybin) 249, 257*t*
hams and glutes
  daily activity for 126
  strengthening and stretching 127
happiness, principles bringing 15
Harvard alumni study 17
HCV (HIV and hepatitis C) 252
HDL-C (high-density lipoprotein cholesterol) 323-324
health 40, 54, 76, 189, 272-273
health and fitness categories, %fat 158-159
health span 5, 5*f*
Healthways 7
Healthy Children 279
healthy eating 20, 170-184, 185-195
healthy habits 36*f*
Healthy People 2020 (HP 2020) 6
Healthy People 2030 (HP 2030) 6, 368
healthy vegetarian eating pattern 187, 188
heart 61-62, 61*f*, 79
heart attack 317, 319*f*, 321*t*, 326*f*
heart failure 321
heart rate 253, 256, 265
height, altered 158
hemorrhagic stroke 317
heroin 246, 249, 251

herpes simplex virus (HSV) 290, 293
HHS Physical Activity Guidelines 27
high blood pressure 322, 323
high-density lipoprotein cholesterol (HDL-C) 323-324
high-intensity interval training (HITT) 70, 82-83
hip abductors
  daily activity and 132
  strengthening and stretching 133
hip adductors 132-133
  daily activity and 134
  strengthening and stretching 135
Hippocrates 330
HITT. *See* high-intensity interval training (HITT)
HIV/AIDS 291-292, 292*f*
HIV and hepatitis C (HCV) 252
homesickness 329
hookahs 265
hormonal birth control methods 285-287
hormonal disorders, osteoporosis and 162
hormones 166, 206, 231
HPA axis (hypothalamus-pituitary-adrenal axis) 221
HPV. *See* human papilloma virus (HPV)
HSV (herpes simplex virus) 290, 293
hubble-bubble. *See* hookahs
human body 87-89
human immunodeficiency virus (HIV). *See* HIV/AIDS
human movement paradigm 27, 27*f*
human papilloma virus (HPV) 293, 294, 295*f*
hydration 57*f*, 181, 183, 185
hydrodensitometry (underwater weighing) 152
hydrogenated oil 175
hydrogenation, of dietary fat 174-175
hymen 276
hypercholesterolemia 323
hyperglycemia 311
hyperlipidemia 323
hypertension 322-323
hypertrophy, muscle 91-92
hypothalamus 221
hypothalamus-pituitary-adrenal axis (HPA axis) 221

I
Iceberg model 8
identity, transition to independence and 229
"identity capital" 9
illegal drugs 250-255
illicit drugs 244, 245, 245*f*, 246
Illness-wellness model, Travis 8, 8*f*
imaging, to detect cancer 339*t*
immune function, cardiorespiratory fitness and 74
implant (Nexplanon) 281, 282*f*, 286, 286*f*
incomplete protein 177-178
inflammatory response 310
inhalants 249, 250, 252-253

injuries 56-57
insoluble fiber 173-174
Institute of Medicine 172, 173, 174, 177, 183, 185
intellectual wellness 12, 16
intensity
  building 82
  as factor in cardiorespiratory fitness 78
  in flexibility training 110
  muscular fitness and 97-98
  of training 77, 99-100
intentional exercise practices, history of 28
intermuscular adipose tissue 153
International Diabetes Federation 308, 309
internet addiction 243
interval training 81-82
intoxication 259*f*
intra-abdominal fat. *See* visceral fat
intrahepatic bile cancer of 335
intrauterine devices (IUDs) 279, 281, 287*f*
iron 182*t*, 192
ischemic stroke 317
isometric muscle contraction 89, 90
isotonic concentric muscle contraction 89, 90
isotonic eccentric muscle contraction 89, 90
It's On Us campaign 303
IUDs. *See* intrauterine devices (IUDs)

J
Jay, Meg 9
joint action 92
joint injury or repair, flexibility and 107
joints, preventing injury of 102
joint structure, flexibility and 106

K
Kaiser Permanente 32
Kaposi's sarcoma 291
ketamine 249, 257*t*
kidneys 171, 178, 311, 335
kilocalorie (kcal) 65, 171

L
labia majora 275*f*, 276, 277*f*
labia minora 275*f*, 276, 277*f*
laboratory methods, for assessing body composition 151-157
lacto-ovo vegetarians 187
lacto-vegetarians 187
latissimus dorsi 140-141
lats and middle back
  daily activity and 140
  strengthening and stretching 141
LDL-C (low-density lipoprotein cholesterol) 323-324
lean mass 150
lean or muscle mass, as component of weight 148
lean soft tissue 165
legalization of marijuana 251
licensed dietitian 180, 194
Life, Be in It! 23

life, managing 232-234
life expectancy 3-4, 4*f*, 5, 26
life span 2-3, 5, 30, 356-357
lifestyles. *See also* wellness
  active, physically 26
  body composition changes and 150
  cancer and 344-349
  diabetes and changes in 314
  evaluating 23
  healthy 18-19, 22-23
  managing 211
  poor choices of 201
lignin (noncarbohydrate substance) 173
limberness 106
linoleic acid 174
liver
  cancer 335
  fatty 159
location ranking 6
Longevity Project, The (Friedman and Martin) 118
low back pain, preventing 116-118, 117*f*
low-density lipoprotein cholesterol (LDL-C) 323-324
lower back
  daily activity and 130
  strengthening and stretching 131
LSD 249, 257*t*
lung cancer 335, 350*t*, 351*t*

M
macronutrient balance 209*t*
macronutrients 66, 170, 171*f*, 174*f*
magnesium 182*t*
magnetic resonance imaging (MRI) 153, 339*t*
maintenance stage of change 40, 44*f*
major depressive disorder 237
Making Learning Whole: How Seven Principles of Teaching Can Transform Education (Perkins) 23
Male Athletes Against Violence 303
male circumcision 279, 289
male condom 282*f*, 284*f*
malignant tumor 332, 332*f*
mammary glands (breasts) 277, 277*f*
mammogram, to detect cancer 339*t*
mantra 232
marijuana 241, 245, 249, 250-251, 250*f*
maximal heart rate (MHR) 78, 84
maximal oxygen consumption 72, 72*f*
maximal oxygen uptake ($\dot{V}O_2$ max) 72
MDMA 249, 257*t*
meal timing 209*t*
mechanics, using proper, as strategy in injury prevention 57*f*
medical evaluation, in weight changes 216
medical model 2
medical procedures, osteoporosis and 162
medications
  osteoporosis and 162
  for prediabetes 314

medications *(continued)*
  side effects of 238
  sleep and 235
  for treating addictions 242, 244
meditation 232
Mediterranean-style eating pattern 187, 188
melanoma 347
men
  addiction and 245
  beer belly 160
  body composition of 150
  energy expenditure and exercise modes 207t
  essential fat for 149
  hormones and 166
  most diagnosed cancers in 334f
  %fat for 158, 159t
  recommendations of alcohol for 184
  recommended intake of fluid 183
mental alertness, sleep and 235
mental health issues, addiction and 245
men who have sex with men (MSM) 290, 300
mescaline 57t, 249
mesomorph 151
metabolic cart 72
metabolic equivalents (METs) 78
metabolic syndrome (MetS) 308-309, 310, 311f
metabolism 65
metastasis 342
meth. *See* methamphetamine
methadone 254
methamphetamine 249, 250, 254
meth labs and future life plans 255
METs (metabolic equivalents) 78
MetS (metabolic syndrome) 308-309, 310, 311f
MHR (maximal heart rate) 78, 84
micronutrients 170, 180-181
middle age 76, 157, 160, 163, 185, 210, 255
mindfulness mediation 232
minerals 180-181, 182t
monounsaturated fats (MUFAs) 174, 175t
mons pubis 276
mortality rates 12, 266f, 333f, 336f, 337
movement 54, 71, 82
  bone loading and 165
  energy systems 69t
  into everyday life, fitting 34, 35f
  habitual 236
  SMART goals for fitness and 36-37
  type of, choosing 98-99
  in weight management 210
moving safely, challenges to 56
MRI (magnetic resonance imaging) 153, 339t
MSM (men who have sex with men) 290, 300
MUFAs (monounsaturated fats) 174, 175t
muffin top 160
multijoint or compound exercises 99
muscle balance 118-119

muscle dysmorphia disorder 214
muscle groups, opposing 99, 99f
muscle imbalances, common 100t
muscle mass 150, 214
muscle movement. *See* thermic effect of activity (TEA)
muscles, protein and 177
muscle size, flexibility and 107
muscle spindles 112-113, 113f
muscular endurance 100
muscular fitness
  adaptation to muscular overload 91
  analyzing fitness choices 101-102
  aspects of 86
  benefits to daily life 95
  designing your program for 95-101
  following FITT 96-98, 97f
  human body and 87-89
  incorporating movements into daily life 102
  muscle capacity and assessment 91-94
  muscle contractions 89-90
  muscle fibers 88, 88f
  muscle hypertrophy 91-92
  muscle learning 91
  muscle size and tone 94
  muscular endurance 86, 86f, 91, 93, 100
  muscular power 86, 86f, 94
  muscular strength 86, 86f, 91, 93, 98
  overloading options 96-97, 96t
  personal plan and goals 96
  safety while training 102-103
  volume, pattern, and progression and 99-101, 100t
mutation 332-333
myocardial infarction 317
MyPlate 186, 187f, 189

N

naltrexone 254
Narcotics Anonymous 243
narghile. *See* hookahs
National Athletic Training Association (NATA) 56, 103
National Cancer Act 331
National Cancer Institute (NCI) 268, 335, 337, 343, 346
National Commission for Certifying Agencies (NCCA) 216
National Council on Alcoholism and Drug Dependence 249
National Council on Sexual Addiction Compulsivity 242f
National Domestic Violence Hotline 305
National Eating Disorders Association 215
National Institute on Alcohol Abuse and Alcoholism 257, 260, 262
National Institute on Drug Abuse 241, 242, 245, 246, 250, 251, 252, 253, 254, 256, 257, 262
National Institute on Drug Abuse for Teens 252, 253
National Institutes of Health 232
National Institutes of Mental Health 237, 238

National Institutes of Neurological Orders and Strokes 116
National Osteoporosis Foundation 162
National Physical Activity Plan (NPAP) 31-33, 52, 52t
National Sexual Assault Hotline 305
National Survey on Drug Use and Health 258
natural family planning 288
nature, nurture and 151, 201
NCCA. *See* National Commission for Certifying Agencies (NCCA)
NCI. *See* National Cancer Institute (NCI)
needle exchange program 252
neuromotor exercise 106, 113-114, 119
neuromotor fitness 86, 114-116
neuromotor movements, introducing 120
neuromotor training
  for abdominals 129
  for back of upper arm 145
  for chest and front of shoulder 137
  for claves 123
  destabilization and 115
  for front of upper arm 143
  for hams and glutes 127
  for hip abductors 133
  for hip adductors 135
  introducing 120
  for lats and middle back 141
  for lower back 131
  for quads 125
  for upper back and shoulders 139
neuromuscular training. *See* neuromotor exercise
neuropathy 311
nicotine 265, 267, 268
nitrites 252
non-GMO food 194
nonoxidative (anaerobic) energy system 69t, 70, 88
noradrenaline. *See* norepinephrine
norepinephrine 221
NPAP. *See* National Physical Activity Plan (NPAP)
nutrients 170, 188-189
nutrition 57f, 162, 165, 185-195

O

obesity 357, 358f
  American adults and 198-199, 198f
  bariatric surgery of 211
  binging and 214
  BMI and 157, 157t
  food and eating addictions and 242f
  link to other diseases 199
  morbid 211
  prevention of 202-203
  quality of life and 200
  staying active to avoid 199f
obesogenic environment 201
obliques, external and internal 128
occupational wellness 9, 14
Office of Disease Prevention and Health 120, 236

Office of Disease Prevention and Health Promotion 2018 32
older adults 95, 115, 149, 192, 200, 334
one-repetition maximum (1RM) 93, 98
oocytes 274, 275
opiate addiction 249
opioids 249, 256
opium 249
organic food 194
organized sport participation 52*t*
osteoporosis 161-162, 161*f*, 181
ovaries 275, 275*f*
overweight 159*f*, 198-199, 198*f*, 316*f*, 346, 346*f*
ovulation 275
oxidative (aerobic) system 69*t*, 70, 88
OxyContin (opioids) 256

P

PAD (peripheral artery disease) 320
PAG (Physical Activity Guidelines) 31, 32-33
panic disorder 237
Pap smear 293
parasympathetic nervous system 220, 221
PAR-Q+ (Physical Activity Readiness Questionnaire for Everyone) 56
patch 282*f*, 286, 286*f*
pathophysiology 310
pattern, muscular fitness and 100
PCP 249
pectorals 136, 137
pelvic inflammatory disease (PID) 274, 276, 298, 298*f*
penis 278, 278*f*
perceived behavioral control 47, 48
%fat health and fitness categories 158-159, 159*t*
percent body fat 150
perfect use 281
performance, fuel quality and hydration and 185
peripheral artery disease (PAD) 320
personal diet plan 194*f*
personal fitness, movement history and 34
personality 222-223
personal measurement of weight status, body composition and 155
Personal Movement Program, starting with 55-56
personal trainers 365-367
pescatarian 187
Physical Activity Guidelines (PAG) 31, 32-33
physical activity(ies) 52*f*, 76
    blood pressures and 323
    body composition changes and 150
    cancer and 346, 347
    cholesterol and 325
    daily patterns of 18, 18*f*
    energy expenditure during 207*t*
    movement mode matters 164-165
    osteoporosis and 162
    prediabetes and 314

reduced 158
    resting metabolic rate and 206
    sleep and 235
    steps per day and 45
    as stress management strategy 230-231
    understanding recommendations of 27-31
Physical Activity Readiness Questionnaire for Everyone (PAR-Q+) 56
physical fitness. *See* wellness
physical function, energetic 164
physical signs, of excessive stress 227*t*
physical tasks, daily, cardiorespiratory fitness and 74
physical wellness 11, 16
Physicians Committee for Responsible Medicine 249
physiological response to stress 221-221, 221*f*
physiological stress response system 220-221, 221*f*, 224
physiological teamwork 114-116
physiological vs. chronological age 359
physiology, of stretch reflex 112-113
PID. *See* pelvic inflammatory disease (PID)
pituitary gland 221
plastic surgery addiction 243
PNF (proprioceptive neuromotor facilitation) 111
polycystic ovary syndrome 316*f*
polyps 340
polyunsaturated fats (PUFAs) 174
polyunsaturated:omega-3 175*t*
polyunsaturated: omega-6 175*t*
portable options, for body composition assessment 154
portion sizes 209*t*
posterior deltoids 138-139
posture 117-118
potassium 182*t*
Pott, Percivall 330-331
precontemplation stage of change 41, 44, 44*f*
prediabetes 312-314
PrEP (pre-exposure prophylaxis) 292
preparation stage of change 40, 44-45, 44*f*
preparticipation screening questionnaire 56, 58
prescription, defined 28
prescription medications 211, 246, 249
preteens 294
processed foods 170, 176, 209*t*
Prochaska's transtheoretical model (TTM) 40, 42, 43, 44-45
procrastination 367-368
professional counselor, in weight management behaviors 215
professional help, for weight management 215-216
prognosis 340
program design, for muscular fitness 95-101
progression 81-82, 101
progress slowly 81, 103

proprioceptive neuromotor facilitation (PNF) 111
proprioceptors, flexibility and 107
prostate cancer 335, 350*t*, 351*t*
prostate gland 278
protein 67, 171*f*, 177-179, 179*t*, 180, 193
protein isolates 193
psilocybin 249
psychoactive drugs 249-257
psychological challenges, stress and 218
psychological concerns regarding 213-214
psychologist, in weight management behaviors 215
psychosocial stress, roles in health and society 211
psychosocial support, for treating behavioral addictions 244
psychosocial well-being, cardiorespiratory fitness and 75-76
psyllium 173-174
PUFAs (polyunsaturated fats) 174

Q

qigong 362
quadriceps 124-125
quads
    daily activity and 124
    strengthening and stretching 124-125
quality of life 192, 200
quality resources and services, body composition and 155
QuitLine 268

R

race 158, 159*f*, 162, 316*f*
radiation therapy, for treating cancer 343
Ramazzini, Bernardino 330
range of motion 57*f*, 103, 111. *See also* flexibility
rape 303
rapid eye movement (REM) 233
rating of perceived exertion (RPE) 78, 79*t*
RD (registered dietitian) 194
RDA (recommended dietary allowance) 185
RDN. *See* registered dietitian nutritionist (RDN)
recommended dietary allowance (RDA) 185
rectus abdominis 128
refined carbohydrates 172-173
refined grains 173
registered dietitian (RD) 194
registered dietitian nutritionist (RDN) 180, 194, 215
Registered Student Organizations 231
relationships 229, 231
relaxation techniques, calming the mind and body by 232
REM (rapid eye movement) 233
repetitions and sets 99-101, 120-121
reproductive system 274*f*, 275-278
    female 275-277, 275*f*
    male 277-278, 278*f*
resistance training 95, 99-100, 210, 212

respiratory system 64-65, 64f, 65f. *See also* cardiorespiratory system
resting heart rate (RHR) 77
resting metabolic rate (RMR) 203, 205, 206, 211, 212
rhomboids 138-139
RHR (resting heart rate) 77
rhythmic aerobic exercise 79-80
RICE (rest, ice, compression, and elevation) principle 56
risky behavior addiction 243
Ritalin 246, 256
Ritalin Abuse Health 256
RMR. *See* resting metabolic rate (RMR)
Rohypnol 249, 257t
RPE (rating of perceived exertion) 78, 79t
run/walk tests 72-73

S

safety, Personal Movement Program and 55-56
safety while training 102-103
SAID principle (specific adaptation to imposed demands) 11
Sapolsky, Robert 224
sarcopenia, preventing 159-160
satiety 203
saturated fatty acids 174, 175t, 176
scrotum 277, 278, 278f
sedentarism 28, 31-32, 33-34
sedentary behavior 52t. *See also* sedentarism
sedentary living 18-19, 53f
self-confidence 46-47, 95
self-detection techniques, for cancer 340, 340f
self-efficacy 46
self-efficacy theory 45, 46-47
self-esteem 164
self-image 164, 229
semen 278
seminal vesicles 278, 278f
seminiferous tubules 277, 278f
sense of place 13
sex 107, 150, 158, 159t, 162, 337t
sexual addiction 242f, 243
sexual assault 302-305, 302f
sexual health 272-273
sexually transmitted infections (STIs)
  abstinence and 282
  bacterial 274, 296-299
  as common disease 290-291, 291f
  reducing the risks and prevention of 299-302, 301f
  symptoms of 299
  viral, most common 291-295
shisha. *See* hookahs
shot (Depo-Provera) 282f, 287
simple carbohydrates 172
sitting 33-34, 210
"sitting time" 18-19. *See also* sedentarism
sit-to-stand desks 34
skin cancer 347, 348
skinfold thickness, for assessing body composition 154
skippy. *See* Adderall; Ritalin

sleep
  devices and 236
  implications of 211
  improved, cardiorespiratory fitness and 75-76
  managing stress through 232
  poor, health risks associated with 234-235
  quantity and quality 232-234, 235f
  social life, stress and 235-236
  stages of 233-234
  strategies for enhancing 235
slow dynamic stretching 111
slow-twitch fibers 88, 89
SMART goals, for fitness and movement 36-37, 58, 367-368
smarties. *See* Adderall; Ritalin
smoking 117, 265, 266f, 267, 268, 324
Smoking and Health: Report of the Advisory Committee of the Surgeon General of the Public Health Services (Centers for Disease Control and Prevention) 345
social anxiety disorder 237
social ecological model 48-49, 48f, 49f
social life, sleep, stress and 235-236
social roles, transition to independence and 229
social support, for reduction of stressors 231
social wellness 12, 16
society and health 5-6
sodium 182t, 188
soleus 123
soluble or viscous fiber 173
specificity of training 71, 88
sperm 274, 278
spermicides 289
spiritual wellness 15, 16
sport performance 74, 86, 164
squat 92
staging of cancer 340
stairs vs. escalator 28
starches 172t
static stretching 110-111
steps per day, physical activity and 45, 81
step tests 73
sterilization 281, 289, 289f
steroids, osteoporosis and 162
stimulants 247, 247f, 249, 256
STIs. *See* sexually transmitted infections (STIs)
Stop Medicine Abuse 256
street names for drugs 257t
strength, interaction of flexibility and 107, 109
strength training 98. *See also* muscular endurance; muscular fitness
stress. *See also* stress management; stressors
  and aging process, before and after office 226
  defined 219
  excessive, signs and symptoms of 227, 227t
  experience, contemporary 218-225

hypertension and 323
  implications of 211
  managing through sleep 232
  personality and 223
  social life, sleep and 235-236
  transition to independence and 229
stress eating 231
stress management 218-238
stressors 219, 222, 225-230
stress response 220, 221-224, 225, 225f, 238
stretching 108, 111, 121. *See also* flexibility
stretch reflex 112-113, 113f
stroke 315, 317-318, 319f
subcutaneous fat 149
subjective norm 47-48
substance abuse (drug addiction) 241, 244-246, 248-249
Substance Abuse and Mental Health Services Administration 240, 241, 242, 245, 249, 250, 251, 252, 253, 256, 258, 263
substance addiction 240, 241-242
sugar-glucose 70
sun exposure, cancer and 347
supplements 192-193
surgery, for treating cancer 343
surgical treatment 211
sweating 67
sympathetic nervous system 220
syphilis 298-299, 299f
systole 61, 63

T

T2D. *See* Type 2 diabetes (T2D)
Take-a-Stand Project 34
talk test 78-79
TBP (theory of planned behavior) 47-48
TEA. *See* thermic effect of activity (TEA)
TEM. *See* thermic effect of meals (TEM)
testes 277
testicles 277, 278f
testicular self-exam 342f
theory of planned behavior (TBP) 47-48
thermic effect of activity (TEA) 203, 205, 206
thermic effect of meals (TEM) 205, 206-208
three-legged stool, for body composition management 164, 164f, 167
time 79, 97, 110
time management 230, 230f, 232, 233
  college students and 230, 230f
  definitions and steps to 232, 233
TNM system 342
tobacco 263f, 264-268, 265f, 266f, 345-346
to-do list, managing life and 232
training. *See also* high-intensity interval training (HITT); neuromotor training
  conventional endurance 82
  core muscle 99
  cross- 77, 80
  eccentric 103

intensity of 77, 99-100
interval 81-82
muscle learning and 91
proprioceptive 86
resistance 95, 99-100, 210, 212
safety while 102-103
specificity of 71, 88
strength and endurance 98
volume 98
transcendental meditation 232
trans fats (trans fatty acids) 174, 175*t*, 176
trans fatty acids (trans fats) 174, 175*t*, 176
transportation, active 82
transtheoretical model. *See* Prochaska's transtheoretical model (TTM)
transversus abdominis 128
Travis, Jack 8-9
triceps 144
triceps stretch 107, 107*f*
triglycerides 324
TTM. *See* Prochaska's transtheoretical model (TTM)
12-step facilitation therapy 242
"two elephants on a seesaw" model 224, 224*f*
type 79-80, 98-99, 110-111
type 2 diabetes (T2D) 73, 199, 200, 225, 310, 315, 316*f*. *See also* prediabetes
typical use 281

U
ultrasound, to detect cancer 339*t*
underweight, BMI classification of 157*t*
United States
    cancer death rates by race and ethnicity 336*f*
    cancer in 333, 335
    causes of death in 3, 3*f*, 331, 331*f*
    chlamydia and gonorrhea infections in 297*f*
    deaths from excessive drinking in 257
    drugs and alcohol in 240
    happiest and saddest states in 7, 7*f*
    illegal drugs in 250, 251
    meth labs in 2014 255*t*
    people with HIV 290
    survival rates for cancers 338*f*
    syphilis rates in 299*f*
University of South Florida 232
unsaturated fat 174
unsaturated fatty acids 174
upper arm, back of
    daily activity and 144
    strengthening and stretching 145
upper arm, front of
    daily activity and 142
    strengthening and stretching 143
upper back and shoulders
    daily activity and 138
    strengthening and stretching 139
upper intake level, tolerable 185
urethra 278, 278*f*
U.S. Burden of Disease collaborators 2013 26

U.S. Department of Agriculture (USDA) 172, 173, 174, 176, 177, 178, 181, 184, 186, 187, 188, 189
U.S. Department of Health and Human Services (USDHHS) 31, 76, 79, 172, 173, 174, 178, 184, 186, 187, 188, 265, 267, 285, 289, 345, 346
U.S. Department of Justice 303
U.S. National Prevention Health Promotion and Public Health Council 5
USP Dietary Supplement Verification Services 192
U.S. Surgeon General 267
uterus 275, 275*f*, 276

V
vagina 275, 275*f*, 276
vaginal ring 286, 286*f*
Valliant, George 49
vaping 267
variable resistance machine, for strengthening and stretching
    abdominals 129
    back of upper arm 145
    calves 123
    chest and front of shoulder 137
    hams and glutes 127
    hip abductors 133
    hip adductors 135
    lats and middle back 141
    lower back 131
    positives and negatives of 96, 96*t*
    quads 123
    upper back and shoulders 139
vas deferens 278, 278*f*
venules 63
video or computer game addiction 243
viral STIs, most common 291-295
visceral fat 149
vitamin R. *See* Adderall; Ritalin
vitamins 180-181, 182*t*, 191-192
volatile solvents 252
volume 80-81, 98, 99-100
volume, pattern, and progression (VPP) 99-101, 100*t*, 112
vulva 276-277

W
waistline, managing 160
Waldinger, Robert 49
walking activity 80, 82
Walking Revolution, The 32
warm-up 57*f*, 102, 120
Washington, D.C. 7*f*
water-soluble vitamins 181
weather, checking 84
WebMD 56, 103
weight. *See also* weight management; weight status
    BMI classification of 157*t*
    change 150, 206
    factors influencing change in 150
    gain 19, 203, 207, 210, 212
    loss 203, 207, 208, 210, 212-213
    major components of 148
    %fat 159*t*

weight management 185-186
    blood pressure and 323
    cardiorespiratory fitness and 73-74
    daily movement and 212-213
    energy balance math 203-207
    general principles for 208
    modern health challenge of 198-203
    movement and healthy food in 210
    professional help in 215-216
    psychological concerns regarding 213-214
    strategies of 207-212
weight status 155, 157-159, 199
wellness 8-9, 10*f*, 11-17, 20, 24, 363, 369. *See also* emotional wellness; environmental wellness
wellness model 2
Well People 2011 8
whole foods 194
whole grains 172-173, 173*f*
Whole Grains Council 173
"Why Exercise?" (Åstrand) 16
Why Zebras Don't Get Ulcers (Sapolsky) 224
withdrawal 279, 282*f*, 289
women
    blood alcohol level in 261
    body composition of 150
    energy expenditure and common exercise modes 207*t*
    essential fat for 149
    fat distribution and genetics 151
    fluid recommendations for 183
    folate or folic acid for 192
    hormones and 166
    most diagnosed cancers in 334*f*
    muffin top for 160
    %fat for 158, 159*t*
    recommendations of alcohol for 184
    regular strength routine of
    syphilis diagnosis of 290
World Health Organization (WHO) 157, 161, 277, 317

X
x-rays, detecting cancers by 339

Y
young adults
    addiction in 240
    blood cholesterol levels for 324*t*
    common activities to promote cardiorespiratory fitness for 80*f*
    fitness categories for body composition levels for 159 159*t*
    healthy, muscle mass and 159-160
    key vitamins and minerals in 182*t*
    lean mass, bone mass, and density in 150
    obesity and 200
    prevalence of marijuana among 246-247
    women, fluid recommendations for 183

Z
Zika 294-295, 296*f*
zygote 276

ABOUT THE AUTHORS

Carol K. Armbruster, PhD, is a senior lecturer in the department of kinesiology in the School of Public Health at Indiana University (IU) at Bloomington. During her more than 35 years of teaching college students and training fitness leaders, she has served on the American College of Sports Medicine (ACSM) and American Council on Exercise (ACE) credentialing committees, and she is a fellow of ACSM. She is also an ACSM-certified exercise physiologist, holds the level 2 Exercise Is Medicine credential, and has level 1 Functional Movement Screening certification.

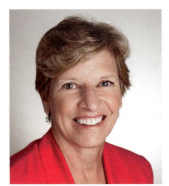

Courtesy of Indiana University School of Public Health-Bloomington.

She previously served as a program director of fitness and wellness for the IU Division of Recreational Sports, where she managed a program that offered more than 100 group exercise sessions per week. Prior to working at IU, Armbruster worked at the University of Illinois, Colorado State University, Rocky Mountain Health Club, the Loveland (Colorado) Parks and Recreation Department, and the Sheboygan (Wisconsin) School District.

Armbruster enjoys combining her interests of teaching, community engagement, and translational research. Her doctoral work focused on translational research of active-duty military in the over-40 age population. She is especially interested in functional movement, worksite wellness outcomes, safe and effective movement instruction, and evaluating safe and effective outcome-based physical activity and movement program delivery methods in order to encourage healthy lifestyles and focus on improved quality of life and prevention of illness.

Ellen M. Evans, PhD, is a professor in the department of kinesiology, associate dean for research and graduate education, and director of the Center for Physical Activity and Health in the College of Education at the University of Georgia (UGA). She was a postdoctoral research fellow in geriatrics and gerontology and applied physiology at Washington University School of Medicine and was on faculty at the University of Illinois at Urbana-Champaign prior to joining the faculty at UGA.

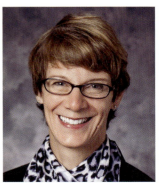

Photo courtesy of University of Georgia.

Evans has been named a fellow of the American College of Sports Medicine (ACSM) and the National Academy of Kinesiology (NAK).

At UGA, Evans embraces the land-grant institution's mission by integrating her teaching, research, and public service work. The goal of her research is to create and disseminate knowledge regarding the importance of exercise and physical activity, and nutrition for optimal body composition, with a special interest in women's health. Her primary populations of interest are older adults and college students. Evans teaches courses ranging from a freshman seminar to core and elective undergraduate courses to graduate-level courses in the areas of clinical exercise physiology, aging, and obesity.

Catherine M. Laughlin, HSD, MPH, is a clinical professor and assistant department chair of the department of applied health science in the School of Public Health at Indiana University (IU) at Bloomington. Her research interests include sexual health education, cancer prevention and education, program planning, and implementation and evaluation in community-based organizations. She is regularly interviewed by media outlets as a human sexuality and sexual health education expert.

Laughlin has won numerous teaching and service awards throughout her more than 25 years of service at IU. In 2017, she received the Distinguished Service Award from IU. In 2015, she was the recipient of the Founding Dean's Medallion and the Outstanding Service Award from IU's School of Public Health. In 2014, she earned the Tony and Mary Hulman Health Achievement Award for Innovative Public Health Programming from the Indiana Public Health Association.

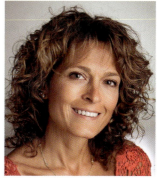

Courtesy of Indiana University School of Public Health-Bloomington.

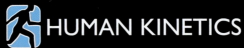
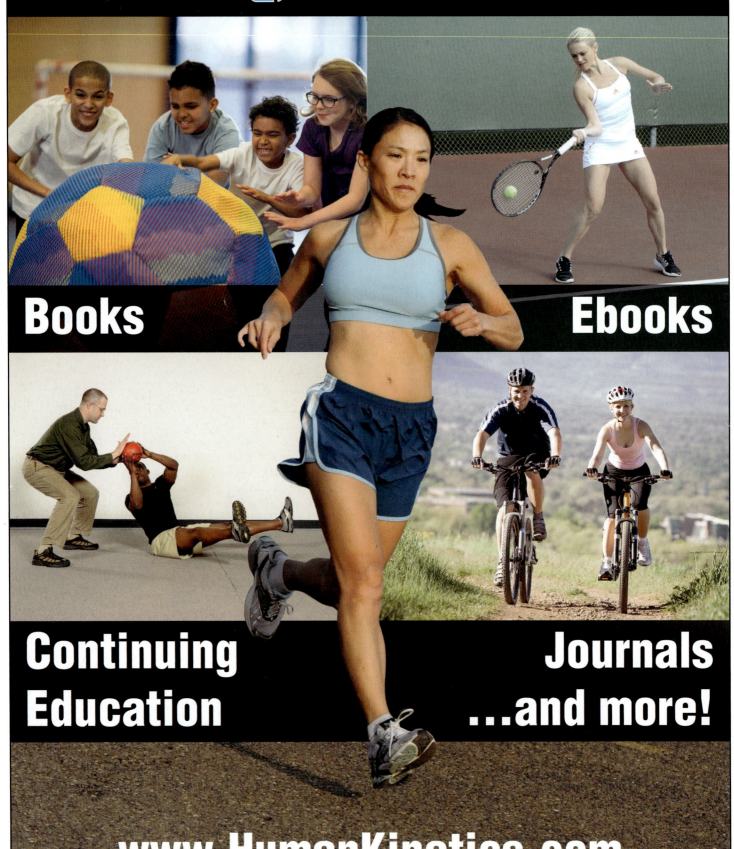